# Handbook of Neuronal Signaling

# Handbook of Neuronal Signaling

Editor: Christian Manning

AMERICAN
MEDICAL PUBLISHERS
www.americanmedicalpublishers.com

AMERICAN
MEDICAL PUBLISHERS
www.americanmedicalpublishers.com

**Cataloging-in-Publication Data**

Handbook of neuronal signaling / edited by Christian Manning.
p. cm.
Includes bibliographical references and index.
ISBN 979-8-88740-153-9
1. Neural transmission. 2. Neurotransmitter receptors. 3. Neurons.
4. Neuroglia. I. Manning, Christian.
QP364.5 .H36 2023
599.018 8--dc23



American Medical Publishers,
41 Flatbush Avenue,
1st Floor, New York,
NY 11217, USA

ISBN 979-8-88740-153-9 (Hardback)

# Contents

# Preface

Neurons are largest cells, which have polarized and complex morphologies. They are divided into pre- and post-synaptic regions, synapse, dendrite, soma, and axon, all of which are necessary for their functions. Their typical process lengths in many species range from millimeters to centimeters, and axons can even reach meters in large mammals. Signaling inside and between neuronal compartments needs the positioning of sophisticated mechanisms for setting basal conditions, which allows processing of information and ensures transmission of encoded data to the end destination. Molecular processes are involved in the origin, variation, and death of cell in the nervous system. These molecular processes comprise lipid mediators, lipid-binding proteins, protein-lipid interactions, protein misfolding and not fully characterized membrane-protein receptors. Bioactive lipids and transcription factors trigger signal transduction. Deregulation of lipid-mediated processes results in neurodegenerative diseases, such as retinopathies, Alzheimer's and Parkinson's. It can also cause proliferative disorders like diabetic retinopathy and brain cancer. This book explores all the important aspects of neuronal signaling in the present day scenario. It will help the readers in keeping pace with the rapid changes in this field. This book is a resource guide for experts as well as students.

Significant researches are present in this book. Intensive efforts have been employed by authors to make this book an outstanding discourse. This book contains the enlightening chapters which have been written on the basis of significant researches done by the experts.

Finally, I would also like to thank all the members involved in this book for being a team and meeting all the deadlines for the submission of their respective works. I would also like to thank my friends and family for being supportive in my efforts.

**Editor**

# 1

# The Impact of Frequency Scale on the Response Sensitivity and Reliability of Cortical Neurons to $1/f^{\beta}$ Input Signals

*Guojie Qu†, Boqiang Fan†, Xin Fu and Yuguo Yu**

*State Key Laboratory of Medical Neurobiology, School of Life Science, Human Phenome Institute, Institute of Brain Science, Institute of Science and Technology for Brain-Inspired Intelligence, Fudan University, Shanghai, China*

***Correspondence:**
*Yuguo Yu*
*yuyuguo@fudan.edu.cn*

*†These authors have contributed equally to this work*

What type of principle features intrinsic inside of the fluctuated input signals could drive neurons with the maximal excitations is one of the crucial neural coding issues. In this article, we examined both experimentally and theoretically the cortical neuronal responsivity (including firing rate and spike timing reliability) to input signals with different intrinsic correlational statistics (e.g., white-type noise, showed $1/f^0$ power spectrum, pink noise 1/f, and brown noises $1/f^2$) and different frequency ranges. Our results revealed that the response sensitivity and reliability of cortical neurons is much higher in response to 1/f noise stimuli with long-term correlations than $1/f^0$ with short-term correlations for a broad frequency range, and also higher than $1/f^2$ for all frequency ranges. In addition, we found that neuronal sensitivity diverges to opposite directions for 1/f noise comparing with $1/f^0$ white noise as a function of cutoff frequency of input signal. As the cutoff frequency is progressively increased from 50 to 1,000 Hz, the neuronal responsiveness increased gradually for 1/f noise, while decreased exponentially for white noise. Computational simulations of a general cortical model revealed that, neuronal sensitivity and reliability to input signal statistics was majorly dominated by fast sodium inactivation, potassium activation, and membrane time constants.

**Keywords: $1/f^{\beta}$ noise, cortical neurons, patch clamp recording, long-term correlation, Hodgkin-Huxley model, response reliability**

## INTRODUCTION

For a signal, the inherent frequency structure shown in the Fourier frequency domain characterizes its second-order statistics. The power spectrum of various natural signals typically exhibits the power law $1/f^{\beta}$ in the frequency domain, with $\beta$ close to one (Voss and Clarke, 1978; Gilden et al., 1995; Musha and Yamamoto, 1997; De Coensel et al., 2003). Moreover, this 1/f property within a specific frequency range is widely observed in neural activities at all levels, as evidenced in recordings of the membrane potential and current (Diba, 2004; Jacobson et al., 2005; Bédard et al., 2006; Yaron-Jakoubovitch, 2008; El Boustani et al., 2009), EEG (Novikov et al., 1997; Bhattacharya and Petsche, 2001; Bédard et al., 2006; Dehghani et al., 2010; Voytek et al., 2015), MEG (Novikov et al., 1997; Dehghani et al., 2010), LFPs (Bédard and Destexhe, 2009; Bedard et al., 2017; Maex, 2018), and fMRI signals (Bullmore et al., 2001; He, 2011; Ciuciu et al., 2014). In practice, the white noise (the power law $1/f^0$) with generally low cutoff frequencies is widely used to detect neuronal input-and-output functions (Sakai, 1992; Fairhall et al., 2001; Cook et al., 2007; Vilela and Lindner, 2009). Besides, $1/f^2$ noise is also observed in neural field potentials (Freeman and Zhai, 2009; Miller et al., 2009; Milstein et al., 2009; He et al., 2010; Halnes et al., 2016) and membrane currents under special conditions (Diba, 2004).

Mammalian sensory neural systems exhibit better responses to naturalistic signals rather than white-type noise signals in a specific frequency domain (Aertsen and Johannesma, 1981; Baddeley et al., 1997; de Ruyter van Steveninck et al., 1997; Yu et al., 2005; Garcia-Lazaro et al., 2006, 2011). It has been speculated that the 1/f property might be the key in shaping the neuronal function preference to the naturalistic input (Yu et al., 2005; Garcia-Lazaro et al., 2006, 2011); this preference may extend to the atomic level of neural organization, namely the single neuronal input-output function (Gal and Marom, 2013).

In addition, white and colored noises with various cutoff frequencies enhance the detection of weak signals by neuronal systems via stochastic resonance (SR) (Nozaki and Yamamoto, 1998,?; Nozaki et al., 1999b; Hutcheon and Yarom, 2000; Jia et al., 2001; Ruszczynski et al., 2001; Chizhov and Graham, 2008; Mino and Durand, 2008; Gutkin et al., 2009; Higgs and Spain, 2009; Sekine et al., 2009; Guo and Li, 2011; Sobie et al., 2011; Duan et al., 2014; Zhao et al., 2017). However, previous studies have regarded the signals with $1/f^\beta$ statistics as mere background noise. In particular, although the signal frequency range has been confirmed to significantly affect neuronal excitability (Nozaki et al., 1999b; Higgs and Spain, 2009), the exact role of the frequency range in neuronal responsiveness to the $1/f^\beta$ statistic remains unclear. As neurons generally encode information according to the rate and/or the precise timing of spikes (Nowak et al., 1997; Reinagel and Reid, 2000; Fellous et al., 2001; Brette and Guigon, 2003; Avissar et al., 2007; Freund and Cerquera, 2012), we sought to examine the neuronal firing rate and spike-timing reliability to input statistics. In this study, we focus on the effects of the signal frequency range to identify the neuronal responsiveness to $1/f^\beta$ ($\beta = 0$, 1, and 2) noises with respect to the firing rate and spike-timing reliability. Specifically, we reveal the mechanism underlying neuronal responsivity to $1/f^\beta$ and the frequency range using theoretical experiments, as this mechanism has not been clearly determined in previous model-based studies (Nozaki and Yamamoto, 1998; Nozaki et al., 1999b; Brunel and Latham, 2003; Mino and Durand, 2008; Sekine et al., 2009; Sobie et al., 2011; Ostojic et al., 2015; Schwalger et al., 2015; Zhao et al., 2017). We conducted *in vitro* whole-cell patch clamp recording experiments on mouse cortical pyramidal neurons to examine the neuronal firing rate and reliability to 1/f, $1/f^0$, and $1/f^2$ noises with various cutoff frequencies ($F_{cut}$). We have also carried out a set of computational simulations of a general Hodgkin-Huxley neuronal model (Yu et al., 2012) to reproduce our experimental observations, and revealed the critical factors underlying the neuronal responsiveness to second-order statistics at the cellular level.

# METHODS

## Signal Production

Input noise stimuli of each type of $1/f^\beta$–white noise ($1/f^0$), pink noise (1/f), and brown noise ($1/f^2$) were first generated digitally by computer programming. The noise stimuli were then filtered by different low-pass filter with aimed cutoff frequency range. Each signal intensity [represented by the standard deviation (SD)] was set to the defined value. All the above were done in Matlab R2017a software (Mathworks, USA), and then the signal was loaded to Micro 1401 (CED, UK), where the signals were converted from digital to analog. In the experimental study, a unique set of noise stimuli with designed cutoff frequencies and noise intensities were used as the input signals to recorded neurons. The three signal types have different slopes in PSDs (the white noise has a slope of 0 and 1/f noise has a slope of −1, while $1/f^2$ noise has a slope of −2), as shown in **Figure 1A**. The 1/f and $1/f^2$ noises have more power in the low frequency components and less power in the high frequency components, while white noise has equal energy at each frequency interval. All three types of signals have equal total power within the examined frequency range.

## Brain Slice Preparation

The experimental procedures involving animal experiments in this study were approved by Animal Ethics Committee of Fudan University School of Life Science. Using 0.7% chloral hydrate, 14–28 day-old mice were anesthetized and brain slices prepared by a protective slicing and recovery method reported previously (Ting et al., 2014). Briefly, anesthetized mice were perfused intracardially with ice-cold oxygenated (95% $O_2$, 5% $CO_2$) NMDG-based cutting solution containing (in mM) 93 mM NMDG, 2.5 mM KCl, 1.2 mM $NaH_2PO_4$, 30 mM $NaHCO_3$, 20 mM HEPES, 25 mM glucose, 5 mM sodium ascorbate, 2 mM thiourea, 3 mM sodium pyruvate, 10 mM $MgSO_4$, 2 mM $CaCl_2$, and 12 mM NAC (pH 7.3–7.4, 300–305 mOsm). Brains were carefully removed from the skull and cut coronally at a thickness of 300 μm with a vibratome VT1000S (Leica, Germany) in chilled oxygenated (95% $O_2$, 5% $CO_2$) NMDG-based cutting solution. Slices were initially recovered in NMDG-based cutting solution at 32°C for 10 min. Slices were then incubated in oxygenated (95% $O_2$, 5% $CO_2$) HEPES-modified solution containing (in mM) 94 mM NaCl, 2.5 mM KCl, 1.2 mM $NaH_2PO_4$, 30 mM $NaHCO_3$, 20 mM HEPES, 25 mM glucose, 5 mM sodium ascorbate, 2 mM thiourea, 3 mM sodium pyruvate, 2 mM $MgSO_4$, 2 mM $CaCl_2$, and 6 mM NAC (pH 7.3–7.4, 300–305 mOsm) at room temperature for 30 min. Finally, slices were incubated in oxygenated (95% $O_2$, 5% $CO_2$) ACSF at room temperature for at least 1 h before recording. The ACSF contained 126 mM NaCl, 2.5 mM KCl, 2 mM $MgSO_4$, 2 mM $CaCl_2$, 26 mM $NaHCO_3$, 1.25 mM $NaH_2PO_4$, and 12.5 mM dextrose (pH 7.3–7.4, 300–305 mOsm).

## Electrophysiological Recordings

Whole-cell slice recordings were performed on the cell body of layer 5 pyramidal neurons in the prefrontal cortex (**Figure 1B**). In total, 12 neurons in 12 slices of six mice were examined.

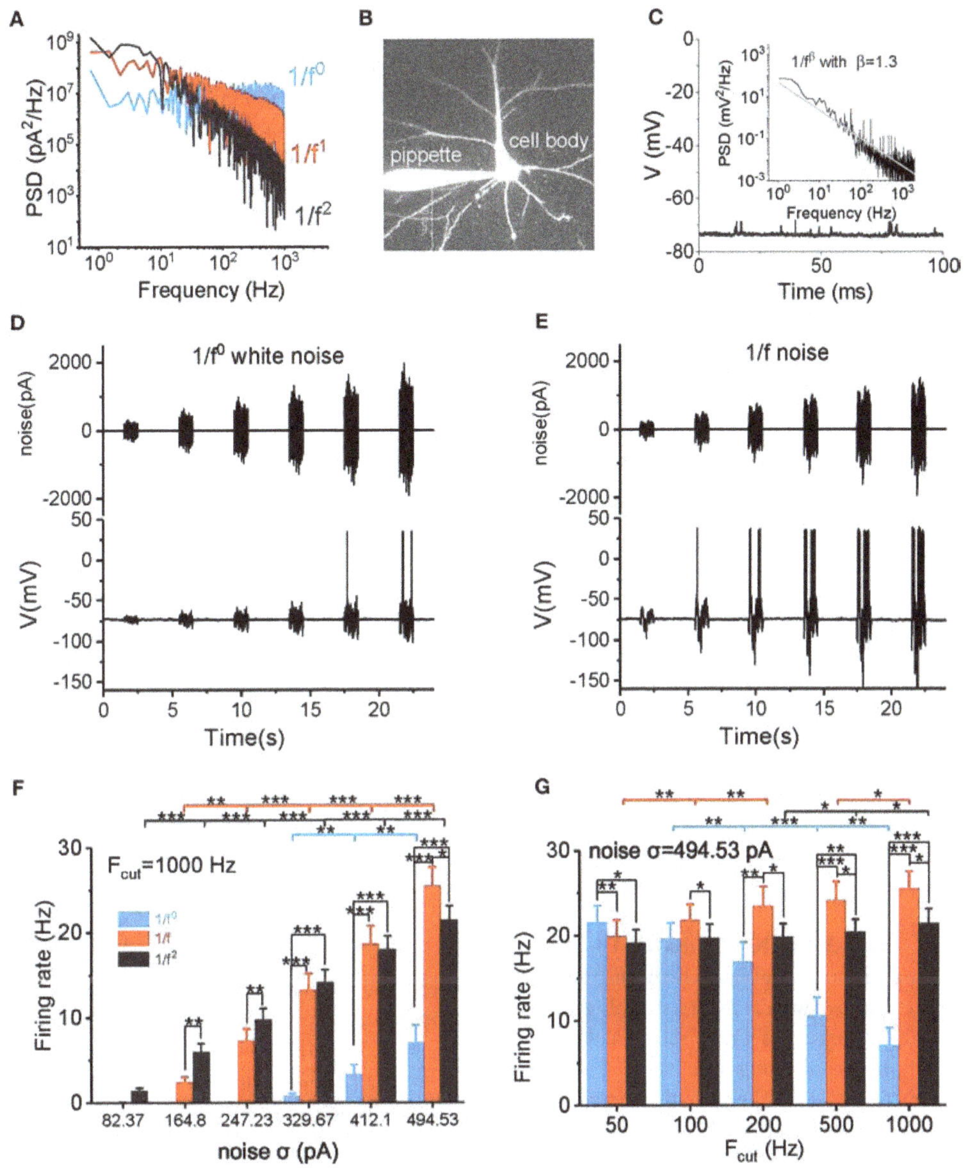


**FIGURE 1 |** Neuronal firing rate in response to different types of input signal. **(A)** The PSD plots for white noise (blue), 1/f noise (red), and $1/f^2$ noise (black) are shown. Noises with a 1,000 Hz cutoff frequency are shown here. **(B)** *In vitro* patch clamp recording of a pyramidal cell. The scale bar indicates 50 μm. **(C)** Plot of the recorded membrane potentials in the resting state vs. time. Inset: The power spectrum density (PSD) plot of the resting potentials shows a 1/f property in a log-log plot. **(D,E)** Representative trace of input $1/f^0$ white noise **(D)** and 1/f noise **(E)** with different intensities over time. The signal produced at each intensity lasted for 1 s, followed by a 3 s no-stimulus interval. The bottom panel shows the membrane potential and action potential produced by a recorded pyramidal cell in response to the input signal shown in the top panel. **(F)** Neuronal responsive firing rate for white noise (blue), 1/f (red), and $1/f^2$ noise (black) with various intensities (82.37, 164.80, 247.23, 329.67, 412.10, and 494.53 pA) and a cutoff frequency of 1000 Hz. $F_{cut}$, cutoff frequency. **(G)** Neuronal responsive firing rate for white noise (blue), 1/f (red), and $1/f^2$ noise (black) at various cutoff frequencies (50, 100, 200, 500, and 1,000 Hz) with a intensity of 494.53 pA.

Oxygenated (95% $O_2$, 5% $CO_2$) ASCF was used as the recording solution. Recordings were conducted on an upright infrared-differential interference contrast (IR-DIC) microscope (Zeiss Axioskop 2 FS plus) with a recording solution temperature of 36 °C. Cortical slices were suspended on a net to allow an oxygenated solution to flow over both the upper and lower surfaces at a rate of 3–4 ml/min. The membrane potential in the whole-cell recordings was corrected for Donnan liquid junction potentials of 15 mV. The temperature was regulated by a Warner Instruments Corporation two channel temperature regulator (Model TC344B).

Whole-cell recordings from the soma were achieved with the help of a Multiclamp 700B amplifier (Axon Instruments, Union City, CA) and Micro 1401 converter. Pipettes had an impedance of 5-6 MΩ and were filled with an intracellular solution that contained 140 mM K-gluconate, 3 mM KCl, 2 mM

$MgCl_2$, 2 mM $Na_2ATP$, 10 mM HEPES, and 0.2 mM EGTA, and the pH was adjusted to 7.3 with KOH–(270 mOsm). The sample rate of the membrane potential data was 25 kHz for both experiments and computational simulations. Those recorded neurons with input resistance within 100–200 MΩ were saved for analysis in this paper while others were discarded so that the studied neurons have the similar biophysical membrane properties.

## Stimulation Mode

To experimentally examine the responsive firing rate to the input signal, the current signal with each intensity ($\sigma = 82.37$, 164.80, 247.23, 329.67, 412.10, and 494.53 pA) and each cutoff frequency ($F_{cut} = 50$, 100, 200, 500, and 1,000 Hz) was injected into neurons three times (**Figures 1D,E**). The signals ($\sigma = 494.53$ pA; $F_{cut} =$ 50, 200, 500, and 1,000 Hz) in firing rate detection were also used for spike reliability examination, in which 50 repetitions of signals were injected into neurons. Every neuron in our study received all types of input signal, with its firing rate and reliability for each signal cutoff frequency examined. In the model simulation, the neuron received input signals ($\sigma = 1.5$, 3, 4.5, 6, 7.5, 9 $\mu A/cm^2$; Fcut = 50, 200, 500, and 1,000 Hz) thrice for firing rate detection. The signal ($\sigma = 9$ pA; $F_{cut} =$ 50, 200, 500, and 1,000 Hz) was also injected 50 times for the spike reliability examination. In each test, to simulate the background noise from external or intrinsic fluctuations of the neuron itself, a 1/f noise with 500 Hz cutoff frequency and an intensity of 0.2169 $\mu A/cm^2$ was added to the input signal. The duration of stimuli signal of each cutoff frequency and intensity was 1 s.

## Firing Rate and Spike Time Reliability

For each neuron under an input signal of each cutoff frequency and intensity, the spike number within the 1s stimuli duration was the firing rate. We averaged the firing rates in the three repetitions to get each neuronal firing rate value. For spike time reliability, 50 repetitions of a 1 s stimuli were injected into neurons, and cross covariance was calculated between all pair-wise combinations of trials (within stimulus size) within each neuron, on binary spike timing trains (with "1" representing an action potential with a 2 ms time bin and "0" representing a non-spiking neuron). The black-covariance function estimates the mean-removed cross-correlation between the two sequences of random processes, thus avoiding the contribution of the mean firing rate to the spike timing reliability. The resulting cross-covariance values at zero-lag (normalized by the average autocovariance function) for each neuron were used to quantify the spike reliability for each input signal statistic (Haider et al., 2010).

## Hodgkin-Huxley-Style Cortical Neuronal Model

Three major ionic voltage-dependent currents were used in our cortical model: fast $Na^+$, $I_{Na}$, fast $K^+$, $I_K$, and a leak current, $I_L$. The equations describing the voltage and time dependence of the $Na^+$ and $K^+$ conductance have been reported in previous publications (McCormick and Huguenard, 1992) and the channel kinetics were modified based on models of cortical neurons (Mainen et al., 1995; Mainen and Sejnowski, 1996; Yu et al., 2008) and experimental studies (Huguenard et al., 1989; Colbert and Pan, 2002; Yu et al., 2008; Schmidt-Hieber and Bischofberger, 2010). The following equations describe the cortical axon single compartment model:

$$
\begin{aligned}
C\frac{dV}{dt} &= I_{stim} - g_{Na}^{max} \cdot m^3 \cdot h \cdot (V - V_{Na}) \\
&\quad - g_K^{max} \cdot n \cdot (V - V_K) - g_L \cdot (V - V_L), \\
\tau m\frac{dm}{dt} &= -m + m_\infty, \ \tau m = \frac{1}{\alpha_m + \beta_m}, \ m_\infty = \frac{\alpha_m}{\alpha_m + \beta_m} \\
\tau h\frac{dh}{dt} &= -h + h_\infty, \ \tau h = \frac{1}{\alpha_h + \beta_h}, \ h_\infty = \frac{1}{1 + e^{(V+60)/6.2}} \\
\tau n\frac{dn}{dt} &= -n + n_\infty, \ \tau_n = \frac{1}{\alpha_n + \beta_n}, \ n_\infty = \frac{\alpha_n}{\alpha_n + \beta_n} \\
\alpha_m(V) &= \varnothing \cdot \frac{0.182 \cdot (V + 30)}{1 - e^{-(V+30)/8}} \\
\beta_m(V) &= -\varnothing \cdot \frac{0.124 \cdot (V + 30)}{1 - e^{(V+30)/8}} \\
\alpha_h(V) &= \varnothing \cdot \frac{0.028 \cdot (V + 45)}{1 - e^{-(V+45)/6}} \\
\beta_h(V) &= -\varnothing \cdot \frac{0.0091 \cdot (V + 70)}{1 - e^{(V+70)/6}} \\
\alpha_n(V) &= \varnothing \cdot \frac{0.01 \cdot (V - 30)}{1 - e^{-(V-30)/9}} \\
\beta_n(V) &= -\varnothing \cdot \frac{0.0005 \cdot (V - 30)}{1 - e^{(V-30)/9}} \\
\varnothing &= Q_{10}{}^{(T-23)/10}
\end{aligned}
$$

where the $Q_{10}$ effect is described by $\Phi$ on regulating the temperature dependence of the biochemical reaction rate with $Q_{10} = 2.3$ (Frankenhaeuser and Moore, 1963; Matteson and Armstrong, 1982). The relationships between temperature and $I_{Na}$ and $I_K$ activation and inactivation are not monotonic and vary in different species (Fohlmeister et al., 2010). The reverse potentials for $Na^+$ and $K^+$ currents were adjusted for change in temperature according to the Nernst equation (not shown). Similar results were obtained with a variety of values for $Q_{10}$. For example, the use of a $Q_{10}$ of 3 yielded similar results for spike efficiency and changes in spike rate with temperature. In our cortical model, $Na^+$ kinetics were determined based on recent experimental observations (Kole et al., 2008). The parameters used were: membrane capacitance = 0.75 $\mu F/cm^2$, $g_{Na} = 1950$ $pS/\mu m^2$, density of $g_K = 40$ $pS/\mu m^2$, and $g_{leak} = 0.25$ $pS/\mu m^2$, based on recent experimental results (Mainen and Sejnowski, 1995; Colbert and Pan, 2002; Kole et al., 2008; Hu et al., 2009; Fleidervish et al., 2010; Schmidt-Hieber and Bischofberger, 2010). The reversal potentials were $V_L = -70$ mV, $V_{Na} =$ 60 mV, and $V_K = -90$ mV for leak, sodium, and potassium channels, respectively.

## Statistical Analysis

To detect the differential response under various signal intensities, cutoff frequencies, or signal types, we performed paired $t$-test and Wilcoxon rank sum test. First, Kolmogorov-Smirnov goodness-of-fit hypothesis test was done on the paired difference between the two compared data groups. Depending on whether the normality assumption held for the data, we used a paired $t$-test or the Wilcoxon test for statistical significant comparison. A $p < 0.05$ was considered statistically significant. The data presented in the figures are reported as the mean ± standard error, and the significant level are labeled by $^{*}p < 0.05$, $^{**}p < 0.01$, and $^{***}p < 0.001$, respectively.

# RESULTS

## Neuronal Responsiveness to Input Stimuli

In the absence of external stimuli, neuronal resting membrane potentials (~-75 to −70 mV) showed fluctuating synaptic potentials that were received from somatic and dendritic synapses (**Figure 1C**). A power spectrum density (PSD) analysis of resting potentials displayed a typical 1/f property in a log-log plot (see the inset in **Figure 1C**), suggesting that the membrane potentials observed *in vitro* in neurons with synaptic inputs also exhibit a similar statistical property as neurons *in vivo*.

First, we examined the neuronal firing rate in response to the input signal (**Figures 1D,E**). As shown in **Figure 1F** and **Supplementary Figure S1**, the neuronal firing rate increases non-linearly as the noise intensity increases within a firing rate of 0–30 Hz. When the noise cutoff frequency is within 50 Hz, neurons are sensitive to white noise, firing with a high frequency at high noise intensities (**Figure 1G** and **Supplementary Figure S1A**). However, as the cutoff frequency increases, neurons lose their responsiveness to the white noise (**Figure 1G** and **Supplementary Figure S1**) and produce a low firing rate, even at a very high noise intensity levels and when the cutoff frequency is 1,000 Hz (**Figures 1F,G**). The neuronal firing rate increases minimally at a cutoff frequency of $1/f^2$ noise (**Figure 1G**). In contrast, the firing rate increases gradually with the cutoff frequency for 1/f noise (**Figure 1G**). When the cutoff frequency is >200 Hz, firing rates for 1/f and $1/f^2$ noise are higher than for the white noise (**Figures 1F,G**, and **Supplementary Figures S1C,D**). At low intensities, 1/f noise evokes lower firing rates than the $1/f^2$ noise; but at high intensities, 1/f noise evokes higher firing rates than the $1/f^2$ noise. The switch in firing rates emerges under various cutoff frequencies (**Figure 1F** and **Supplementary Figure S1**). Notably, at $\sigma$ = 494.53 pA and a 1,000 Hz cutoff frequency, 1/f noise evokes the highest firing rate (25.47 ± 2.24 Hz) in all our recordings. Overall, 1/f noise evokes relatively high firing rates under all conditions, particularly at high input intensities, and high cutoff frequencies.

We next examined spike reliability (**Figure 2A**) at four cutoff frequencies ($F_{cut}$ = 50, 200, 500, and 1,000 Hz). The neuronal responses are shown in the post-stimulus time histogram (PSTH) and raster plot (**Figure 2A**). **Figures 2B,C** show the spike-timing reliability, which quantifies the extent of repeatability of spike timing in response to the input signal (Mainen and Sejnowski, 1995; Haider et al., 2010) (calculated from the representative data shown in **Figure 1A**). As the cutoff frequency increases to above 200 Hz, the reliability of the response to white noise decreases significantly (**Figure 2B**). For both the 1/f and $1/f^2$ noises, the reliability increases as the cutoff frequency increases (**Figure 2B**). When the cutoff frequency is 50 Hz, the reliability for the 1/f noise is greater than the $1/f^2$ noise and less than that for the white noise (**Figure 2B** and **Supplementary Figure S2A**). When the cutoff frequency increases to 200 Hz, the reliability for white noise remains greater than for the 1/f and $1/f^2$ noises (**Figure 2B** and **Supplementary Figure S2B**). Interestingly, at 500 and 1,000 Hz, the 1/f noise evokes the greatest reliability (**Figures 2B,C**, and **Supplementary Figure S2C**), suggesting that neurons respond with relatively high reliability to the 1/f property in signals, particularly when the input signal has a high cutoff frequency.

Our data demonstrate that neurons respond to white noise with low sensitivity and reliability, except when the noise is composed of low frequency components only. When the noise intensity is weak, $1/f^2$ noise more readily evokes neuronal firing, but high firing rate is difficult to evoke. For the 1/f noise, neurons respond with relatively high sensitivity and high reliability under all conditions. In particular, at high cutoff frequencies or high input intensities, the 1/f noise evokes the highest firing rate and the most reliable neuronal response among all signal types tested. These findings indicate a clear neuronal preference for responses to 1/f noise with high cutoff frequencies.

## Computer Simulations of Hodgkin-Huxley Model

A cortical Hodgkin-Huxley-type neuronal model was constructed to study the key factors and dynamic mechanisms underlying neuronal responsiveness to signals with different statistics. We only considered the fast sodium and potassium channels in the model and ignored other subtypes of sodium/potassium and calcium channels to identify the common mechanism underlying the neuronal preference for 1/f statistics.

The model neuron first reproduced the similar responses to input signals with various noise intensities described in our experimental study (**Figure 3A**). For cutoff frequency of 1,000 Hz, the firing rates of neuronal model to white noise is significantly lower than that of 1/f and $1/f^2$ noise, and 1/f noise evokes the highest firing rate for the high intensities (**Figures 3B,C**). When the cutoff frequency increases from 50 to 1,000 Hz, the neuronal firing rate of model to input white noise decreases gradually. However, it increases slightly for 1/f noise, while it keeps almost invariant for $1/f^2$ noise (**Figure 3C**).

We also evaluated the spike reliability of the model neuron based on the evoked spike trains by repeatedly feeding the model neuron with each type of input signal with the different cutoff frequencies. Neuronal reliability for white noise is high only at a low cutoff frequency, while it decreases significantly with an increase in cutoff frequency (**Figure 3D**). On the contrary, neuronal response reliability to 1/f noise keeps at a much higher reliability level for almost the whole range of cutoff frequency (**Figure 3D**). In addition, the neuronal response reliability to $1/f^2$ noise is lower than the other two type of inputs (**Figure 3E**). However, its reliability increases as the cutoff frequency of $1/f^2$

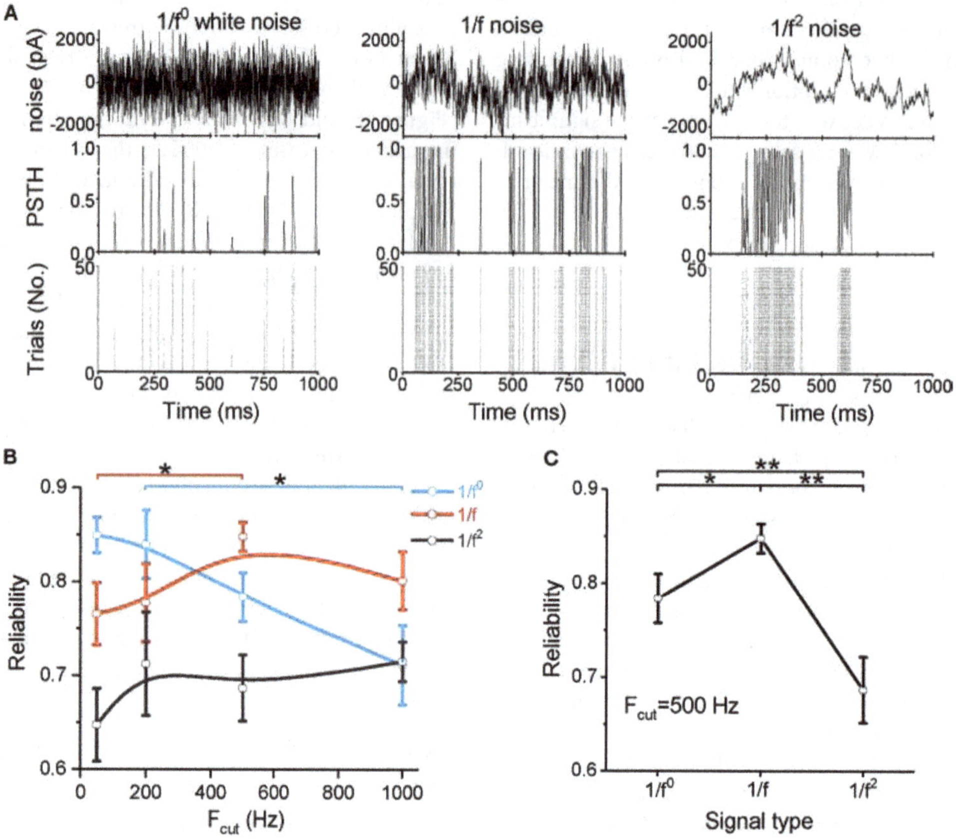


**FIGURE 2 |** Neuronal spike reliability to different types of input signal. **(A)** Raster plot of the responses from 50 trials (bottom panel) and PSTH (middle panel) for the repeated input stimulus (top panel) reflecting the reliability of cortical neuron firing patterns evoked by white noise (left panel), 1/f noise (middle panel), and $1/f^2$ noise (right panel). **(B)** Plot of reliability vs. cutoff frequencies for the three signal types. $F_{cut}$, cutoff frequency. **(C)** Plot of reliability vs. β for the three types of $1/f^{\beta}$ input signals with a cutoff frequency of 500 Hz.

noise increases (**Figure 3D**). These model simulation results are consistent with the experimental observations.

Next, we investigated the critical factors of neurons affecting the neuronal preference to 1/f signals. Considering that the responseness of neuronal model is dominated by the sodium and potassium channel kinetics, especially the channel opening velocity constant (e.g., $\alpha_m$, $\alpha_h$, $\alpha_n$) and channel closing velocity constant (e.g., $\beta_m$ $\beta_h$, and $\beta_n$) (Yu et al., 2012), we systematically changed the values of these parameters to study their effects on neuronal preference to inputs. We have also varied the values of membrane input resistance $R_{input}$ and the membrane capacitance $C_m$ to understand the effect of the passive membrane property on the neuronal responseness. First we examined the effect of open ($\alpha_m$) and close ($\beta_m$) velocity constants of sodium activation variable. Although neuronal firing rate could be significantly affected by an increase or decrease of the values of $\alpha_m$ and $\beta_m$, the changing amount of the firing rate is almost same for all the three signal types (**Supplementary Figures S3A,B**).

However, when the value of $\alpha_h$ is halved, the neuronal firing rate as a function of noise intensity (**Figure 4A1**) or cutoff frequency (**Figure 4A2**) decreases dramatically for both 1/f and $1/f^2$ noise, but slightly for white noise. **Figure 4A3** summarizes the contribution effect. When the$\alpha_h$ value increases, the neuronal firing rate increases gradually to a saturation level for both 1/f and $1/f^2$ noises while keeps invariant for white noise input. This suggests that $\alpha_h$ plays a role in the neuronal preference to 1/f signals. Next, we varied the value of $\beta_h$ and observed almost no effect on neuronal firing rate (please see **Supplementary Figure S3C**).

Next, we examined the effect of $\alpha_n$ and $\beta_n$ for the potassium channel activation variable. When the value of $\alpha_n$ was doubled (**Figures 4B1,B2**), the neuronal firing rate as a function of noise intensity (**Figure 4B1**) or cutoff frequency (**Figure 4B2**) decreased dramatically for both 1/f and $1/f^2$ noise, but slightly for white noise. **Figure 4B3** summarizes the contribution effect, and shows that the firing rates of neuronal model decrease gradually when the $\alpha_n$ value increased for both 1/f and $1/f^2$ noises while deceased slightly for the white noise input. This suggests that $\alpha_n$ also contributes to the neuronal preference to 1/f signals.

Moreover, when $\beta_n$ is increased, firing rate for $1/f^2$ noise increases greater than for 1/f noise, much more than for white noise, at each noise intensity (**Figure 4C1**) as well as for cutoff frequency (**Figure 4C2**). As a result, in the case of large $\beta_n$,

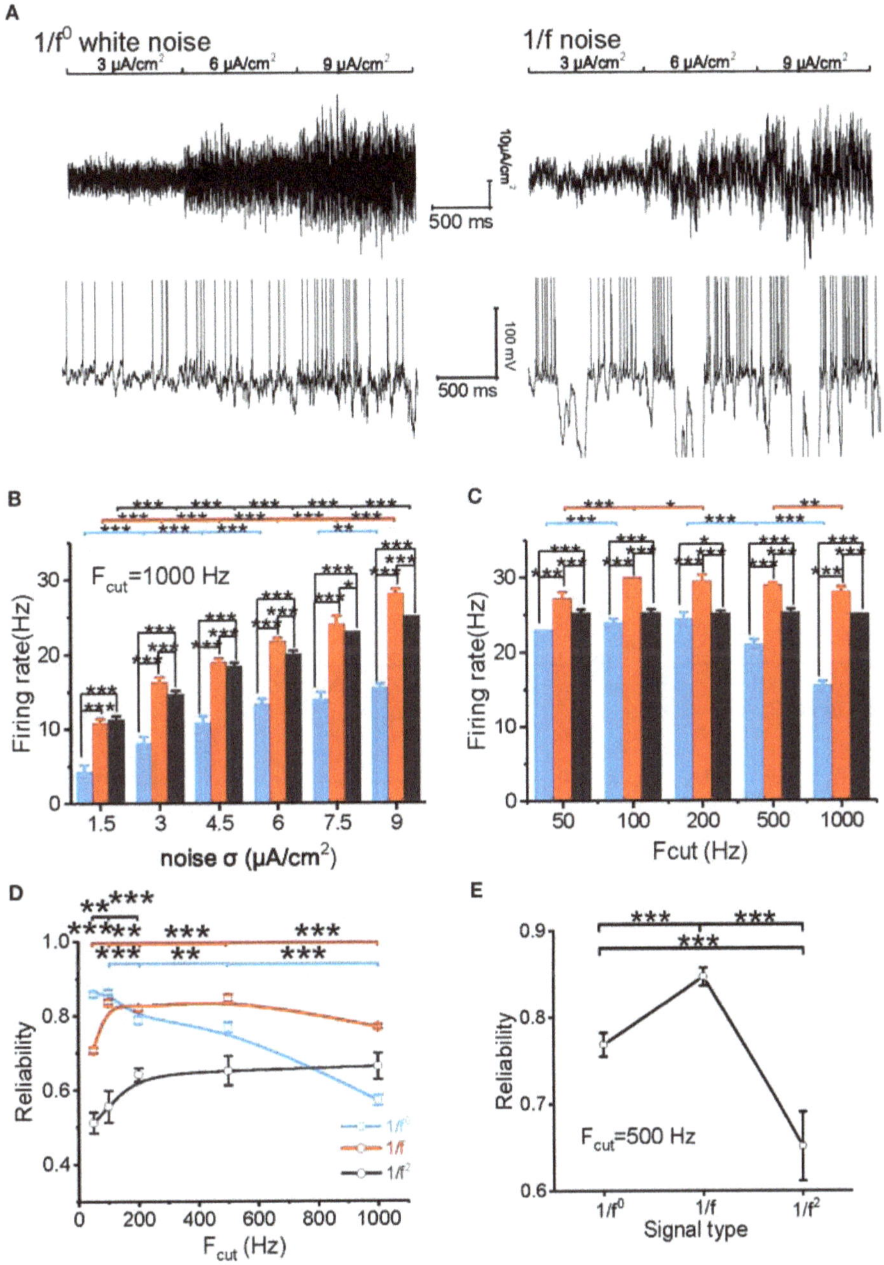


**FIGURE 3 |** Model neuronal response to different types of input signal. **(A)** The top panel shows white noise (left) and 1/f noise (right) with step-changed variance introduced into the neuronal model. The bottom panel shows the membrane potentials of the model neuron in response to the input. The noise intensity shown here is 3, 6, and 9 $\mu A/cm^2$. **(B)** Histogram of the neuronal firing rate vs. input signal SD for white noise (blue), 1/f noise (red), and $1/f^2$ noise (black) at the cutoff frequency of 1,000 Hz. **(C)** Histogram of the neuronal firing rate vs. cutoff frequencies (50, 100, 200, 500, and 1,000 Hz) for white noise (blue), 1/f (red), and $1/f^2$ noise (black) when the noise SD was 9 $\mu A/cm^2$. **(D)** Plot of model neuronal reliability vs. cutoff frequencies (50, 100, 200, 500, and 1,000 Hz) for white noise (blue), 1/f (red), and $1/f^2$ noise (black). $F_{cut}$, cutoff frequency. **(E)** Plot of reliability vs. β for the three types of $1/f^\beta$ input signals with a cutoff frequency of 500 Hz.

neuronal firing rate for $1/f^2$ noise is larger than 1/f noise, while in the case of small $\beta_n$, neuronal firing rate for $1/f^2$ noise is lower than 1/f noise (**Figure 4C3**). This indicated that relatively large $\beta_n$ value may dominate the neuronal preference to 1/f and $1/f^2$ noise. For the much small $\beta_n$ value, neuronal preference to 1/f noise decreases dramatically.

Based on the equation, the membrane time constant $\tau_c = R_{input} * C_m$, $\tau_c$ could be changed by either changing $R_{input}$ or $C_m$. Halved $R_{input}$ increased neuronal firing rate to all the three type of input, and the neuronal sensitivity reached the maximum to white noise in the low cutoff frequency around 200 Hz, which is higher than to 1/f and $1/f^2$ noise stimuli (**Figures 5A1,A2**).

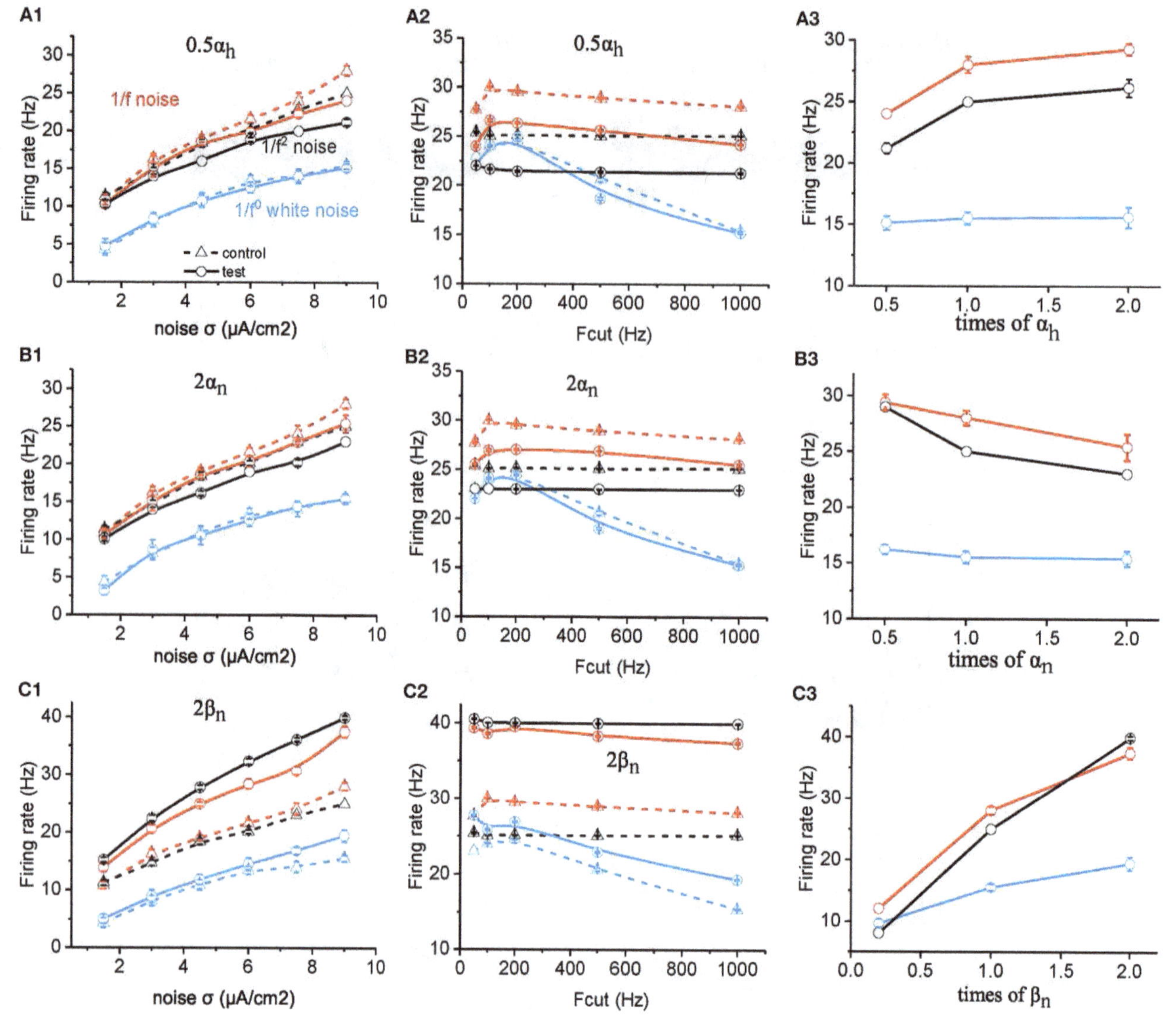


**FIGURE 4 |** Effects of ionic channel kinetic constants on the responsive firing rate of model neurons. **(A1–C1)** Plots of firing rate vs. intensity for white noise (blue), 1/f (red), and $1/f^2$ noise (black) for a normal neuron (dotted line) compared with the results from the model neuron in the case of 0.5 $\alpha_h$ (solid line, **A1**), 2 $\alpha_n$ (solid line, **B1**), 2 $\beta_n$ (solid line, **C1**). Fcut = 1,000 Hz. **(A2–C2)** Plots of firing rate vs. cutoff frequency for white noise (blue), 1/f (red), and $1/f^2$ noise (black) for a normal neuron (dotted line) compared with the results from the model neuron in the case of 0.5 $\alpha_h$ (solid line, **A2**), 2 $\alpha_n$ (solid line, **B2**), 2 $\beta_n$ (solid line, **C2**). Noise $\sigma = 9\ \mu A/cm^2$. **(A3–C3)** Plots of firing rate vs. times of $\alpha_h$ (solid line, **A3**), $\alpha_n$ (solid line, **B3**), and $\beta_n$ (solid line, **C3**) for white noise (blue), 1/f (red), and $1/f^2$ noise (black) for a normal neuron (dotted line) compared with the results from the model neuron. $F_{cut}$ = 1,000 Hz. Noise $\sigma = 9\ \mu A/cm^2$.

Doubled $C_m$ decreases the firing rate and makes the neuronal firing rate for $1/f^2$ noise larger than for 1/f noise at various noise intensity (**Figure 5B1**) and each cutoff frequency, respectively (**Figure 5B2**). As shown in **Figures 5A,B**, both $C_m$ and $R_{input}$ changed the neuronal firing rate for white noise more than for 1/f noise, while the change for $1/f^2$ noise is not that strong. This is contrary to the situation of changing $\beta_n$. As $\beta_{nand}$ $R_{input}$ or $C_m$ have different weighted effect on neuronal response, they may act together to support the neuronal preferential response to 1/f noise with a broad frequency range. So we concluded $\beta_n$, $R_{input}$ and $C_m$ play important roles in neuronal responsive firing rate to $1/f^{\beta}$ noises.

We also examined changes in the spike reliability in response to noises with altered neuronal biophysical parameters. As shown in **Figure 6A**, an increased value of$\beta_m$ results in a significant decreased spike reliability for both 1/f noise (in all frequency range) and white noise (mainly with cutoff frequency higher than 200 Hz). On the contrary, increased $\beta_m$ results in significantly increased spike reliability for $1/f^2$ noise. With doubled $\alpha_h$, $\alpha_n$, and $\beta_n$ (**Figures 6B–D**) and decreased $R_{input}$ (**Figure 6E**), neuronal spike reliability for $1/f^2$ noise decreases significantly for most of frequency range. These effects for $1/f^2$ noise are stronger than for 1/f noise, and much stronger for white noise. On the contrary, doubled $C_m$

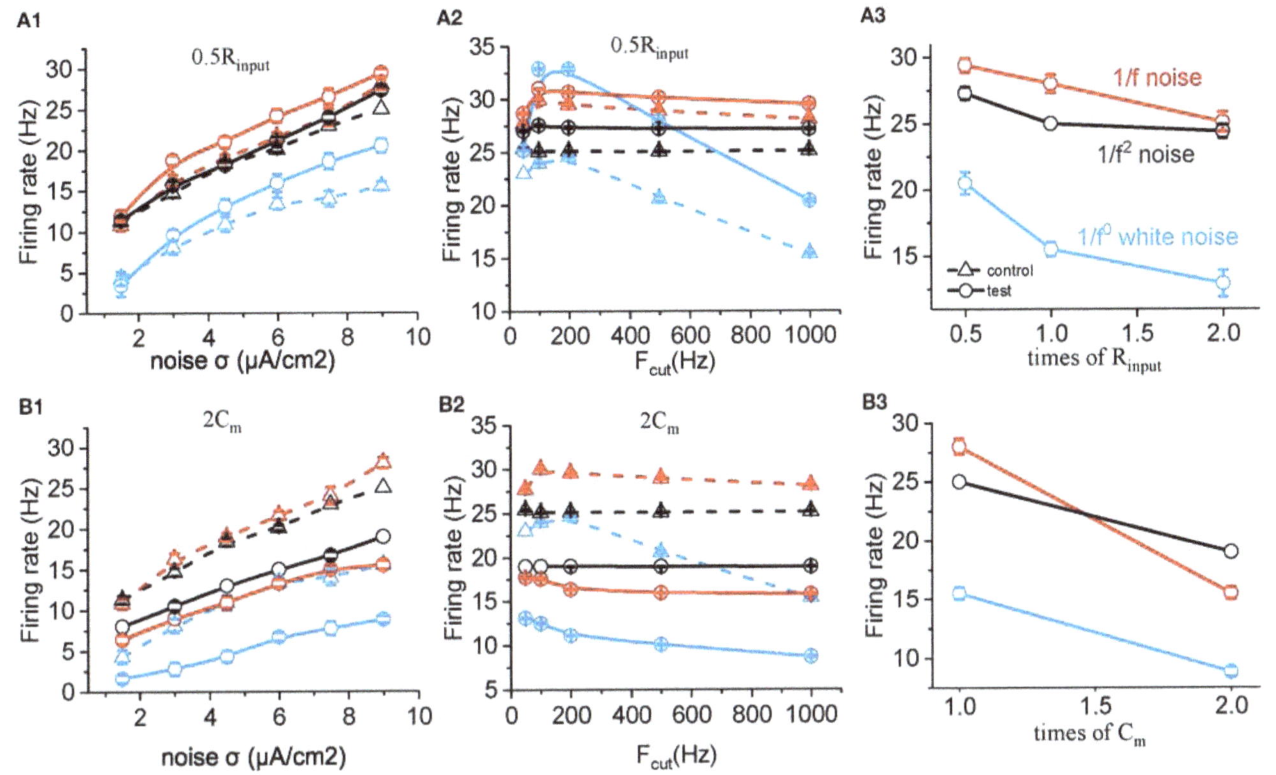


**FIGURE 5 |** Effects of membrane time constants on the responsive firing rate of model neurons. **(A1,B1)** Plots of firing rate vs. intensity for white noise (blue), 1/f (red), and $1/f^2$ noise (black) for a normal neuron (dotted line) compared with the results from the model neuron in the case of 0.5 $R_{input}$ (solid line, **A1**), 2 $C_m$ (solid line, **B1**). Fcut = 1,000 Hz. **(A2,B2)** Plots of firing rate vs. cutoff frequency for white noise (blue), 1/f (red), and $1/f^2$ noise (black) for a normal neuron (dotted line) compared with the results from the model neuron in the case of 0.5 $R_{input}$ (solid line, **A2**), 2 $C_m$ (solid line, **B2**). Noise $\sigma = 9\ \mu A/cm^2$. **(A3,B3)** Plots of firing rate vs. times of $R_{input}$ (solid line, **A3**), and $C_m$ (solid line, **B3**) for white noise (blue), 1/f (red), and $1/f^2$ noise (black) for a normal neuron (dotted line) compared with the results from the model neuron. $F_{cut}$ = 1000 Hz. Noise $\sigma = 9\ \mu A/cm^2$.

decreases the reliability significantly for each type of input, especially for the white noise (**Figure 6F**). Noted here, there is no clear change observed for the other rate constants (i.e., $\alpha_m$ and $\beta_h$).

## DISCUSSION

Recordings of neuronal membranes exhibit time-dependent voltage fluctuations (Destexhe et al., 2003; El Boustani et al., 2009), which have not been extensively studied in the last few decades due to the lack of a functional understanding of the underlying noise composition. In addition, $1/f^\beta$ noise has mainly been considered as background noise in previous studies (Mainen and Sejnowski, 1995; Nozaki and Yamamoto, 1998; Nozaki et al., 1999b; Jia et al., 2001; Ruszczynski et al., 2001; Richardson et al., 2003; Chizhov and Graham, 2008; Köndgen et al., 2008; Mino and Durand, 2008; Gutkin et al., 2009; Higgs and Spain, 2009; Sekine et al., 2009; Guo and Li, 2011; Sobie et al., 2011; Duan et al., 2014; Zhao et al., 2017). Here, for the first time, we directly examine cortical pyramidal neuronal responsiveness to $1/f^\beta$ ($\beta$ = 0, 1, and 2) input signals. Our results shed light on the mechanism by which the statistical structure of input signals affects the dynamics of spike generation in cortical pyramidal cells.

### The Effect of the Frequency Range on the $1/f^\beta$ Noise Response

We compared neuronal responses to $1/f^0$, 1/f, and $1/f^2$ noises with various cutoff frequencies (50–1,000 Hz) and observed that cortical pyramidal cells exhibit a substantial loss of reliability and sensitivity to white noise when the cutoff frequency exceeds 200 Hz. Neuronal responsiveness to 1/f is also better than $1/f^2$ at various cutoff frequencies. In previous studies, white noise has been widely utilized to detect neuronal input and output functions (Sakai, 1992; Fairhall et al., 2001; Cook et al., 2007; Vilela and Lindner, 2009). Based on our results, 1/f noise should be a much better probe for determining the response properties of neurons at various input frequency ranges, instead of white noise or $1/f^2$ noise, and the signal cutoff frequency should be carefully established in future studies.

Our work suggests that the neuronal firing rate and reliability for 1/f noise are both enhanced with an increase in the cutoff frequency. Thus, each frequency interval has an effect on neuronal responses, and future work should examine the

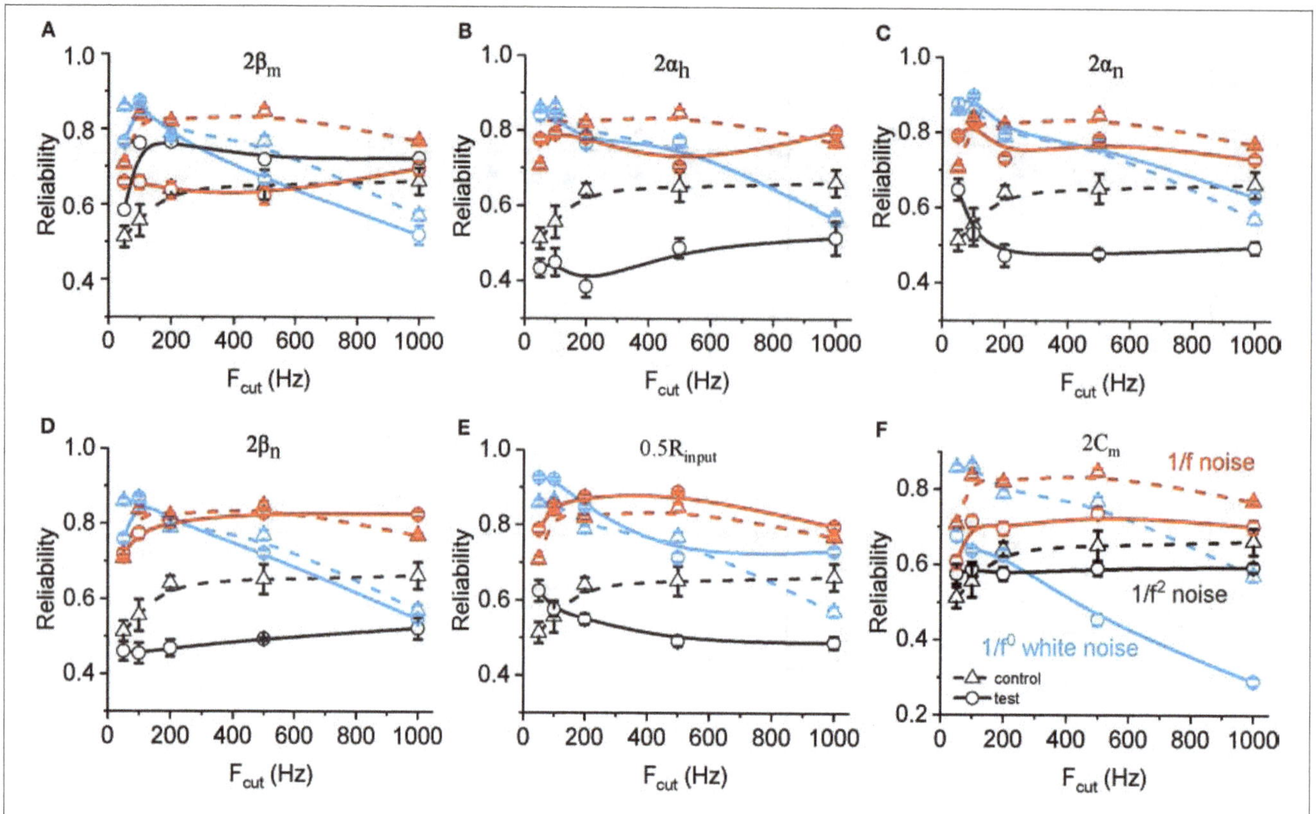


**FIGURE 6 |** Effects of ionic and membrane time constants on the spike reliability of model neurons. **(A–F)** Plots of reliability vs. cutoff frequency for white noise (blue), 1/f (red) and $1/f^2$ noise (black) for a normal neuron (dotted line, **A–F**) compared with the results from the model neuron in the case of 2 $\beta_m$ (solid line, **A**), 2 $\alpha_h$ (solid line, **B**), 2 $\alpha_n$ (solid line, **C**), 2 $\beta_n$ (solid line, **D**), 0.5 $R_{input}$ (solid line, **E**), and 2 $C_m$ (solid line, **F**). $F_{cut}$, cutoff frequency. $R_{input}$, membrane input resistance. $C_m$, membrane capacitance.

optimum signal frequency range for neuronal responsiveness and derive the neuronal input-output function for each frequency interval. Although a previous study has found that injecting white noise to the DC component increases neuronal spike reliability (Mainen and Sejnowski, 1995), our findings with zero mean signals imply that neuronal excitability may determine the effects of signal frequency range, and ultimately modulate neuronal response.

## Preferential Neuronal Response to 1/f Noise With a Large Frequency Range

The 1/f noise is a common phenomenon in nature (Bak et al., 1987; Gilden et al., 1995; Musha and Yamamoto, 1997; Novikov et al., 1997; De Coensel et al., 2003; Bédard et al., 2006; He, 2014). In the brain, EEG and ECoG recordings reveal that when neuronal populations exhibit the 1/f characteristic, the neural network is capable of highly efficient information processing (Soma et al., 2003; Lin and Chen, 2005; Shew and Plenz, 2013; Wood et al., 2016). At the cellular level, 1/f noise was found to originate from intact network inputs (El Boustani et al., 2009), and can enhance neuronal excitability and the stochastic resonanGarciace effect (Nozaki and Yamamoto, 1998; Nozaki et al., 1999a,b; El Boustani et al., 2009). Based on neuronal sensitivity to low-frequency sine wave signals (Hutcheon et al., 1996; Hunter et al., 1998; Volgushev et al., 1998; Fellous et al., 2001; Yu et al., 2001; Brumberg, 2002; Richardson et al., 2003; Köndgen et al., 2008; Levi et al., 2015), an individual neuron uses signals with a low frequency range to process information. However, recent experiments have observed high frequency components in the recorded membrane potentials of cortical neurons *in vivo* (El Boustani et al., 2009; Bedard et al., 2017).

Our results, for the first time, show that neurons respond preferentially to the 1/f noise in large frequency ranges, with respect to the firing rate and spike timing reliability. Because the rate and temporal encoding are two major encoding methods for neurons (Nowak et al., 1997; Reinagel and Reid, 2000; Fellous et al., 2001; Brette and Guigon, 2003; Avissar et al., 2007; Freund and Cerquera, 2012) and neuronal activities at all levels show 1/f characteristics *in vivo* (Bédard et al., 2006; El Boustani et al., 2009; Freeman and Zhai, 2009; Milstein et al., 2009; Dehghani et al., 2010; He et al., 2010; Ciuciu et al., 2012; Pettersen et al., 2014; Voytek et al., 2015), our results may indicate the positive effects of the 1/f property and large frequency range on the neuronal responses for normal physiological functioning. In addition, since the 1/f type of signal substantially drives neuronal response, our findings suggest new operating rules for synaptic transmission, neuronal plasticity and other activities relying on neuronal firing. It is likely that future studies of neuronal interactions and network activities will discover additional distinct effects of 1/f probe signals on neural information process and neural computation.

## Neuronal Dynamics Underlying the 1/f Preference

Given the low-pass filter property of neuronal membrane, once the signal contain more power in low frequency range, it may induce more neuronal firing, as seen from the neuronal response to 1/f compared with to white noise (Fellous et al., 2001; Brumberg, 2002; Levi et al., 2015). However, this is in contradiction with our finding that 1/f noise evokes higher firing rate than $1/f^2$ noise in a large frequency rage. Especially, we observed that neuronal firing rate for 1/f noise increases with the cutoff frequency of 1/f noise increases. In addition, it was reported previously that the refractory period endows neuron with high-pass filtering (Nozaki et al., 1999a), increasing the response complexity. We performed numerical simulations by using the Hodgkin-Huxley model to gain deep insights into the mechanism underlying the neuronal responsive preference for the 1/f noise. We found that $\beta_n$, $R_{input}$, and $C_m$ determine the neuronal preference to input signal with different type of statistics. **Figure 4** shows that the effect of changing $\beta_n$ on the neuronal firing rate to $1/f^2$ is larger to 1/f, much larger than to $1/f^0$ noise. On the contrary, the effects of changing $R_{input}$ or $C_m$ on the neuronal firing rate is stronger to $1/f^0$ noise than 1/f, even stronger than to $1/f^2$ inputs. Here, close rate constant of potassium activation $\beta_n$ seems to form a high-pass filter effect, while both $R_{input}$ and $C_m$ act as low-pass filter effect. Their appropriately combined action may result in neuronal responsive preference for 1/f noise with a broad frequency range.

In addition, we found the neuronal responsive reliability for $1/f^\beta$ signal types is majorly dominated by several key factors of ion channels and membrane time constants, respectively. Specifically, as shown in results section, the spike reliability for white noise is mainly determined by $C_m$. Spike reliability for 1/f and $1/f^2$ noise is mainly dominated by sodium activation close rate constant ($\alpha_m$), inactivation open rate constant ($\alpha_h$) and both open ($\alpha_n$), and close ($\beta_n$) rate constants of potassium channel, as well as membrane time constant. With doubled $\alpha_h$, $\alpha_n$, and $\beta_n$ (**Figures 6B–D**) and decreased $R_{input}$ (**Figure 6E**), neuronal spike reliability for $1/f^2$ noise decreases significantly for most of frequency range. These effects for $1/f^2$ noise are stronger than for 1/f noise, and much stronger for white noise. These results revealed that the membrane capacitance dominates the neuronal preference to low frequency component, while the combined ion channel kinetics dominates the neuronal preference to high frequency components in the $1/f^\beta$ type noise stimuli.

A prevailing hypothesis in neuronal response is that the stochastic opening and closing of individual ion channels endows cortical neurons an inherent noise. When the correlation time of the external input matches the time scale of the inherent noise, the neuronal responsiveness is maximized. Indeed, previous studies have demonstrated the existence of the optimum time scale of input signals for neuronal spiking reliability (Galán et al., 2008; McGinley et al., 2015). The neuron-preferred 1/f signal in our finding is consistent with this hypothesis.

In addition, cortical neurons are also enriched in other subtypes of sodium, potassium, and calcium channels, which may play important roles in precisely controlling the cellular sensitivity to the input signals with different temporal correlations (Wang et al., 2003). Additionally, a balance between excitatory and inhibitory synaptic inputs may adjust neuronal excitability to different signal statistics (Brunel et al., 2001; Chance et al., 2002; Wang, 2010). The dendritic morphology of the cell may even enhance the neuronal sensitivity to some frequency components within input signals (Eyal et al., 2014; Ostojic et al., 2015). Future studies should examine how the synaptic balance and the interaction between the neuronal intrinsic dynamics and modulations from the recurrent network contribute to the neuronal responses to input signals with various higher order statics and cutoff frequencies.

In summary, as the signal cutoff frequency progressively increases from 50 to 1,000 Hz, the neuronal responsive firing rate and reliability increase for 1/f noise, but decrease for white noise. Ion channel kinetic and membrane time constants endow neurons with a preferential response for 1/f noise with high cutoff frequencies. These results suggest that the 1/f noise is important in determining the computational rules and operating principles of cortical circuits.

## AUTHOR CONTRIBUTIONS

YY supervised the research. YY, GQ, and BF designed the research. GQ and XF performed the experimental research. GQ and YY wrote the paper. All authors performed data analysis and reviewed the manuscript.

## FUNDING

YY thanks for the support from the National Natural Science Foundation of China (81761128011, 31571070), Shanghai Science and Technology Committee support (16410722600), the program for the Professor of Special Appointment (Eastern Scholar SHH1140004) at Shanghai Institutions of Higher Learning, the Research Fund for the Doctoral Program of Higher Education of China (1322051), and Omics-based precision medicine of epilepsy entrusted by the Key Research Project of the Ministry of Science and Technology of China (Grant No. 2016YFC0904400) for their support.

## REFERENCES


Aertsen, A. M., and Johannesma, P. I. (1981). A comparison of the spectro-temporal sensitivity of auditory neurons to tonal and natural stimuli. *Biol. Cybern.* 42, 145–156. doi: 10.1007/BF00336732

Avissar, M., Furman, A. C., Saunders, J. C., and Parsons, T. D. (2007). Adaptation reduces spike-count reliability, but not spike-timing precision, of auditory nerve responses. *J. Neurosci.* 27, 6461–6472. doi: 10.1523/JNEUROSCI.5239-06.2007

Baddeley, R., Abbott, L. F., Booth, M. C., Sengpiel, F., Freeman, T., Wakeman, E. A., et al. (1997). Responses of neurons in primary and inferior temporal visual cortices to natural scenes. *Proc. Biol. Sci.* 264, 1775–1783. doi: 10.1098/rspb.1997.0246.

Bak, P., Tang, C., and Wiesenfeld, K., (1987). Self-organized criticality: An explanation of the 1/f noise. *Phys. Rev. Lett.* 59, 381–384. doi: 10.1103/PhysRevLett.59.381

Bédard, C., and Destexhe, A. (2009). Macroscopic models of local field potentials and the apparent 1/f noise in brain activity. *Biophys. J.* 96, 2589–2603. doi: 10.1016/j.bpj.2008.12.3951

Bedard, C., Gomes, J.-M., Bal, T., and Destexhe, A. (2017). A framework to reconcile frequency scaling measurements, from intracellular recordings, local-field potentials, up to EEG and MEG signals. *J. Integr. Neurosci.* 16, 3–18. doi: 10.3233/JIN-160001

Bédard, C., Kröger, H., and Destexhe, A. (2006). Does the 1/f frequency scaling of brain signals reflect self-organized critical states? *Phys. Rev. Lett.* 97:118102. doi: 10.1103/PhysRevLett.97.118102

Bhattacharya, J., and Petsche, H. (2001). Universality in the brain while listening to music. *Proc. Biol. Sci.* 268, 2423–2433. doi: 10.1098/rspb.2001.1802

Brette, R., and Guigon, E. (2003). Reliability of spike timing is a general property of spiking model neurons. *Neural Comput.* 15, 279–308. doi: 10.1162/089976603762552924

Brumberg, J. C. (2002). Firing pattern modulation by oscillatory input in supragranular pyramidal neurons. *Neuroscience* 114, 239–246. doi: 10.1016/S0306-4522(02)00252-X

Brunel, N., Chance, F. S., Fourcaud, N., and Abbott, L. F. (2001). Effects of synaptic noise and filtering on the frequency response of spiking neurons. *Phys. Rev. Lett.* 86, 2186–2189. doi: 10.1103/PhysRevLett.86.2186

Brunel, N., and Latham, P. E. (2003). Firing rate of the noisy quadratic integrate-and-fire neuron. *Neural Comput.* 15, 2281–2306. doi: 10.1162/089976603322362365

Bullmore, E., Long, C., Suckling, J., Fadili, J., Calvert, G., Zelaya, F., et al. (2001). Colored noise and computational inference in neurophysiological (fMRI) time series analysis: resampling methods in time and wavelet domains. *Hum. Brain Mapp.* 12, 61–78. doi: 10.1002/1097-0193(200102)12:23.0.CO;2-W.3.0.CO;2-W

Chance, F. S., Abbott, L. F., and Reyes, A. D. (2002). Gain modulation from background synaptic input. *Neuron* 35, 773–782. doi: 10.1016/S0896-6273(02)00820-6

Chizhov, A. V., and Graham, L. J. (2008). Efficient evaluation of neuron populations receiving colored-noise current based on a refractory density method. *Phys. Rev. E Stat. Nonlin. Soft Matter Phys.* 77:011910. doi: 10.1103/PhysRevE.77.011910

Ciuciu, P., Abry, P., and He, B. J. (2014). Interplay between functional connectivity and scale-free dynamics in intrinsic fMRI networks. *NeuroImage* 95, 248–263. doi: 10.1016/j.neuroimage.2014.03.047

Ciuciu, P., Varoquaux, G., Abry, P., Sadaghiani, S., and Kleinschmidt, A. (2012). Scale-free and multifractal time dynamics of fMRI signals during rest and task. *Front. Physiol.* 3:186. doi: 10.3389/fphys.2012.00186

Colbert, C. M., and Pan, E. (2002). Ion channel properties underlying axonal action potential initiation in pyramidal neurons. *Nat. Neurosci.* 5, 533–538. doi: 10.1038/nn857

Cook, E. P., Wilhelm, A. C., Guest, J. A., Liang, Y., Masse, N. Y., and Colbert, C. M. (2007). The neuronal transfer function: contributions from voltage- and time-dependent mechanisms. *Prog. Brain Res.* 165, 1–12. doi: 10.1016/S0079-6123(06)65001-2

De Coensel, B., Botteldooren, D., De Muer, T. (2003). "1/f noise in rural and urban soundscapes. *Acta Acustica United Acustica* 89, 287–295. doi: 10.1134/1.1560388

de Ruyter van Steveninck, R. R., Lewen, G. D., Strong, S. P., Koberle, R., and Bialek, W. (1997). Reproducibility and variability in neural spike trains. *Science* 275, 1805–1808. doi: 10.1126/science.275.5307.1805

Dehghani, N., Bédard, C., Cash, S. S., Halgren, E., and Destexhe, A. (2010). Comparative power spectral analysis of simultaneous elecroencephalographic and magnetoencephalographic recordings in humans suggests non-resistive extracellular media. *J. Comput. Neurosci.* 29, 405–421. doi: 10.1007/s10827-010-0263-2

Destexhe, A., Rudolph, M., and Paré, D. (2003). The high-conductance state of neocortical neurons *in vivo*. *Nat. Rev. Neurosci.* 4, 739–751. doi: 10.1038/nrn1198

Diba, K. (2004). Intrinsic noise in cultured hippocampal neurons: experiment and modeling. *J. Neurosci.* 24, 9723–9733. doi: 10.1523/JNEUROSCI.1721-04.2004

Duan, F., Chapeau-Blondeau, F., and Abbott, D. (2014). Stochastic resonance with colored noise for neural signal detection. *PLoS ONE* 9:e91345. doi: 10.1371/journal.pone.0091345

El Boustani, S., Marre, O., Béhuret, S., Baudot, P., Yger, P., Bal, T., et al. (2009). Network-state modulation of power-law frequency-scaling in visual cortical neurons. *PLoS Comput. Biol.* 5:e1000519. doi: 10.1371/journal.pcbi.1000519

Eyal, G., Mansvelder, H. D., de Kock, C. P. J., and Segev, I. (2014). Dendrites impact the encoding capabilities of the axon. *J. Neurosci. Off. J. Soc. Neurosci.* 34, 8063–8071. doi: 10.1523/JNEUROSCI.5431-13.2014

Fairhall, A. L., Lewen, G. D., Bialek, W., and de Ruyter Van Steveninck, R. R. (2001). Efficiency and ambiguity in an adaptive neural code. *Nature* 412, 787–792. doi: 10.1038/35090500

Fellous, J. M., Houweling, A. R., Modi, R. H., Rao, R. P., Tiesinga, P. H., and Sejnowski, T. J. (2001). Frequency dependence of spike reliability in cortical pyramidal cells and interneurons. *J. Neurophysiol.* 85, 1782–1787. doi: 10.1152/jn.2001.85.4.1782

Fleidervish, I. A., Lasser-Ross, N., Gutnick, M. J., and Ross, W. N. (2010). Na+ imaging reveals little difference in action potential-evoked Na+ influx between axon and soma. *Nat. Neurosci.* 13, 852–860. doi: 10.1038/nn.2574

Fohlmeister, J. F., Cohen, E. D., and Newman, E. A. (2010). Mechanisms and distribution of ion channels in retinal ganglion cells: using temperature as an independent variable. *J. Neurophysiol.* 103, 1357–1374. doi: 10.1152/jn.00123.2009

Frankenhaeuser, B., and Moore, L. E. (1963). The effect of temperature on the sodium and potassium permeability changes in myelinated nerve fibres of xenopus laevis. *J. Physiol.* 169, 431–437. doi: 10.1113/jphysiol.1963.sp007269

Freeman, W. J., and Zhai, J. (2009). Simulated power spectral density (PSD) of background electrocorticogram (ECoG). *Cogn. Neurodyn.* 3, 97–103. doi: 10.1007/s11571-008-9064-y

Freund, J. A., and Cerquera, A. (2012). How spurious correlations affect a correlation-based measure of spike timing reliability. *Neurocomputing* 81, 97–103. doi: 10.1016/j.neucom.2011.10.014

Gal, A., and Marom, S. (2013). Entrainment of the intrinsic dynamics of single isolated neurons by natural-like input. *J. Neurosci.* 33, 7912–7918. doi: 10.1523/JNEUROSCI.3763-12.2013

Galán, R. F., Ermentrout, G. B., and Urban, N. N. (2008). Optimal time scale for spike-time reliability: theory, simulations, and experiments. *J. Neurophysiol.* 99, 277–283. doi: 10.1152/jn.00563.2007

Garcia-Lazaro, J. A., Ahmed, B., and Schnupp, J. W. (2006). Tuning to natural stimulus dynamics in primary auditory cortex. *Curr. Biol. CB* 16, 264–271. doi: 10.1016/j.cub.2005.12.013

Garcia-Lazaro, J. A., Ahmed, B., and Schnupp, J. W. (2011). Emergence of tuning to natural stimulus statistics along the central auditory pathway. *PLoS ONE* 6:e22584. doi: 10.1371/journal.pone.0022584

Gilden, D. L., Thornton, T., and Mallon, M. W. (1995). 1/f noise in human cognition. *Science* 267, 1837–1839. doi: 10.1126/science.7892611

Guo, D., and Li, C. (2011). Signal propagation in feedforward neuronal networks with unreliable synapses. *J. Comput. Neurosci.* 30, 567–587. doi: 10.1007/s10827-010-0279-7

Gutkin, B. S., Jost, J., and Tuckwell, H. C. (2009). Inhibition of rhythmic neural spiking by noise: the occurrence of a minimum in activity with increasing noise. *Naturwissenschaften* 96, 1091–1097. doi: 10.1007/s00114-009-0570-5

Haider, B., Krause, M. R., Duque, A., Yu, Y., Touryan, J., Mazer, J. A., et al. (2010). Synaptic and network mechanisms of sparse and reliable visual cortical activity during nonclassical receptive field stimulation. *Neuron* 65, 107–121. doi: 10.1016/j.neuron.2009.12.005

Halnes, G., Mäki-Marttunen, T., Keller, D., Pettersen, K. H., Andreassen, O. A., and Einevoll, G. T. (2016). Effect of ionic diffusion on extracellular potentials in neural tissue. *PLoS Comput. Biol.* 12:e1005193. doi: 10.1371/journal.pcbi.1005193

He, B. J. (2011). Scale-free properties of the functional magnetic resonance imaging signal during rest and task. *J. Neurosci. Off. J. Soc. Neurosci.* 31, 13786–13795. doi: 10.1523/JNEUROSCI.2111-11.2011

He, B. J. (2014). Scale-free brain activity: past, present, and future. *Trends Cogn. Sci.* 18, 480–487. doi: 10.1016/j.tics.2014.04.003

He, B. J., Zempel, J. M., Snyder, A. Z., and Raichle, M. E. (2010). The temporal structures and functional significance of scale-free brain activity. *Neuron* 66, 353–369. doi: 10.1016/j.neuron.2010.04.020

Higgs, M. H., and Spain, W. J. (2009). Conditional bursting enhances resonant firing in neocortical layer 2-3 pyramidal neurons. *J. Neurosci.* 29, 1285–1299. doi: 10.1523/JNEUROSCI.3728-08.2009

Hu, W., Tian, C., Li, T., Yang, M., Hou, H., and Shu, Y. (2009). Distinct contributions of Nav1.6 and Nav1.2 in action potential initiation and backpropagation. *Nat. Neurosci.* 12, 996–1002. doi: 10.1038/nn.2359

Huguenard, J. R., Hamill, O. P., and Prince, D. A. (1989). Sodium channels in dendrites of rat cortical pyramidal neurons. *Proc. Natl. Acad. Sci. U. S. A.* 86, 2473–2477. doi: 10.1073/pnas.86.7.2473

Hunter, J. D., Milton, J. G., Thomas, P. J., and Cowan, J. D. (1998). Resonance effect for neural spike time reliability. *J. Neurophysiol.* 80, 1427–1438. doi: 10.1152/jn.1998.80.3.1427

Hutcheon, B., Miura, R. M., and Puil, E. (1996). Subthreshold membrane resonance in neocortical neurons. *J. Neurophysiol.* 76, 683–697. doi: 10.1152/jn.1996.76.2.683

Hutcheon, B., and Yarom, Y. (2000). Resonance, oscillation and the intrinsic frequency preferences of neurons. *Trends Neurosci.* 23, 216–222. doi: 10.1016/S0166-2236(00)01547-2

Jacobson, G. A., Diba, K., Yaron-Jakoubovitch, A., Oz, Y., Koch, C., Segev, I., et al. (2005). Subthreshold voltage noise of rat neocortical pyramidal neurones. *J. Physiol.* 564, 145–160. doi: 10.1113/jphysiol.2004.080903

Jia, Y., Zheng, X., Hu, X., and Li, J. (2001). Effects of colored noise on stochastic resonance in a bistable system subject to multiplicative and additive noise. *Phys. Rev. E Stat. Nonlin. Soft Matter Phys.* 63:031107. doi: 10.1103/PhysRevE.63.031107

Kole, M. H., Ilschner, S. U., Kampa, B. M., Williams, S. R., Ruben, P. C., and Stuart, G. J. (2008). Action potential generation requires a high sodium channel density in the axon initial segment. *Nat. Neurosci.* 11, 178–186. doi: 10.1038/nn2040

Köndgen, H., Geisler, C., Fusi, S., Wang, X.-J., Lüscher, H.-R., and Giugliano, M. (2008). The dynamical response properties of neocortical neurons to temporally modulated noisy inputs *in vitro*. *Cereb. Cortex* 18, 2086–2097. doi: 10.1093/cercor/bhm235

Levi, R., Akanyeti, O., Ballo, A., and Liao, J. C. (2015). Frequency response properties of primary afferent neurons in the posterior lateral line system of larval zebrafish. *J. Neurophysiol.* 113, 657–668. doi: 10.1152/jn.00414.2014

Lin, M., and Chen, T. (2005). Self-organized criticality in a simple model of neurons based on small-world networks. *Phys. Rev. E Stat. Nonlin. Soft Matter Phys.* 71:016133. doi: 10.1103/PhysRevE.71.016133

Maex, R. (2018). An interneuron circuit reproducing essential spectral features of field potentials. *Neural Comput.* 30, 1296–1322. doi: 10.1162/NECO_a_01068

Mainen, Z. F., Joerges, J., Huguenard, J. R., and Sejnowski, T. J. (1995). A model of spike initiation in neocortical pyramidal neurons. *Neuron* 15, 1427–1439. doi: 10.1016/0896-6273(95)90020-9

Mainen, Z. F., and Sejnowski, T. J. (1995). Reliability of spike timing in neocortical neurons. *Science* 268, 1503–1506. doi: 10.1126/science.7770778

Mainen, Z. F., and Sejnowski, T. J. (1996). Influence of dendritic structure on firing pattern in model neocortical neurons. *Nature* 382, 363–366. doi: 10.1038/382363a0

Matteson, D. R., and Armstrong, C. M. (1982). Evidence for a population of sleepy sodium channels in squid axon at low temperature. *J. Gen. Physiol.* 79, 739–758. doi: 10.1085/jgp.79.5.739

McCormick, D. A., and Huguenard, J. R. (1992). A model of the electrophysiological properties of thalamocortical relay neurons. *J. Neurophysiol.* 68, 1384–1400. doi: 10.1152/jn.1992.68.4.1384

McGinley, M. J., David, S. V., and McCormick, D. A. (2015). Cortical membrane potential signature of optimal states for sensory signal detection. *Neuron* 87, 179–192. doi: 10.1016/j.neuron.2015.05.038

Miller, K. J., Sorensen, L. B., Ojemann, J. G., and den Nijs, M. (2009). Power-law scaling in the brain surface electric potential. *PLoS Comput. Biol.* 5:e1000609. doi: 10.1371/journal.pcbi.1000609

Milstein, J., Mormann, F., Fried, I., and Koch, C. (2009). Neuronal shot noise and Brownian 1/f2 behavior in the local field potential. *PLoS ONE* 4:e4338. doi: 10.1371/journal.pone.0004338

Mino, H., and Durand, D. M. (2008). Stochastic resonance can induce oscillation in a recurrent Hodgkin-Huxley neuron model with added Gaussian noise. *Conf Proc IEEE Eng Med Biol Soc.* 2008, 2457–2460. doi: 10.1109/IEMBS.2008.4649697

Musha, T., and Yamamoto, M. (1997). "1/f fluctuations in biological systems," in *Proceedings of the 19th Annual International Conference of the IEEE Engineering in Medicine and Biology Society. 'Magnificent Milestones and Emerging Opportunities in Medical Engineering' (Cat. No. 97CH36136)*, Vol. 6 (Chicago, IL: IEEE), 2692–2697. doi: 10.1109/IEMBS.1997.756890

Novikov, E., Novikov, A., Shannahoff-Khalsa, D., and Schwartz, B. (1997). Scale-similar activity in the brain. *Phys. Rev.* 56, R2387–R2389. doi: 10.1103/PhysRevE.56.R2387

Nowak, L. G., Sanchez-Vives, M. V., and McCormick, D. A. (1997). Influence of low and high frequency inputs on spike timing in visual cortical neurons. *Cereb. Cortex* 7, 487–501. doi: 10.1093/cercor/7.6.487

Nozaki, D., Collins, J. J., and Yamamoto, Y. (1999a). Mechanism of stochastic resonance enhancement in neuronal models driven by 1/f noise. *Phys. Rev. E Stat. Phys. Plasmas Fluids Relat. Interdiscip. Top.* 60, 4637–4644. doi: 10.1103/PhysRevE.60.4637

Nozaki, D., Marder, D. J., Grigg, P., and Collins, J. J. (1999b). Effects of colored noise on stochastic resonance in sensory neurons. *Phys. Rev. Lett.* 82, 2402–2405. doi: 10.1103/PhysRevLett.82.2402

Nozaki, D., and Yamamoto, Y. (1998). Enhancement of stochastic resonance in a FitzHugh-Nagumo neuronal model driven by colored noise. *Phys. Lett. A* 243, 281–287. doi: 10.1016/S0375-9601(98)00247-3

Ostojic, S., Szapiro, G., Schwartz, E., Barbour, B., Brunel, N., and Hakim, V. (2015). Neuronal morphology generates high-frequency firing resonance. *J. Neurosci. Off. J. Soc. Neurosci.* 35, 7056–7068. doi: 10.1523/JNEUROSCI.3924-14.2015

Pettersen, K. H., Lindén, H., Tetzlaff, T., and Einevoll, G. T. (2014). Power laws from linear neuronal cable theory: power spectral densities of the soma potential, soma membrane current and single-neuron contribution to the EEG. *PLoS Comput. Biol.* 10:e1003928. doi: 10.1371/journal.pcbi.1003928

Reinagel, P., and Reid, R. C. (2000). Temporal coding of visual information in the thalamus. *J. Neurosci. Off. J. Soc. Neurosci.* 20, 5392–5400. doi: 10.1523/JNEUROSCI.20-14-05392.2000

Richardson, M. J., Brunel, N., and Hakim, V. (2003). From subthreshold to firing-rate resonance. *J. Neurophysiol.* 89, 2538–2554. doi: 10.1152/jn.00955.2002

Ruszczynski, P. S., Kish, L. B., and Bezrukov, S. M. (2001). Noise-assisted traffic of spikes through neuronal junctions. *Chaos Woodbury N.* 11, 581–586. doi: 10.1063/1.1379308

Sakai, H. M. (1992). White-noise analysis in neurophysiology. *Physiol. Rev.* 72, 491–505. doi: 10.1152/physrev.1992.72.2.491

Schmidt-Hieber, C., and Bischofberger, J. (2010). Fast sodium channel gating supports localized and efficient axonal action potential initiation. *J. Neurosci. Off. J. Soc. Neurosci.* 30, 10233–10242. doi: 10.1523/JNEUROSCI.6335-09.2010

Schwalger, T., Droste, F., and Lindner, B. (2015). Statistical structure of neural spiking under non-Poissonian or other non-white stimulation. *J. Comput. Neurosci.* 39, 29–51. doi: 10.1007/s10827-015-0560-x

Sekine, M., Mino, H., and Durand, D. M. (2009). Noise induced oscillations in recurrent neural networks. *Conf. Proc. IEEE Eng. Med. Biol. Soc.* 2009, 1521–1524. doi: 10.1109/IEMBS.2009.5333069

Shew, W. L., and Plenz, D. (2013). The functional benefits of criticality in the cortex. *Neuroscientist* 19, 88–100. doi: 10.1177/1073858412445487

Sobie, C., Babul, A., and de Sousa, R. (2011). Neuron dynamics in the presence of 1/f noise. *Phys. Rev. E Stat. Nonlin. Soft Matter Phys.* 83:051912. doi: 10.1103/PhysRevE.83.051912

Soma, R., Nozaki, D., Kwak, S., and Yamamoto, Y. (2003). 1/f noise outperforms white noise in sensitizing baroreflex function in the human brain. *Phys. Rev. Lett.* 91:078101. doi: 10.1103/PhysRevLett.91.078101

Ting, J. T., Daigle, T. L., Chen, Q., and Feng, G. (2014). "Acute brain slice methods for adult and aging animals: application of targeted patch clamp analysis and optogenetics," in *Patch-Clamp Methods and Protocols*, eds. M. Martina and S. Taverna (New York, NY: Springer New York), 221–242. Available online at: http://link.springer.com/10.1007/978-1-4939-1096-0_14 (accessed April 24, 2016). doi: 10.1007/978-1-4939-1096-0_14

Vilela, R. D., and Lindner, B. (2009). Are the input parameters of white noise driven integrate and fire neurons uniquely determined by rate and CV? *J. Theor. Biol.* 257, 90–99. doi: 10.1016/j.jtbi.2008.11.004

Volgushev, M., Chistiakova, M., and Singer, W. (1998). Modification of discharge patterns of neocortical neurons by induced oscillations of the membrane potential. *Neuroscience* 83, 15–25. doi: 10.1016/S0306-4522(97)00380-1

Voss, R. G., and Clarke, J. (1978). "1/f noise"in music: music from 1/f noise. *J. Acoust. Soc. Am.* 63, 258–263. doi: 10.1121/1.381721

Voytek, B., Kramer, M. A., Case, J., Lepage, K. Q., Tempesta, Z. R., Knight, R. T., et al. (2015). Age-related changes in 1/f neural electrophysiological noise. *J. Neurosci. Off. J. Soc. Neurosci.* 35, 13257–13265. doi: 10.1523/JNEUROSCI.2332-14.2015

Wang, X.-J. (2010). Neurophysiological and computational principles of cortical rhythms in cognition. *Physiol. Rev.* 90, 1195–1268. doi: 10.1152/physrev.00035.2008

Wang, X.-J., Liu, Y., Sanchez-Vives, M. V., and McCormick, D. A. (2003). Adaptation and temporal decorrelation by single neurons in the primary visual cortex. *J. Neurophysiol.* 89, 3279–3293. doi: 10.1152/jn.00242.2003

Wood, T., Osredkar, D., Puchades, M., Maes, E., Falck, M., Flatebø, T., et al. (2016). Treatment temperature and insult severity influence the neuroprotective effects of therapeutic hypothermia. *Sci. Rep.* 6:23430. doi: 10.1038/srep 23430

Yaron-Jakoubovitch, A. (2008). A paradoxical isopotentiality: a spatially uniform noise spectrum in neocortical pyramidal cells. *Front. Cell. Neurosci.* 2:3. doi: 10.3389/neuro.03.003.2008

Yu, Y., Hill, A. P., and McCormick, D. A. (2012). Warm body temperature facilitates energy efficient cortical action potentials. *PLoS Comput. Biol.* 8:e1002456. doi: 10.1371/journal.pcbi.1002456

Yu, Y., Liu, F., Wang, J., and Wang, W. (2001). Spike timing precision for a neuronal array with periodic signal. *Phys. Lett.* 282, 23–30. doi: 10.1016/S0375-9601(01)00167-0

Yu, Y., Romero, R., and Lee, T. S. (2005). Preference of sensory neural coding for 1/f signals. *Phys. Rev. Lett.* 94:108103. doi: 10.1103/PhysRevLett.94.108103

Yu, Y., Shu, Y., and McCormick, D. A. (2008). Cortical action potential backpropagation explains spike threshold variability and rapid-onset kinetics. *J. Neurosci.* 28, 7260–7272. doi: 10.1523/JNEUROSCI.1613-08.2008

Zhao, J., Deng, B., Qin, Y., Men, C., Wang, J., Wei, X., et al. (2017). Weak electric fields detectability in a noisy neural network. *Cogn. Neurodyn.* 11, 81–90. doi: 10.1007/s11571-016-9409-x

# 2

# Attenuates Spinal Cord Ischemia-Reperfusion Injury via Anti-oxidative Activity and Inhibition of Mitochondrial Dysfunction in Rabbits

*Jie Zhu†, Li-Kun Yang†, Wei-Liang Chen, Wei Lin, Yu-Hai Wang* and Tao Chen**

*Department of Neurosurgery, The 101th Hospital of PLA, School of Medicine, Anhui Medical University, Wuxi, China*

****Correspondence:***
*Yu-Hai Wang*
*prof_wyh101@163.com*
*Tao Chen*
*fmmuchentao@163.com*

*† These authors have contributed equally to this work*

Spinal cord ischemia-reperfusion injury (SCI/R) is a rare but devastating disorder with a poor prognosis. Small conductance calcium-activated $K^+$ ($SK/K_{Ca}$) channels are a family of voltage-independent potassium channels that are shown to participate in the pathological process of several neurological disorders. The aim of this study was to investigate the role of $SK/K_{Ca}$ channels in experimental SCI/R in rabbits. The expression of $SK/K_{Ca}1$ protein significantly decreased in both cytoplasm and mitochondria in spinal cord tissues after SCI/R. Treatment with 2 mg/kg NS309, a pharmacological activator for $SK/K_{Ca}$ channel, attenuated SCI/R-induced neuronal loss, spinal cord edema and neurological dysfunction. These effects were still observed when the administration was delayed by 6 h after SCI/R initiation. NS309 decreased the levels of oxidative products and promoted activities of antioxidant enzymes in both serum and spinal cord tissues. The results of ELISA assay showed that NS309 markedly decreased levels of pro-inflammatory cytokines while increased anti-inflammatory cytokines levels after SCI/R. In addition, treatment with NS309 was shown to preserve mitochondrial respiratory complexes activities and enhance mitochondrial biogenesis. The results of western blot analysis showed that NS309 differentially regulated the expression of mitochondrial dynamic proteins. In summary, our results demonstrated that the $SK/K_{Ca}$ channel activator NS309 protects against SCI/R via anti-oxidative activity and inhibition of mitochondrial dysfunction, indicating a therapeutic potential of NS309 for SCI/R.

**Keywords: $SK/K_{Ca}$ channels, NS309, spinal cord ischemia and reperfusion, mitochondrial dysfunction, mitochondrial dynamic**

## INTRODUCTION

Spinal cord ischemia-reperfusion injury (SCI/R) is a rare but devastating disorder induced by a period of deterioration of the spinal cord blood supply. SCI/R is associated with several pathophysiological states, while thoracoabdominal surgery and atherosclerotic disease are the most frequent causes (New and McFarlane, 2012). It has been shown that approximately 32% of patients with thoracic or thoracoabdominal aortic repair surgery suffered from SCI/R, and the incidence of paraplegia was up to 5% (LeMaire et al., 2012; Panthee and Ono, 2015). Many neuroprotective drugs, such as mannitol, corticosteroids and naloxone, have been demonstrated to be beneficial to function recovery in experimental SCI/R models, but none of them was convincingly confirmed in clinical trials (Griepp and Griepp, 2007).

Small conductance calcium-activated $K^+$ (SK/$K_{Ca}$) channels are a family of voltage-independent potassium channels that are activated solely by intracellular $Ca^{2+}$. SK/$K_{Ca}$ channels are extensively expressed throughout the central nervous system, including the brain and spinal cord tissues (Kuiper et al., 2012). They are encoded by the *KCNN* gene family, and three different subtypes of SK/$K_{Ca}$ channels, including SK/$K_{Ca}$1, SK/$K_{Ca}$2, and SK/$K_{Ca}$3, have been cloned in mammals (Stocker, 2004). SK/$K_{Ca}$ channels are activated by increases in intracellular $Ca^{2+}$, and they not only contribute to the after-hyperpolarization that follows action potentials, but also play key roles in regulating dendritic excitability, synaptic transmission and synaptic plasticity (Faber and Sah, 2007). Three decades of research has shown that SK/$K_{Ca}$ channels are involved in multiple neurological diseases caused by neuronal excitotoxicity and dysfunction of $Ca^{2+}$ homeostasis (Kuiper et al., 2012). By using pharmacological inhibitors and activators, Dolga and colleagues found that SK/$K_{Ca}$ channels participated in the pathological process of stroke, Parkinson's disease (PD), Alzheimer's disease (AD) and schizophrenia (Anderson et al., 2006; Dolga et al., 2011, 2012; Dolga and Culmsee, 2012). A previous study showed that activation of the SK/$K_{Ca}$ channel protected against glutamate-induced oxytosis through inhibiting mitochondrial dysfunction (Dolga et al., 2013). More importantly, activation of the SK/$K_{Ca}$ channel in the spinal cord was shown to reduce the NMDA receptor antagonist dose needed to produce anti-nociception in an inflammatory pain model (Hipolito et al., 2015). In the present study, we investigated the role of SK/$K_{Ca}$ channels in a SCI/R model in rabbits. Previous studies have demonstrated that SK/$K_{Ca}$ channels were also located in mitochondrial-enriched fraction, and this type of subcellular expression of SK/$K_{Ca}$ channels was associated with normal mitochondrial function in dopaminergic neurons (Dolga et al., 2014). Thus, we also determined the underlying mechanism with focus on oxidative stress and mitochondrial function.

## MATERIALS AND METHODS

### Animals and Agents

Adult New Zealand white rabbits (2.5–3.0 kg) were obtained from the Laboratory Animal Center of Anhui Medical University. All rabbits were kept in standard laboratory conditions with free access to rabbit chow and tap water. All experimental procedures were performed in compliance with the NIH guidelines for the use of experimental animals and approved by the Ethics Review Committee of Anhui Medical University. The mitochondrial isolation kit, malondialdehyde (MDA) assay kit, 8-iso-prostaglandin F2α (8-iso-PGF2α) assay kit, superoxide dismutase (SOD) assay kit and catalase (CAT) assay kit was purchased from Jiancheng Biotech Company (Nanjing, Jiangsu, China). The anti-SK/$K_{Ca}$1 (ab66624), anti-COX IV (ab66739), and anti-Tubulin (ab56676) antibodies were obtained from abcam (CA, United States). The anti-Opa-1 (sc-30573), anti-Mfn-1 (sc-166644), anti-Drp-1 (sc-101270), anti-Fis-1 (sc-376447), and anti-β-actin (sc-47778) antibodies were purchased from Santa Cruz Biotechnology (Santa Cruz, CA, United States).

### SCI/R Model

SCI/R was established by infrarenal aortic occlusion as previously described (Zhou et al., 2013). The animals were anesthetized by intramuscular administration of 25 mg/kg ketamine and 0.10 mg/kg atropine. The right femoral artery was catheterized for measuring distal blood pressure and ear artery was used to collect blood sample. A 5-cm-long midline incision was made to expose abdominal aorta, and aortic clamping was performed using artery clips just below renal artery after administration of 200 units of heparin. After 20 min occlusion, the clips were removed to restore the blood flow. Then, the incision was sutured layer-by-layer, and the rabbits were allowed to recover. During the operation process, the body temperature was maintained close to 38.2°C using a heating lamp.

### Experimental Design

#### Experimental 1

To investigate the effect of SCI/R on the expression of SK/$K_{Ca}$1 and mitochondrial dynamic proteins, forty animals were randomly divided into sham ($n$ = 8) and SCI/R ($n$ = 32) group. The animals in sham group were given operation without artery occlusion. The animals in SCI/R group were treated with SCI/R and spinal cord tissues were obtained at 3, 6, 12, and 24 h.

#### Experimental 2

To investigate the protective effect of NS309 against SCI/R, thirty-two animals were randomly divided into vehicle ($n$ = 16) and NS309 ($n$ = 16) group. The animals in NS309 group were treated with 2 mg/kg NS309 by intraperitoneal injection at the time of spinal cord ischemia initiation, and the animals in vehicle group were treated with saline (0.9%) with 1% DMSO. Eight animals in each group were used to measure neurological function and H&E staining, and the other 8 animals were used to measure spinal cord edema.

#### Experimental 3

To investigate the therapeutic time window of NS309, sixty-four animals were randomly divided into vehicle ($n$ = 16), NS309 at 3 h ($n$ = 16), NS39 at 6 h ($n$ = 16) and NS309 at 9 h ($n$ = 16) group. The animals in vehicle group were treated with saline (0.9%) with 1% DMSO, and the animals in NS309 groups were treated with 2 mg/kg NS309 by intraperitoneal injection at 3, 6, or 9 h after spinal cord ischemia initiation, respectively. Eight animals in each group were used to measure neurological function and H&E staining, and the other 8 animals were used to measure spinal cord edema.

### Experimental 4

To investigate the effect of NS309 on oxidative stress, and mitochondrial dysfunction, sixteen animals were randomly divided into vehicle ($n$ = 8) and NS309 ($n$ = 8) group. The animals in NS309 group were treated with 2 mg/kg NS309 by intraperitoneal injection at the time of spinal cord ischemia initiation, and the animals in vehicle group were treated with saline (0.9%) with 1% DMSO. The blood samples were collected at 0, 3, 6, 12, 24, and 48 h after spinal cord ischemia initiation, and the spinal cord tissues were collected at 72 h.

## Mitochondrial Isolation

After treatments, the spinal cord tissues were removed and homogenized, and mitochondria was isolated using the mitochondrial isolation kit following the manufacturer's suggested protocol. Mitochondrial pellets were resuspended, and the protein content was quantified using a BCA method. The mitochondrial and cytosolic fractions were used to detect SK/$K_{Ca}$1 expression, and the total protein was used to detect the expression of mitochondrial dynamic proteins.

## Hematoxylin and Eosin (H&E) Staining

After various treatments, the spinal cord tissues were removed, and the paraffin embedded blocks were made. The 5 μm sections from each group was subjected to standard H&E staining and evaluated microscopically. The number of normal motor neurons was counted by an investigator blinded to the grouping.

## Spinal Cord Edema Measurement

Spinal cord edema was evaluated by spinal cord water content using the wet-dry method at 72 h after SCI/R. Briefly, after the animals were sacrificed, the spinal cord tissues (L4-6 segments) were quickly removed. Tissue samples were weighed immediately to get wet weight. After drying in an oven for 48 h at 100°C, the tissues were re-weighed to get the dry weight. Spinal cord water content was then calculated using the following formula: % $H_2O$=(1-dry weight/wet weight) × 100%.

## Neurological Function Assay

The hind-limb motor function was determined by the modified Tarlov criteria: no voluntary hind-limb function as score 0; only perceptible joint movement as score 1; active movement but unable to stand as score 2; able to stand but unable to walk as score 3; and complete normal hind-limb motor function as score 4.

## Sample Collection

At 0, 3, 6, 12, 24, and 48 after SCI/R, 2 mL of blood was collected from auricular vein, and the serum was separated by centrifugation at 3,000 × $g$ for 15 min at 4°C. At 72 h after reperfusion, the animals were sacrificed, the spinal cord tissues (L4-6 segments) were removed. The spinal cord samples were homogenized in chilled PBS, and then centrifuged at 10,000 × $g$ at 4°C for 10 min. The protein concentration was quantified using a BCA method.

## Quantification of Oxidative Products and Antioxidant Enzymes

The levels MDA and 8-iso-PGF2α and the enzymatic activities of SOD and CAT in the serum and spinal cord samples were measured by commercial kits following the manufacturer's suggested protocol.

## Quantification of Inflammatory Cytokines

To detect the levels of inflammatory cytokines, animals were sacrificed at 12, 24, or 48 h after SCI/R, and the spinal cord homogenates were obtained. The concentrations of tumor necrosis factor-α (TNF-α), IL-1β, IL-10 and transforming growth factor-β1 (TGF-β1) were measured using specific ELISA kits according to the manufacturers' instructions (Boster Biological Technology, Wuhan, China).

## Determination of Mitochondrial Complexes Activities

After treatment with NS309 or vehicle, spinal cord mitochondria were isolated from each group and the enzymatic activities of mitochondrial complexes were assayed using the following methods: NADH dehydrogenase for complex I, succinate dehydrogenase for complex II, ubiquinol cytochrome c oxidase for complex III, and cytochrome c oxidase for complex IV as previously described (Ye et al., 2011).

## Real-Time RT-PCR

Total RNA was extracted from the spinal cord tissues using the Trizol reagent (Invitrogen, Carlsbad, CA, United States). Reverse transcription was performed according to the manufacturer's instructions of the real-time PCR kit (BioTNT Co., Ltd., Shanghai, China). The primers sequences used are shown in **Table 1**. The mRNA levels were normalized using GAPDH as an internal control.

## Western Blot Analysis

Total proteins from spinal cord tissues were extracted and the protein concentration was determined using a BCA assay kit (Jiancheng Biotech Company, Jiangsu, China). Equivalent proteins (60 μg per sample) were separated using 10 or 12% sodium dodecyl sulfate (SDS)-PAGE, and then electro-transferred onto polyvinylidene fluoride (PVDF) membranes.

**TABLE 1** | Primers sequences used in real-time PCR.

| Gene | Forward sequences | Reverse sequences |
|---|---|---|
| D-loop | 5′-AGGCATCTGGTTCTTACTTC-3′ | 5′-TGACGGCTATGTTGAGGA-3′ |
| ATP8 | 5′-CTTCCCAAACCTTTCCTG-3′ | 5′-GGTAATGAAAGAGGCA AATAGA-3′ |
| PGC-1 | 5′-GTGCAGCCAAGACTCTG TATGG-3′ | 5′-GTCCAGGTCATTCACAT CAAGTTC-3′ |
| NRF-1 | 5′-GAGTGACCCAAACCGAACA-3′ | 5′-GGAGTTGAGTATGTCC GAGT-3′ |
| TFAM | 5′-GGTGTATGAAGCGGATTT-3′ | 5′-CTTTCTTCTTTAGGCGTTT-3′ |
| GAPDH | 5′-ATGTATCCGTTGTGGAT CTGAC-3′ | 5′-CCTGCTTCACCACCTT CTTG-3′ |

The membranes were incubated with the following primary antibodies: SK/$K_{Ca}$1 (1:500), COX IV (1:800), Tubulin (1:1000), Opa-1 (1:500), Mfn-1 (1:800), Drp-1 (1:800), Fis-1 (1:500), and β-actin (1:2000). After incubation with secondary antibodies for 1 h, the bands were visualized by using chemiluminescent detection system. Image J (Scion Corporation) was used to quantify the optical density of each band. The expression of each protein was calculated from the optical density of each band normalized against the optical density of β-actin, tubulin or COX IV, and expressed as the fold of control levels.

## Statistical Analysis

Each experiment was repeated at least three times. Statistical analysis was performed using SPSS. Statistical evaluation of the data was performed by the Student's *t*-test between two groups. A value of $p < 0.05$ referred to the statistical difference.

# RESULTS

## SCI/R Decreases the Expression of SK/$K_{Ca}$1 Subtype

The changes of arterial pH, $PaO_2$, $PaCO_2$, and blood glucose levels in vehicle or 2 mg/kg NS309 treated rabbits were measured at 10 min before ischemia, 10 min after ischemia initiation and 10 min after reperfusion, respectively. As shown in **Table 2**, no significant differences in blood pH, $PaO_2$, $PaCO_2$, or glucose were observed among all groups. The results of distal blood pressure (DBP) showed that an approximate 90% reduction in DBP was observed during the time when artery was clamped. The value of DBP was recovered to 90–95% of the baseline within 10 min after reperfusion.

To investigate the effect of SCI/R on SK/$K_{Ca}$ channels expression, western blot analysis was used to detect the changes of SK/$K_{Ca}$1 subtype at 3, 6, 12, or 24 h after reperfusion (**Figure 1A**). The results showed that the expression of SK/$K_{Ca}$1 protein significantly decreased at 12 and 24 h after reperfusion. To determine the subcellular localization of SK/$K_{Ca}$1 after SCI/R, the expression of SK/$K_{Ca}$1 protein was assayed after mitochondria isolation (**Figure 1B**). The results showed an enrichment of SK/$K_{Ca}$1 from whole cell extracts to cytoplasm, as well as in mitochondrial fractions, and the decreased expression of SK/$K_{Ca}$1 protein was also observed in isolated mitochondria after SCI/R (**Figure 1C**).

## The SK/$K_{Ca}$ Channel Activator NS309 Protects Against SCI/R

To investigate the effect of SK/$K_{Ca}$ channel activation on SCI/R, rabbits were treated with 2 mg/kg NS309, a pharmacological activator for SK/$K_{Ca}$ channel, at the time of spinal cord ischemia

**TABLE 2** | Physiological parameters.

| | Rectal temperature (°C) | pH | $PaO_2$ (mm Hg) | $PaCO_2$ (mm Hg) | Glucose (mg/dl) | DBP (mm Hg) |
|---|---|---|---|---|---|---|
| *10 min before ischemia* | | | | | | |
| Vehicle | 38.3 ± 0.2 | 7.41 ± 0.13 | 124.2 ± 11.4 | 34.4 ± 3.8 | 157 ± 17 | 106 ± 5.7 |
| NS309 2 mg/kg | 38.1 ± 0.2 | 7.39 ± 0.09 | 129.5 ± 13.9 | 31.1 ± 4.6 | 168 ± 19 | 104 ± 7.1 |
| *10 min after ischemia* | | | | | | |
| Vehicle | 38.3 ± 0.3 | 7.35 ± 0.19 | 133.4 ± 15.3 | 34.3 ± 2.5 | 154 ± 18 | 13 ± 2.9* |
| NS309 2 mg/kg | 38.2 ± 0.2 | 7.38 ± 0.17 | 127.9 ± 15.2 | 32.7 ± 4.3 | 164 ± 23 | 17 ± 4.3* |
| *10 min after reperfusion* | | | | | | |
| Vehicle | 38.0 ± 0.1 | 7.37 ± 0.10 | 125.9 ± 11.4 | 36.8 ± 3.3 | 153 ± 19 | 100 ± 10.4 |
| NS309 2 mg/kg | 38.4 ± 0.4 | 7.41 ± 0.18 | 131.6 ± 12.3 | 38.3 ± 3.1 | 160 ± 22 | 98 ± 9.3 |

*Data are presented as mean ± SEM. *p < 0.05 vs. 10 min before ischemia.*

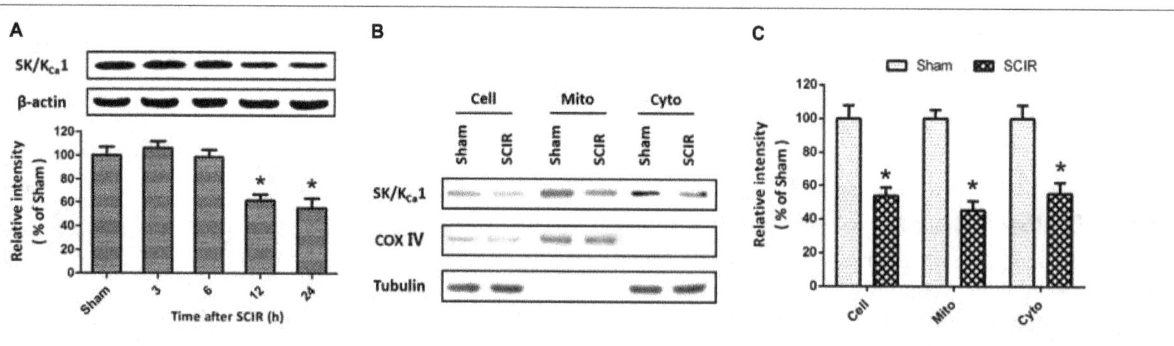


**FIGURE 1** | SCI/R decreases the expression of SK/$K_{Ca}$1 subtypes. The animals were exposed to spinal I/R, and the expression of SK/$K_{Ca}$1 protein in spinal cord tissues was detected by western blot analysis at 3, 6, 12, or 24 h after reperfusion **(A)**. Immunoblot analysis of whole-cell extract (depicted as "Cell"), cytosol supernatant (depicted as "Cyto") or crude mitochondrial pellets (depicted as "Mito") were also performed **(B)**, and calculated **(C)** to determine subcellular expression of SK/$K_{Ca}$1 protein. Data are shown as mean ± SEM ($n$ = 8). *$p < 0.05$ vs. Sham.

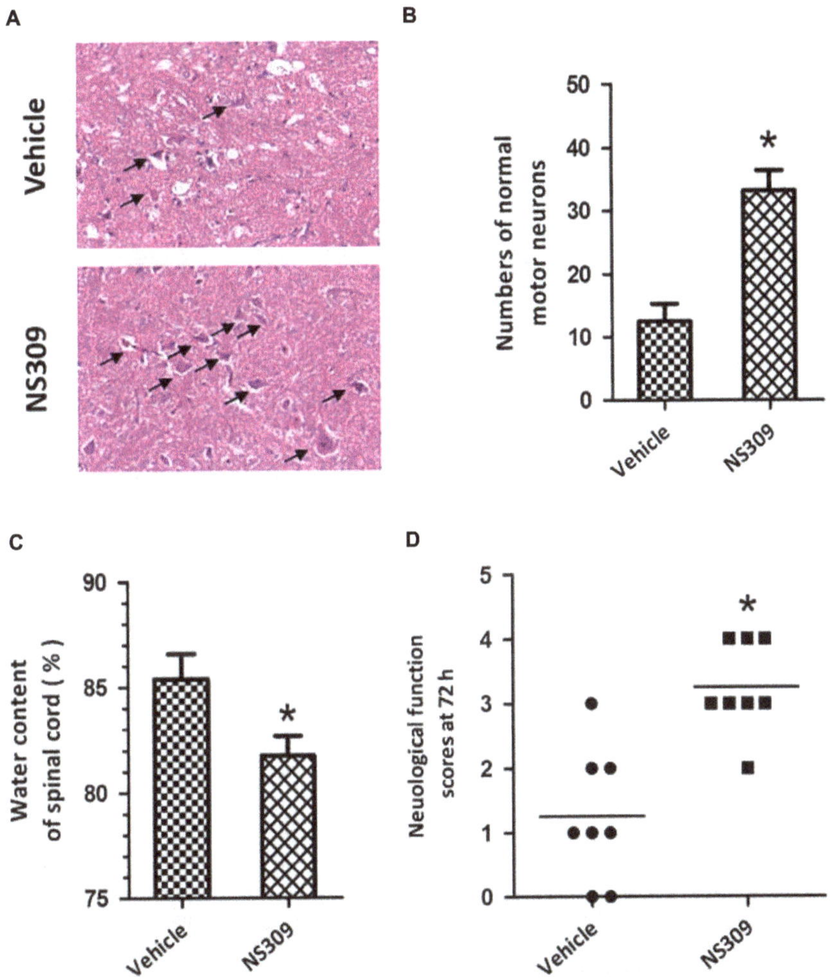


**FIGURE 2 |** The SK/$K_{Ca}$ channel activator NS309 protects against SCI/R. The animals were treated with 2 mg/kg NS309 or vehicle at the beginning of SCI/R operation. Hematoxylin and eosin staining was performed in the ventral horn of L4 spinal cord segment at 72 h after reperfusion **(A)**, and the number of normal motor neurons was countered **(B)**. The spinal cord edema was assayed by measuring spinal cord water content at 72 h **(C)**. Neurological function scores were assessed at 72 h after reperfusion by an independent observer **(D)**. Arrowheads indicate normal neurons. The data were represented as means ± SEM ($n$ = 8). $^*p < 0.05$ vs. Vehicle.

initiation. The representative micrographs of H&E staining in the ventral horn of L4 spinal cord segment at 72 h after reperfusion are shown in **Figure 2A**. The number of normal motor neurons in NS309 group was higher than that in vehicle group (**Figure 2B**). We also determined spinal cord edema by measuring water content of spinal cord tissues at 72 h after injury, and a marked decrease in spinal cord water content was observed in NS309 treated animals as compared with vehicle group (**Figure 2C**). Next, we measured hind-limb motor function scores at 72 h after injury. As shown in **Figure 2D**, treatment with NS309 significantly improved neurological outcome of SCI/R challenged rabbits.

To determine the therapeutic time window of NS309-induced protective effects, the post-injury administration pattern was used, and the rabbits were treated with 2 mg/kg NS309 at different time points (3, 6, or 9 h after ischemia initiation). A significant reduction in spinal cord water content (**Figure 3A**) and increased numbers of normal motor neurons (**Figure 3B**) were observed when NS309 was administrated 3 or 6 h after ischemia initiation but not when the administration was delayed by 9 h. In consistent with these results, a significant improvement of neurologic outcome was still detected when NS309 treatment was started 3 or 6 h, but not 9 h after ischemia initiation (**Figure 3C**).

## NS309 Reduces Oxidative Stress and Regulates Inflammation After SCI/R

The levels of MDA and 8-iso-PGF2α, two classic oxidative products, in serum and spinal cord tissues were measured after SCI/R. The results showed that the levels of MDA (**Figure 4A**) and 8-iso-PGF2α (**Figure 4B**) in serum significantly increased after SCI/R in a time-dependent manner, but these increases were attenuated by NS309 treatment. The levels of MDA (**Figure 4C**) and 8-iso-PGF2α (**Figure 4D**) in spinal cord tissues from

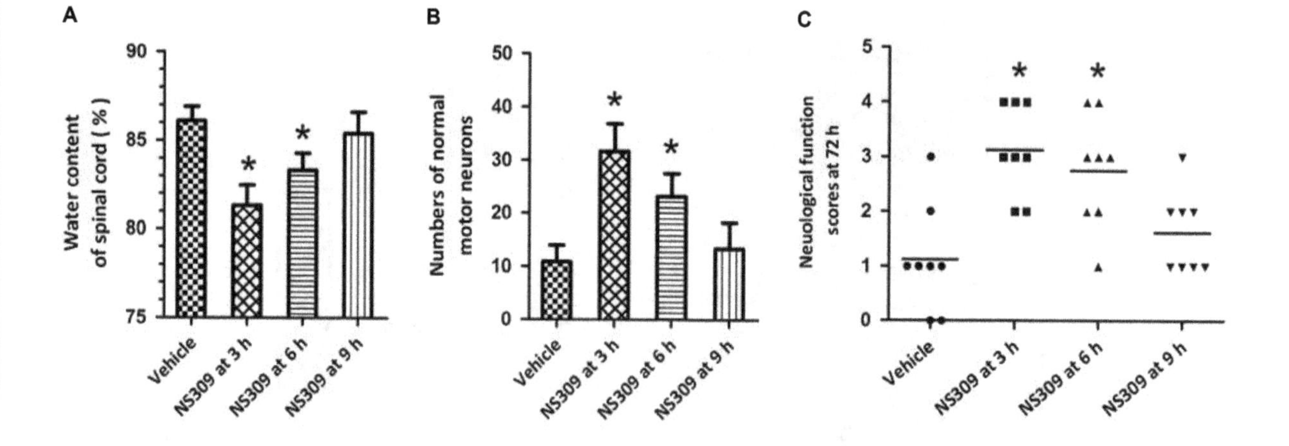


**FIGURE 3 |** Time window of NS309-induced neuroprotection. The animals were exposed to SCI/R and treated with 2 mg/kg NS309 at different time points (3, 6, or 9 h after SCI/R beginning). The spinal cord water content **(A)**, number of normal motor neurons **(B)** and neurological function scores **(C)** were measured 72 h later. The data were represented as means ± SEM ($n$ = 8). *$p$ < 0.05 vs. Vehicle.

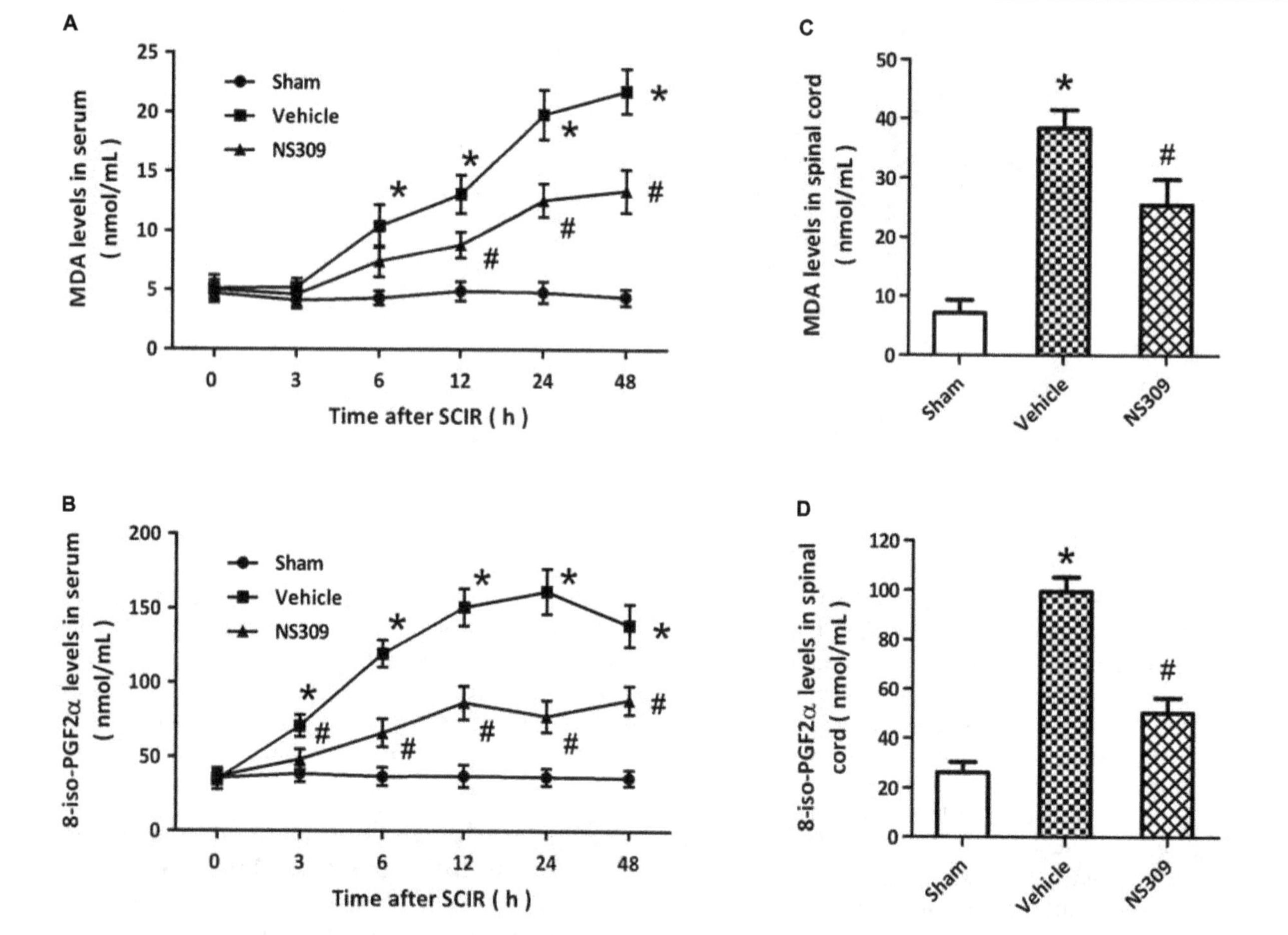


**FIGURE 4 |** NS309 reduces the expression of oxidative products after SCI/R. The animals were treated with 2 mg/kg NS309 or vehicle at the beginning of SCI/R. The expression levels of MDA **(A)** and 8-iso-PGF2α **(B)** in serum were measured at different time points (0, 3, 6, 12, 24, and 48 h). The expression levels of MDA **(C)** and 8-iso-PGF2α **(D)** in spinal cord tissues were detected at 72 h after reperfusion. The data were represented as means ± SEM ($n$ = 8). *$p$ < 0.05 vs. Sham. #$p$ < 0.05 vs. Vehicle.

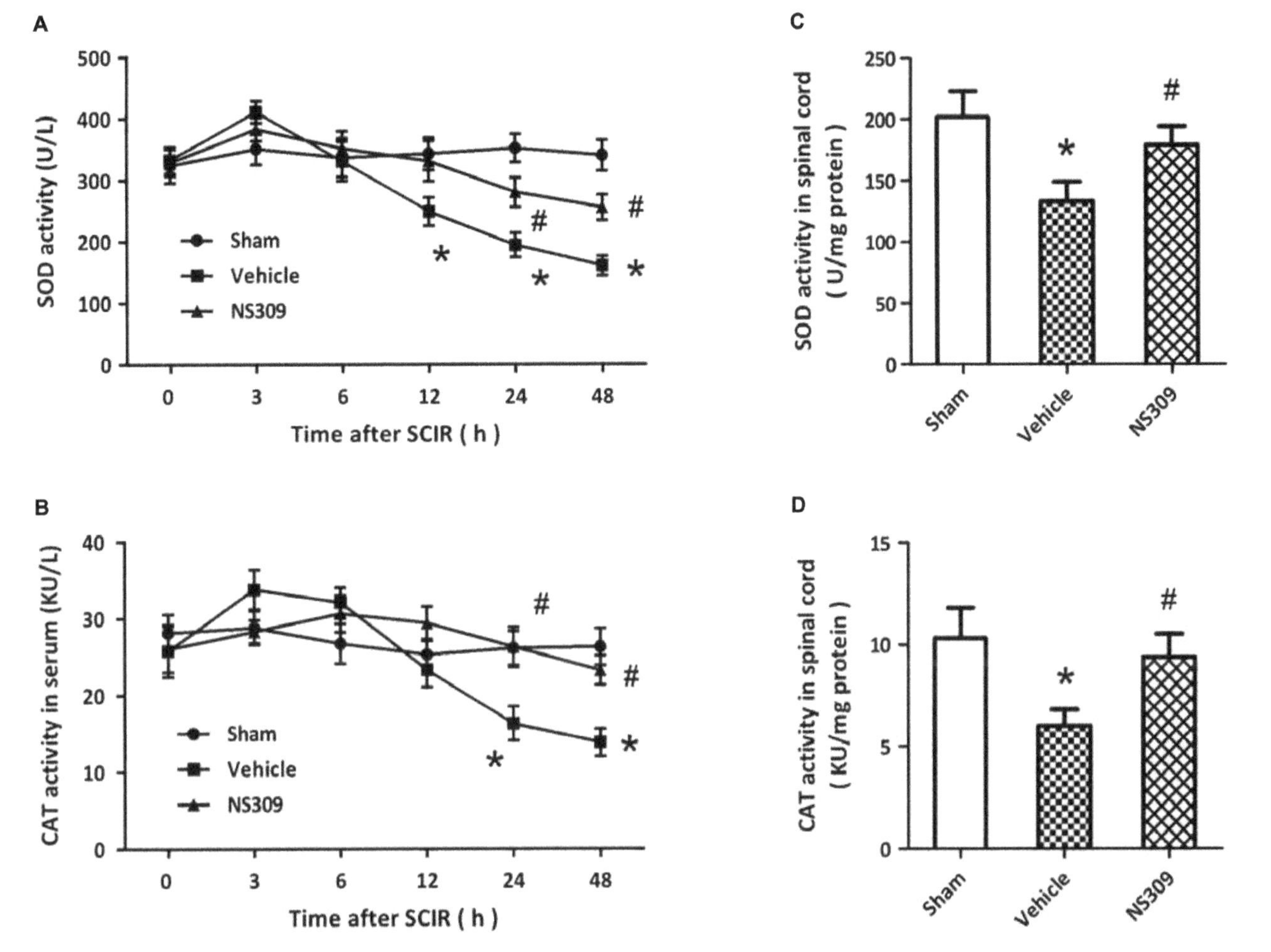


**FIGURE 5 |** NS309 preserves the activity of antioxidant enzymes after SCI/R. The animals were treated with 2 mg/kg NS309 or vehicle at the beginning of SCI/R. The enzymatic activities of SOD **(A)** and CAT **(B)** in serum were measured at different time points (0, 3, 6, 12, 24, and 48 h). The enzymatic activities of SOD **(C)** and CAT **(D)** in spinal cord tissues were detected at 72 h after reperfusion. The data were represented as means ± SEM ($n$ = 8). *$p$ < 0.05 vs. Sham. #$p$ < 0.05 vs. Vehicle.

NS309-treated animals was lower than that in vehicle group. In addition, we also detected the activities of SOD and CAT, two endogenous antioxidant enzymes. The results showed that the activities of SOD (**Figure 5A**) and CAT (**Figure 5B**) in serum from NS309-treated animals was higher than that in vehicle group from 12 to 48 h after SCI/R. As shown in **Figures 5C,D**, NS309 also markedly increased SOD and CAT activities in spinal cord tissues.

To investigate the effect of NS309 on inflammatory responses after SCI/R, the levels of inflammatory cytokines were determined in spinal cord tissues at different time points. The results showed that SCI/R significantly increased the levels of TNF-α (**Figure 6A**) and IL-1β (**Figure 6B**), two pro-inflammatory cytokines. However, application of NS309 significantly reduced the levels of these two cytokines in spinal cord tissues at 12, 24 and 48 h. Furthermore, we also measured the levels of IL-10 and TGF-β1, two anti-inflammatory cytokines. We found that NS309 markedly increased the levels of IL-10 at 24 and 48 h, but not at 12 h after SCI/R (**Figure 6C**). The TGF-β1 levels in NS309-treated group were higher than that in vehicle group at all time points measured (**Figure 6D**).

## NS309 Inhibits Mitochondrial Dysfunction After SCI/R

Mitochondrial function plays a key role in regulating oxidative stress under ischemia and reperfusion injury. Thus, we detected the activities of mitochondrial complexes in spinal cord tissues. The results showed that SCI/R significantly decreased the activities of all four mitochondrial complexes, and the activities of complex I (**Figure 7A**), complex III (**Figure 7C**) and complex IV (**Figure 7D**), but not complex II **Figure 7B**), were preserved by NS309 treatment. In addition, we investigated the effect of NS309 on mitochondrial biogenesis. NS309 increased mtDNA levels (**Figure 7E**) and elevated the levels of NRF-1 and PGC-1 mRNA after SCI/R (**Figure 7F**).

Mitochondrial dynamics are also involved in mitochondrial dysfunction under oxidative stress. As shown in **Figure 8A**, we

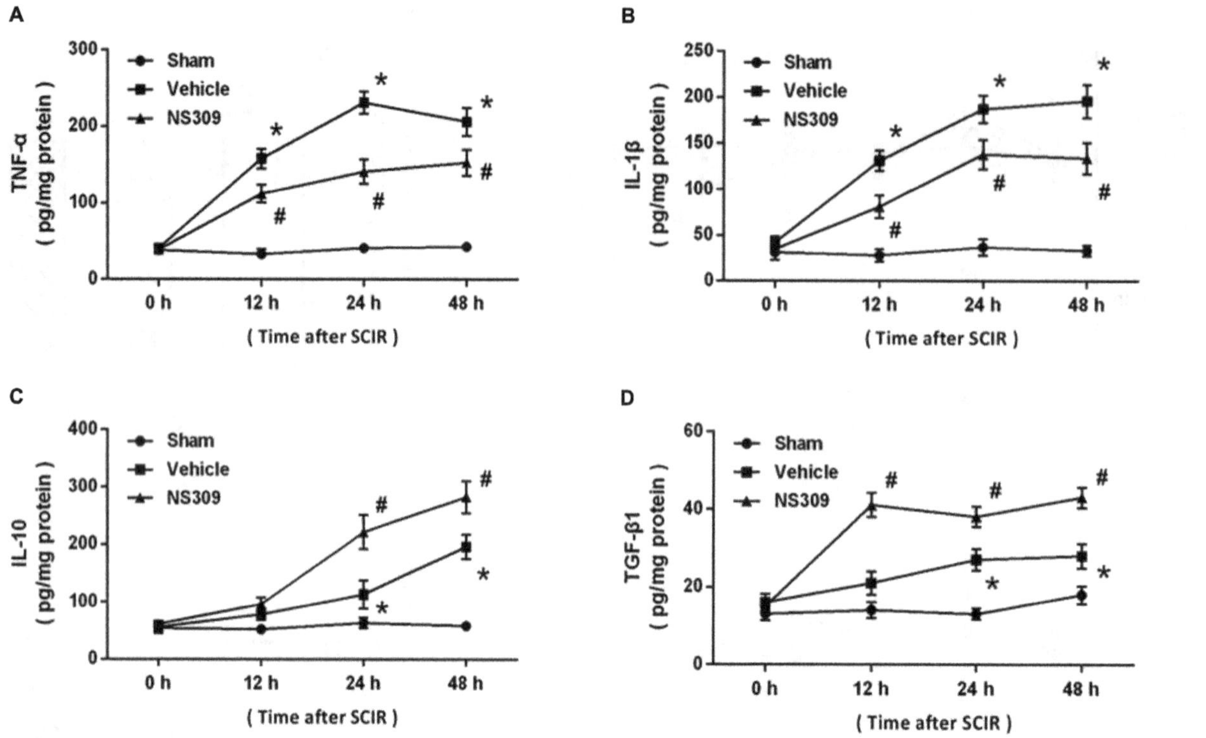


**FIGURE 6 |** NS309 regulates inflammatory cytokines after SCI/R. The animals were treated with 2 mg/kg NS309 or vehicle at the beginning of SCI/R. The levels of TNF-α **(A)**, IL-1β **(B)**, IL-10 **(C)**, and TGF-β1 **(D)** in spinal cord tissues were determined at different time points (0, 12, 24, and 48 h). The data were represented as means ± SEM (*n* = 8). $^{*}p < 0.05$ vs. Sham. $^{\#}p < 0.05$ vs. Vehicle.

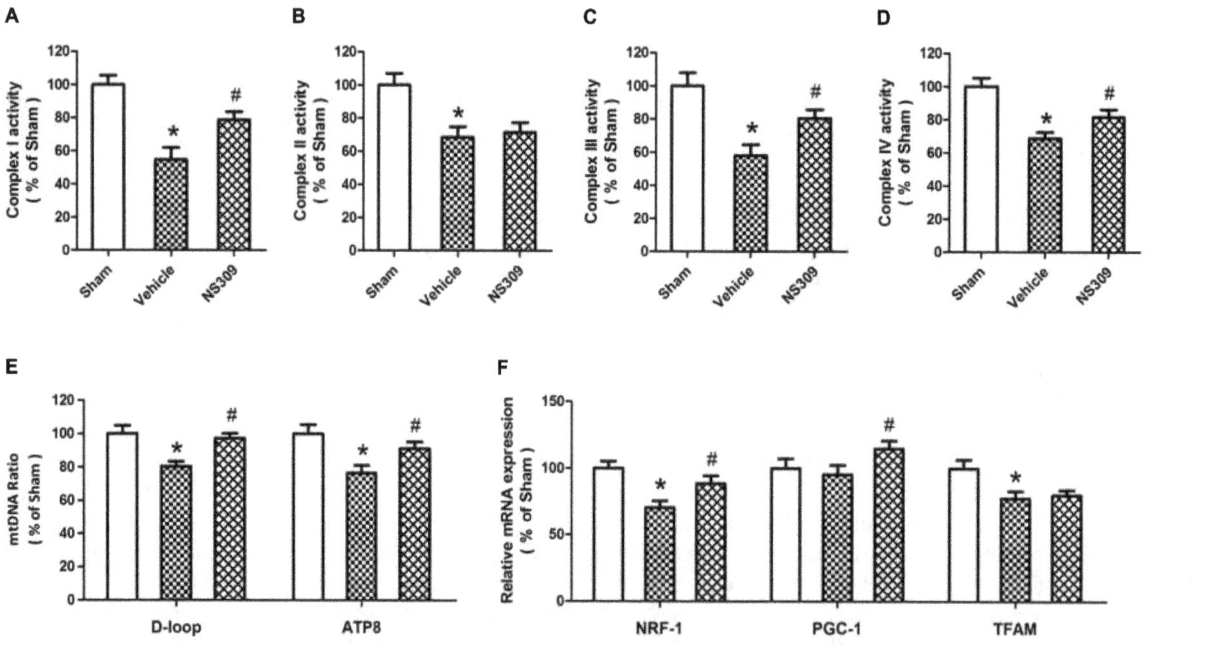


**FIGURE 7 |** NS309 preserves mitochondrial complex activity and mitochondrial biogenesis after SCI/R. The animals were treated with 2 mg/kg NS309 or vehicle at the beginning of SCI/R. The activities of mitochondrial complex I **(A)**, II **(B)**, III **(C)**, and IV **(D)** were observed in spinal cord, respectively. Real-time RT-PCR was used to detect mtNDA ratio **(E)** and the expression of mitochondrial biogenesis factors **(F)**. The data were represented as means ± SEM (*n* = 8). $^{*}p < 0.05$ vs. Sham. $^{\#}p < 0.05$ vs. Vehicle.

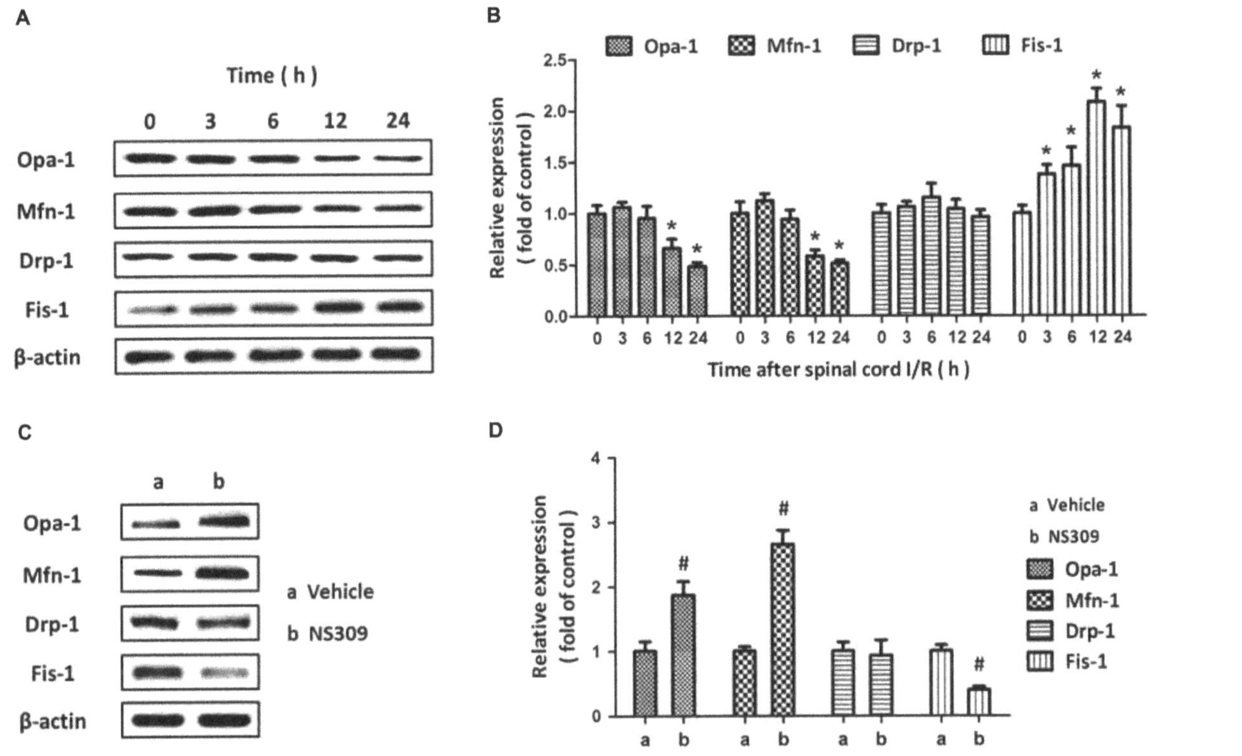


**FIGURE 8 |** NS309 differently regulates the expression of mitochondrial dynamic proteins. The animals were treated with 2 mg/kg NS309, and the expression of Opa-1, Mfn-1, Drp-1, and Fis-1 at different time points (0, 3, 6, 12, and 24 h) was detected by western blot analysis **(A,B)**. The animals were treated with 2 mg/kg NS309 or vehicle at the beginning of SCI/R. The expression of Opa-1, Mfn-1, Drp-1, and Fis-1 was detected by western blot analysis **(C)** and calculated **(D)**. The data were represented as means ± SEM ($n$ = 8). $^*p < 0.05$ vs. Sham. $^\#p < 0.05$ vs. Vehicle.

detected the expression of mitochondrial dynamic proteins in spinal cord tissues after SCI/R at different time points. The results showed that SCI/R decreased the expression of Opa-1 and Mfn-1 at 12 and 24 h but increased the expression of Fis-1 from 3 to 24 h, with no effect on Drp-1 expression (**Figure 8B**). Furthermore, we detected the expression of these proteins after NS309 treatment (**Figure 8C**). We found that the decreased expression of Opa-1 and Mfn-1, as well as increased expression of Fis-1 after SCI/R, were all partially prevented by NS309 treatment (**Figure 8D**).

## DISCUSSION

Due to the lack of data from randomized controlled clinical trials, contemporary concepts about SCI/R protection are mainly adapted from guidelines for brain ischemia, cardiovascular ischemia and spinal cord trauma (Nardone et al., 2016). This study provides evidence that NS309, a pharmacological activator for SK/$K_{Ca}$ channel, protects against experimental SCI/R in rabbits. Our results showed that (a) SCI/R decreases SK/$K_{Ca}$1 protein expression in spinal cord tissues; (b) NS309 attenuates neuronal loss and neurological dysfunction after SCI/R; (c) NS309 reduces oxidative stress and regulates the levels of inflammatory cytokines after SCI/R; (d) NS309 preserves mitochondrial function and promotes mitochondrial biogenesis; and (e) NS309 differently regulates mitochondrial dynamic proteins.

The SK/$K_{Ca}$ channels are extensively expressed throughout the central nervous system, but the three subtypes are differentially expressed. SK/$K_{Ca}$1 can be found in cortex, hippocampus, midbrain, cerebellum and spinal cord; SK/$K_{Ca}$2 is localized in cortex, amygdala, medial habenula and the inferior olivary complex; SK/$K_{Ca}$3 is expressed in olfactory bulbs, dentate gyrus thalamus and the locus coeruleus (Sailer et al., 2004). Thus, we detected the expression of SK/$K_{Ca}$1 protein to investigate the effect of SCI/R on SK/$K_{Ca}$ channels. Significant decrease in SK/$K_{Ca}$1 expression was observed at 12 and 24 h after SCI/R, and this decrease was detected in both cytosolic and mitochondrial fractions. In neuronal cells, SK/$K_{Ca}$ channels were originally thought to be predominantly presented in the plasma membrane where they regulates $K^+$ efflux (Honrath et al., 2017). However, a previous study showed that SK/$K_{Ca}$ channels were also located in the inner mitochondrial membrane of neuronal mitochondria (Dolga et al., 2013). In addition, Dolga et al. demonstrated that the SK/$K_{Ca}$2 subtype expressed in mitochondrial-enriched fractions and co-localized with the mitochondrial markers in neuronal dopaminergic cells (Dolga et al., 2014). Our results here demonstrated that SK/$K_{Ca}$1 was also localized in mitochondria in spinal cord, and was downregulated after SCI/R, indicating a potential role in mitochondrial function after SCI/R.

Activation of SK/$K_{Ca}$ channels has been demonstrated to exert protective effects in many *in vitro* neuronal models, and is considered as an emerging therapeutic approach for the treatment of several neurological diseases (Anderson et al., 2006; Dolga et al., 2011, 2012, 2013, 2014; Dolga and Culmsee, 2012). NS309 is a selective and potent SK/$K_{Ca}$ channel opener that activates SK/$K_{Ca}$ channels via increasing their $Ca^{2+}$ sensitivity (Strobaek et al., 2006). The $EC_{50}$ of NS309 to SK/$K_{Ca}$ channels is 30 nM, and it has been demonstrated to be safe and could activate SK/$K_{Ca}$ channels in both *in vitro* and *in vivo* experimental models (Hipolito et al., 2015; Honrath et al., 2017). In this study, we found that NS309 treatment reduced spinal cord edema and spinal cord neuronal loss after SCI/R, which were accompanied by preserved neurological function. Our data extended the neuroprotective effects of SK/$K_{Ca}$ channels activation into SCI/R. Importantly, we found that the protective effects of NS309 were still observed when it was administrated at 6 h after ischemia initiation. One of the serious problems of preclinical experiments is that many neuroprotective agents are administrated prior to injury initiation (Menon, 2009). It is of little clinical relevance due to the difficulty in obtaining informed consent. Our results showed that the therapeutic time window of NS309 was up to 6 h after ischemia initiation, which is useful for future clinical trials. This time window of administration makes it possible to treat SCI/R with NS309 associated neuroprotective agents. Considering the safety of NS309 treatment in previous experimental animal models, NS309 might be an ideal candidate for clinical drug research for SCI/R.

Free radicals-associated oxidative damage is one of the most important mechanisms underlying secondary injury after SCI/R, especially in the reperfusion phase (Chen X.P. et al., 2011). The overproduced ROS causes protein and lipid peroxidation, thereby leading to loss of membrane potential and corruption of membrane fluidity, which eventually results in the release of organelle content. In this study, increased levels of MDA and 8-iso-PGF2α, two oxidative products that correlate with the extent of ROS-mediated damage, was observed in both serum and spinal cord tissues after SCI/R, which were reduced by NS309. Neuronal fate under oxidative stress is dependent on the balance between ROS and the anti-oxidative defense mechanisms within the cell (Jia et al., 2012). SOD and CAT are two endogenous antioxidant enzymes, that can scavenge the superoxide radicals by changing the $O_2^-$ into less damaging species (Rodrigo et al., 2011). At 24 and 48 h after SCI/R, reduced activities of SOD and CAT was found to be preserved by NS309, indicating the anti-oxidative activity of NS309 in our model. Thus, the effects of NS309 on prevention of oxidative stress after SCI/R might be the direct result of the increased activity of antioxidant enzymes, which needs to be further determined in the future. Inflammation is a subsequent event of SCI/R, and inflammatory cell infiltration and release of inflammatory cytokines were observed in spinal cords (Zhu et al., 2013). The pro-inflammatory cytokines, such as TNF-α and IL-1β, and anti-inflammatory cytokines, including IL-10 and TGF-β1, play opposite roles in inflammation regulation (Spitzbarth et al., 2012). Here, NS309 treatment was shown to upregulate anti-inflammatory cytokines but downregulate pro-inflammatory cytokines in the spinal cord tissues. Thus, inhibition of inflammatory responses via differentially regulating inflammatory cytokines might also contribute to NS309-induced protection against SCI/R.

Considering that the SK/$K_{Ca}$1 subtype was found in spinal cord mitochondria, and that NS309 alleviated oxidative stress after SCI/R, we speculated that activation of SK/$K_{Ca}$ channels could regulate mitochondrial function in the spinal cord. Thus, we further measured mitochondrial complexes activity. It has been demonstrated that dysfunction of mitochondrial complexes occurred within 4–6 h after reperfusion and resulted in permanent mitochondrial damage (Sims and Muyderman, 2010). As expected, we found that the reduced activities of mitochondrial complexes after SCI/R, except for complex II, were all partially prevented by NS309. In addition, these effects were accompanied by the changes in mitochondrial biogenesis factors. Mitochondrial biogenesis is defined as the regulation of mitochondrial mass and turnover, a mechanism aimed to maintain diverse homeostatic demands under physiological and pathological conditions (Chen S.D. et al., 2011). It requires exquisite communication between the mitochondrial genome and the nuclear genome, and can be measured by the copy number and integrity of mtDNA, as well as the levels of many transcription factors, such as NRF-1, PGC-1, and TFAM (Kelly and Scarpulla, 2004). Previous studies have shown that these candidate mitochondrial biogenesis regulatory proteins correlate with mitochondrial respiratory capacity and could augment tolerance to ischemic injury via activating antioxidant system (McLeod et al., 2005). Thus, our results strongly indicate that NS309 might promote mitochondrial biogenesis, leading to inhibition of oxidative stress, and thereby induce protection against SCI/R.

Dynamic structural changes of the mitochondrial network, named as mitochondrial dynamics, are governed by the delicate balance between frequent fusion and fission events, and can adapt mitochondrial function to meet energy demand under stress (Otera et al., 2013). Impaired regulation of mitochondrial dynamic proteins contributes to ischemic injury via reducing energy production and promoting ROS generation (Calo et al., 2013). Multiple mitochondrial guanosine triphosphates hydrolases (GTPases) that regulate mitochondrial networking have been identified, among which DRP-1 and Fis-1 are related to mitochondrial fission, whereas mitochondrial fusion is mediated by Opa-1 and Mfn-1 (Karbowski et al., 2002; Hoppins et al., 2007). We found that SCI/R decreased the expression of Opa-1 and Mfn-1 but increased the levels of Fis-1 rather than Drp-1, indicating the induction of mitochondrial fragmentation in spinal cord after injury. In addition, the changes of these proteins after SCI/R were significantly prevented by NS309 treatment. Previous studies have shown that Opa-1 and Mfn-1 functionally interact to promote mitochondrial elongation, while Fis-1 was required in the recruitment of Drp-1 to mitochondria during mitochondrial fission (Cipolat et al., 2004; De Palma et al., 2010). However, no significant changes in Drp-1 expression after SCI/R and/or NS309 treatment was observed in this study. Thus, a Drp-1-independent mechanism after SCI/R might exist, which need to be further determined.

In conclusion, our present study demonstrated the neuroprotective effects of NS309, a pharmacological activator for SK/$K_{Ca}$ channel, against SCI/R in rabbits, which may involve an integrated process of the suppression of oxidative stress and the preservation of mitochondrial function.

## AUTHOR CONTRIBUTIONS

TC and Y-HW conceived and designed the experiments. JZ, L-KY, and W-LC performed the experiments. WL analyzed the data. TC and JZ wrote the paper.

## FUNDING

This work was supported by the National Natural Science Foundation of China (Nos. 81701932, 81601719, and 81871589).

## REFERENCES


Anderson, N. J., Slough, S., and Watson, W. P. (2006). In vivo characterisation of the small-conductance KCa (SK) channel activator 1-ethyl-2-benzimidazolinone (1-EBIO) as a potential anticonvulsant. *Eur. J. Pharmacol.* 546, 48–53. doi: 10.1016/j.ejphar.2006.07.007

Calo, L., Dong, Y., Kumar, R., Przyklenk, K., and Sanderson, T. H. (2013). Mitochondrial dynamics: an emerging paradigm in ischemia-reperfusion injury. *Curr. Pharm. Des.* 19, 6848–6857. doi: 10.2174/138161281939131127110701

Chen, S. D., Yang, D. I., Lin, T. K., Shaw, F. Z., Liou, C. W., and Chuang, Y. C. (2011). Roles of oxidative stress, apoptosis, PGC-1alpha and mitochondrial biogenesis in cerebral ischemia. *Int. J. Mol. Sci.* 12, 7199–7215. doi: 10.3390/ijms12107199

Chen, X. P., Fu, W. M., and Gu, W. (2011). Spinal cord stimulation for patients with inoperable chronic critical leg ischemia. *World J. Emerg. Med.* 2, 262–266. doi: 10.5847/wjem.j.1920-8642.2011.04.003

Cipolat, S., Martins de Brito, O., Dal Zilio, B., and Scorrano, L. (2004). OPA1 requires mitofusin 1 to promote mitochondrial fusion. *Proc. Natl. Acad. Sci. U.S.A.* 101, 15927–15932. doi: 10.1073/pnas.0407043101

De Palma, C., Falcone, S., Pisoni, S., Cipolat, S., Panzeri, C., Pambianco, S., et al. (2010). Nitric oxide inhibition of Drp1-mediated mitochondrial fission is critical for myogenic differentiation. *Cell Death Differ.* 17, 1684–1696. doi: 10.1038/cdd.2010.48

Dolga, A. M., and Culmsee, C. (2012). Protective roles for potassium SK/K(Ca)2 channels in microglia and neurons. *Front. Pharmacol.* 3:196. doi: 10.3389/fphar.2012.00196

Dolga, A. M., de Andrade, A., Meissner, L., Knaus, H. G., Hollerhage, M., Christophersen, P., et al. (2014). Subcellular expression and neuroprotective effects of SK channels in human dopaminergic neurons. *Cell Death Dis.* 5:e999. doi: 10.1038/cddis.2013.530

Dolga, A. M., Letsche, T., Gold, M., Doti, N., Bacher, M., Chiamvimonvat, N., et al. (2012). Activation of KCNN3/SK3/K(Ca)2.3 channels attenuates enhanced calcium influx and inflammatory cytokine production in activated microglia. *Glia* 60, 2050–2064. doi: 10.1002/glia.22419

Dolga, A. M., Netter, M. F., Perocchi, F., Doti, N., Meissner, L., Tobaben, S., et al. (2013). Mitochondrial small conductance SK2 channels prevent glutamate-induced oxytosis and mitochondrial dysfunction. *J. Biol. Chem.* 288, 10792–10804. doi: 10.1074/jbc.M113.453522

Dolga, A. M., Terpolilli, N., Kepura, F., Nijholt, I. M., Knaus, H. G., D'Orsi, B., et al. (2011). KCa2 channels activation prevents [Ca2+]i deregulation and reduces neuronal death following glutamate toxicity and cerebral ischemia. *Cell Death Dis.* 2:e147. doi: 10.1038/cddis.2011.30

Faber, E. S., and Sah, P. (2007). Functions of SK channels in central neurons. *Clin. Exp. Pharmacol. Physiol.* 34, 1077–1083. doi: 10.1111/j.1440-1681.2007.04725.x

Griepp, R. B., and Griepp, E. B. (2007). Spinal cord perfusion and protection during descending thoracic and thoracoabdominal aortic surgery: the collateral network concept. *Ann. Thorac. Surg.* 83, S865–S869; discussion S890–S892. doi: 10.1016/j.athoracsur.2006.10.092

Hipolito, L., Fakira, A. K., Cabanero, D., Blandon, R., Carlton, S. M., Moron, J. A., et al. (2015). In vivo activation of the SK channel in the spinal cord reduces the NMDA receptor antagonist dose needed to produce antinociception in an inflammatory pain model. *Pain* 156, 849–858. doi: 10.1097/j.pain.0000000000000124

Honrath, B., Krabbendam, I. E., Culmsee, C., and Dolga, A. M. (2017). Small conductance Ca(2+)-activated K(+) channels in the plasma membrane, mitochondria and the ER: pharmacology and implications in neuronal diseases. *Neurochem. Int.* 109, 13–23. doi: 10.1016/j.neuint.2017.05.005

Hoppins, S., Lackner, L., and Nunnari, J. (2007). The machines that divide and fuse mitochondria. *Annu. Rev. Biochem.* 76, 751–780. doi: 10.1146/annurev.biochem.76.071905.090048

Jia, Z., Zhu, H., Li, J., Wang, X., Misra, H., and Li, Y. (2012). Oxidative stress in spinal cord injury and antioxidant-based intervention. *Spinal Cord* 50, 264–274. doi: 10.1038/sc.2011.111

Karbowski, M., Lee, Y. J., Gaume, B., Jeong, S. Y., Frank, S., Nechushtan, A., et al. (2002). Spatial and temporal association of Bax with mitochondrial fission sites, Drp1, and Mfn2 during apoptosis. *J. Cell Biol.* 159, 931–938. doi: 10.1083/jcb.200209124

Kelly, D. P., and Scarpulla, R. C. (2004). Transcriptional regulatory circuits controlling mitochondrial biogenesis and function. *Genes Dev.* 18, 357–368. doi: 10.1101/gad.1177604

Kuiper, E. F., Nelemans, A., Luiten, P., Nijholt, I., Dolga, A., and Eisel, U. (2012). K(Ca)2 and k(ca)3 channels in learning and memory processes, and neurodegeneration. *Front. Pharmacol.* 3:107. doi: 10.3389/fphar.2012.00107

LeMaire, S. A., Price, M. D., Green, S. Y., Zarda, S., and Coselli, J. S. (2012). Results of open thoracoabdominal aortic aneurysm repair. *Ann. Cardiothorac. Surg.* 1, 286–292. doi: 10.3978/j.issn.2225-319X.2012.08.16

McLeod, C. J., Pagel, I., and Sack, M. N. (2005). The mitochondrial biogenesis regulatory program in cardiac adaptation to ischemia–a putative target for therapeutic intervention. *Trends Cardiovasc. Med.* 15, 118–123. doi: 10.1016/j.tcm.2005.05.001

Menon, D. K. (2009). Unique challenges in clinical trials in traumatic brain injury. *Crit. Care Med.* 37, S129–S135. doi: 10.1097/CCM.0b013e3181921225

Nardone, R., Pikija, S., Mutzenbach, J. S., Seidl, M., Leis, S., Trinka, E., et al. (2016). Current and emerging treatment options for spinal cord ischemia. *Drug Discov. Today* 21, 1632–1641. doi: 10.1016/j.drudis.2016.06.015

New, P. W., and McFarlane, C. L. (2012). Retrospective case series of outcomes following spinal cord infarction. *Eur. J. Neurol.* 19, 1207–1212. doi: 10.1111/j.1468-1331.2012.03702.x

Otera, H., Ishihara, N., and Mihara, K. (2013). New insights into the function and regulation of mitochondrial fission. *Biochim. Biophys. Acta* 1833, 1256–1268. doi: 10.1016/j.bbamcr.2013.02.002

Panthee, N., and Ono, M. (2015). Spinal cord injury following thoracic and thoracoabdominal aortic repairs. *Asian Cardiovasc. Thorac. Ann.* 23, 235–246. doi: 10.1177/0218492314548901

Rodrigo, R., Miranda, A., and Vergara, L. (2011). Modulation of endogenous antioxidant system by wine polyphenols in human disease. *Clin. Chim. Acta* 412, 410–424. doi: 10.1016/j.cca.2010.11.034

Sailer, C. A., Kaufmann, W. A., Marksteiner, J., and Knaus, H. G. (2004). Comparative immunohistochemical distribution of three small-conductance Ca2+-activated potassium channel subunits, SK1, SK2, and SK3 in mouse brain. *Mol. Cell Neurosci.* 26, 458–469. doi: 10.1016/j.mcn.2004.03.002

Sims, N. R., and Muyderman, H. (2010). Mitochondria, oxidative metabolism and cell death in stroke. *Biochim. Biophys. Acta* 1802, 80–91. doi: 10.1016/j.bbadis.2009.09.003

Spitzbarth, I., Baumgartner, W., and Beineke, A. (2012). The role of pro- and anti-inflammatory cytokines in the pathogenesis of spontaneous canine CNS diseases. *Vet. Immunol. Immunopathol.* 147, 6–24. doi: 10.1016/j.vetimm.2012.04.005

Stocker, M. (2004). Ca(2+)-activated K+ channels: molecular determinants and function of the SK family. *Nat. Rev. Neurosci.* 5, 758–770. doi: 10.1038/nrn1516

Strobaek, D., Hougaard, C., Johansen, T. H., Sorensen, U. S., Nielsen, E. O., Nielsen, K. S., et al. (2006). Inhibitory gating modulation of small conductance Ca2+-activated K+ channels by the synthetic compound (R)-N-(benzimidazol-2-yl)-1,2,3,4-tetrahydro-1-naphtylamine (NS8593) reduces afterhyperpolarizing current in hippocampal CA1 neurons. *Mol. Pharmacol.* 70, 1771–1782. doi: 10.1124/mol.106.027110

Ye, R., Zhang, X., Kong, X., Han, J., Yang, Q., Zhang, Y., et al. (2011). Ginsenoside Rd attenuates mitochondrial dysfunction and sequential apoptosis after transient focal ischemia. *Neuroscience* 178, 169–180. doi: 10.1016/j.neuroscience.2011.01.007

Zhou, L., Wang, X., Xue, W., Xie, K., Huang, Y., Chen, H., et al. (2013). Beneficial effects of hydrogen-rich saline against spinal cord ischemia-reperfusion injury in rabbits. *Brain Res.* 1517, 150–160. doi: 10.1016/j.brainres.2013.04.007

Zhu, P., Li, J. X., Fujino, M., Zhuang, J., and Li, X. K. (2013). Development and treatments of inflammatory cells and cytokines in spinal cord ischemia-reperfusion injury. *Med. Inflamm.* 2013:701970. doi: 10.1155/2013/701970

# 3

# A Defective Crosstalk Between Neurons and Müller Glial Cells in the *rd1* Retina Impairs the Regenerative Potential of Glial Stem Cells

*Yanel A. Volonté[1], Harmonie Vallese-Maurizi[1†], Marcos J. Dibo[1†], Victoria B. Ayala-Peña[1], Andrés Garelli[1], Samanta R. Zanetti[1], Axel Turpaud[1], Cheryl Mae Craft[2,3], Nora P. Rotstein[1], Luis E. Politi[1*] and Olga L. German[1*]*

[1] *Instituto de Investigaciones Bioquímicas de Bahía Blanca, Departamento de Biología, Bioquímica y Farmacia, Universidad Nacional del Sur – National Research Council of Argentina (CONICET), Bahía Blanca, Argentina,* [2] *Department of Ophthalmology, USC Roski Eye Institute, Keck School of Medicine of the University of Southern California, Los Angeles, CA, United States,* [3] *Department of Integrative Anatomical Sciences, Keck School of Medicine of the University of Southern California, Los Angeles, CA, United States*

***Correspondence:**
*Luis E. Politi*
*inpoliti@criba.edu.ar*
*Olga L. German*
*olgerman@criba.edu.ar*

*† These authors have contributed equally to this work*

Müller glial cells (MGC) are stem cells in the retina. Although their regenerative capacity is very low in mammals, the use of MGC as stem cells to regenerate photoreceptors (PHRs) during retina degenerations, such as in retinitis pigmentosa, is being intensely studied. Changes affecting PHRs in diseased retinas have been thoroughly investigated; however, whether MGC are also affected is still unclear. We here investigated whether MGC in *retinal degeneration 1* (*rd1*) mouse, an animal model of retinitis pigmentosa, have impaired stem cell properties or structure. *rd1* MGC showed an altered morphology, both in culture and in the whole retina. Using mixed neuron-glial cultures obtained from newborn mice retinas, we determined that proliferation was significantly lower in *rd1* than in *wild type (wt)* MGC. Levels of stem cell markers, such as *Nestin* and *Sox2*, were also markedly reduced in *rd1* MGC compared to *wt* MGC in neuron-glial cultures and in retina cryosections, even before the onset of PHR degeneration. We then investigated whether neuron-glial crosstalk was involved in these changes. Noteworthy, *Nestin* expression was restored in *rd1* MGC in co-culture with *wt* neurons. Conversely, *Nestin* expression decreased in *wt* MGC in co-culture with *rd1* neurons, as occurred in *rd1* MGC in *rd1* neuron-glial mixed cultures. These results imply that MGC proliferation and stem cell markers are reduced in *rd1* retinas and might be restored by their interaction with "healthy" PHRs, suggesting that alterations in *rd1* PHRs lead to a disruption in neuron-glial crosstalk affecting the regenerative potential of MGC.

**Keywords: Müller glial cells, stem cells, retinal degeneration, retinal regeneration, photoreceptors**

## INTRODUCTION

Retinitis pigmentosa constitutes a group of inherited diseases that have as a common feature the degeneration and loss of rod and cone photoreceptors (PHRs). Although the genetic mutations leading to this disease are well-established, it has still no cure or effective treatments. The use of stem cells to replace neuronal loss in the injured retina is now being actively investigated as a promising new treatment for this disease. The discovery that Müller glial cells (MGC) can regenerate retina neurons following diverse insults (Karl et al., 2008) makes these cells potentially useful candidates for replacement therapies. MGC have multiple key roles in the retina, such as providing nutrients and trophic factors required for PHR survival (Bringmann et al., 2009; Vecino et al., 2016). Fischer and Reh (Fischer and Reh, 2003) have shown that MGC are stem cells that effectively regenerate the eye in fish and lower vertebrates. However, their regenerative potential is extremely low in vertebrates; generation of a few novel neurons in the murine retina was only possible because of the use of multiple exogenous stimuli (Fischer and Reh, 2003). *Notch* and *Wnt* signaling have been proposed to regulate the mechanisms by which MGC promote retina regeneration (Das et al., 2006). We previously showed that MGC express several stem cell markers and can transform PHR progenitor cells into multipotent stem cells, which in turn differentiate as functional PHRs (Insua et al., 2008; Simón et al., 2012). Nevertheless, MGC are inefficient in regenerating the retina in humans, such as in patients suffering from retinitis pigmentosa, and in the *rd1* mice, a frequently used animal model for this disease.

About 100 gene mutations have been identified to cause PHR cell death in retinitis pigmentosa (Hartong et al., 2006; Huang et al., 2017), most of them affecting PHRs. In the *rd1* mice, the occurrence of a mutation in the beta-subunit of rod cGMP phosphodiesterase gene, which mainly affects PHRs, is responsible for the disease (Pittler and Baehr, 1991). By contrast, only a few mutations causing the disease have been found in MGC; one of them, affecting a gene encoding CRALBP in an autosomal recessive form of retinitis pigmentosa, may disturb Vitamin A metabolism (Maw et al., 1997). Little is known regarding the role of MGC in this disease. Following neuronal damage in the injured retina, MGC show a reactive gliosis, characterized by an increase in glial cell proliferation, preceded by downregulation of the cell cycle blocker, $p27^{kip1}$ (Dyer and Cepko, 2000; Bringmann et al., 2006). Defects in MGC have been reported in another ocular disorder, Retinal Telangiectasia; a mutation in *Crb1* gene delocalizes the cellular connections at retinal MGC/PHR junctions (Zhao et al., 2015). Even when these alterations in MGC may not be the main cause of retinal degenerations, they might disrupt the normal crosstalk between MGC and PHRs, thus contributing to the degenerative process (Dong et al., 2017).

Retinal degeneration in the *rd1* mice occurs much faster than in humans. In the healthy mouse retina, most PHRs are "born" between PN days (PND) 0 and 2; soon after, their progenitors exit the cell cycle and begin their differentiation; a small peak in their apoptosis is detected by PND 7 and 8, and no cell death is detectable thereafter (Young, 1984). In the *rd1* retina, significant PHR cell death starts by PND 11, peaking by PND 15 and 16 (Lolley et al., 1994; Portera-Cailliau et al., 1994); after 4 weeks, while in the healthy mice PHRs become differentiated and functional, in the *rd1* mice the PHR cell layer completely disappears (Farber and Lolley, 1974; Politi and Adler, 1988).

The finding of the group of Canto Soler that human induced pluripotent stem cells (iPS) differentiate into retinal progenitors that originate retinal tissue containing the major retinal cell types, including functional PHRs (Zhong et al., 2014), underscores the therapeutic potential of stem cells. However, whether MGC are adequate sources of stem cells for retina regeneration in mammals remains to be established. In particular, alterations in PHRs in retinitis pigmentosa might change their normal interactions with MGC, disturbing neuron-glial crosstalk; in turn, this would lead to a deficient release of survival factors by MGC and contribute to a generalized retinal damage. Hence, understanding the significance of the alterations in MGC and in neuron-glial crosstalk during retina degeneration is particularly relevant when considering the use of MGC as a source of stem cells in regenerative therapies.

To establish whether MGC isolated from diseased retinas are a viable option for replacement therapies it is necessary to ascertain if these cells differ in their regenerative potential and in their cellular interactions with PHRs in healthy and degenerating retinas. For this purpose, we first analyzed stem cell characteristics of MGC in whole retinas and neuron-glial cultures from *rd1* and *wt* animals. Then, we separately prepared pure neuronal and MGC cultures to obtain co-cultures and investigated the interactions of *rd1* MGC with either *rd1* or *wt* neurons. We determined that proliferation and the levels of stem cell markers decreased in *rd1* MGC compared to their *wt* counterparts, and that these markers were partially restored when *rd1* MGC were co-cultured with *wt* neurons, suggesting that an impaired neuron-glial crosstalk affects the stem cell potential of *rd1* MGC.

## MATERIALS AND METHODS

### Materials

Two-day-old C57BL/6J (*wt*) or C57BL/6J-Pde6brd1-2J/J (*rd1*) mice bred in our own colony were used in all experiments. All proceedings concerning animal use were in accordance with the guidelines published in the NIH *Guide for the care and use of laboratory animals* and following the protocols approved by the Institutional Committee for the Care of Laboratory Animals from the Universidad Nacional del Sur (Argentina). Plastic 35-mm-diameter and 60-mm-diameter culture dishes were purchased from Greiner Bio-One (GBO). Fetal bovine serum (FBS) was from Natocor (Córdoba, Argentina). Dulbecco's modified Eagle's medium (DMEM) was purchased from Life Technologies (Grand Island, NY, United States). Trypsin, trypsin inhibitor, transferrin, hydrocortisone, putrescine, insulin, polyornithine, selenium, gentamycin, 4,6-diamidino-2-phenylindole (DAPI), poly-ornithine, paraformaldehyde (PF) and primers for RQ-PCR were from Sigma (St. Louis, MO, United States). Fluorescein-conjugated secondary antibodies were from Jackson InmunoResearch (West Grove, PA, United States). Type 2 collagenase was purchased from Invitrogen. Monoclonal antibodies against BrdU (clone G3G4) and VIMENTIN (clone 40E-C) were from DSHB (developed under the auspices of the NICHD and maintained by the University of Iowa, Department of Biological Sciences), NESTIN was from DSHB and from ABCAM (clone Rat-401), anti-Glutamine Synthetase (GS) and anti-SOX2 (SRY, sex determing region Y-box 2) were from ABCAM. Polyclonal goat anti-SOX2 (Santa Cruz # sc-17320) was a generous gift from Valeria Levi and Alejandra Guberman (University of Buenos Aires, Argentina). Polyclonal rabbit anti-CRX was from Cheryl M. Craft's laboratory (Zhu and Craft, 2000). CellTracer® Green CMFDA Dye, Alexa Fluor™ 555 Phalloidin, TO-PRO™-3 Iodide, terminal deoxynucleotidyl transferase (Tdt), BrdUTP (5-Bromo-2′-Deoxyuridine 5′-Triphosphate) and TdT Buffer were from Molecular Probes, Invitrogen (Carlsbad, CA, United States). Quick-zol RNA Isolation Reagent was from Kalium technologies (Embiotec). The Moloney Murine Leukemia Virus Reverse Transcriptase (M-MLV RT) and RNasin® Ribonuclease Inhibitors were from Promega. KAPPA SYBRs FAST qPCR Kit were from Biosystems S.A. (Buenos Aires, Argentina). The IntraStain, Two-step fixation and permeabilization for Flow Cytometry was from Agilent Dako. OCT Embedding Compound Cryoplast® was from Biopack®. Solvents were HPLC grade, and all other reagents were analytical grade.

## Retina Cultures

### Müller Glial Cell Cultures

Purified cultures of Müller glial cells were prepared following protocols previously described (Hicks and Courtois, 1990). Briefly, newborn mouse eyes were excised and incubated overnight in DMEM at room temperature and then treated with trypsin (1 mg/ml) and type 2 collagenase (2 mg/ml). Retinas were then dissected, chopped into small pieces, and seeded onto 35-mm-diameter plastic dishes, in culture medium supplemented with 10% FBS. The medium was routinely replaced every 3–4 days. After 8–10 days, pure Müller glial cells became confluent and were used for neuron-glial co-cultures (**Figures 1a–e**).

### Neuronal Cultures

Neuronal cultures from 2-day mouse retinas were obtained following previously described procedures, with slight modifications (Politi et al., 1996; Rotstein et al., 1996, 1997). In brief, after dissection and dissociation of the retinas, the cells were resuspended in a chemically defined medium (Politi et al., 1988) and seeded onto 35-mm-diameter plastic dishes, pretreated with poly-ornithine and schwannoma-conditioned medium (Adler, 1982). Cultures were incubated at 36°C in a humidified atmosphere of 5% $CO_2$. Immediately after seeding, nearly all cells were undifferentiated retinal progenitor cells, which were still in the cell cycle; many of them underwent their last mitotic division during the first day *in vitro*. Soon after exiting the cell cycle, cells began to differentiate into PHRs and amacrine neurons (**Figures 1f–j**).

### Mixed Neuron–Glial Cultures

To analyze the interactions between MGC and neurons from either *wt* or *rd1* retinas, we obtained long-term mixed cultures of MGC and retina neurons, following previously described protocols (Politi et al., 1996; Simón et al., 2012), with slight modifications. Briefly, retinas from 2-day-old mice were chemically and mechanically dissociated with trypsin [250 μl of 0.25% trypsin in 6 ml of calcium- and magnesium-free Hanks (CMF)] for 6 min. Cells were then resuspended in DMEM medium supplemented with 10% FBS and seeded onto 35-mm-diameter plastic dishes with no previous treatment. Analysis of

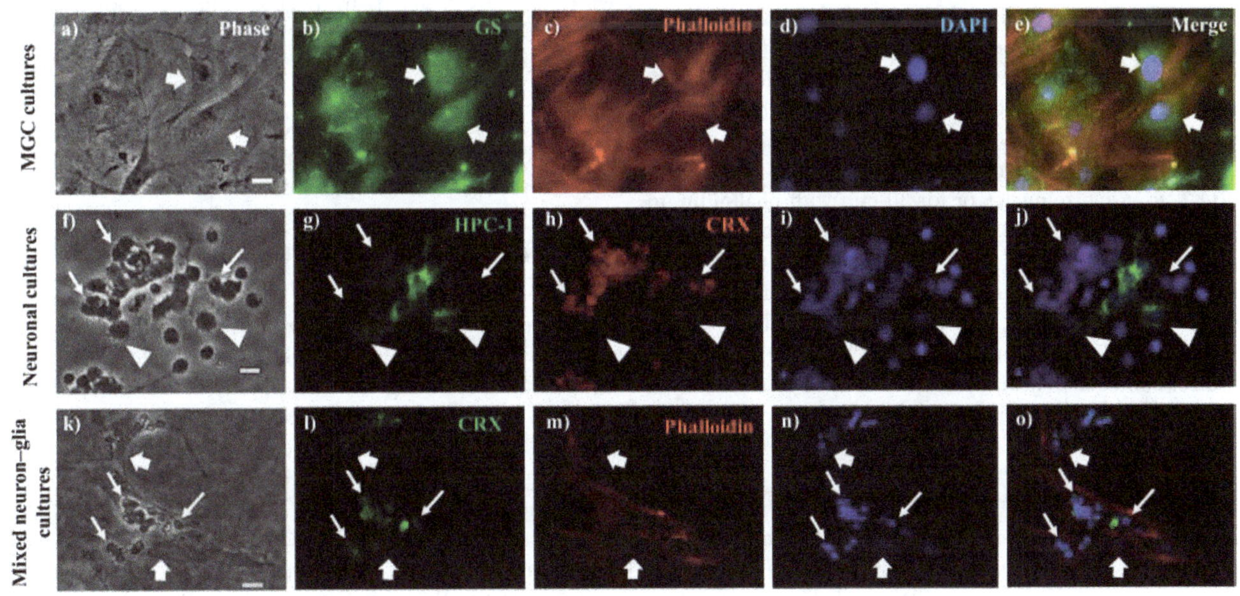


**FIGURE 1** | Identification of neurons and Müller glial cells (MGC) in glial, neuronal and mixed neuron-glial cultures. Phase **(a,f,k)** and fluorescence **(b–e,g–j,l–o)** photomicrographs of *wt* MGC culture **(a–e)**, 2-day *wt* neuronal cultures **(f–j)** and 6-day *wt* mixed neuron-glial cultures **(k–o)**, showing MGC (thick arrows) identified by their anti-Glutamine Synthase (GS) labeling **(b)**, with their actin cytoskeleton visualized by phalloidin labeling **(c,m)**; photoreceptors (thin arrows) labeled with anti-CRX **(h,l)** and amacrine neurons (arrowheads) labeled with HPC-1 **(g)** antibodies. Cell nuclei were visualized with the DNA probe DAPI **(d,i,n)**. Note that cell nuclei were markedly smaller in neurons than in MGC **(n)**. Merge images **(e,j,o)**. Scale bars: 20 μm.

MGC began at day 6, since only after this time *in vitro*, MGC are clearly recognizable and begin to express most of their markers. This time *in vitro* is equivalent to 8 days *in vivo*, when the retina has a maximum of gliogenic factors and cues that signal and stabilize glial fate (Nelson et al., 2011; **Figures 1k–o**).

### Neuron-Glial Co-cultures

To investigate whether the crosstalk between neurons and glial cells might modulate the stem cell potential of MGC, we prepared neuron-glial co-cultures combining *rd1* and *wt* neurons with either *rd1* or *wt* MGC. Pure neuronal cultures from *wt* or *rd1* retinas were initially labeled with the fluorescent dye CellTracer® following the manufacturer's specifications and after 3 days *in vitro* they were co-cultured with unlabeled *rd1* or *wt* MGC for 24 h. For this purpose, confluent (8–10 days) *rd1* or *wt* MGC were detached from their substrata and reseeded over the pre-labeled pure neuronal cultures. As the dye fluorescence persists during the whole culture time, even after mitosis, unlabeled MGC and their newly generated daughter cells were easily recognized from the pre-labeled neurons. Cells were then fixed and analyzed by immunocytochemical methods and RQ-PCR.

In the diverse cellular culture protocols described above, the number of cells seeded in each culture dish was standardized; in each experiment we seeded about 700,000 cells per dish (700,979 cells/dish; +/−49,755), so the starting points were comparable.

## Immunocytochemical and Immunohistochemical Methods

To prepare retina cryosections, PND 9, PND 14 and PND30 (adult) *wt* and *rd1* mice were sacrificed, their eyes were enucleated, and then fixed for 3 h. in PBS-2% PF at 4°C. After lens removal, eyes were immersed in PBS-30% sucrose until sunk, mounted in OCT blocks, frozen first at −20°C and then stored at −70°C until they were cut with a Leica CM1860 cryostat. Cultures were fixed for 1 h. with PBS-4%PF, followed by permeation with 0.1% Triton X-100. The cultures and slices were then stained at room temperature for 10 min with DAPI, TOPRO-3, to visualize nuclei, or for 30 min with phalloidin, to label the actin cytoskeleton. Alternatively, immunohistological staining of cells was carried out using an anti-CRX rabbit antibody (1:800), anti-NESTIN mouse antibody (1:100), anti-GS rabbit antibody (1:100), anti-BrdU mouse antibody (1:00), and anti-opsin (Rho4D2) mouse antibody (1:100). Secondary antibodies, conjugated with Cy2 or Cy3 (1:200 dilution) were then used. Background labeling was removed by washing with PBS prior to microscopy.

## Cell Identification

Müller glial cells were identified by their flat and irregular morphology and by immunocytochemistry, with polyclonal antibodies against GS (Simón et al., 2012, 2015; **Figures 1a–e,k–o** and **Supplementary Figures S1f–j**). PHRs and amacrine cells were the two main neuronal types present in neuronal cultures; they represented more than 98% of the cells and were identified by their morphology using phase-contrast microscopy, and by immunocytochemistry with monoclonal antibodies against CRX and syntaxin (HPC-1), respectively. Controls for immunocytochemistry were done by omitting the primary or secondary antibodies. PHRs have a round cell body of about 5–10 μm, and a short and single axon, which usually ends in a conspicuous synaptic "spherule"; sometimes these cells display a connecting cilium at the opposite end, but they fail to develop their characteristic outer segments (**Figures 1f–j,k–o** and **Supplementary Figures S1a–e, S2b,f**); all of them express CRX, the PHR specific transcription factor, and were identified by using a CRX antibody (Cheryl M. Craft's laboratory; University of Southern California, Los Angeles, CA, United States), (Garelli et al., 2006; **Figures 1h,l**). Amacrine cells are larger than PHRs (10–30 μm) and have multiple neurites; they all show anti-syntaxin immunoreactivity (Barnstable, 1980), which starts at early stages of development, and is retained even after undergoing degenerative changes that alter their morphology (Politi et al., 2001; **Figure 1g**).

## Evaluation of Cell Proliferation

To identify cells that were replicating their DNA, mixed neuron-glial cultures were incubated with 50 μM BrdU (final concentration in culture) for the final 24 h. before fixation, at days 6 and 11 in culture. After fixation, BrdU uptake was analyzed by immunocytochemistry using an anti- BrdU monoclonal antibody.

## Flow Cytometry

For quantitative evaluation of NESTIN expression, MGC from 11-day neuron–glial mixed cultures were analyzed by flow cytometry. Single cell suspensions, previously filtered using a 32-μm pore-size nylon mesh, were fixed and then permeated with solutions A and B from Dako IntraStain kit. Cells were then successively stained with primary (NESTIN 1/100) and secondary (Cy2 anti-mouse 1/200) antibodies. Flow cytometry analyses were done with a FACSCalibur flow cytometer (BD Biosciences). Quantification of NESTIN-positive MGC by FACS was performed using FACSComp. A minimum of 10,000 events was analyzed for each sample.

## Real-Time Quantitative Polymerase Chain Reaction (RQ-PCR)

*Wild type* and *rd1* mice were sacrificed at PND 0 (birth), PND 2, PND 4, PND 8, PND 10 (when all cell types have been generated and early signs of degeneration appear), PND 20 (progressive stages of PHR degeneration), PND 40 (complete loss of PHR), and PND 180. Retinas from three different mice were used for each stage. Retinas were dissected, and total RNA was extracted with Quick-Zol reagent (Kalium Technologies), according to the manufacturer's instructions. The amount of RNA was measured by spectrophotometry. Reverse transcription of total RNA was performed using the High-Capacity cDNA Reverse Transcription Kit. Quantitative PCR was done by SYBR Green real-time PCR methods. The relative mRNA expression was calculated using the quantification cycle method (Cq-method) (Bustin et al., 2009), with *Eef2* (Eukaryotic elongation factor) for normalization. All experimental conditions were processed in triplicate.

RQ-PCR primers were specifically designed to amplify the following cDNAs:

m-*Bax* F(5′TACTCCCGTCCTACCTCAGC 3′) R(5′CGCGG GTACTAAATGAACGC 3′),
m-*Nes* F(5′CCCTTAGTCTGGAAGTGGCTAC 3′) R(5′GTGC TGGTCCTCTGGTATCC 3′),
m-*Sox2* F(5′TGGATAACTGTTCAGCCACCAA 3′) R(5′GGC GCAGTATCTCATCTGCT 3′),
m-*Vim* F(5′ATGCTTCTCTGGCACGTCTT 3′) R(5′AGCCA CGCTTTCATACTGCT 3′),
m-*Eef2* F(5′GACTCTGAGAATCCGTCGCC 3′) R(5′CACAC AAGGGAGTCGGTCAG 3′).

The efficiency was about 90% for each pair of primers.

## Quantitative Image Analysis

After performing immunocytochemical labeling, cultures and tissue cryosections were analyzed by phase contrast and epifluorescence microscopy, using a Nikon Eclipse E600 microscope with a C-C Phase Contrast Turret Condenser and a Y-FL Epi-Fluorescence Attachment or with a laser scanning confocal microscope (Leica DMIRE2) with a 63X-water objective. Phase photomicrographs were processed using the XnView image processor to give a differential interference contrast effect. Fluorescence intensities of the 8- or 16-bit image were analyzed after manually outlining regions of interest (ROI) with the software Fiji-Image J (NIH, Bethesda, MD, United States) (Schindelin et al., 2012). The average fluorescence intensity of a given ROI was measured within the stained positive regions of the cell, and the average fluorescence intensity of an area of the same size positioned over a region outside the cell was subtracted. In cryosections, the measurements were carried out on randomly chosen cells, selected from phase-contrast images obtained from three PND 14 mice per each condition. We then calculated the *Corrected Total Cell Fluorescence* (CTCF) as *Integrated Density - (Area of selected cells x Mean fluorescence of background readings.* To evaluate morphological changes of radial processes of MGC during the time course of the degeneration, we measured and compared the thickness of NESTIN-immunolabeled radial processes in both *wt* and *rd1* mice at PND 14. Ten measurements were performed for each condition. Data were evaluated by Student's $t$-test and differences were considered significant at $p < 0.05$.

## Statistical Analysis

The results represent the average of at least three experiments ( ± SEM), unless specifically indicated, and each experiment was performed in triplicate. For cytochemical studies, 10 fields per sample, randomly chosen, were analyzed in each case. Each value represents the average of at least three experiments, with three or four dishes for each condition ± SEM, unless otherwise indicated. Statistical significance was determined by Student's two-tailed $t$-test or by ANOVA followed by Tukey's test with $p < 0.05$ considered significant.

# RESULTS

## The Course of *rd1* Neuronal Death Was Similar *in vivo* and *in vitro*

We first compared the structure of *rd1* and *wt* retinas, at 9, 14, and 30 days of development *in vivo*. As expected, at PND 9 the outer nuclear layer (ONL) of both *wt* and *rd1* retinas had almost the same width and showed a similar pattern of opsin labeling (**Figures 2Aa–f**). In contrast, by PND 14 the ONL in *rd1* retinas was significantly reduced and showed a decrease in opsin labeling, which was below detectable levels after 4 weeks of development (Adult). In contrast, ONL width and opsin labeling were preserved in *wt* retinas (**Figures 2Ag–r**).

To investigate interactions between neurons and MGC, we prepared neuron-glial cultures (**Figures 2Ba–h**). Analysis of CRX labeling at 6 and 11 days *in vitro* revealed that most neurons in these mixed cultures were PHRs. In mixed *wt* cultures, PHRs amounted to 96 ± 29% and 94 ± 18.5%, respectively, of total neurons; similarly, in *rd1* cultures, these values were 94.5 ± 37% and 96 ± 20%, respectively, **Supplementary Figure S2**). The course of PHR death in mixed neuro-glial cultures was in close correspondence with the observed in whole retinas. By day 11 in culture (equivalent to 13 days *in vivo*), a marked increase in the amount of TUNEL-positive neurons (**Figures 2Bb,f**) and of pyknotic nuclei (**Figures 2Bc,g**, white arrowheads) was observed in *rd1* compared to *wt* neuronal cultures. Whereas at day 6 in culture (equivalent to 8 days *in vivo*) both *wt* and *rd1* cultures had similar percentages of pyknotic or fragmented neuronal nuclei, by day 11 the percentage of fragmented nuclei remained at 18 ± 3% in *wt* cultures but increased to 32.5 ± 1.7% in *rd1* cultures (**Figure 2Bi**). Consistently, the percentages of TUNEL-positive PHRs by day 11 were 7.5 ± 3.8% and 23.9 ± 5.4% in *wt* and *rd1*cultures, respectively (**Figure 2Bj**). In contrast, no TUNEL-positive MGC were observed at either time in culture; in addition, MGC had intact nuclei in the *rd1* and in the *wt* cultures (**Figures 2Bb,c,f,g** empty arrowheads). Quantitative analysis showed that the percentage of surviving *rd1* and *wt* MGC in each case was 100% ± 0.0%; (**Figure 2Bk**). We then evaluated the expression level of the Bcl-2 pro-apoptotic protein BAX in mixed neuron-glia cultures. The translocation of this protein to the outer mitochondrial membrane is crucial for triggering the intrinsic apoptotic pathway. Analysis of *Bax* mRNA levels by RQ-PCR showed they significantly increased (in arbitrary units) in *rd1* compared to *wt* cultures, with a 3.7 ± 0.4 fold-increase at day 6 and 1.3 ± 0.2 fold-increase at day 11 (**Figure 2Bl**).

## Cell Cycle Progression Decreased in *rd1* MGC

Since one of the hallmarks of stem cells is their proliferative capacity, we evaluated whether it was affected in *rd1* MGC in mixed neuron-glial cultures (**Figures 3a–j**). Evaluation of BrdU uptake in mixed cultures showed that this uptake was lower in *rd1* than in *wt* MGC. By day 11, less BrdU-labeled MGC were visible in *rd1* than in *wt* cultures (**Figures 3a,f**). Quantitative analysis established that the percentages of BrdU-labeled MGC were significantly lower in *rd1* than in *wt* MGC (**Figure 3k**), both

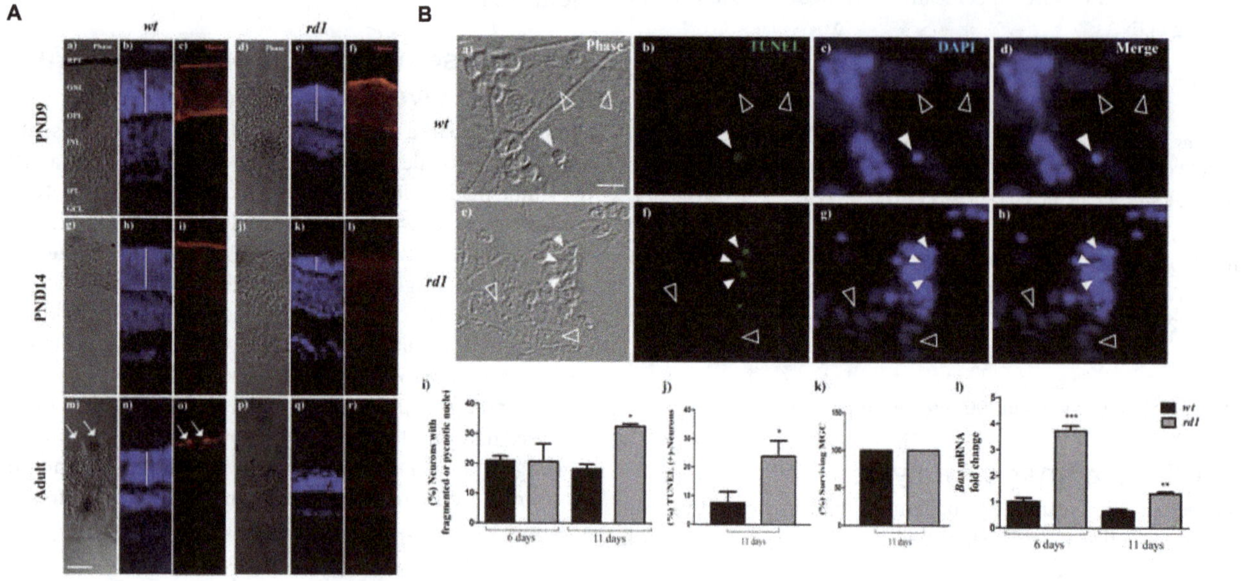

**FIGURE 2 |** Selective degeneration of photoreceptors in the *rd1* mice retina and in mixed *rd1* neuron-glial cultures. Panel **(A)** phase **(a,d,g,j,m,p)** and fluorescence **(b,c,e,f,h,i,k,l,n,o,q,r)** photomicrographs of retinal cryosections from *wt* PND 9 **(a–c)**, PND 14 **(g–i)** and Adult **(m–o**, PND30); and *rd1* PND 9 **(d–f)**, PND 14 **(j–l)**, and Adult **(p–r)**. Photoreceptors were labeled with an anti-opsin, Rho4-D2, antibody **(c,f,i,l,o,r)** and cell nuclei were stained with the nuclear probe TOPRO-3 **(b,e,h,k,n,q)**. White vertical bars show the thickness of the Outer Nuclear Layer (ONL) in *wt* and *rd1* retinas. Opsin immunolabeling was evident in *wt* and *rd1* retinas at PND 9 **(c,f)**, and concentrated in photoreceptor outer segments of *wt* retinas at PND 14 and 30 **(i,o)**; in contrast, it was barely visible in *rd1* retinas at PND 14 **(l)** and completely disappeared by PND 30 **(r)**. White arrows in **(m,o)** show outer segments in *wt* photoreceptors at PND 30. Panel **(B)** phase **(a,e)** and fluorescence **(b–d,f–h)** photomicrographs of mixed neuron-glial cultures from *wt* **(a–d)** and *rd1* **(e–h)** mice after 11 days in culture showing apoptotic neurons (white arrowheads) detected by TUNEL labeling **(b,f)**. Nuclei were stained with DAPI **(c,g)**. Note that MGC nuclei (empty arrowheads in **a–h**) remained intact in *wt* and *rd1* cultures. Bars in **(i)** show the percentage of neurons with fragmented or pyknotic nuclei, **(j)** depict the percentage of TUNEL-positive neurons, **(k)** show the percentage of surviving MGC and **(l)** represent the fold-change in Bax mRNA levels relative to these levels in wt cultures at day 6. In Panel **(A)** scale bar: 50 μm. In Panel **(B)** scale bar: 5 μm. Results represent the mean ± SEM of three experiments ($n = 3$). Statistical analysis was performed using a two-tailed Student *t*-test [Panel **(B) j,k**] and a One-way ANOVA with a *post hoc* Tukey test [Panel **(B) i,l**]. $^{*}p < 0.05$, $^{**}p < 0.01$, $^{***}p < 0.001$.

after 6 and 11 days in culture. By day 11, when *wt* cultures still had 37.36 ± 5.4% BrdU-positive cells, this percentage was only 5.2 ± 1.7% in *rd1* cultures (**Figure 3k**).

A reduction in proliferation in *rd1* MGC would lead to a progressive decrease in their number. Quantification of *rd1* and *wt* MGC evidenced that the number of *rd1* MGC was approximately half of that observed in *wt* cultures by day 6 (**Table 1**). This difference decreased with time in culture and tended to disappear by day 11; this might be a consequence of the cells reaching confluence in *wt* cultures, which posed additional restrictions to their proliferation. As a whole, the above results suggest that proliferation, a critical parameter of stem cells, was reduced in *rd1* MGC.

**TABLE 1 |** Number of MGC per dish.

| Days in culture | MGC/dish | |
|---|---|---|
| | *wt* | *rd1* |
| 6 | 32375 ± 7249 | 16720 ± 1747* |
| 11 | 104110 ± 15110 | 95297 ± 14693 |

*Number of rd1 and wt MGC per 35 mm dish after 6 and 11 in vitro. One-tailed Student t-test, *p < 0.05.*

## Stem Cell Markers Decreased in *rd1* MGC

To investigate whether the stem cell potential of MGC in *rd1* retinas was affected, we evaluated the expression of *Nestin*, a neuroectodermal stem cell marker that is expressed in many different, mitotically active cell types during development (Lendahl et al., 1990; Park et al., 2010). By day 11, nearly all MGC in *wt* neuron-glial cultures had an intense NESTIN labeling, with a widespread, radial distribution toward the edges of the cells; by contrast, *rd1* MGC showed weaker NESTIN labeling, which remained close to the nucleus or formed fiber bundles (**Figures 4Aa–h**). Further analysis of NESTIN expression by flow cytometry showed that at day 11 the number of MGC expressing NESTIN was similar in both *wt* and *rd1* cultures (**Figure 4Ai**); however, evaluation of mean fluorescence intensity (MFI) evidenced that this intensity, i.e., NESTIN expression, was lower in *rd1* than in *wt* MGC (**Figures 4Aj,k**). This implies that although the amount of MGC expressing NESTIN remained similar in *rd1* and *wt* cultures, individual *rd1* MGC expressed less NESTIN than their *wt* counterparts.

We then evaluated the levels of *Nestin* mRNA in *rd1* and *wt* mixed neuron-glial cultures at days 6 and 11. At day 6, *Nestin* mRNA levels were similar in *rd1* and *wt* cultures; however, by

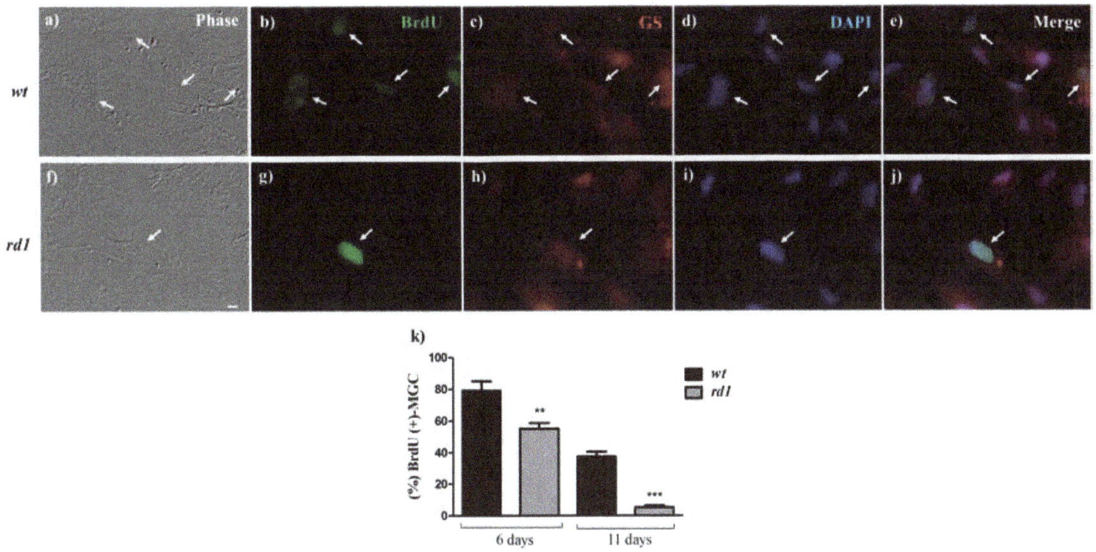


**FIGURE 3 |** Decreased proliferation of *rd1* Müller glial cells in neuron-glial cultures. Phase **(a,f)** and fluorescence photomicrographs of 11-day *wt* **(a–e)** and *rd1* **(f–j)** mixed neuron-glial cultures showing BrdU uptake by MGC, determined with a monoclonal anti-BrdU antibody **(b,g**, arrows). MGC were identified by their labeling with an anti-GS antibody **(c,h)**. Nuclei were labeled with DAPI **(d,i)**. Merge **(e,j)**. Bars in **(k)** represent the percentage of BrdU-positive at days 6 and 11. Scale bar: 30 μm. Results represent the mean ± SEM of three experiments (*n* = 3). Statistical analysis was performed using a One-way ANOVA with a *post hoc* Tukey test. $^{**}p < 0.01$, $^{***}p < 0.001$.

day 11, they were significantly reduced in *rd1* compared with *wt* cultures (**Figure 4Al**).

Since NESTIN participates in the organization of intermediate filaments (Boraas et al., 2016), we also analyzed the expression of *Vimentin*, a type III intermediate filament protein. *Vimentin* mRNA levels showed a significant fold-reduction in *rd1* neuron-glial cultures compared with *wt* cultures, both by days 6 and 11 (**Figure 4Am**).

Similar changes in NESTIN expression were observed in MGC *in vivo.* Since the reduction in NESTIN expression was more evident at day 11 *in vitro,* we analyzed NESTIN distribution in cryosections from *wt* and *rd1* retinas at PND 14, an equivalent time of development *in vivo*. MGC showed an intense NESTIN labeling throughout the *wt* retina, which overlapped with GS labeling (**Figures 4Ba–d**). In contrast, NESTIN labeling was reduced and lost its fibrillary pattern in MGC in *rd1* retinas (**Figures 4Be–h**), and the number of NESTIN-labeled MGC per area decreased in *rd1* compared to *wt* retinas (**Figure 4Bk**). Quantitative analysis of fluorescence intensity evidenced a remarkable decrease in NESTIN immunolabeling in *rd1* retinas, which was reduced to half of that observed in *wt* retinas (**Figure 4Bl**). Conspicuous morphological changes were also evident in MGC in *rd1* retinas. The basal regions of MGC projections were thicker in *rd1* than in *wt* retinas, as observed when analyzing equivalent areas and positions in retinal sections (**Figures 4Bi,j,m**).

A maximum peak of mitosis occurs in newborn mice between PND 0 to PND 3 (Livesey and Cepko, 2001). As NESTIN has been proposed to play a role in the transition from proliferating stem cells to postmitotic neurons (Zimmerman et al., 1994), *Nestin* expression would be expected to increase at PND 3, the timepoint at which most proliferating stem cells in the retina become postmitotic and begin to differentiate as neurons (Livesey and Cepko, 2001). Analysis of the changes in *Nestin* mRNA levels in *wt* and *rd1* retinas at different developmental times evidenced that in *wt* retinas *Nestin* mRNA increased 4.1 ± 2.1 and 6.3 ± 0.01 fold at PND 2 and PND 4, respectively, compared to PND 0 (**Figure 4Bn**). By contrast, in *rd1* retinas *Nestin* mRNA at PND 2 remained at PND 0 levels, and by PND 4, its fold increase was lower than that observed in *wt* retinas (**Figure 4Bn**). By PND 8, the fold change in *Nestin* levels was below PND0 levels, both in *rd1* and *wt,* and remained lower than PND0 levels from PND 10 to adulthood.

Expression of *Sox2,* a transcription factor involved in self-renewal of stem cells was also affected in *rd1* retinas. In *wt* retinas, *Sox2* mRNA levels peaked at PND 2, rapidly decreased at PND 4 and were below PND 0 levels beyond PND 8 (**Figure 5h**) whereas in *rd1* retinas, *Sox2* mRNA levels were significantly lower than in *wt* retinas at PND 2 and 4 (**Figure 5h**).

When PND 14 retina cryosections were analyzed, SOX2 expression was reduced in *rd1* compared to *wt* retinas (**Figures 5a–f**, arrowheads). At this time of development, *rd1* retinas had fewer SOX2-positive nuclei than *wt* retinas (**Figure 5g**). Whereas *wt* retinas had SOX2-positive cells in the ganglion cell layer, virtually no SOX2-positive cells were detectable in this layer in *rd1* retinas.

## Interaction With *wt* Neurons Restored *Nestin* Expression in *rd1* MGC

As a whole, the above results show that proliferation and stem cell markers were decreased in *rd1* MGC, even before the

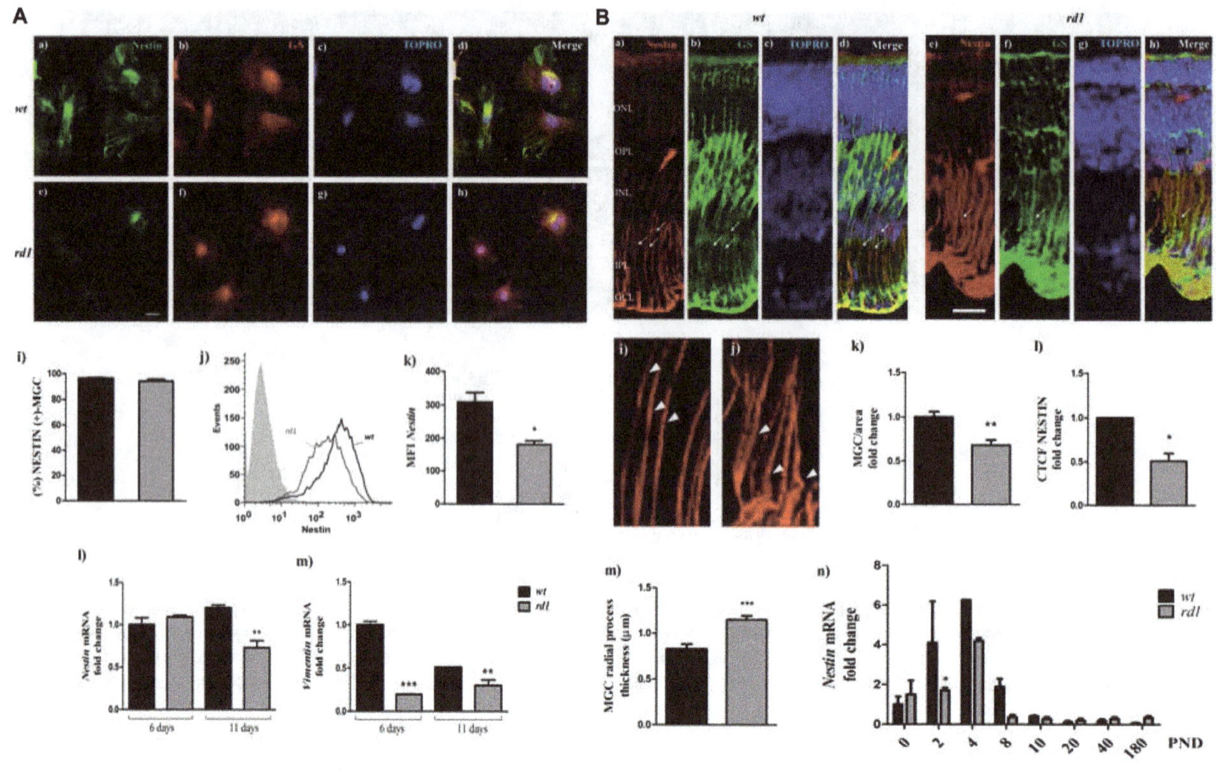


**FIGURE 4** | *Nestin* expression decreased in *rd1* retinas. Panel **(A)** fluorescence photomicrographs of 11-day *wt* **(a–d)** and *rd1* **(e–h)** mixed neuron-glial cultures showing NESTIN **(a,e)**; GS **(b,f)** and TOPRO-3 **(c,g)** labeling. Merge pictures are shown in **(d,h)**. Bars in **(i)** depict the percentage of NESTIN-expressing MGC, determined by flow cytometry. The histogram **(j)** shows the distribution of the intensity of NESTIN expression in MGC and bars in **(k)** show the medium fluorescence intensity of NESTIN labeling in *wt* and *rd1* MGC. Bars represent the fold-change in *Nestin* **(l)** and *Vimentin* mRNA levels **(m)** in *rd1* and *wt* cultures, relative to their levels in *wt* cultures at day 6. Scale bar: 40 μm. Results represent the mean ± SEM of three experiments ($n = 3$). Panel **(B)** Fluorescence photomicrographs of *wt* **(a–d)** and *rd1* **(e–h)** PND 14 retina cryosections showing MGC labeling with NESTIN **(a,e)** and GS **(b,f)**; MGC projections are indicated with thin arrows. Nuclei were stained with TOPRO-3 **(c,g)**. Merge pictures are shown in **(d,h)**. Confocal optical sections of retinas show the regular nestin filament distribution in MGC radial processes in *wt* retinas (**i**, arrowheads) and the conspicuous thickening and disorganization of radial processes at their basal ends in the *rd1* retinas (**j**, arrowheads). Bars in **(k)** show the fold change in the number of NESTIN-expressing MGC per area. Bars **(l)** depict the *Corrected Total Cell Fluorescence* (CTCF) as *Integrated Density– (Area of selected cells x Mean fluorescence of background readings,* analyzed after manually outlining regions of interest (ROI) with the software Fiji-Image J (see section "Materials and Methods"). Bars in **(m)** depict the thickness of MGC radial processes in *wt* and *rd1* retinas [shown with thin arrows in Panel **(B) a,b,d,e,f,h**; arrowheads in **i,j**]. Bars in **(n)** represent the fold changes in *Nestin* mRNA levels at PND 0-180 in *rd1* and *wt* mice retinas relative to their levels at PND 0 in *wt* retinas. Scale bar: 20 μm. Results in **k–m** represents the mean ± SEM of ten separate measures. Results in **(n)** represent the mean ± SEM of three mice per condition at each PND day analyzed. Statistical analysis was performed using a two-tailed Student *t*-test [Panels **(A) i,k** and **(B) k–m]** and a One-way ANOVA with a *post hoc* Tukey test [Panels **(A) l,m and (B) n]**. $^{*}p < 0.05$, $^{**}p < 0.01$, $^{***}p < 0.001$.

PHR degeneration peak, suggesting a deficiency in the stem cell potential of these cells. We reasoned that the alterations in *rd1* neurons might impair neuron-glial crosstalk and affect the normal functions of *rd1* MGC, thus contributing to this deficiency. If this was the case, the interaction of healthy *wt* neurons with *rd1* MGC would, at least partially, reestablish their stem cell potential. Our culture systems allow us to prepare purified neuronal and MGC cultures, from developing *rd1* or *wt* retinas, and then seed them together to obtain co-cultures with different combinations of *rd1* and *wt* cells. To investigate the influence of neuronal cells on the stem cell capability of MGC, we separately cultured pure *rd1* and *wt* retinal neurons, labeled them with CellTracer® for 3 days and then seeded unlabeled *wt* or *rd1* MGC over these neuronal cultures, to analyze NESTIN expression in the different neuron-glial co-cultures. *rd1* MGC co-cultured with *rd1* neurons had a faint NESTIN labeling (**Figures 6Aa–d**). Noteworthy, interaction with *wt* neurons (**Figures 6Ae–h**) increased NESTIN expression in *rd1* MGC. Quantitative analysis evidenced that NESTIN-positive *rd1* MGC significantly increased in *rd1* MGC-*wt* neuron co-cultures compared to *rd1* pure MGC cultures; in contrast, no significant change was observed in *rd1* MGC-*rd1* neuron co-cultures compared to *rd1* pure MGC cultures (**Figure 6Ai**). To further assess the effect of neuron-glial interactions on *Nestin* levels, we analyzed the levels of *Nestin* mRNA. In *rd1* MGC-*wt* neuron co-cultures, *Nestin* mRNA levels increased almost 50-fold relative to *rd1* pure MCG cultures; in contrast, no increase was observed in *rd1* MGC- *rd1* neuron co-cultures (**Figure 6Aj**).

If neuron-glial interactions were responsible for modulating the levels of stem cell markers such as *Nestin*, *rd1* neurons

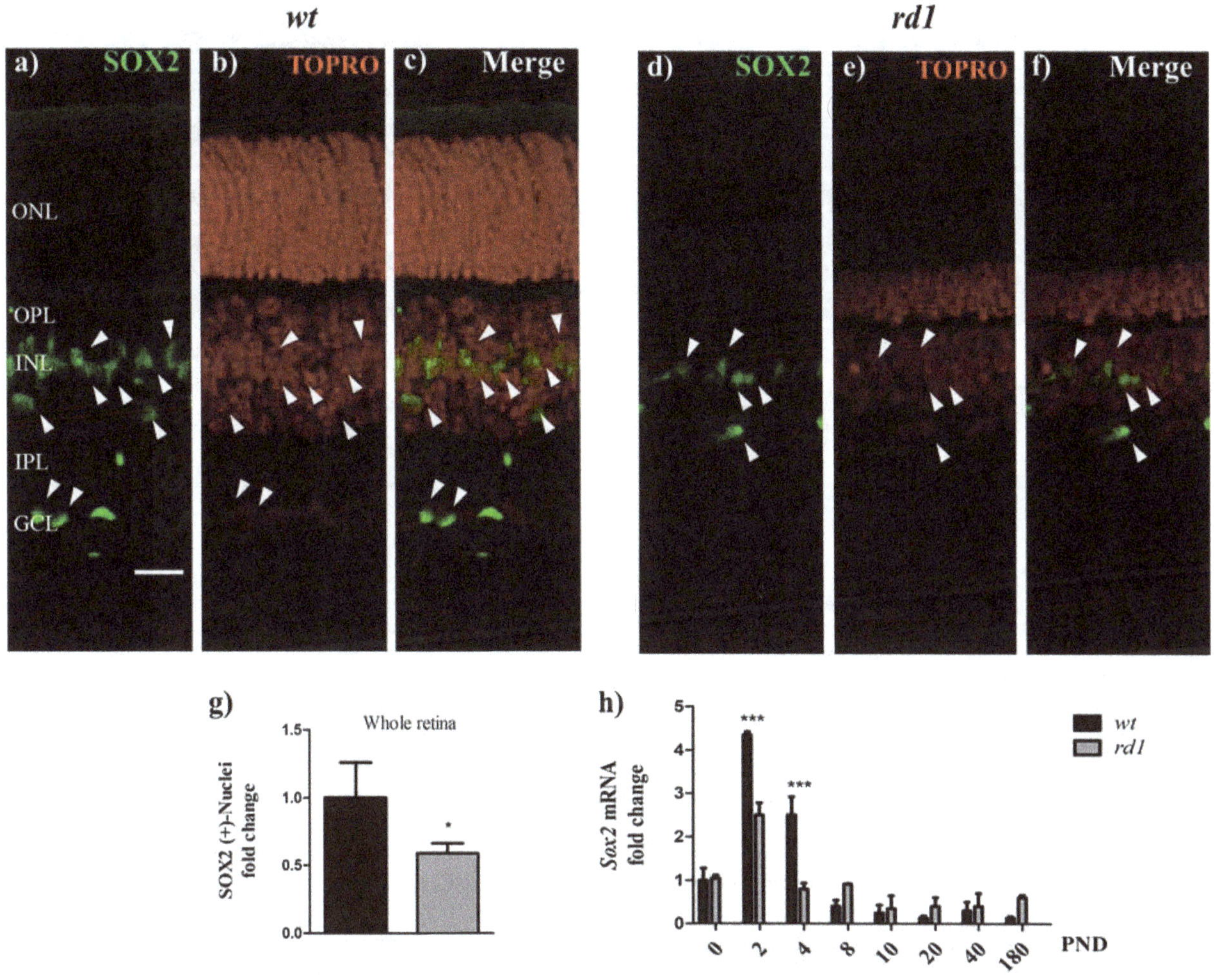


**FIGURE 5 |** SOX2 expression decreased in *rd1* retinas. Fluorescence photomicrographs show SOX2 expression **(a,d,** arrowheads) in retina cryosections obtained from *wt* **(a–c)** and *rd1* **(d–f)** mice at PND14, determined with an anti-SOX2 polyclonal antibody. Nuclei were stained with DAPI **(b,e)** and merge pictures are shown in **(c,f)**. Bars **(g)** show the fold change of total SOX2-positive nuclei in *rd1* retinas relative to *wt* retinas. Bars **(h)** represent the fold changes in *Sox2* mRNA levels at PND 0-180 in *rd1* and *wt* mice retinas relative to their levels at PND 0 in *wt* retinas. Scale bar: 20 μm. Results in **(g)** represent the mean ± SEM of ten measures. Results in **(h)** represent the mean ± SEM of three mice per condition. Statistical analysis was performed using a two-tailed Student *t*-test **(g)**, and a One-way ANOVA with a *post hoc* Tukey test **(h)**. $^*p < 0.05$, $^{***}p < 0.001$.

would downregulate these levels in *wt* MGC in co-culture. This reduction in NESTIN expression was evident when *wt* MGC were co-cultured with *rd1* neurons. Whereas *wt* MGC showed a bright NESTIN expression when co-cultured with *wt* neurons (**Figures 6Ba–d**), their NESTIN expression was noticeably reduced when co-cultured with *rd1* neurons (**Figures 6Be–h**). The fold change in NESTIN-positive *wt* MGC, relative to their number in *wt* pure MGC cultures, was reduced by half when co-cultured with *rd1* neurons; in contrast, NESTIN positive-*wt* MGC were the same in pure *wt* MGC cultures and in co-culture with *wt* neurons (**Figure 6Bi**). Noteworthy, the levels of *Nestin* mRNA were dramatically reduced in *wt* MGC-*rd1* neuron co-cultures relative to pure *wt* MGC cultures, and significantly increased, up to nearly 3.3 ± 1 times in *wt* MGC-*wt* neuron co-cultures (**Figure 6Bj**).

As a whole, these results suggest that the crosstalk between neurons and MGC is crucial for regulating Nestin expression in MGC, and interactions with *wt* neurons can restore this expression in *rd1* MGC.

## MGC Had a Distorted Morphology and Were Overloaded With Neurons in *rd1* Cultures

We finally analyzed whether the changes in the levels of intermediate filaments, as NESTIN and VIMENTIN, in *rd1* MGC correlated with changes in MGC morphology. Analysis of their actin cytoskeleton revealed that *rd1* MGC had remarkable alterations in their morphology. By day 6, *wt* cultures had many MGC, which exhibited an extended actin cytoskeleton (**Figures 7a,b,d**). In contrast, *rd1* cultures showed fewer

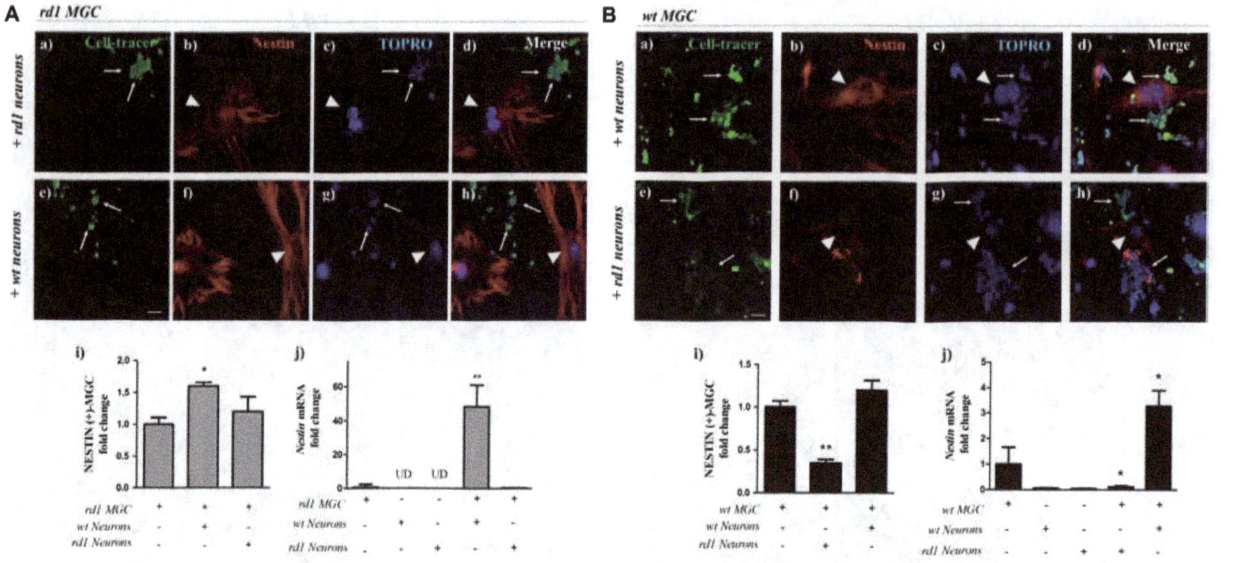


**FIGURE 6 |** Changes in *Nestin* expression in MGC when co-cultured with *wt* or *rd1* neurons. Neuron-glial co-cultures were prepared seeding unlabeled *rd1* MGC (Panel **A**) or *wt* MGC (Panel **B**) over 3-day cultures of either *rd1* or *wt* neurons labeled with the green fluorescent CellTracer probe (thin arrows), and were then incubated for 24 h. Fluorescence photomicrographs show Cell-Trace labeled neurons (green in **a,e**) and NESTIN-labeled MGC (red in **b,f**, arrowheads); nuclei were stained with TOPRO-3 (blue in **c,g**). Merge pictures are shown in **(d,h)**. Bars in Panels **A (i)** and **B (i)** show the fold change in NESTIN-positive *rd1 MGC* (Panel **A**) *or wt MGC* (Panel **B**) when co-cultured with either *wt* neurons or *rd1* neurons, relative to pure *rd1* or *wt* MGC cultures, respectively. Bars in Panels **A (j)** and **B (j)** depict the fold change *in Nestin* mRNA levels in *rd1* MGC (Panel **A**) or *wt* MGC (Panel **B**) when co-cultured with either *wt* or *rd1* neurons, relative to pure *rd1 or wt* MGC cultures, respectively. Scale bar: 40 μm. Results represent the mean ± SEM of three experiments ($n = 3$). UD, undetected. Statistical analysis was performed using a One-way ANOVA with a *post hoc* Tukey test. *$p < 0.05$, **$p < 0.01$.

MGC, which evidenced a marked retraction in their actin cytoskeleton and almost a complete loss of their lamellipodia, leading to a decrease in cell body size and a distorted morphology (**Figures 7e,f,h**).

In addition, the neuron:MGC ratio was markedly different in *wt* and *rd1* neuro-glial cultures. Whereas in *wt* cultures few neurons were observed growing on MGC (**Figures 7a–d**), their number markedly increased in *rd1* cultures by day 6 (**Figures 7e–h**). This difference might result from the reduction in the number of MGC in *rd1* cultures compared with *wt* cultures at this time of development, due to the decrease in their proliferation, as described above (**Table 1**). Quantitative analysis showed that the ratio of neurons per glial cell at day 6 was almost three-fold higher in *rd1* than in *wt* cultures (**Table 2**). This implies that individual *rd1* MGC supported significantly more neurons than their *wt* counterparts.

**TABLE 2 |** MGC: neuron ratio.

| Days in culture | G:N | |
|---|---|---|
| | *wt* | *rd1* |
| 6 | 1 : 2.3 ± 0.5 | 1 : 6.6 ± 2.5* |
| 11 | 1 : 1 ± 0.3 | 1 : 2 ± 0.5 |

*MGC: neuron ratios in wt and rd1 mixed neuron-glial cultures at 6 and 11 days in vitro. One-way ANOVA with a post hoc Tukey test, *p < 0.05.*

## DISCUSSION

The major conclusions from the present work are that *rd1* MGC have a significant decrease in their stem cell markers even before the degeneration of PHR started in *rd1* retinas. Furthermore, at least one of their stem cell characteristics was restored by their interaction with *wt* neurons in co-culture, suggesting that a defective cross talk between neurons and MGC is at least partially responsible for this decrease.

The mechanisms regulating the neurogenic potential of MGC remain enigmatic. Their regenerative capacity is remarkably dissimilar among vertebrates. Although in the zebrafish, MGC can efficiently regenerate the retina after different lesions (Sherpa et al., 2008, 2014; Lenkowski and Raymond, 2014; Ranski et al., 2018), these cells are unable to function as retinal progenitors in mammals (Goldman, 2014). Intriguingly, cumulative evidence suggests that mammalian MGC have the molecular mechanisms to accomplish retina regeneration. Different injuries trigger their proliferation; activation of MGC following oxidative damage induces their dedifferentiation and re-entry in the cell cycle (Abrahan et al., 2009); neurotoxic damage promotes proliferation and the expression of progenitor markers in retina MGC (Ooto et al., 2004), which differentiate as specific neuronal types (Das et al., 2006). A human embryonic stem cell line (hESC) can differentiate into retinal amacrine neurons and ganglion cells, and integration of the hESC-derived retinal progenitors with a degenerated mouse retina increases the expression of specific PHR markers (Lamba et al., 2006). Human induced

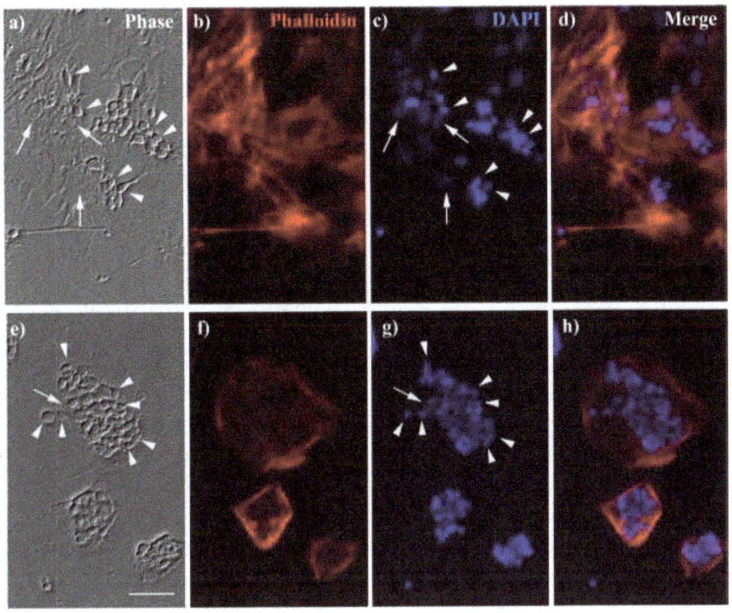


**FIGURE 7 |** MGC morphology and neuron:glial ratio was altered in *rd1* mixed neuron-glial cultures. Phase **(a,e)** and fluorescence photomicrographs **(b–d,f–h)** of 6-day *wt* **(a–d)** and *rd1* **(e–h)** mixed neuron glial cultures showing neuronal cells (arrowheads) growing on top of MGC (arrows). Actin cytoskeleton was stained with phalloidin **(b,f)** and nuclei with DAPI **(c,g)**. Merge pictures are shown in **(d,h)**. Scale bar: 50 μm.

pluripotent stem cells (hiPSC) have been shown to differentiate into retinal progenitors and recapitulate retinal development to form three-dimensional retina cups containing major retinal cell types, including PHR with an advanced differentiation and photosensitivity (Zhong et al., 2014), implying that the generation of functional PHR from stem cells is feasible in mammals. Stem cells in mammalian retinas, such as MGC, can be assumed to replace neurons lost during the life span of healthy retinas. However, the substantial differences in the genetic setup of hiPSCs and mature MGC likely contribute to the incapacity of the latter to regenerate PHRs during retina degeneration. The inability of MGC to regenerate the retina has been suggested to result from either intrinsic features of mammalian MGC or extrinsic properties of their "niche," which interfere with the reprograming process of these cells (Xia and Ahmad, 2016). Analysis of cultured MGC from *rd1* retinas revealed that their cell cycle was downregulated, compared to *wt* MGC. By day 6, prior to the onset of PHR degeneration, the number of *rd1* MGC was about half of that of *wt* MGC in mixed neuron-glial cultures and their BrdU-uptake was markedly reduced; this uptake was virtually negligible at day 11 *in vitro* in *rd1* MGC, whereas *wt* MGC still retained their proliferative capacity at this time in culture. This is in close agreement with previous findings showing that there are significantly less MGC in the *rd1* retinas than in the corresponding *wt* retinas (Chua et al., 2013). The significant reduction in the mitotic cycle in *rd1* MGC might further diminish the already limited regenerative capacity of healthy MGC.

Expression of stem cell markers was also reduced in *rd1* MGC. NESTIN is a well-established stem cell marker; its levels increase in most stem cells in the central nervous system (Lendahl et al., 1990) and it is downregulated upon differentiation (Sahlgren et al., 2006). The levels and distribution of NESTIN were affected in *rd1* MGC compared to *wt* MGC. *Nestin* was down regulated in *rd1* MGC, which had lower mRNA levels than *wt* MGC by day 11. Even when a similar number of MGC expressed NESTIN in *rd1* and *wt* neuron-glial cultures, the level of NESTIN expression was significantly lower in *rd1* cultures. This was consistent with the significant reduction in NESTIN-positive MGC in whole *rd1* retinas compared to *wt* retinas by PND 14. Early during development, the rodent retina is enriched in NESTIN-expressing progenitors, which later differentiate as neuronal progenitors and, further during development, as MGC. PND 2 is a critical point in development, corresponding with the highest mitotic peak of PHR progenitors and with the onset of MGC differentiation, which reaches its maximum levels between PND 5 and 8 (Cepko et al., 1996; Nelson et al., 2011). Interestingly, the largest difference in the level of *Nestin* mRNA between *rd1* and *wt* retinas was visible at PND2, suggesting a reduction in the number of progenitors in *rd1* retinas. SOX2 is a critical transcription factor for reprograming MGC toward a proliferative mode, for inducing their transformation into pluripotent stem cells and for the maintenance of neural stem cells (Favaro et al., 2009; Gorsuch et al., 2017). *Sox2* was also downregulated in *rd1* retinas; the levels of *Sox2* mRNA were lower in *rd1* than in *wt* retinas early during development. *Sox2* changes were similar to those described for *Nestin*. In *wt* retinas, the fold changes in *Sox2* mRNA levels relative to PND 0 showed a peak at PND 2, and rapidly decreased thereafter. In the *rd1* retinas the pattern of changes in *Sox2* mRNA was similar to the observed in *wt* retinas, but their increase at PND 2 and 4 was significantly lower than in *wt* retinas. Consistently, *rd1* retinas had remarkably less SOX2-expressing nuclei than *wt* retinas by PND 14. VIMENTIN is also considered a stem cell marker, although less specific than *Nestin*, since its expression has been found not only in developing tissues, but also in differentiated tissues (Traub et al., 1985; Lendahl et al., 1990). *Vimentin* is expressed in human stem cells when cultured on mouse PA6 stromal cells (Gong et al., 2008), and in cells derived from stem cell spheres when acquiring a Müller glial phenotype (Coles et al., 2004). VIMENTIN is closely linked to NESTIN, which is required for its polymerization (Park et al., 2010); in turn, NESTIN, along with the mitosis promoting factor (MPF), are important for the phosphorylation-mediated disassembly of VIMENTIN during mitosis (Chou et al., 2003). Noteworthy, *Vimentin* mRNA levels were significantly lower in *rd1* than in *wt* neuron-glial cultures by days 6 and 11 in culture. As a whole, our present findings that *wt* MGC expressed stem cell markers like *Nestin*, *Sox2* and *Vimentin*, and proliferated in culture are consistent with previous work from our laboratory evidencing that cultured rat MGC proliferate actively and express PAX6 and NESTIN (Insua et al., 2008; Simón et al., 2012). Our results also suggest that the regenerative capacity still preserved by MGC in *wt* retinas was further decreased in *rd1* retinas. *Nestin*, *Sox2* and *Vimentin* levels were reduced in *rd1* retinas, particularly in MGC, and these cells also evidenced a decreased proliferation rate. These findings support a decline in the stem cell potential of MGC in *rd1* retinas.

Little is known regarding the alterations that *rd1* MGC undergo during retinal degeneration (Roesch et al., 2012). Most studies on retinitis pigmentosa, including those using the *rd1* mice, focus mainly on the alterations affecting PHRs, such as genetic mutations, cell death, or abnormal development or functionality (Pittler and Baehr, 1991; Arikawa et al., 1992; Chen et al., 1996). Moreover, among the over 100 mutations leading to retinitis pigmentosa, most affect PHRs. Only a few reported mutations are known to affect MGC, such as a mutation in *Cralbp*, altering retinoid association/dissociation to its ligand binding pocket, and consequently the visual cycle (Golovleva et al., 2003), and no evidences of mutations affecting the regenerative capacity of MGC have been reported for this pathology. Our data strongly suggests that a defective neuron-glial crosstalk is responsible for the impaired stem cell capacity of *rd1* MGC. *Nestin* levels dramatically increased when *rd1* MGC were co-cultured with *wt* neurons. In contrast, when *wt* MGC were co-cultured with *rd1* neurons, *Nestin* levels were markedly reduced. These experiments strongly suggest that the crosstalk with neurons regulates *Nestin* expression in MGC and the interaction with healthy PHR progenitors is crucial for regulating MGC stem cell potential. To our knowledge, this is the first report highlighting the relevance of neuron-glial crosstalk in supporting the stem cell potential of MGC. This is consistent with the hypothesis that the "niche," i.e., the environment surrounding MGC, might be modified in the retina during neurodegenerative diseases. MGC and neurons are known to maintain an active crosstalk, or "molecular dialogue" in the retina. The occurrence of gliosis in MGC in the beta-PDE model, *rd10* mice, before the beginning of retinal degeneration, suggests this crosstalk between PHR and MGC starts very early during development (Dong et al., 2017). Many of the factors involved in this "dialogue" have been identified; MGC release several molecules, such as FGF, GDNF, DHA, and LIF, that rescue PHRs in different models of retinal degeneration (Faktorovich et al., 1990, 1992; LaVail et al., 1992, 1998; Rotstein et al., 1996; Cayouette et al., 1998; Chong et al., 1999; Frasson et al., 1999; Harada et al., 2002; Miranda et al., 2009; German et al., 2013). MGC also release molecular cues that regulate their own regenerative responses, reducing proliferation (Fischer et al., 2004; Zhao et al., 2014). In turn, PHRs regulate MGC functions, even while undergoing degeneration. PHR degeneration modulates the expression of *Neurotrophin* receptor genes in retinal MGC (Harada et al., 2000). PHRs have also been reported to release stress signals, the damage-associated molecular patterns (DAMPs) during degenerative processes of the retina, that orchestrate a broad neuroprotective response in MGC, including release of Leukemia Inhibitory Factor (LIF), a critical PHR survival factor (Hooper et al., 2018). A further putative signal might be glutamate, which PHRs release as a neurotransmitter; activation of NMDA receptors has been shown to increase proliferation and differentiation of hippocampal neural progenitor cells (Joo et al., 2007) and might have a similar effect on retinal MGC. The progressive degeneration of PHRs in the *rd1* mice might lead to a shortage of glutamate, among other factors, which might affect MGC stem cell capability. Further research is required to establish how neuron-glial crosstalk is regulated and modified along development or after retinal injuries to regulate MGC regenerative capacity.

## CONCLUSION

Replacement therapies using stem cells are currently intensely investigated for retina neurodegenerations and establishing the most adequate source of these stem cells is crucial for these therapies. Our results imply that the limited capacity of mammalian MGC for restoring lost PHRs is further impaired in degenerated retinas. This capacity might be improved by their crosstalk with "healthy" PHR partners, suggesting that it is possible to manipulate these stem cells to recover their proliferative potential by creating an adequate "niche." Identifying the molecular cues required for this manipulation is an exciting challenge that deserves further investigation.

## AUTHOR CONTRIBUTIONS

All authors contributed intellectually to the manuscript. YV, HV-M, MD, OG, VA-P, SZ, and AG performed the experiments and analyzed the data. YV involved in the all experiments. YV, OG, HV-M, and AT performed the cultures. HV-M and AT involved in the immunocytochemistry imaging. MD involved in the immunohistochemistry and image processing. VA-P involved in the RQ-PCR assays. SZ and MD involved in the Flow Cytometry assays. AG involved in the preparation of retina cryosections. CC interpreted and analyzed the data and reviewed the manuscript. YV, OG, and LP elaborated strategies for the experiments. YV, OG, NR, and LP interpreted the data and elaborated the manuscript. LP and OG conducted the research and wrote the manuscript.

## FUNDING

This work was supported by the National Research Council of Argentina (CONICET) (PIP 11220-1101-00827, to LP); the National Agency for Science and Technology (ANPCYT), (PICT-201-0475 to OG, PICT-2016-0353 to LP); from the Secretary of Science and Technology, UNS (24/ZB68 to OG, 24-B190 to LP); from P30EY029220 from the NIH and unrestricted Grant to the Department of Ophthalmology, Keck School of Medicine of USC from the Research to Prevent Blindness, New York, NY, United States to CC.

## ACKNOWLEDGMENTS

YV has a postdoctoral fellowship from the Argentina National Research Council (CONICET). HV-M, MD, and AT have doctoral fellowships from the CONICET. VA-P and SZ are assistant researchers, OG and AG are adjunct researchers and NR and LP are principal researchers from the CONICET. We thank Beatriz De los Santos and Edgardo Buzzi for their excellent technical assistance. We are very grateful to Valeria Levi and Alejandra Guberman (Facultad de Ciencias Exactas y Naturales, Universidad de Buenos Aires, Buenos Aires, Argentina) for the kind gift of anti-SOX2.

## SUPPLEMENTARY MATERIAL

**FIGURE S1** | Specificity of photoreceptors and glial markers in culture. Phase **(a,f)** and fluorescence **(b–e,g–j)** photomicrographs of *wt* neuronal cultures **(a–e)**, showing photoreceptors labeled with an anti-CRX antibody **(c,h)**, and of *rd1* MGC cultures **(f–j)**, showing MGC labeled with an anti-GS antibody **(b,g)**. Nuclei were visualized with DAPI **(d,i)**. Merge images **(e,j)**. Scale bar: 20 μm.

**FIGURE S2** | CRX-positive neurons in mixed neuron-glial cultures. Phase **(a,e)** and fluorescence **(b–d,f–h)** photomicrographs of 6-day mixed *wt* **(a–d)** and *rd1* **(e–h)** neuron-glial cultures showing photoreceptors labeled with anti-CRX antibody **(b f)**. Cell nuclei were visualized with DAPI **(c,g)**. Merge images **(d,h)**. Bars in **(i)** represent the percentage of CRX-positive neurons (photoreceptors) at days 6 and 11 in *wt* and *rd1* mixed neuron-glial cultures. Scale bar: 20 μm. Statistical analysis was performed using a One-way ANOVA with a *post hoc* Tukey test. No significant differences were observed between conditions.

## REFERENCES

Abrahan, C. E., Insua, M. F., Politi, L. E., German, O. L., and Rotstein, N. P. (2009). Oxidative stress promotes proliferation and dedifferentiation of retina glial cells in vitro. *J. Neurosci. Res.* 87, 964–977. doi: 10.1002/jnr.21903

Adler, R. (1982). Regulation of neurite growth in purified retina neuronal cultures: effects of PNPF, a substratum-bound, neurite-promoting factor. *J. Neurosci. Res.* 8, 165–177. doi: 10.1002/jnr.490080207

Arikawa, K., Molday, L. L., Molday, R. S., and Williams, D. S. (1992). Localization of peripherin/rds in the disk membranes of cone and rod photoreceptors: relationship to disk membrane morphogenesis and retinal degeneration. *J. Cell Biol.* 116, 659–667. doi: 10.1083/jcb.116.3.659

Barnstable, C. J. (1980). Monoclonal antibodies which recognize different cell types in the rat retina. *Nature* 286, 231–235. doi: 10.1038/286231a0

Boraas, L. C., Guidry, J. B., Pineda, E. T., and Ahsan, T. (2016). Cytoskeletal expression and remodeling in pluripotent stem cells. *PLoS One* 11:e0145084. doi: 10.1371/journal.pone.0145084

Bringmann, A., Pannicke, T., Biedermann, B., Francke, M., Iandiev, I., Grosche, J., et al. (2009). Role of retinal glial cells in neurotransmitter uptake and metabolism. *Neurochem. Int.* 54, 143–160. doi: 10.1016/j.neuint.2008.10.014

Bringmann, A., Pannicke, T., Grosche, J., Francke, M., Wiedemann, P., Skatchkov, S. N., et al. (2006). Müller cells in the healthy and diseased retina. *Prog. Retin. Eye Res.* 25, 397–424. doi: 10.1016/j.preteyeres.2006.05.003

Bustin, S. A., Benes, V., Garson, J. A., Hellemans, J., Huggett, J., Kubista, M., et al. (2009). The MIQE guidelines: minimum information for publication of quantitative real-time PCR experiments. *Clin. Chem.* 55, 611–622. doi: 10.1373/clinchem.2008.112797

Cayouette, M., Behn, D., Sendtner, M., Lachapelle, P., and Gravel, C. (1998). Intraocular gene transfer of ciliary neurotrophic factor prevents death and increases responsiveness of rod photoreceptors in the retinal degeneration slow mouse. *J. Neurosci* 18, 9282–9293. doi: 10.1523/jneurosci.18-22-09282.1998

Cepko, C. L., Austin, C. P., Yang, X., Alexiades, M., and Ezzeddine, D. (1996). Cell fate determination in the vertebrate retina. *Proc. Natl. Acad. Sci. U.S.A.* 93, 589–595.

Chen, J., Flannery, J. G., LaVail, M. M., Steinberg, R. H., Xu, J., and Simon, M. I. (1996). bcl-2 overexpression reduces apoptotic photoreceptor cell death in three different retinal degenerations. *Proc. Natl. Acad. Sci. U.S.A.* 93, 7042–7047. doi: 10.1073/pnas.93.14.7042

Chong, N. H., Alexander, R. A., Waters, L., Barnett, K. C., Bird, A. C., and Luthert, P. J. (1999). Repeated injections of a ciliary neurotrophic factor analogue leading to long-term photoreceptor survival in hereditary retinal degeneration. *Invest. Ophthalmol. Vis. Sci.* 40, 1298–1305.

Chou, Y.-H., Khuon, S., Herrmann, H., and Goldman, R. D. (2003). Nestin promotes the phosphorylation-dependent disassembly of vimentin intermediate filaments during mitosis. *Mol. Biol. Cell* 14, 1468–1478. doi: 10.1091/mbc.E02-08-0545

Chua, J., Nivison-Smith, L., Fletcher, E. L., Trenholm, S., Awatramani, G. B., and Kalloniatis, M. (2013). Early remodeling of Müller cells in the rd/rd mouse model of retinal dystrophy. *J. Comp. Neurol.* 521, 2439–2453. doi: 10.1002/cne.23307

Coles, B. L. K., Angénieux, B., Inoue, T., Del Rio-Tsonis, K., Spence, J. R., McInnes, R. R., et al. (2004). Facile isolation and the characterization of human retinal stem cells. *Proc. Natl. Acad. Sci. U.S.A.* 101, 15772–15777. doi: 10.1073/pnas.0401596101

Das, A. V., Mallya, K. B., Zhao, X., Ahmad, F., Bhattacharya, S., and Thoreson, W. B. (2006). Neural stem cell properties of Müller glia in the mammalian retina: regulation by Notch and Wnt signaling. *Dev. Biol.* 299, 283–302. doi: 10.1016/j.ydbio.2006.07.029

Dong, E., Bachleda, A., Xiong, Y., Osawa, S., and Weiss, E. R. (2017). Reduced phosphoCREB in Müller glia during retinal degeneration in rd10 mice. *Mol. Vis.* 23, 90–102.

Dyer, M. A., and Cepko, C. L. (2000). Control of Müller glial cell proliferation and activation following retinal injury. *Nat. Neurosci.* 3, 873–880. doi: 10.1038/78774

Faktorovich, E. G., Steinberg, R. H., Yasumura, D., Matthes, M. T., and LaVail, M. M. (1990). Photoreceptor degeneration in inherited retinal dystrophy delayed by basic fibroblast growth factor. *Nature* 347, 83–86. doi: 10.1038/347083a0

Faktorovich, E. G., Steinberg, R. H., Yasumura, D., Matthes, M. T., and LaVail, M. M. (1992). Basic fibroblast growth factor and local injury protect photoreceptors from light damage in the rat. *J. Neurosci* 12, 3554–3567. doi: 10.1523/jneurosci.12-09-03554.1992

Farber, D. B., and Lolley, R. N. (1974). Cyclic guanosine monophosphate: elevation in degenerating photoreceptor cells of the C3H mouse retina. *Science* 186, 449–451. doi: 10.1126/science.186.4162.449

Favaro, R., Valotta, M., Ferri, A. L. M., Latorre, E., Mariani, J., Giachino, C., et al. (2009). Hippocampal development and neural stem cell maintenance require Sox2-dependent regulation of Shh. *Nat. Neurosci.* 12, 1248–1256. doi: 10.1038/nn.2397

Fischer, A. J., and Reh, T. A. (2003). Potential of Müller glia to become neurogenic retinal progenitor cells. *Glia* 43, 70–76. doi: 10.1002/glia.10218

Fischer, A. J., Schmidt, M., Schmidt, M., Omar, G., and Reh, T. A. (2004). BMP4 and CNTF are neuroprotective and suppress damage-induced proliferation of Müller glia in the retina. *Mol. Cell. Neurosci.* 27, 531–542. doi: 10.1016/j.mcn.2004.08.007

Frasson, M., Picaud, S., Léveillard, T., Simonutti, M., Mohand-Said, S., Dreyfus, H., et al. (1999). Glial cell line-derived neurotrophic factor induces histologic and functional protection of rod photoreceptors in the rd/rd mouse. *Invest. Ophthalmol. Vis. Sci.* 40, 2724–2734.

Garelli, A., Rotstein, N. P., and Politi, L. E. (2006). Docosahexaenoic acid promotes photoreceptor differentiation without altering Crx expression. *Investig. Ophthalmol. Vis. Sci.* 47, 3017–3027. doi: 10.1167/iovs.05-1659

German, O. L., Monaco, S., Agnolazza, D. L., Rotstein, N. P., and Politi, L. E. (2013). Retinoid X receptor activation is essential for docosahexaenoic acid protection of retina photoreceptors. *J. Lipid Res.* 54, 2236–2246. doi: 10.1194/jlr.M039040

Goldman, D. (2014). Müller glial cell reprogramming and retina regeneration. *Nat. Rev. Neurosci.* 15, 431–442. doi: 10.1038/nrn3723

Golovleva, I., Bhattacharya, S., Wu, Z., Shaw, N., Yang, Y., Andrabi, K., et al. (2003). Disease-causing mutations in the cellular retinaldehyde binding protein tighten and abolish ligand interactions. *J. Biol. Chem.* 278, 12397–12402. doi: 10.1074/jbc.M207300200

Gong, J., Sagiv, O., Cai, H., Tsang, S. H., and Del Priore, L. V. (2008). Effects of extracellular matrix and neighboring cells on induction of human embryonic stem cells into retinal or retinal pigment epithelial progenitors. *Exp. Eye Res.* 86, 957–965. doi: 10.1016/j.exer.2008.03.014

Gorsuch, R. A., Lahne, M., Yarka, C. E., Petravick, M. E., Li, J., and Hyde, D. R. (2017). Sox2 regulates Müller glia reprogramming and proliferation in the regenerating zebrafish retina via Lin28 and Ascl1a. *Exp. Eye Res.* 161, 174–192. doi: 10.1016/j.exer.2017.05.012

Harada, T., Harada, C., Kohsaka, S., Wada, E., Yoshida, K., Ohno, S., et al. (2002). Microglia-Müller glia cell interactions control neurotrophic factor production during light-induced retinal degeneration. *J. Neurosci* 22, 9228–9236. doi: 10.1523/jneurosci.22-21-09228.2002

Harada, T., Harada, C., Nakayama, N., Okuyama, S., Yoshida, K., Kohsaka, S., et al. (2000). Modification of glial-neuronal cell interactions prevents photoreceptor apoptosis during light-induced retinal degeneration. *Neuron* 26, 533–541. doi: 10.1016/s0896-6273(00)81185-x

Hartong, D. T., Berson, E. L., and Dryja, T. P. (2006). Retinitis pigmentosa. *Lancet* 368, 1795–1809. doi: 10.1016/S0140-6736(06)69740-7

Hicks, D., and Courtois, Y. (1990). The growth and behaviour of rat retinal Müller cells in vitro. 1. An improved method for isolation and culture. *Exp. Eye Res.* 51, 119–129. doi: 10.1016/0014-4835(90)90063-z

Hooper, M. J., Wang, J., Browning, R., and Ash, J. D. (2018). Damage-associated molecular pattern recognition is required for induction of retinal neuroprotective pathways in a sex-dependent manner. *Sci. Rep.* 8, 9115. doi: 10.1038/s41598-018-27479-x

Huang, L., Zhang, Q., Huang, X., Qu, C., Ma, S., Mao, Y., et al. (2017). Mutation screening in genes known to be responsible for retinitis pigmentosa in 98 small han chinese families. *Sci. Rep.* 7:1948. doi: 10.1038/s41598-017-00963-6

Insua, M. F., Simón, M. V., Garelli, A., de los Santos, B., Rotstein, N. P., and Politi, L. E. (2008)). Trophic factors and neuronal interactions regulate the cell cycle and Pax6 expression in Müller stem cells. *J. Neurosci. Res.* 86, 1459–1471. doi: 10.1002/jnr.21606

Joo, J.-Y., Kim, B.-W., Lee, J.-S., Park, J.-Y., Kim, S., Yun, Y.-J., et al. (2007). Activation of NMDA receptors increases proliferation and differentiation of hippocampal neural progenitor cells. *J. Cell Sci.* 120, 1358–1370. doi: 10.1242/jcs.002154

Karl, M. O., Hayes, S., Nelson, B. R., Tan, K., Buckingham, B., and Reh, T. A. (2008). Stimulation of neural regeneration in the mouse retina. *Proc. Natl. Acad. Sci.* 105, 19508–19513. doi: 10.1073/pnas.0807453105

Lamba, D. A., Karl, M. O., Ware, C. B., and Reh, T. A. (2006). Efficient generation of retinal progenitor cells from human embryonic stem cells. *Proc. Natl. Acad. Sci. U.S.A.* 103, 12769–12774. doi: 10.1073/pnas.0601990103

LaVail, M. M., Unoki, K., Yasumura, D., Matthes, M. T., Yancopoulos, G. D., and Steinberg, R. H. (1992). Multiple growth factors, cytokines, and neurotrophins rescue photoreceptors from the damaging effects of constant light. *Proc. Natl. Acad. Sci. U.S.A.* 89, 11249–11253. doi: 10.1073/pnas.89.23.11249

LaVail, M. M., Yasumura, D., Matthes, M. T., Lau-Villacorta, C., Unoki, K., Sung, C. H., et al. (1998). Protection of mouse photoreceptors by survival factors in retinal degenerations. *Invest. Ohthalmol. Vis. Sci.* 39, 592–602.

Lendahl, U., Zimmerman, L. B., and McKay, R. D. (1990). CNS stem cells express a new class of intermediate filament protein. *Cell* 60, 585–595. doi: 10.1016/0092-8674(90)90662-x

Lenkowski, J. R., and Raymond, P. A. (2014). Müller glia: stem cells for generation and regeneration of retinal neurons in teleost fish. *Prog. Retin. Eye Res.* 40, 94–123. doi: 10.1016/j.preteyeres.2013.12.007

Livesey, F. J., and Cepko, C. L. (2001). Vertebrate neural cell-fate determination: lessons from the retina. *Nat. Rev. Neurosci.* 2, 109–118. doi: 10.1038/35053522

Lolley, R. N., Rong, H., and Craft, C. M. (1994). Linkage of photoreceptor degeneration by apoptosis with inherited defect in phototransduction. *Invest. Ophthalmol. Vis. Sci.* 35, 358–362.

Maw, M. A., Kennedy, B., Knight, A., Bridges, R., Roth, K. E., Mani, E. J., et al. (1997). Mutation of the gene encoding cellular retinaldehyde-binding protein in autosomal recessive retinitis pigmentosa. *Nat. Genet.* 17, 198–200. doi: 10.1038/ng1097-198

Miranda, G. E., Abrahan, C. E., Politi, L. E., and Rotstein, N. P. (2009). Sphingosine-1-phosphate is a key regulator of proliferation and differentiation in retina photoreceptors. *Invest. Ophthalmol. Vis. Sci.* 50, 4416–4428. doi: 10.1167/iovs.09-3388

Nelson, B. R., Ueki, Y., Reardon, S., Karl, M. O., Georgi, S., Hartman, B. H., et al. (2011). Genome-wide analysis of Müller glial differentiation reveals a requirement for Notch signaling in postmitotic cells to maintain the glial fate. *PLoS One* 6:e22817. doi: 10.1371/journal.pone.0022817

Ooto, S., Akagi, T., Kageyama, R., Akita, J., Mandai, M., Honda, Y., et al. (2004). Potential for neural regeneration after neurotoxic injury in the adult mammalian retina. *Proc. Natl. Acad. Sci. U.S.A.* 101, 13654–13659. doi: 10.1073/pnas.0402129101

Park, D., Xiang, A. P., Mao, F. F., Zhang, L., Di, C. G., Liu, X. M., et al. (2010). Nestin is required for the proper self-renewal of neural stem cells. *Stem Cells* 28, 2162–2171. doi: 10.1002/stem.541

Pittler, S. J., and Baehr, W. (1991). Identification of a nonsense mutation in the rod photoreceptor cGMP phosphodiesterase beta-subunit gene of the rd mouse. *Proc. Natl. Acad. Sci. U.S.A.* 88, 8322–8326. doi: 10.1073/pnas.88.19.8322

Politi, L., and Adler, R. (1988). Selective failure of long-term survival of isolated photoreceptors from both homozygous and heterozygous rd (retinal degeneration) mice. *Exp. Eye Res.* 47, 269–282. doi: 10.1016/0014-4835(88)90010-3

Politi, L. E., Bouzat, C., de los Santos, E. B., and Barrantes, F. J. (1996). Heterologous retinal cultured neurons and cell adhesion molecules induce clustering of acetylcholine receptors and polynucleation in mouse muscle BC3H-1 clonal cell line. *J. Neurosci. Res.* 43, 639–651. doi: 10.1002/(sici)1097-4547(19960315)43:6<639::aid-jnr1>3.0.co;2-f

Politi, L. E., Lehar, M., and Adler, R. (1988). Development of neonatal mouse retinal neurons and photoreceptors in low density cell culture. *Invest. Ophthalmol. Vis. Sci.* 29, 534–543.

Politi, L. E., Rotstein, N. P., and Carri, N. G. (2001). Effect of GDNF on neuroblast proliferation and photoreceptor survival: additive protection with docosahexaenoic acid. *Invest. Ophthalmol. Vis. Sci.* 42, 3008–3015.

Portera-Cailliau, C., Sung, C. H., Nathans, J., and Adler, R. (1994). Apoptotic photoreceptor cell death in mouse models of retinitis pigmentosa. *Proc. Natl. Acad. Sci. U.S.A.* 91, 974–978. doi: 10.1073/pnas.91.3.974

Ranski, A. H., Kramer, A. C., Morgan, G. W., Perez, J. L., and Thummel, R. (2018). Characterization of retinal regeneration in adult zebrafish following multiple rounds of phototoxic lesion. *PeerJ* 6:e5646. doi: 10.7717/peerj.5646

Roesch, K., Stadler, M. B., and Cepko, C. L. (2012). Gene expression changes within Müller glial cells in retinitis pigmentosa. *Mol. Vis.* 18, 1197–1214.

Rotstein, N. P., Aveldaño, M. I., Barrantes, F. J., and Politi, L. E. (1996). Docosahexaenoic acid is required for the survival of rat retinal photoreceptors in vitro. *J. Neurochem.* 66, 1851–1859. doi: 10.1046/j.1471-4159.1996.66051851.x

Rotstein, N. P., Aveldaño, M. I., Barrantes, F. J., Roccamo, A. M., and Politi, L. E. (1997). Apoptosis of retinal photoreceptors during development in vitro: protective effect of docosahexaenoic acid. *J. Neurochem.* 69, 504–513. doi: 10.1046/j.1471-4159.1997.69020504.x

Sahlgren, C. M., Pallari, H.-M., He, T., Chou, Y.-H., Goldman, R. D., and Eriksson, J. E. (2006). A nestin scaffold links Cdk5/p35 signaling to oxidant-induced cell death. *EMBO J.* 25, 4808–4819. doi: 10.1038/sj.emboj.7601366

Schindelin, J., Arganda-Carreras, I., Frise, E., Kaynig, V., Longair, M., Pietzsch, T., et al. (2012). Fiji: an open-source platform for biological-image analysis. *Nat. Methods* 9, 676–682. doi: 10.1038/nmeth.2019

Sherpa, T., Fimbel, S. M., Mallory, D. E., Maaswinkel, H., Spritzer, S. D., Sand, J. A., et al. (2008). Ganglion cell regeneration following whole-retina destruction in zebrafish. *Dev. Neurobiol.* 68, 166–181. doi: 10.1002/dneu.20568

Sherpa, T., Lankford, T., McGinn, T. E., Hunter, S. S., Frey, R. A., Sun, C., et al. (2014). Retinal regeneration is facilitated by the presence of surviving neurons. *Dev. Neurobiol.* 74, 851–876. doi: 10.1002/dneu.22167

Simón, M. V., De Genaro, P., Abrahan, C. E., de los Santos, B., Rotstein, N. P., and Politi, L. E. (2012). Müller glial cells induce stem cell properties in retinal progenitors in vitro and promote their further differentiation into photoreceptors. *J. Neurosci. Res.* 90, 407–421. doi: 10.1002/jnr.22747

Simón, M. V., Prado Spalm, F. H., Politi, L. E., and Rotstein, N. P. (2015). Sphingosine-1-phosphate is a crucial signal for migration of retina müller glial cells. *Investig. Ophthalmol. Vis. Sci.* 56, 5808–5815. doi: 10.1167/iovs.14-16195

Traub, P., Perides, G., Scherbarth, A., and Traub, U. (1985). Tenacious binding of lipids to vimentin during its isolation and purification from Ehrlich ascites tumor cells. *FEBS Lett.* 193, 217–221. doi: 10.1016/0014-5793(85)80155-1

Vecino, E., Rodriguez, F. D., Ruzafa, N., Pereiro, X., and Sharma, S. C. (2016). Glia–neuron interactions in the mammalian retina. *Prog. Retin. Eye Res.* 51, 1–40. doi: 10.1016/j.preteyeres.2015.06.003

Xia, X., and Ahmad, I. (2016). Unlocking the neurogenic potential of mammalian Müller Glia. *Int. J. stem cells* 9, 169–175. doi: 10.15283/ijsc16020

Young, R. W. (1984). Cell death during differentiation of the retina in the mouse. *J. Comp. Neurol.* 229, 362–373. doi: 10.1002/cne.902290307

Zhao, M., Andrieu-Soler, C., Kowalczuk, L., Paz Cortés, M., Berdugo, M., Dernigoghossian, M., et al. (2015). A new CRB1 rat mutation links Müller glial cells to retinal telangiectasia. *J. Neurosci.* 35, 6093–6106. doi: 10.1523/JNEUROSCI.3412-14.2015

Zhao, X.-F., Wan, J., Powell, C., Ramachandran, R., Myers, M. G., and Goldman, D. (2014). Leptin and IL-6 family cytokines synergize to stimulate Müller Glia reprogramming and retina regeneration. *Cell Rep.* 9, 272–284. doi: 10.1016/j.celrep.2014.08.047

Zhong, X., Gutierrez, C., Xue, T., Hampton, C., Vergara, M. N., Cao, L.-H., et al. (2014). Generation of three-dimensional retinal tissue with functional photoreceptors from human iPSCs. *Nat. Commun.* 5:4047. doi: 10.1038/ncomms5047

Zhu, X., and Craft, C. M. (2000). ). Modulation of CRX transactivation activity by phosducin isoforms. *Mol. Cell. Biol.* 20, 5216–5226. doi: 10.1128/mcb.20.14.5216-5226.2000

Zimmerman, L., Parr, B., Lendahl, U., Cunningham, M., McKay, R., Gavin, B., et al. (1994). Independent regulatory elements in the nestin gene direct transgene expression to neural stem cells or muscle precursors. *Neuron* 12, 11–24. doi: 10.1016/0896-6273(94)90148-1

4

# Lipids at the Crossroad of α-Synuclein Function and Dysfunction: Biological and Pathological Implications

*Natalia P. Alza[1,2], Pablo A. Iglesias González[1†], Melisa A. Conde[1,3†], Romina M. Uranga[1,3] and Gabriela A. Salvador[1,3]**

*[1] Instituto de Investigaciones Bioquímicas de Bahía Blanca, Consejo Nacional de Investigaciones Científicas y Técnicas, Universidad Nacional del Sur, Bahía Blanca, Argentina, [2] Departamento de Química, Universidad Nacional del Sur, Bahía Blanca, Argentina, [3] Departamento de Biología, Bioquímica y Farmacia, Universidad Nacional del Sur, Bahía Blanca, Argentina*

***Correspondence:**
*Gabriela A. Salvador*
*salvador@inibibb-conicet.gob.ar;*
*salvador@criba.edu.ar*

*† These authors have contributed equally to this work*

Since its discovery, the study of the biological role of α-synuclein and its pathological implications has been the subject of increasing interest. The propensity to adopt different conformational states governing its aggregation and fibrillation makes this small 14-kDa cytosolic protein one of the main etiologic factors associated with degenerative disorders known as synucleinopathies. The structure, function, and toxicity of α-synuclein and the possibility of different therapeutic approaches to target the protein have been extensively investigated and reviewed. One intriguing characteristic of α-synuclein is the different ways in which it interacts with lipids. Though in-depth studies have been carried out in this field, the information they have produced is puzzling and the precise role of lipids in α-synuclein biology and pathology and *vice versa* is still largely unknown. Here we provide an overview and discussion of the main findings relating to α-synuclein/lipid interaction and its involvement in the modulation of lipid metabolism and signaling.

**Keywords: α-synuclein, lipids, lipid metabolism, lipid signal transduction, membrane lipids**

## INTRODUCTION

α-Synuclein is a cytosolic protein of 140 amino acids which was discovered in 1988 together with β- and γ-synucleins by Maroteaux et al. (1988). The name α-synuclein derives from the fact that it was originally described as being located in presynaptic endings and also as being associated with nuclear envelopes. In the central nervous system, α-synuclein is abundantly expressed in neurons of different brain areas such as the neocortex, hippocampus, SN, thalamus, and cerebellum (Iwai et al., 1995; Asi et al., 2014). α-Synuclein is also present in the peripheral nervous system, muscle, liver, heart, lungs, kidney, hematopoietic cells of the bone marrow, and circulating blood cells

---

**Abbreviations:** AA, arachidonic acid; Chol, cholesterol; DHA, docosahexaenoic acid; FFA, free fatty acids; HMG-CoA, 3-hydroxy-3-methylglutaryl coenzyme A; LB, Lewy bodies; LD, lipid droplet; PA, phosphatidic acid; PC, phosphatidylcholine; PD, Parkinson's disease; PE, phosphatidylethanolamine; PI, phosphatidylinositol; PL, phospholipid; PLA2, phospholipases A2; PLC, phospholipase C; PLD, phospholipase D; PS, phosphatidylserine; PUFA, polyunsaturated fatty acids; SN, *substantia nigra pars compacta*; TAGs, triacylglycerols.

(Gardai et al., 2013; Burré et al., 2018; Mohamed Badawy et al., 2018). β-Synuclein is also located at presynaptic terminals in the central nervous system (Jakes et al., 1994; Wilhelm et al., 2014) while γ-synuclein is primarily expressed in the peripheral nervous system, and the ocular and adipose tissues (Buchman et al., 1998; Surguchov et al., 2001). It has been reported that γ-synuclein is overexpressed in different human tumors (Bruening et al., 2000; Guo et al., 2007; Hibi et al., 2009).

Though numerous studies have been carried out on the biology of α-synuclein, its physiological function remains a matter of debate. The search for a fuller understanding of this function is driven by the fact that it has been linked with several devastating diseases known as synucleinopathies, including neurodegenerative disorders such as: PD, Lewy body dementia, neurodegeneration with brain iron accumulation, Krabbe disease, dementia with LB, diffuse Lewy body disease, Lewy body variant of Alzheimer's disease, among others (Burré, 2015; Burré et al., 2018).

Parkinson's disease is the second most prevalent neurodegenerative age-associated disorder after Alzheimer's disease and is mainly characterized by movement impairments such as resting tremor, bradykinesia, and rigidity. The loss of dopaminergic neurons in the SN has been identified as the cause of the typical motor disablement (Dunnett and Björklund, 1999). Current therapies focus on the reestablishment of the neurotransmitter dopamine for controlling motor symptoms, but specific treatments are still not available owing mainly to a lack of knowledge of the molecular mechanisms that trigger neuronal degeneration and death (Oertel and Schulz, 2016). Since diagnosis occurs when the loss of dopaminergic neurons is massive, a better understanding of the molecular events involved in the neurodegenerative process would undoubtedly help in the discovery of specific treatments.

Parkinson's disease is a multifactorial neurodegenerative disorder whose etiopathogenesis is still largely unknown, though a common finding in patients' brain is the abnormal accumulation, and aggregation of α-synuclein. Intracellular aggregates of α-synuclein, named LB, constitute the histological hallmark of the PD brain. LB are also the main histopathological findings in the above-mentioned synucleinopathies. The role of α-synuclein as one of the leading causes of dopaminergic cell death was described after the identification of the first missense mutations (A30P, E46K, and A53T) in the SNCA gene (Polymeropoulos et al., 1997; Krüger et al., 1998; Zarranz et al., 2004). The involvement of α-synuclein mutants in familial inherited PD has been confirmed by genome-wide association studies (Chang et al., 2017). In addition, SNCA duplication and triplication causing elevated levels of the protein are associated with early-onset PD (Singleton et al., 2003; Chartier-Harlin et al., 2004). Although the α-synuclein protein does not display any mutations in sporadic PD and LB dementia, its involvement in neuronal damage is widely recognized. Of the several mechanisms that could be responsible for the association of α-synuclein with PD pathogenesis, there is an overall consensus that its aggregation leading to the formation of oligomers is a central event related to neuronal dysfunction (Ingelsson, 2016; Bengoa-Vergniory et al., 2017). These α-synuclein oligomeric forms are considered the most toxic species, disrupting cellular homeostasis and triggering neuronal death. Moreover, α-synuclein can exert a deleterious effect by spreading from cell to cell and thus contributing to progressive neurodegeneration (Desplats et al., 2009). Identification of the factors promoting the toxic conversion of mutated or wild-type forms of α-synuclein is a topic of intense interest. Deeper insight into the physiological function and pathological features of α-synuclein would not only contribute toward a better understanding of the pathogenesis but also help to develop biomarkers for early disease detection and progression and to design specific disease-modifying therapies for synucleinopathies.

The α-synuclein protein is composed of three well-described regions that confer the biological and functional characteristics that implicate it in PD pathology. The N-terminal domain comprises residues 1–60 and bestows lipid binding properties on the protein, in particular, the ability to interact with membranes and lipid micelles. This distinctive feature of α-synuclein is explained by the presence of amphipathic repeats of 11 amino acids, predominantly with the highly conserved KTKEGV motif, similar to that present in apolipoprotein domains (Bussell and Eliezer, 2003). This structural characteristic is shared with β- and γ-synucleins (Clayton and George, 1998). The missense mutations A53T, A30P, H50Q, G51D, A53E, and E46K reside in the N-terminal domain of α-synuclein (Polymeropoulos et al., 1997; Krüger et al., 1998; Zarranz et al., 2004; Flagmeier et al., 2016). The central hydrophobic region (residues 61–95) called NAC (non-amyloid β component) is essential for the conformational change of α-synuclein from random coil to β-sheets, leading to aggregation, and fibrillation (El-Agnaf et al., 1998; Rodriguez et al., 2015). Giasson et al. (2001) demonstrated through different assays that amino acids 71–82 represent the specific sequence of the NAC core which is necessarily involved in α-synuclein fibrillation. Biophysical studies using methods like nuclear magnetic resonance, electron paramagnetic resonance, circular dichroism and transmission electron microscopy,with recombinant proteins of α-synuclein and synthetic fragments of NAC were the first and are still used to demonstrate the importance of this region in the fibrillation pathway (El-Agnaf et al., 1998; Giasson et al., 2001; Der-Sarkissiant et al., 2003; Tashiro et al., 2008; Waxman et al., 2009; Shaltiel-Karyo et al., 2010). The elimination of the NAC region or its targeting with antibodies showed to inhibit aggregation and toxicity in cell culture (Lynch et al., 2008; Luk et al., 2009). *In vivo* models were also used to evaluate the pathological effects of this region. For instance, the deletion of amino acids 71–82 in *Drosophila* prevents α-synuclein aggregation and neurotoxicity, thus testifying to the importance of this region in the pathogenicity of the protein (Periquet et al., 2007). Differences in the amino acid sequence of the NAC region have been attributed to be responsible for the non-fibrillation feature of β-synuclein (Uversky and Fink, 2002). The third region of α-synuclein, enriched in glutamate, aspartate, and proline residues, is the acidic C-terminal domain (residues 96–140). It constitutes the main site of post-translational modifications, such as phosphorylation and nitration, although other modifications (ubiquitination, glycation, and methionine oxidation) also occur in the N-terminal domain (Chen et al., 2019). These modifications alter α-synuclein structure and provoke changes in hydrophobicity and protein-protein and protein-lipid interactions (Burré et al., 2018). Oxidation, nitration and phosphorylation are thought to contribute to different extents to α-synuclein aggregation and fibrillation (Barrett and Timothy Greenamyre, 2015). Phosphorylation is the most relevant post-translational modification related to synucleinopathies. Increased levels of the phosphorylated protein at serine 87 have been found in human brains from LB dementia patients (Paleologou et al., 2010) and at serine 129 in LB from PD patients (Fujiwara et al., 2002). Although this latter has been widely investigated, its role on the pathogenesis of PD has not been determined yet. Some authors propose that it is implicated in α-synuclein pathological aggregation (Fujiwara et al., 2002) whereas others suggest that it has a protective role on the aggregation and toxicity (Oueslati et al., 2010; Chen et al., 2019). The protein also suffers C-terminal truncation linked to an increase of α-synuclein aggregation *in vitro* (Murray et al., 2003); the loss of SN neurons in transgenic mice overexpressing this form has been reported (Wakamatsu et al., 2008). Both the N- and C-terminal domains have also been involved in the interaction with proteins and metal ions (Miotto et al., 2014; Carboni and Lingor, 2015; Billings et al., 2016).

From a conformational point of view, under physiological conditions α-synuclein is considered to be an intrinsically unstructured protein. The soluble α-synuclein in the cytosol is natively unfolded (Burré et al., 2013). Conformational flexibility is largely attributed to the α-synuclein structure because it can adopt a range of conformations depending on its interactions with membranes or proteins (Lashuel et al., 2013). When α-synuclein/PL interaction occurs, the N-terminal domain takes on an α-helical configuration that occurs physiologically in a dynamic equilibrium with the soluble state (Eliezer et al., 2001). An α-helical homo-tetramer of the protein has recently been identified in neurons and other cells (Bartels et al., 2011; Wang et al., 2011; Fanning et al., 2018), occurring in equilibrium with α-synuclein monomers. As the tetramer is resistant to pathological aggregation, the promotion of its formation could be protective against α-synuclein oligomerization (Bartels et al., 2011; Dettmer et al., 2013, 2015a,b, 2017). Moreover, under pathological conditions, the induction of α-synuclein aggregation results in the formation of an initial population of oligomers enriched in insoluble cross-β-sheets (Conway et al., 2000; Pineda and Burré, 2017). These species may act as nuclei for the next steps of elongation and assembly into fibrils, which are finally deposited in LB (Wood et al., 1999; Lashuel et al., 2013). Another proposed mechanism for the formation of fibrillar aggregates is the lateral association of the oligomeric granules without nuclei formation (Bhak et al., 2009; Makwana and Sundd, 2016). Oxidative stress, post-translational modifications, accumulation of α-synuclein and changes in the levels of metal ions, PL, and fatty acids have been proposed as modulators of the aggregation process (Ruipérez et al., 2010; Lashuel et al., 2013; Galvagnion, 2017).

This review focuses on the intriguing characteristic of α-synuclein to pleiotropically interact with and modulate a variety of lipids and on how these interactions participate in the protein's biological and pathological functions.

## FUNCTIONS OF α-SYNUCLEIN

The physiological cellular functions of α-synuclein are still a matter of intense debate, despite continuous efforts over the last 30 years to clarify the issue. Since it is highly concentrated in presynaptic terminals, where it is associated with synaptic vesicles (Maroteaux et al., 1988), the involvement of α-synuclein in neurotransmission, and synaptic plasticity has been extensively investigated (Burré, 2015; Zaltieri et al., 2015). Although there is disagreement as to whether it promotes or inhibits neurotransmitter release, it is well-established that α-synuclein mediates this process by regulating the availability of synaptic vesicles in different pools, facilitating their clustering, recycling, and docking to the cell membrane (Chandra et al., 2005; Burré et al., 2010; Zaltieri et al., 2015; Miraglia et al., 2018). The involvement of α-synuclein in synaptic vesicle endocytosis has been demonstrated (Vargas et al., 2014). In addition, α-synuclein can act as a chaperone molecule thus contributing to the assembly of the SNARE complex (Bonini and Giasson, 2005; Diao et al., 2013; Burré et al., 2014). The modulation of dopamine levels by α-synuclein has been demonstrated as a consequence of the inhibition of the neurotransmitter synthesis through the regulation of tyrosine hydroxylase activity (Abeliovich et al., 2000; Peng, 2005) and the inhibition of the vesicular monoamine transporter-2 (Guo et al., 2008). It also has a regulatory effect on the targeting and activity of the dopamine transporter DAT (Swant et al., 2011; Oaks et al., 2013; Butler et al., 2015).

α-Synuclein also has roles which are unrelated to synaptic functions. Surguchev and Surguchov have reviewed recent findings focused on its implication in the regulation of gene expression (Surguchev and Surguchov, 2017). A plethora of other biological functions have been attributed to α-synuclein such as regulation of apoptosis, modulation of glucose and calmodulin levels, and neuronal differentiation (Emamzadeh, 2016). Even though these latter functions have not been explored in depth, they provide evidence for proposing α-synuclein as a pleiotropic molecule.

β- and γ-synucleins have not been linked to the pathogenesis of PD. However, several reports have shown that β-synuclein has an inhibitory effect on the aggregation of α-synuclein (Brown et al., 2016) suggesting a neuroprotective role against synucleinopathies. Otherwise, it has been proposed that γ-synuclein is involved in cancer progression and metastasis (Hibi et al., 2009; Hua et al., 2009; Dunn et al., 2015).

## α-SYNUCLEIN AND MEMBRANE LIPIDS

Although the native α-synuclein three-dimensional conformation is still under discussion, differential folding states for physiological and pathological conditions have been assigned.

One of the cutting-edge questions is the role of membrane lipids in α-synuclein conformation since protein-membrane binding has been associated with both normal and pathological functions. It has been reported that the α-synuclein/membrane interaction induces different α-helix states that could participate in protein function or drive aggregation (Bodner et al., 2010; Dikiy and Eliezer, 2012; Fares et al., 2014; Ysselstein et al., 2015; Burré et al., 2018; O'Leary et al., 2018). At the same time, the targeting of α-synuclein in its different conformations at the membrane surface can alter lipid composition, thus promoting pathological effects (van Rooijen et al., 2009; Reynolds et al., 2011; Tosatto et al., 2012; Hellstrand et al., 2013). A significant body of experimental evidence reinforces the hypothesis that oligomers, the initial state of protein aggregation, are the most neurotoxic species because of their ability, after interaction, to disrupt biological membranes (Danzer et al., 2007; Winner et al., 2011; Fusco et al., 2017; Galvagnion, 2017).

The nature of the interactions between α-synuclein and PLs has been extensively reviewed in several papers that mainly address this topic through biophysical studies (Dikiy and Eliezer, 2012; Pineda and Burré, 2017; Burré et al., 2018; O'Leary and Lee, 2018). Here we will discuss the most biologically relevant findings. One of the points included in this section is how specific PLs participate in the induction of conformational changes of α-synuclein and how this affects its biological and/or pathological functions.

After adipose tissue, the brain is the organ with the highest lipid content. PL content in the brain is approximately 6% of dry weight and is represented by two main classes of molecules: glycerophospholipids and sphingolipids (Lahiri and Futerman, 2007). A glycerophospholipid molecule consists of two fatty acids, one saturated and one unsaturated, esterified in sn-1 and sn-2 of the glycerol backbone, respectively. The brain is particularly enriched in two PUFA: arachidonic acid (AA, 20:4-ω-6) and docosahexaenoic acid (DHA, 22:6-ω-3) (Chen et al., 2008). PLs are the main constituents of cellular membranes and because of their amphipathic nature, they provide the necessary biophysical environment for ensuring the proper functioning of structural proteins, receptors, enzymes, and ion channels located at the cell surface or in intracellular membranes.

The plasma and organelle membranes are asymmetric; this characteristic determines specific and differential lipid composition in the inner and the outer leaflets. PC, PE, sphingomyelin, and Chol are the most abundant lipids in the outer hemimembranes. PS and PI are acidic PLs and are predominantly located in the inner hemimembranes. This particular lipid composition is determinant for the formation of lipid rafts, specific membrane liquid-ordered microdomains that govern protein recruitment (van Meer et al., 2008; Marquardt et al., 2015).

In native conditions, α-synuclein can be mainly found in two states: a soluble unfolded monomeric form or a membrane-associated multimeric form. The pathological state of the protein is composed of predominantly β-sheet oligomers and amyloid fibrils (Burré, 2015). PLs have been reported to participate in and modulate the different states of α-synuclein. Originally, α-synuclein was described as a monomer in equilibrium between the cytosol and the membrane fraction (i.e., plasma membrane or vesicles). The occurrence of these two physiological states has generated some controversy, but consensus has now been reached that α-synuclein mainly occurs as an intrinsically disordered monomer (Burré et al., 2013). Very recently, a helically folded tetramer of the soluble protein has been described in equilibrium with the monomer (Bartels et al., 2011; Wang et al., 2011; Fanning et al., 2018). Soluble α-synuclein exists as a random coil three dimensional structure that increases α-helical conformation after interacting with membrane PLs, suggesting that protein/PL interaction triggers structural changes that could modulate biological function (Davidson et al., 1998; Zhu et al., 2003). Furthermore, biophysical studies using tryptophan- and spin-labeled determinations demonstrated that the portion of the protein that interacts with the membrane adopts an α-helix conformation which is entirely buried within the depth of the membrane whereas the rest of the segments present lower membrane penetration and higher flexibility (Bussell, 2005; Wietek et al., 2013).

The preferred PLs for α-synuclein membrane binding are those with an acidic head group such as PS and PI (Shvadchak et al., 2011). The charged nature of these PLs makes lysine residues candidates for α-synuclein binding sites (Jo et al., 2000; Perrin et al., 2000). The interaction between the N-terminal of α-synuclein and PS seems to be critical for C-terminal SNARE-dependent vesicle docking (Lou et al., 2017). Since SNARE-dependent vesicle docking is necessary for calcium-mediated neurotransmitter release, it is reasonable to assume that α-synuclein/PS interaction is critical to the neurotransmission process at the synapse. Indeed, as previously mentioned, one of the best characterized biological functions of α-synuclein is its participation in vesicle recycling (Scott and Roy, 2012; Wang et al., 2014). Experiments performed in giant unilamellar vesicles composed of different proportions of dioleoyl-PC and several anionic PLs demonstrated that wild-type α-synuclein binding is dependent on the presence of negatively charged head groups. Binding to anionic PLs is also dependent of the liquid-ordered state of the vesicles, thus indicating that protein/membrane interactions are governed not only by electrostatic forces but also by lipid packaging and hydrophobic forces (O'Leary and Lee, 2018). The interaction of β- and γ-synucleins with membranes depends on the presence of PL acidic head group and is also determined by the curvature of the binding surface (Ducas and Rhoades, 2012).

A fact that argues in favor of the role of α-synuclein/lipid interaction in the etiopathogenesis of synucleinopathies is that all missense mutations responsible for familial PD are localized in the 11-residue repeat domain that has membrane-binding properties; indeed, these mutations alter the lipid binding properties (Jo et al., 2002; Fares et al., 2014; Ghosh et al., 2014; Robotta et al., 2017). A30P and E46K mutants display altered binding to anionic PLs, thus suggesting that membrane interaction could be disrupted in the familial forms of PD (Stöckl et al., 2008).

Binding to PS has been shown to induce an increase in α-synuclein oligomerization, thus providing evidence of the role of protein/PL interaction in the modulation of the pathological aggregation of the protein (Hu et al., 2016). After interacting with PLs, the impairing effects of α-synuclein on biological membranes could be explained by the increase in membrane tension and lipid extraction that promote pore formation and membrane lysis (Jo et al., 2000; Zhu et al., 2003; Tosatto et al., 2012; Braun and Sachs, 2015; Pan et al., 2018). In line with this, it has been proposed that the interaction between acidic PLs and α-synuclein plays a role during nuclear extrusion in erythroblast differentiation (Araki et al., 2018).

Phosphatidic acid (PA), another anionic PL, differs from PS, and PI mainly in terms of the small size of its head group; this particular characteristic allows its localization very close to the hydrophobic core of the lipid bilayer. PA is also an α-synuclein partner for membrane targeting (Perrin et al., 2000). Specifically, PA esterified with saturated/monounsaturated fatty acids is the preferred molecular species for α-synuclein binding and also induces an enhancement in protein aggregation through the induction of changes in the secondary structure (Mizuno et al., 2017). It has been reported that α-synuclein overexpression is also able to modulate enzyme pathways that produce PA (Dikiy and Eliezer, 2012) (see the section "α-Synuclein and Lipid Signaling").

α-Synuclein has also been shown to be associated with mitochondrial membranes (Ghio et al., 2016). Binding of α-synuclein to mitochondrial membranes has been detected in SN dopaminergic neurons from mice and human brain (Li et al., 2007; Devi et al., 2008). The nature of protein association with mitochondria was determined by using liquid-disordered membranes enriched in cardiolipin, an essential PL very abundant in the inner mitochondrial membrane and also essential for organelle function. Cardiolipin-mediated binding of α-synuclein could represent a mechanism by which the cytosolic protein is targeted to mitochondria (Ghio et al., 2016). Once attached to the membrane surface, the protein is also able to extract lipids, which could explain the loss of mitochondrial integrity during dopaminergic neuronal degeneration (Pozo Devoto and Falzone, 2017).

The structural changes that α-synuclein undergoes after interacting with PLs in membranes and how these changes contribute to amyloidogenesis is nevertheless still under debate. There is agreement that acidic PLs are the preferred lipids for membrane targeting and that the protein/lipid ratio could be determinant for both biological function and amyloidogenic propensity. Very recently, it has been shown that the conformational state of α-synuclein depends on the protein/lipid ratio. A high α-synuclein/lipid ratio would promote protein/protein interaction and in consequence increase the propensity to form oligomers enriched in β-sheet conformation which in turn could also fibrillate and induce amyloid aggregation (Powers et al., 2017; Terakawa et al., 2018). A low α-synuclein/lipid ratio, on the other hand, would establish a condition of protein dilution, thus blocking amyloid fibrillation, and indeed maintaining physiological interactions with the membrane (Terakawa et al., 2018). Previously mentioned evidence describes the interaction of α-synuclein with membranes in the absence of post-translational modifications; however, it has been shown that post-translational modifications such as phosphorylated or acetylated forms of the protein would interact in a different way (Burré et al., 2018). One of the physiologically relevant post-translational modifications of α-synuclein is its acetylation in the N-terminal, which enhances binding to PC, a zwitterionic PL presented in micelles and small unilamellar vesicles with high curvature (r~16–20 nm). Chol, another important membrane constituent, has been shown to reduce N-acetylated α-synuclein-PC binding. These *in vitro* results reported by O'Leary and coworkers suggest that N-acetylation promotes the binding of α-synuclein to highly curved membranes and that Chol interferes with this interaction (O'Leary et al., 2018). Moreover, N-acetylated α-synuclein has been shown to diminish the aggregation propensity triggered by ganglioside GM1 binding (Bartels et al., 2014). Phosphorylated α-synuclein in serine 129 has been studied in depth in the last decade, with disparate data being reported in relation to membrane interaction. However, the most accepted theory to emerge from *in vitro* and *in vivo* experiments is that the phosphorylated form has an inhibitory effect on α-synuclein association with the membrane (Fiske et al., 2011; Kuwahara et al., 2012; Nübling et al., 2014; Oueslati, 2016).

Phospholipids also participate in the spreading of α-synuclein, mainly attributed to exosomes, and are thus involved in synucleinopathy propagation. Mass spectrometry studies show the presence of PC, PE, PI, PS, and the gangliosides GM2 and GM3 in exosomes isolated from neuroblastoma cells (Marie et al., 2015). Moreover, experiments carried out on small unilamellar vesicles to ascertain the role of gangliosides in α-synuclein conformation demonstrated that GM1 and GM3, as well as exosomes, are able to accelerate the aggregation of the protein (Marie et al., 2015).

Despite the mounting evidence mentioned above, the question of how PL interaction intervenes in α-synuclein physiological and pathological function remains unanswered (**Figure 1**). In order to shed further light on the specific role of lipid interactions in α-synuclein biology and pathology and how these interactions occur *in vivo*, it is necessary to carry out additional experiments using models that mimic living cell lipid composition, membrane asymmetry, and the intracellular environment.

## α-SYNUCLEIN AND LIPID DROPLETS

Neutral lipids are part of a large, heterogeneous family of compounds with the distinctive characteristic of being hydrophobic molecules. Another of their particular features is the lack of charged groups. The two main classes of neutral lipids in mammals are TAGs and Chol esters, both of which reside in the cytosol, contained in a simple membrane-surrounded organelle, the LD (Welte, 2015). LD membranes contain PLs, unesterified Chol, and specific anchored proteins with signaling and lipolytic functions (Gao et al., 2017; Sztalryd and Brasaemle, 2017); as highly dynamic storage organelles, they provide a rapidly mobilizable TAG pool to act as an energy source or as a fatty acid donor for lipid remodeling processes.

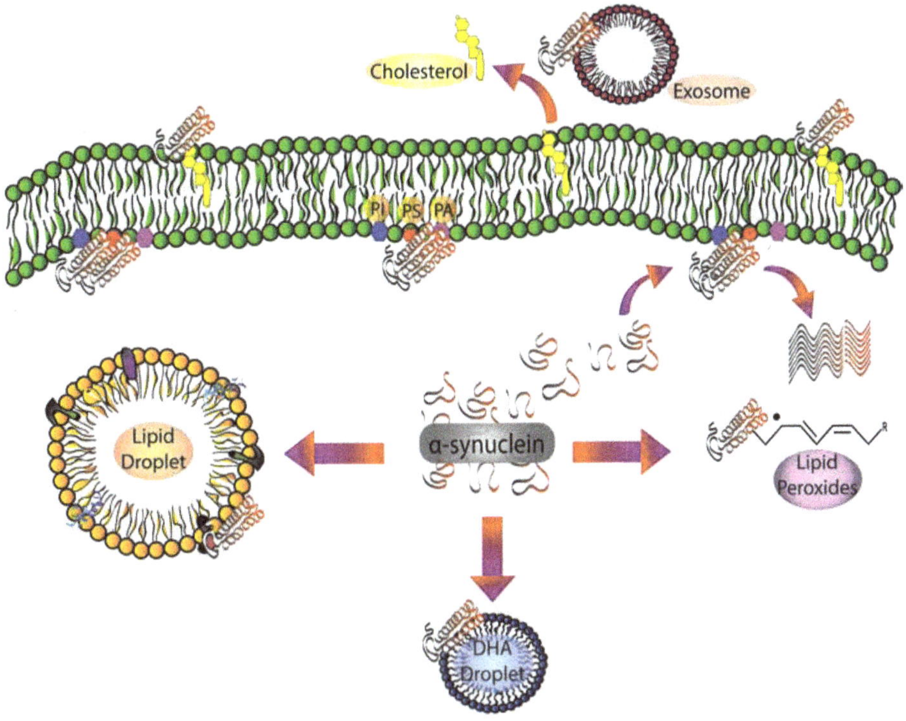


**FIGURE 1 |** α-Synuclein/lipid interactions: from the plasma membrane to intracellular compartments and extracellular vesicles. Soluble α-synuclein exists as a random coil three-dimensional structure. Membrane targeting with acidic PLs (PS and PI) triggers α-helical folding at the N-terminal domain. Protein pathological conformation is predominantly represented by β-sheet oligomers and amyloid fibrils. α-Synuclein pathological aggregation is dependent on the protein/lipid ratio. Spreading of α-synuclein, largely attributed to exosomes, is also regulated by its interaction with the PLs of the extracellular vesicles. Free fatty acids, mainly DHA, are able to induce α-synuclein oligomerization. After the interaction with lipid peroxidation products, α-synuclein is prone to the formation of toxic stable oligomers. α-Synuclein also regulates Chol efflux via ABCA1 transporter. DHA, docosahexaenoic acid; PA: phosphatidic acid; PI, phosphatidylinositol; PS, phosphatidylserine.

Though LDs are present in almost all cell types, their major occurrence is in adipocytes and hepatocytes. They also serve as cellular stress indicators and are associated with pathological states including starvation, infection, cancer, and liver steatosis (Gluchowski et al., 2017; Tirinato et al., 2017). Scarce information on the precise function of LDs on the nervous system is available in the literature. However, recent works correlate the appearance of LDs with pathological situations in neurodegenerative disorders. Glial cells were reported to be LD-positive cells that accumulate neutral lipids in response to the injury of neighbor neurons in several neurodegenerative conditions (Liu et al., 2015; Cabirol-Pol et al., 2018). LDs were detected in Aplysia axons and neuronal primary cultures and neurons of Huntington's disease models (Savage et al., 1987; Martinez-Vicente et al., 2010; Welte, 2015). In addition, iron accumulation, an event intensively described in several neurodegenerative processes and also in PD, has been shown to increase LD formation in dopaminergic neurons (Salvador, 2010; Schneider and Bhatia, 2012; Sánchez Campos et al., 2015).

A large body of evidence points to α-synuclein/LD interaction. Experiments performed *in vitro* demonstrate that α-synuclein binds to artificial 60 nm diameter LDs (Thiam et al., 2013). Moreover, it has been shown that in HeLa cells incubated with a high concentration of fatty acid, wild-type α-synuclein translocates from the cytosol to the surface of LDs (Colebc et al., 2002). α-Synuclein mutants display a different behavior: whereas A53T strongly associates with LDs, A30P remains cytosolic. These findings were corroborated by the heterologous expression of human α-synuclein in *Saccharomyces cerevisiae* (Sere et al., 2010). The biological significance of the α-synuclein-induced increase in LDs observed in yeasts was addressed in a mutant strain unable to synthesize neutral lipids and more tolerant to α-synuclein overexpression (Sere et al., 2010). In line with these findings, we recently reported that A53T α-synuclein overexpression in dopaminergic neurons induces an increase in TAG production and LD accumulation (Sánchez Campos et al., 2018). Fe exposure in A53T α-synuclein-overexpressing neurons increases protein aggregation, thus also augmenting TAG and LD content (Sánchez Campos et al., 2018). The nature of the α-synuclein/LD interaction has been shown to depend on PL packing at the LD membrane, being not fully packed monolayers the preferred surface for protein binding (Thiam et al., 2013). LD surface has been described as a higher hydrophobic environment than the PL bilayer (Thiam et al., 2013; Kory et al., 2016). The need for this highly hydrophobic organelle has been reported in other biological processes such as protein viral assembly (Ogawa et al., 2009; Welte and Gould, 2017).

The relevance of the biological interaction between α-synuclein/LD has not been explored *in vivo*, but it can be proposed that LDs are early markers of neurodegenerative processes and the characteristic of these vesicles make them good candidates for the modulation of α-synuclein conformational changes and pathological aggregation. Further research is required for a deeper understanding of these phenomena and their implications in synucleinopathies (**Figure 1**).

## α-SYNUCLEIN AND FATTY ACIDS

Another interesting discussion is the role of FFA in α-synuclein biology. Brain membranes exclusively contain a high concentration of PUFA, DHA, and AA being the most abundant. DHA is an essential fatty acid that needs to be incorporated from the diet, and disturbances in its metabolism have been reported to be associated with both neurodevelopment and neurodegenerative disorders (Chen et al., 2008). Some years ago, several *in vitro* observations proposed that α-synuclein could act as a fatty acid binding protein in the brain (Sharon et al., 2001). Soon afterward, PUFA were shown to promote the assembly of α-synuclein soluble oligomers (Sharon et al., 2003a; Karube et al., 2008). Both DHA and to a lesser extent AA are able to induce α-synuclein oligomerization as demonstrated by transmission electron microscopy, electrophoresis of native gels, and fluorescence assays with thioflavin T (Broersen et al., 2006). Relative concentrations of α-synuclein and DHA appear to govern the free and bound states of the protein and also its conformational changes, by increasing its α-helix structure (Sharon et al., 2001; Fecchio et al., 2018). Moreover, prolonged exposure to PUFA triggers the formation of α-synuclein fibrils. The establishment of oligomeric or fibrillar conformations in the presence of DHA depends on the protein/FFA ratio. Whereas fibril formation is favored by a 1:10 molar ratio, oligomeric species characterized by lack of seeding properties for fibrillation are stabilized by a 1:50 ratio (De Franceschi et al., 2011). The general consensus among the broad range of studies on the effect of fatty acids on α-synuclein biology is that PUFA elicit the formation of diverse oligomeric forms with differential structural and biological properties (Perrin et al., 2001; Fecchio et al., 2013). Oligomeric species generated *in vitro* by DHA exposure showed a partial α-helical structure, with the capacity to alter the membrane permeability and thus to trigger cytotoxicity (Fecchio et al., 2013). β- and γ-synucleins are also able to interact with PUFA trough their lipid binding domain (Perrin et al., 2001).

A rise in free DHA levels in cytosolic fractions has already been found in brains of patients with PD and LB dementia, and this could be responsible for the oligomerization of α-synuclein and the underlying neuronal damage (Sharon et al., 2003b). Biophysical studies combined with transmission electron microscopy demonstrated that DHA in solution is able to form oil droplets. These oil droplets can be remodeled by α-synuclein, reducing their size and fatty acid concentration (Broersen et al., 2006; De Franceschi et al., 2009; **Figure 1**). In addition, the interaction with DHA droplets promotes differential susceptibility of proteolytic degradation (De Franceschi et al., 2009).

α-Synuclein has been shown not only to form covalent bonds with DHA but also to act as a scavenger of the oxidation products of DHA, mainly through its histidine residue in position 50 (De Franceschi et al., 2017). Moreover, it has been observed that lysine residues, acting as nucleophiles, are able to interact with electrophilic products of lipid peroxidation and that this protective effect is weakened after lysine acetylation. Additionally, α-synuclein binding to liposomes containing PC and PA enriched with PUFA has been reported to have a protective effect against nitration and oxidation (Trostchansky et al., 2006). The interaction of α-synuclein with 4-hydroxy-2-nonenal, one of the main products of PUFA peroxidation, is able to promote the formation of toxic stable oligomers, and also prevent the passage toward the final state of fibrils (Qin et al., 2007; Puspita et al., 2017; Shamoto-Nagai et al., 2018). Furthermore, dopaminergic cells incubated with free PUFA showed decreased viability associated with the presence of oligomeric α-synuclein (Assayag et al., 2007).

The reported findings highlight the connection between oligomeric α-synuclein and fatty acid oxidation in dopaminergic toxicity, suggesting the existence of a positive loop of increased damage when α-synuclein is allowed to interact with PUFA and their oxidation products. One of the most accepted theories for the onset of neurodegenerative diseases associated with aging postulates the increase in oxidative stress as one of the main gating factors. Since the well-described decrease in antioxidant defenses associated with the aging process increases oxidative stress, it is arguable that lipid peroxides could be available for the interaction with α-synuclein thus triggering the generation of toxic oligomeric forms. Moreover, the extensively documented decrease in brain PUFA content during aging could also be responsible for an increase in saturated PLs at the membranes that in turn could decrease the association with α-synuclein and augment the cytosolic levels of the protein available for binding with lipid peroxides (López et al., 1995; Giusto et al., 2002; Mateos et al., 2010; Ledesma et al., 2012). Studies on oligodendroglial cells overexpressing the A53T mutant have shown that oxidative stress exposure after supplementation with DHA is able to promote the genesis of inclusion bodies whose composition includes phosphorylated α-synuclein (serine 129) and ubiquitinated and SUMOylated proteins, all reported to be aggregation inducers (Riedel et al., 2011).

A number of PD animal models have been used to corroborate some of the above-discussed *in vitro* results. The use of transgenic mice overexpressing different α-synuclein forms and subjected to high-DHA diet has served to support some of the earlier findings. Yakunin et al. (2012) showed increased accumulation of soluble and insoluble α-synuclein forms accompanied by astrocytosis and neuritic defects in an A53T transgenic mouse model fed a DHA-enriched diet. Experiments *in vivo* with transgenic mice expressing the A53T α-synuclein mutant demonstrated that a diet with high DHA content reduces lipoxidative damage (Muntané et al., 2010). A very recent report demonstrated that a diet supplemented with n-3 PUFA promotes the accumulation of a 42-kDa oligomeric form of the protein (Yakunin et al., 2012; Coulombe et al., 2018). Analysis of *post-mortem* human brains corroborates some of the previous *in vitro* and *in vivo* experimental findings. Protein profile of synucleinopathy patients was enriched with both soluble and insoluble oligomers and a positive correlation between the accumulation of α-synuclein oligomers and cytosolic DHA content was reported (Sharon et al., 2003a,b).

All these findings postulate DHA in soluble and esterified forms as an important candidate for modulating both the targeting and the biological function of α-synuclein. Thus, the regulation of DHA availability under pathological conditions could be an important event for regulating α-synuclein oligomerization and aggregation processes. In this sense, lipid pathways involved in DHA acylation, and deacylation could constitute a promising strategy for new therapeutic approaches in synucleinopathies (see section "α-Synuclein and Lipid Signaling") (**Figures 1, 3**).

## α-SYNUCLEIN AND LIPID METABOLISM

The clear involvement of a crosstalk between α-synuclein and lipid metabolism was investigated by Murphy's group using protein knock-out mice (Castagnet et al., 2005; Golovko et al., 2006, 2007, 2009; Barceló-Coblijn et al., 2007; Golovko and Murphy, 2008). SNCA (−/−) mice oppositely metabolize the two main brain PUFA, AA, and DHA. The lower intake of AA reported both in neurons and astrocytes from SNCA (−/−) mice was reverted by exogenous wild-type α-synuclein through the modulation of acyl-CoA synthetase activity (Golovko et al., 2006). However, DHA turnover and acylation in PE, PI, and PS was found to be increased in SNCA (−/−) mice when compared with SNCA (+/+) mice (Golovko et al., 2007). This differential effect in AA and DHA metabolism as a consequence of the silencing of α-synuclein argues in favor of compensatory mechanisms associated with PUFA content in brain membranes (**Figure 2**).

Several experimental evidences have demonstrated that both the absence and the overexpression of α-synuclein are able to disturb lipid homeostasis by increasing neutral lipid storage. In astrocytes and whole brain, the absence of α-synuclein switches the distribution of fatty acids to neutral lipid reserves and also increases neutral lipid mass (Castagnet et al., 2005; Barceló-Coblijn et al., 2007). Surprisingly, α-synuclein overexpression gives rise to abnormal lipid metabolism in yeasts, characterized by an increase in LD content (Outeiro and Lindquist, 2003; Su et al., 2010). In line with this, overexpression of wild-type and mutant forms of α-synuclein triggers the accumulation of LDs in HeLa cells, and in human-induced pluripotent stem cell (Colebc et al., 2002; Fanning et al., 2018). Regarding these findings, it can be suggested that physiological levels of α-synuclein are necessary for lipid homeostasis. γ-Synuclein, another member of the synuclein family, has also been implicated in the maintenance of LD formation and in the modulation of lipid composition in adipocytes and the nervous system in mice (Guschina et al., 2011; Voshol et al., 2012).

In harmony with these results, a recent study in our laboratory showed that the overexpression of A53T α-synuclein induces an increase in TAG content and the accumulation of LDs in N27 dopaminergic neurons (Sánchez Campos et al., 2018). The rise in neuronal TAG content was associated with increased fatty acid synthase expression and Acyl-CoA synthetase activity, with no variations in TAG lipase activity or in fatty acid β-oxidation, thus demonstrating that the overexpression of A53T α-synuclein triggers a lipid metabolic switch in dopaminergic neurons. Pharmacological blockage of TAG *de novo* synthesis renders the neurons more susceptible to iron-induced oxidative stress (Sánchez Campos et al., 2018).

α-Synuclein biology and Chol metabolism have been shown to interact in many different ways. Such intersections regulate

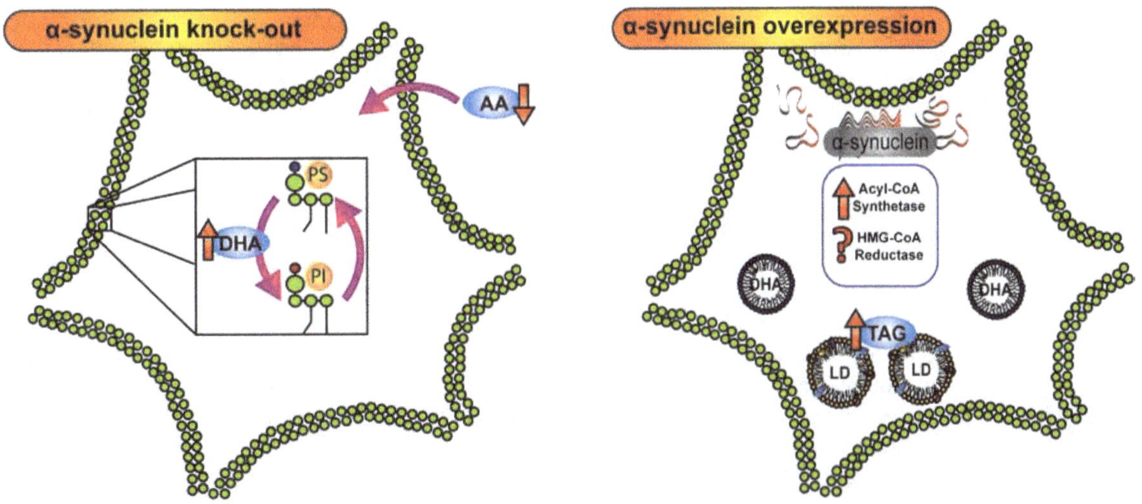


**FIGURE 2** | Crosstalk between α-synuclein and lipid metabolism. Knock-down and overexpression of α-synuclein have demonstrated the involvement of the protein in lipid metabolism. In α-synuclein knock-out mice, AA and DHA, the main polyunsaturated fatty acids in the brain, are oppositely metabolized: whereas AA intake is diminished, DHA turnover and acylation in PI and PS are increased. α-Synuclein overexpression triggers an increase in TAG content and LD accumulation by stimulation of acyl-CoA synthetase activity and probably the modulation of HMG-CoA reductase. AA, arachidonic acid; DHA, docosahexaenoic acid; HMG-CoA, 3-Hydroxy-3-methyl glutaryl coenzyme A; LD, lipid droplet; PI, phosphatidylinositol; PS, phosphatidylserine; TAG, triacylglycerol.

one another in a complex and not yet fully understood manner (Yeger-Lotem et al., 2009; Galvagnion, 2017). Controversial information coexists regarding plasma Chol level since it has been considered as either positive or negative risk factor for PD, or even not being linked at all to PD (Galvagnion, 2017). More concrete evidence links oxidized Chol derivatives with the onset and progression of PD (Bosco et al., 2006; Marwarha and Ghribi, 2015). In this regard, 27-hydroxycholesterol, a product of Chol oxidation, has been found to be increased in the brain, cortex and plasma, of PD patients (Lee et al., 2009; Seet et al., 2010; Cheng et al., 2011). Moreover, exogenous 27-hydroxycholesterol is able to induce the expression and accumulation of α-synuclein in human dopaminergic neurons through a transcriptional mechanism mediated by the transcription factor LXRβ (Marwarha et al., 2011). A possible mechanism that supports these findings could be the regulation of Chol efflux from neuronal cultures via ABCA1 transporter associated with the increased levels of oxidative stress reported in PD (Hsiao et al., 2017).

Regarding Chol biosynthesis, *in silico* analysis from the Yeger-Lotem laboratory identified the ergosterol-mevalonate pathway as a candidate for the cellular response to α-synuclein toxicity. One of the identified genes is Hrd1, a ubiquitin protein ligase related with the regulation of HMG-CoA reductase, the rate-limiting enzyme for the *de novo* Chol synthesis (Yeger-Lotem et al., 2009). They also found that pharmacological inhibition of HMG-CoA reductase by statins makes yeasts more vulnerable to α-synuclein toxicity (Yeger-Lotem et al., 2009).

Our results in dopaminergic neurons and those obtained in yeasts suggest a protective role of neutral lipids (TAG and Chol) during α-synuclein overexpression either against proteotoxicity or against oxidative stress (Yeger-Lotem et al., 2009; Auluck et al., 2010; Sánchez Campos et al., 2018). However, contrasting effects have been reported in primary human neurons treated with statins (Bar-On et al., 2008; Roy and Pahan, 2011). In view of the above, additional studies are needed to understand the biological significance of these controversial experimental evidences. Concerning this matter, the clinical relevance of statins is still under debate and is currently being addressed in a trial with PD patients treated with simvastatin which ends in 2020 (Carroll and Wyse, 2017).

The accumulated data allows us to propose a biological function for α-synuclein as a lipid metabolism modulator. Both at physiological levels and when overexpressed, α-synuclein is able to trigger a metabolic switch involving several aspects of lipid biology (**Figure 2**). The main biological response to α-synuclein overexpression is an increase in neutral lipid content that could be related to a neuroprotective strategy, whereas under physiological conditions the modulation of AA levels by the protein appears to be associated with prostaglandin generation and thus with a role in the inflammatory cascade (Golovko et al., 2007).

The open question is how α-synuclein triggers the above-mentioned metabolic changes. One possibility is that the switch in neutral lipid metabolism in terms of LD accumulation could be a consequence of endoplasmic reticulum stress and autophagy impairment, triggered by proteotoxicity due to the overexpression of α-synuclein (Velázquez et al., 2016; Garcia et al., 2018; Pitcairn et al., 2018). The other possibility is that α-synuclein could be involved in the regulation of gene expression associated with lipid metabolism. This latter possibility relates to the high DNA affinity of amyloidogenic proteins, the nuclear localization of α-synuclein, and its participation in epigenetic modifications through histone acetylation (Ma et al., 2014; Surguchev and Surguchov, 2017). Specifically, it has been described that α-synuclein modulates gene expression related with cell survival by decreasing H3 acetylation (Pavlou et al., 2017) and with ubiquitination (Martins et al., 2011). Additional studies will be required to ascertain which of the above-mentioned mechanisms are biologically and pathologically involved and their link with lipid metabolism.

## α-SYNUCLEIN AND LIPID SIGNALING

Apart from their structural and biophysical role in biological membranes, lipids also serve as reservoirs of intracellular and extracellular messengers. One of the most investigated events in lipid signaling is the action of phospholipases and PL kinases and phosphatases that produce different lipid and non-lipid messengers from membrane PLs.

Phospholipases catalyze the hydrolysis of acyl and phosphate esters and are named according to their hydrolyzed position on the PL molecule. Among them, PLA2 and phospholipases C and D (PLC and PLD) are widely studied and many of them have been implicated in neurodegenerative processes.

Phospholipases A2 catalyzes the hydrolysis of the fatty acid esterified in the sn-2 of the glycerol backbone of PL moieties and releases FFA and a lysophospholipid. There are currently six different known types of PLA2: secreted (groups I, II, III, V, IX, X, XI, XII, XIII, and XIV), cytosolic (cPLA2, group IV), calcium-independent (iPLA2, group VI), lipoprotein (groups VII and VIII), adipose (group XVI) and lysosomal (group XV), together constituting an enzyme superfamily (Dennis et al., 2011; Vasquez et al., 2018). In terms of neurodegenerative processes, and specifically PD, the most studied PLA2 isotypes are cPLA2 and iPLA2. The classical role assigned to iPLA2 enzymes is their active participation in membrane homeostasis through PL remodeling in Lands cycle where phospholipase activity operates coordinately with PL-acyltransferases. Later findings postulate other important functions for iPLA2s: while lysophosphatidyl moieties have been shown to modulate store-operated calcium entry, the released fatty acid, mostly DHA, has been described as the preferred substrate for the production of resolvins, lipid mediators involved in the resolution of inflammatory processes (Bazan, 2005; Serhan and Petasis, 2011). iPLA2 are mainly encoded by the PLA2G6 gene. In the nervous system, iPLA2β has been shown to be essential for remodeling membrane PLs in axons and synapses. Mutations in PLA2G6 have been associated with several neurodegenerative disorders, including adult-onset dystonia-parkinsonism, PARK14. In this regard, PLA2G6 knock-out mice have been widely used for the study of neuronal membrane-associated degeneration (Sumi-Akamaru et al., 2016). Indeed, increased expression of α-synuclein has been associated with mitochondrial injury triggered by iPLA2 dysfunction in PLA2G6 knock-out animals (Sumi-Akamaru et al., 2016). Moreover, the impairment of iPLA2-dependent calcium signaling has recently been implicated in neuronal loss through autophagic dysfunction in dopaminergic neurons derived from fibroblasts from PD patients and PLA2G6 knock-out animals (Zhou et al., 2016).

cPLA2 is mainly associated with the release of AA, the obligate substrate for prostaglandins generation catalyzed by cyclooxygenase-2, which is considered one of the main pathways mediating inflammatory response. Though neuroinflammation is a hallmark of PD, the specific PLA2 isoforms that are activated in dopaminergic neuronal damage have not been fully described. Besides the classical inflammatory process, the exposure to extracellular α-synuclein is able to activate cPLA2 and to promote synapse damage induced by phospholipase-dependent activity (Bate and Williams, 2015).

Upon PLA2 activation, it is important that fatty acid release be properly coupled to PL acylation activity; impairment of the Lands cycle could be responsible for an increase in FFA availability (DHA, AA). This increase in FFA availability, could in turn, be associated with α-synuclein and promote its oligomerization. The rise in cytosolic/soluble DHA content reported by Sharon and coworkers in *post-mortem* brains in PD and LB dementia patients is in agreement with the activation of any specific PLA2 that could consecutively induce α-synuclein oligomerization and aggregation (Sharon et al., 2003a). The workings of this mechanism still lack clarity.

The fact that SNCA knock-out mice present enhanced prostaglandin generation during neuronal injury argues in favor of a biological role for α-synuclein in the regulation of the inflammatory cascade (Golovko and Murphy, 2008). It has been demonstrated that DHA, mainly released from PLs by iPLA2 action, has a long half-life compared with other fatty acids and that its free form is the preferred substrate for neuroprotectin synthesis, and the resolution of the inflammatory process (Murphy, 2013). An important question is whether the dyshomeostasis between cPLA2 and iPLA2 triggered by α-synuclein overexpression could be responsible for a differential AA/DHA ratio and availability, thus modulating the balance between inflammation and resolution processes and promoting the neuroinflammatory phenotype in PD (**Figure 3**).

Among the classical signaling pathways associated with G-protein-coupled receptors is PI-specific PLC. Upon receptor activation, PLC hydrolyzes PI 4,5-bisphosphate to produce the lipid messenger diacylglycerol and the soluble inositol triphosphate. There are now six different families of PLC (β, γ, δ, ε, ζ, and η) described in different tissues, with pleiotropic functions associated with the membrane receptor to which they are coupled (Kadamur and Ross, 2013). It has recently been shown that α-synuclein overexpression interferes with Gq/PLC-β signaling by preventing the rise in cytosolic calcium and ERK 1/2 activation (Volta et al., 2017). α-Synuclein is also able to trigger the impairment of G-protein signaling associated with sphingosine-1-phosphate by promoting the exclusion of the receptor from lipid rafts (Mohamed Badawy et al., 2018).

Phospholipase D signaling impairment has been reported in Alzheimer's disease and the signaling pathway is, therefore, an emerging therapeutic target for this neurodegenerative disorder (Brown et al., 2017). The role of PLD in α-synuclein-associated pathologies, however, still lacks clarity. Classical PLDs, PLD1 and PLD2, catalyze the hydrolysis of the PC head group in order to produce PA. PA has pleiotropic functions both as a lipid messenger, regulating the activity of signaling proteins, and as an important modulator of membrane curvature. Whereas neuronal PLD1 has been associated with cytoskeleton architecture, PLD2 activity is linked to molecular events triggered by the activation of membrane receptors (Watanabe et al., 2011; Comoglio et al., 2014). Both PLD1 and PLD2 have been reported to participate in astroglial differentiation (Burkhardt et al., 2015). Genetic deletion of PLD1 or PLD2 in transgenic mice demonstrates that both

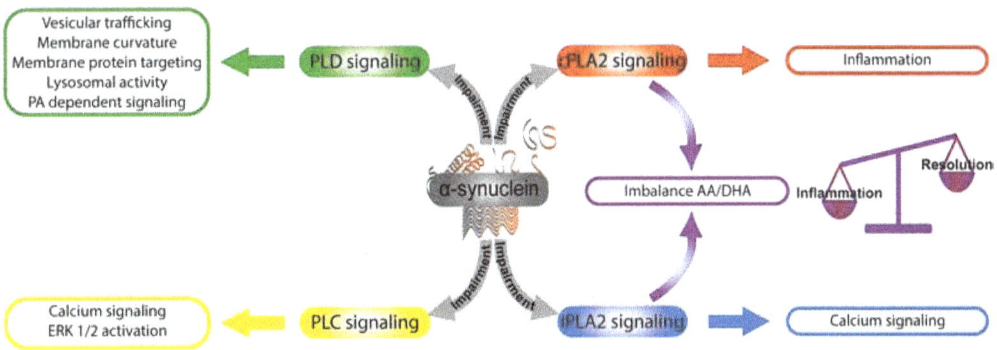


**FIGURE 3 |** α-Synuclein and the modulation of lipid signaling. α-Synuclein is able to intervene lipid signaling by the modulation of phospholipase activities. The α-synuclein -induced impairment of cPLA2 and iPLA2 signaling triggers an imbalance in the AA/DHA ratio that finally could affect the balance of inflammation and resolution processes. Calcium signaling and ERK 1/2 activation are modulated by α-synuclein through PLC pathway impairment. α-Synuclein intervention in PLD signaling impacts on diverse cellular functions as vesicular trafficking, membrane curvature, and membrane protein targeting, lysosomal activity and PA-dependent signaling. AA, arachidonic acid; DHA, docosahexaenoic acid; PA, phosphatidic acid; cPLA2, calcium-sensitive cytosolic phospholipase A2; iPLA2, calcium-independent phospholipase A2; PLC, phospholipase C; PLD, phospholipase D.

enzymes participate in brain development and cognitive function (Burkhardt et al., 2014).

The role of classical PLDs in the several processes of the nervous system has been well-established, but their participation in neurodegenerative processes associated with synucleinopathies is not clear. *In vitro* and *in vivo* assays have given rise to a number of divergent reports of the role of α-synuclein in PLD signaling. *In vivo* experiments have demonstrated that α-synuclein-induced PLD2 inhibition is able to prevent dopaminergic neurodegeneration (Gorbatyuk et al., 2010), whereas *in vitro* assays using recombinant α-synuclein and purified PLD1 and PLD2 have shown no inhibition of PLD activity (Rappley et al., 2009). However, protein profile studies in *post-mortem* brains from PD patients display diminished PLD1 expression (Bae et al., 2014). In yeast, it has been demonstrated that PLD inhibition elicited by α-synuclein was related to dysregulation of lipid metabolism and trafficking (Outeiro and Lindquist, 2003). In line with this, our laboratory has recently described that the overexpression of human α-synuclein in neuroblastoma cells is able to induce a decrease in PLD1 mRNA and protein levels and to impair ERK1/2 signaling (Conde et al., 2018). In this cellular model of synucleinopathy, we demonstrated that the inhibition of PLD1 expression and the impairment of ERK1/2 signaling triggered by α-synuclein overexpression are associated with a decrease in neurofilament light chain expression and in consequence with alteration of the neuronal cytoskeleton. The reported findings highlight the biological significance of PLD regulation exerted by α-synuclein that could modulate PA levels in a compartment-specific manner, thus impacting on different cellular functions: (i) vesicular trafficking, (ii) membrane curvature and membrane protein targeting, (iii) lysosomal activity, and (iv) PA-dependent signaling, among others (**Figure 3**).

It is clear from the above that α-synuclein, mainly when it is overexpressed, is able to disturb lipid signaling. The plethora of lipid messengers (PA, AA, DHA, and diacylglycerol) able to be produced due to α-synuclein could have different impacts on important cellular processes in the nervous system such as vesicular trafficking, autophagy, cytoskeleton architecture, and neuroinflammation. Dissecting the signaling pathways responsible for the production of each lipid messenger and the specific cellular compartment where they work, could contribute to the development of new strategic therapies for synucleinopathies.

## CONCLUDING REMARKS

This review covers the diversity of ways in which α-synuclein interacts and connects with lipid biology. Much of the experimental evidences dealing with the physical interaction of the protein with different lipid moieties derive from biophysical studies performed on artificial membranes. It is clear that the α-synuclein N-terminal domain is able to interact with the majority of PLs and with Chol with different affinities. Further research is required in order to shed more light on precisely which of these α-synuclein/lipid interactions occur *in vivo*; clear findings will undoubtedly contribute to a fuller understanding of both the biological and pathological implications of α-synuclein.

Efforts toward a more detailed characterization of α-synuclein interventions in lipid metabolism and signaling will open the way to a more in-depth assessment of the protein's implications for therapeutic purposes. One hypothesis to be tested is whether α-synuclein pleiotropic properties are able to trigger a lipid metabolic and signaling switch, creating a propensity to interact and aggregate thus establishing a positive feedback. Unraveling this paradigm could provide not only new insights into the biological role of α-synuclein but also innovative ways of devising strategies for the treatment of synucleinopathies.

## AUTHOR CONTRIBUTIONS

GS contributed to conception and design of the study. GS, NA, and PIG organized the database and wrote the sections of the manuscript. MC designed and performed the figures. RU performed the critical reading and editing. All authors contributed to manuscript revision, read, and approved the submitted version.

## FUNDING

GS, NA, and RU are research members of the CONICET. MC and PIG are research fellows of the CONICET. Articles from our laboratory that have been cited in this review were granted by ANPCyT (PICT 2013-0987 and PICT 2017-0224), CONICET (PIP 11220120100251), and UNS (PGI 24/B226).

## REFERENCES

Abeliovich, A., Schmitz, Y., Fariñas, I., Choi-Lundberg, D., Ho, W. H., Castillo, P. E., et al. (2000). Mice lacking α-synuclein display functional deficits in the nigrostriatal dopamine system. *Neuron* 25, 239–252. doi: 10.1016/S0896-6273(00)80886-7

Araki, K., Sugawara, K., Hayakawa, E. H., Ubukawa, K., Kobayashi, I., Wakui, H., et al. (2018). The localization of α-synuclein in the process of differentiation of human erythroid cells. *Int. J. Hematol.* 108, 130–138. doi: 10.1007/s12185-018-2457-8

Asi, Y. T., Simpson, J. E., Heath, P. R., Wharton, S. B., Lees, A. J., Revesz, T., et al. (2014). Alpha-synuclein mRNA expression in oligodendrocytes in MSA. *Glia* 62, 964–970. doi: 10.1002/glia.22653

Assayag, K., Yakunin, E., Loeb, V., Selkoe, D. J., and Sharon, R. (2007). Polyunsaturated fatty acids induce α-synuclein-related pathogenic changes in neuronal cells. *Am. J. Pathol.* 171, 2000–2011. doi: 10.2353/ajpath.2007.070373

Auluck, P. K., Caraveo, G., and Lindquist, S. (2010). α-Synuclein: membrane interactions and toxicity in Parkinson's disease. *Annu. Rev. Cell Dev. Biol.* 26, 211–233. doi: 10.1146/annurev.cellbio.042308.113313

Bae, E. J., Lee, H. J., Jang, Y. H., Michael, S., Masliah, E., Min, D. S., et al. (2014). Phospholipase D1 regulates autophagic flux and clearance of α-synuclein aggregates. *Cell Death Differ.* 21, 1132–1141. doi: 10.1038/cdd.2014.30

Barceló-Coblijn, G., Golovko, M. Y., Weinhofer, I., Berger, J., and Murphy, E. J. (2007). Brain neutral lipids mass is increased in α-synuclein gene-ablated mice. *J. Neurochem.* 101, 132–141. doi: 10.1111/j.1471-4159.2006.04348.x

Bar-On, P., Crews, L., Koob, A. O., Mizuno, H., Adame, A., Spencer, B., et al. (2008). Statins reduce neuronal α-synuclein aggregation in in vitro models of Parkinson's disease. *J. Neurochem.* 105, 1656–1667. doi: 10.1111/j.1471-4159.2008.05254.x

Barrett, P. J., and Timothy Greenamyre, J. (2015). Post-translational modification of α-synuclein in Parkinson's disease. *Brain Res.* 1628(Pt B), 247–253. doi: 10.1016/j.brainres.2015.06.002

Bartels, T., Choi, J. G., and Selkoe, D. J. (2011). α-Synuclein occurs physiologically as a helically folded tetramer that resists aggregation. *Nature* 477, 107–110. doi: 10.1038/nature10324

Bartels, T., Kim, N. C., Luth, E. S., and Selkoe, D. J. (2014). N-alpha-acetylation of α-synuclein increases its helical folding propensity, GM1 binding specificity and resistance to aggregation. *PLoS One* 9:e103727. doi: 10.1371/journal.pone.0103727

Bate, C., and Williams, A. (2015). cAMP-inhibits cytoplasmic phospholipase A2 and protects neurons against amyloid-β-induced synapse damage. *Biology* 4, 591–606. doi: 10.3390/biology4030591

Bazan, N. G. (2005). Neuroprotectin D1 ( NPD1 ): a DHA-derived mediator that protects brain and retina against cell injury-induced oxidative stress. *Brain Pathol.* 15, 159–166. doi: 10.1111/j.1750-3639.2005.tb00513.x

Bengoa-Vergniory, N., Roberts, R. F., Wade-Martins, R., and Alegre-Abarrategui, J. (2017). Alpha-synuclein oligomers: a new hope. *Acta Neuropathol.* 134, 819–838. doi: 10.1007/s00401-017-1755-1

Bhak, G., Lee, J. H., Hahn, J. S., and Paik, S. R. (2009). Granular assembly of α-synuclein leading to the accelerated amyloid fibril formation with shear stress. *PLoS One* 4:e4177. doi: 10.1371/journal.pone.0004177

Billings, J. L., Hare, D. J., Nurjono, M., Volitakis, I., Cherny, R. A., Bush, A. I., et al. (2016). Effects of neonatal iron feeding and chronic clioquinol administration on the Parkinsonian human A53T transgenic mouse. *ACS Chem. Neurosci.* 7, 360–366. doi: 10.1021/acschemneuro.5b00305

Bodner, C. R., Maltsev, A. S., Dobson, C. M., and Bax, A. (2010). Differential phospholipid binding of α-synuclein variants implicated in Parkinson's disease revealed by solution NMR spectroscopy. *Biochemistry* 49, 862–871. doi: 10.1021/bi901723p

Bonini, N., and Giasson, B. (2005). Snaring the function of alpha-synuclein. *Cell* 123, 359–361. doi: 10.1016/j.cell.2005.10.017

Bosco, D. A., Fowler, D. M., Zhang, Q., Nieva, J., Powers, E. T., Wentworth, P., et al. (2006). Elevated levels of oxidized cholesterol metabolites in Lewy body disease brains accelerate α-synuclein fibrilization. *Nat. Chem. Biol.* 2, 249–253. doi: 10.1038/nchembio782

Braun, A. R., and Sachs, J. N. (2015). α-synuclein reduces tension and increases undulations in simulations of small unilamellar vesicles. *Biophys. J.* 108, 1848–1851. doi: 10.1016/j.bpj.2015.03.029

Broersen, K., van den Brink, D., Fraser, G., Goedert, M., and Davletov, B. (2006). Alpha-synuclein adopts an alpha-helical conformation in the presence of polyunsaturated fatty acids to hinder micelle formation. *Biochemistry* 45, 15610–15616. doi: 10.1021/bi061743l

Brown, H. A., Thomas, P. G., and Lindsley, C. W. (2017). Targeting phospholipase D in cancer, infection and neurodegenerative disorders. *Nat. Rev. Drug Discov.* 16, 351–367. doi: 10.1038/nrd.2016.252

Brown, J. W. P., Buell, A. K., Michaels, T. C. T., Meisl, G., Carozza, J., Flagmeier, P., et al. (2016). β-Synuclein suppresses both the initiation and amplification steps of α-synuclein aggregation via competitive binding to surfaces. *Sci. Rep.* 6:36010. doi: 10.1038/srep36010

Bruening, W., Giasson, B. I., Klein-Szanto, A. J. P., Lee, V. M. Y., Trojanowski, J. Q., and Godwin, A. K. (2000). Synucleins are expressed in the majority of breast and ovarian carcinomas and in preneoplastic lesions of the ovary. *Cancer* 88, 2154–2163. doi: 10.1002/(sici)1097-0142(20000501)88%3A9%3C2154%3A%3Aaid-cncr23%3E3.0.co%3B2-9

Buchman, V. L., Hunter, H. J., Pinõn, L. G., Thompson, J., Privalova, E. M., Ninkina, N. N., et al. (1998). Persyn, a member of the synuclein family, has a distinct pattern of expression in the developing nervous system. *J. Neurosci.* 18, 9335–9341. doi: 10.1523/JNEUROSCI.18-22-09335.1998

Burkhardt, U., Beyer, S., and Klein, J. (2015). Role of phospholipases D1 and 2 in astroglial proliferation: effects of specific inhibitors and genetic deletion. *Eur. J. Pharmacol.* 761, 398–404. doi: 10.1016/j.ejphar.2015.05.004

Burkhardt, U., Stegner, D., Hattingen, E., Beyer, S., Nieswandt, B., and Klein, J. (2014). Impaired brain development and reduced cognitive function in phospholipase D-deficient mice. *Neurosci. Lett.* 572, 48–52. doi: 10.1016/j.neulet.2014.04.052

Burré, J. (2015). The synaptic function of α-synuclein. *J. Parkinsons Dis.* 5, 699–713. doi: 10.3233/JPD-150642

Burré, J., Sharma, M., and Südhof, T. C. (2014). α-Synuclein assembles into higher-order multimers upon membrane binding to promote SNARE complex formation. *Proc. Natl. Acad. Sci. U.S.A.* 111, E4274–E4283. doi: 10.1073/pnas.1416598111

Burré, J., Sharma, M., and Südhof, T. C. (2018). Cell biology and pathophysiology of α-synuclein. *Cold Spring Harb. Perspect. Med.* 8:a024091. doi: 10.1101/cshperspect.a024091

Burré, J., Sharma, M., Tsetsenis, T., Buchman, V., Etherton, M. R., and Südhof, T. C. (2010). α-Synuclein promotes SNARE-complex assembly in vivo and in vitro. *Science* 329, 1663–1667. doi: 10.1126/science.1195227

Burré, J., Vivona, S., Diao, J., Sharma, M., Brunger, A. T., and Südhof, T. C. (2013). Properties of native brain α-synuclein. *Nature* 498, E4–E6. doi: 10.1038/nature12125

Bussell, R. (2005). Helix periodicity, topology, and dynamics of membrane-associated α-Synuclein. *Protein Sci.* 14, 862–872. doi: 10.1110/ps.041255905

Bussell, R., and Eliezer, D. (2003). A structural and functional role for 11-mer repeats in α-synuclein and other exchangeable lipid binding proteins. *J. Mol. Biol.* 329, 763–778. doi: 10.1016/S0022-2836(03)00520-5

Butler, B., Saha, K., Rana, T., Becker, J. P., Sambo, D., Davari, P., et al. (2015). Dopamine transporter activity is modulated by α-synuclein. *J. Biol. Chem.* 290, 29542–29554. doi: 10.1074/jbc.M115.691592

Cabirol-Pol, M. J., Khalil, B., Rival, T., Faivre-Sarrailh, C., and Besson, M. T. (2018). Glial lipid droplets and neurodegeneration in a *Drosophila* model of complex I deficiency. *Glia* 66, 874–888. doi: 10.1002/glia.23290

Carboni, E., and Lingor, P. (2015). Insights on the interaction of alpha-synuclein and metals in the pathophysiology of Parkinson's disease. *Metallomics* 7, 395–404. doi: 10.1039/c4mt00339j

Carroll, C. B., and Wyse, R. K. H. (2017). Simvastatin as a potential disease-modifying therapy for patients with Parkinson's disease: rationale for clinical trial, and current progress. *J. Parkinsons Dis.* 7, 545–568. doi: 10.3233/JPD-171203

Castagnet, P. I., Golovko, M. Y., Barceló-Coblijn, G. C., Nussbaum, R. L., and Murphy, E. J. (2005). Fatty acid incorporation is decreased in astrocytes cultured from α-synuclein gene-ablated mice. *J. Neurochem.* 94, 839–849. doi: 10.1111/j.1471-4159.2005.03247.x

Chandra, S., Gallardo, G., Fernández-Chacón, R., Schlüter, O. M., and Südhof, T. C. (2005). α-Synuclein cooperates with CSPα in preventing neurodegeneration. *Cell* 123, 383–396. doi: 10.1016/j.cell.2005.09.028

Chang, D., Nalls, M. A., Hallgrímsdottir, I. B., Hunkapiller, J., Van Der Brug, M., Cai, F., et al. (2017). A meta-analysis of genome-wide association studies identifies 17 new Parkinson's disease risk loci. *Nat. Genet.* 49, 1511–1516. doi: 10.1038/ng.3955

Chartier-Harlin, M. C., Kachergus, J., Roumier, C., Mouroux, V., Douay, X., Lincoln, S., et al. (2004). α-synuclein locus duplication as a cause of familial Parkinson's disease. *Lancet* 364, 1167–1169. doi: 10.1016/S0140-6736(04)17103-1

Chen, C. T., Green, J. T., Orr, S. K., and Bazinet, R. P. (2008). Regulation of brain polyunsaturated fatty acid uptake and turnover. *Prostaglandins Leukot. Essent. Fatty Acids* 79, 85–91. doi: 10.1016/j.plefa.2008.09.003

Chen, H., Zhao, Y.-F., Chen, Y.-X., and Li, Y.-M. (2019). Exploring the roles of post-translational modifications in the pathogenesis of Parkinson's disease using synthetic and semisynthetic modified α-synuclein. *ACS Chem. Neurosci.* 10, 910–921. doi: 10.1021/acschemneuro.8b00447

Cheng, D., Jenner, A. M., Shui, G., Cheong, W. F., Mitchell, T. W., Nealon, J. R., et al. (2011). Lipid pathway alterations in Parkinson's disease primary visual cortex. *PLoS One* 6:e17299. doi: 10.1371/journal.pone.0017299

Clayton, D. F., and George, J. M. (1998). The synucleins: a family of proteins involved in synaptic function, plasticity, neurodegeneration and disease. *Trends Neurosci.* 21, 249–254. doi: 10.1016/S0166-2236(97)01213-7

Colebc, N. B., Murphy, D. D., Grider, T., Rueter, S., Brasaemle, D., and Nussbaum, R. L. (2002). Lipid droplet binding and oligomerization properties of the Parkinson's disease protein α-synuclein. *J. Biol. Chem.* 277, 6344–6352. doi: 10.1074/jbc.M108414200

Comoglio, Y., Levitz, J., Kienzler, M. A., Lesage, F., Isacoff, E. Y., and Sandoz, G. (2014). Phospholipase D2 specifically regulates TREK potassium channels via direct interaction and local production of phosphatidic acid. *Proc. Natl. Acad. Sci. U.S.A.* 111, 13547–13552. doi: 10.1073/pnas.1407160111

Conde, M. A., Alza, N. P., Iglesias González, P. A., Scodelaro Bilbao, P. G., Sánchez Campos, S., Uranga, R. M., et al. (2018). Phospholipase D1 downregulation by α-synuclein: implications for neurodegeneration in Parkinson's disease. *Biochim. Biophys. Acta Mol. Cell Biol. Lipids* 1863, 639–650. doi: 10.1016/j.bbalip.2018.03.006

Conway, K. A., Harper, J. D., and Lansbury, P. T. (2000). Fibrils formed in vitro from α-synuclein and two mutant forms linked to Parkinson's disease are typical amyloid. *Biochemistry* 39, 2552–2563. doi: 10.1021/bi991447r

Coulombe, K., Kerdiles, O., Tremblay, C., Emond, V., Lebel, M., Boulianne, A. S., et al. (2018). Impact of DHA intake in a mouse model of synucleinopathy. *Exp. Neurol.* 301(Pt A), 39–49. doi: 10.1016/j.expneurol.2017.12.002

Danzer, K. M., Haasen, D., Karow, A. R., Moussaud, S., Habeck, M., Giese, A., et al. (2007). Different species of a-synuclein oligomers induce calcium influx and seeding. *J. Neurosci.* 27, 9220–9232. doi: 10.1523/JNEUROSCI.2617-07.2007

Davidson, W. S., Jonas, A., Clayton, D. F., and George, J. M. (1998). Stabilization of α-Synuclein secondary structure upon binding to synthetic membranes. *J. Biol. Chem.* 273, 9443–9449. doi: 10.1074/jbc.273.16.9443

De Franceschi, G., Fecchio, C., Sharon, R., Schapira, A. H. V., Proukakis, C., Bellotti, V., et al. (2017). α-Synuclein structural features inhibit harmful polyunsaturated fatty acid oxidation, suggesting roles in neuroprotection. *J. Biol. Chem.* 292, 6927–6937. doi: 10.1074/jbc.M116.765149

De Franceschi, G., Frare, E., Bubacco, L., Mammi, S., Fontana, A., and de Laureto, P. P. (2009). Molecular insights into the interaction between α-synuclein and docosahexaenoic acid. *J. Mol. Biol.* 394, 94–107. doi: 10.1016/j.jmb.2009.09.008

De Franceschi, G., Frare, E., Pivato, M., Relini, A., Penco, A., Greggio, E., et al. (2011). Structural and morphological characterization of aggregated species of α-synuclein induced by docosahexaenoic acid. *J. Biol. Chem.* 286, 22262–22274. doi: 10.1074/jbc.M110.202937

Dennis, E. A., Cao, J., Hsu, Y. H., Magrioti, V., and Kokotos, G. (2011). Phospholipase A2 enzymes: physical structure, biological function, disease implication, chemical inhibition, and therapeutic intervention. *Chem. Rev.* 111, 6130–6185. doi: 10.1021/cr200085w

Der-Sarkissiant, A., Jao, C. C., Chen, J., and Langen, R. (2003). Structural organization of α-synuclein fibrils studied by site-directed spin labeling. *J. Biol. Chem.* 278, 37530–37535. doi: 10.1074/jbc.M305266200

Desplats, P., Lee, H.-J., Bae, E.-J., Patrick, C., Rockenstein, E., Crews, L., et al. (2009). Inclusion formation and neuronal cell death through neuron-to-neuron transmission of alpha-synuclein. *Proc. Natl. Acad. Sci. U.S.A.* 106, 13010–13015. doi: 10.1073/pnas.0903691106

Dettmer, U., Newman, A. J., Luth, E. S., Bartels, T., and Selkoe, D. (2013). In vivo cross-linking reveals principally oligomeric forms of α-synuclein and β-synuclein in neurons and non-neural cells. *J. Biol. Chem.* 288, 6371–6385. doi: 10.1074/jbc.M112.403311

Dettmer, U., Newman, A. J., Soldner, F., Luth, E. S., Kim, N. C., Von Saucken, V. E., et al. (2015a). Parkinson-causing α-synuclein missense mutations shift native tetramers to monomers as a mechanism for disease initiation. *Nat. Commun.* 6:7314. doi: 10.1038/ncomms8314

Dettmer, U., Newman, A. J., von Saucken, V. E., Bartels, T., and Selkoe, D. J. (2015b). KTKEGV repeat motifs are key mediators of normal α-synuclein tetramerization: their mutation causes excess monomers and neurotoxicity. *Proc. Natl. Acad. Sci. U.S.A.* 112, 9596–9601. doi: 10.1073/pnas.1505953112

Dettmer, U., Ramalingam, N., von Saucken, V. E., Kim, T. E., Newman, A. J., Terry-Kantor, E., et al. (2017). Loss of native α-synuclein multimerization by strategically mutating its amphipathic helix causes abnormal vesicle interactions in neuronal cells. *Hum. Mol. Genet.* 26, 3466–3481. doi: 10.1093/HMG/DDX227

Devi, L., Raghavendran, V., Prabhu, B. M., Avadhani, N. G., and Anandatheerthavarada, H. K. (2008). Mitochondrial import and accumulation of α-synuclein impair complex I in human dopaminergic neuronal cultures and Parkinson disease brain. *J. Biol. Chem.* 283, 9089–9100. doi: 10.1074/jbc.M710012200

Diao, J., Burré, J., Vivona, S., Cipriano, D. J., Sharma, M., Kyoung, M., et al. (2013). Native α-synuclein induces clustering of synaptic-vesicle mimics via binding to phospholipids and synaptobrevin-2/VAMP2. *eLife* 2:e00592. doi: 10.7554/eLife.00592

Dikiy, I., and Eliezer, D. (2012). Folding and misfolding of alpha-synuclein on membranes. *Biochim. Biophys. Acta* 1818, 1013–1018. doi: 10.1016/j.bbamem.2011.09.008

Ducas, V. C., and Rhoades, E. (2012). Quantifying interactions of β-synuclein and γ-synuclein with model membranes. *J. Mol. Biol.* 423, 528–539. doi: 10.1016/j.jmb.2012.08.008

Dunn, T. N., Akiyama, T., Lee, H. W., Kim, J. B., Knotts, T. A., Smith, S. R., et al. (2015). Evaluation of the synuclein-γ (sncg) gene as a PPARγ target in murine adipocytes, dorsal root ganglia somatosensory neurons, and human adipose tissue. *PLoS One* 10:e0115830. doi: 10.1371/journal.pone.0115830

Dunnett, S. B., and Björklund, A. (1999). Prospects for new restorative and neuroprotective treatments in Parkinson's disease. *Nature* 399(Suppl. 6738), A32–A39. doi: 10.1038/399a032

El-Agnaf, O. M. A., Jakes, R., Curran, M. D., Middleton, D., Ingenito, R., Bianchi, E., et al. (1998). Aggregates from mutant and wild-type α-synuclein proteins and NAC peptide induce apoptotic cell death in human neuroblastoma cells by formation of β-sheet and amyloid-like filaments. *FEBS Lett.* 440, 71–75. doi: 10.1016/S0014-5793(98)01418-5

Eliezer, D., Kutluay, E., Bussell, R., and Browne, G. (2001). Conformational properties of α-synuclein in its free and lipid-associated states. *J. Mol. Biol.* 307, 1061–1073. doi: 10.1006/jmbi.2001.4538

Emamzadeh, F. N. (2016). Alpha-synuclein structure, functions, and interactions. *J. Res. Med. Sci.* 21:29. doi: 10.4103/1735-1995.181989

Fanning, S., Haque, A., Imberdis, T., Baru, V., Barrasa, M. I., Nuber, S., et al. (2018). Lipidomic analysis of α-synuclein neurotoxicity identifies stearoyl CoA desaturase as a target for Parkinson treatment. *Mol. Cell* 73, 1001–1014.e8. doi: 10.1016/J.MOLCEL.2018.11.028

Fares, M. B., Ait-Bouziad, N., Dikiy, I., Mbefo, M. K., Jovičić, A., Kiely, A., et al. (2014). The novel Parkinson's disease linked mutation G51D attenuates in vitro aggregation and membrane binding of α-synuclein, and enhances its secretion and nuclear localization in cells. *Hum. Mol. Genet.* 23, 4491–4509. doi: 10.1093/hmg/ddu165

Fecchio, C., De Franceschi, G., Relini, A., Greggio, E., Dalla Serra, M., Bubacco, L., et al. (2013). α-synuclein oligomers induced by docosahexaenoic acid affect membrane integrity. *PLoS One* 8:e82732. doi: 10.1371/journal.pone.0082732

Fecchio, C., Palazzi, L., and Polverino de Laureto, P. (2018). α-Synuclein and polyunsaturated fatty acids: molecular basis of the interaction and implication in neurodegeneration. *Molecules* 23:E1531. doi: 10.3390/molecules23071531

Fiske, M., Valtierra, S., Solvang, K., Zorniak, M., White, M., Herrera, S., et al. (2011). Contribution of alanine-76 and serine phosphorylation in α-synuclein membrane association and aggregation in yeasts. *Parkinsons Dis.* 2011:392180. doi: 10.4061/2011/392180

Flagmeier, P., Meisl, G., Vendruscolo, M., Knowles, T. P. J., Dobson, C. M., Buell, A. K., et al. (2016). Mutations associated with familial Parkinson's disease alter the initiation and amplification steps of α-synuclein aggregation. *Proc. Natl. Acad. Sci. U.S.A.* 113, 10328–10333. doi: 10.1073/pnas.1604645113

Fujiwara, H., Hasegawa, M., Dohmae, N., Kawashima, A., Masliah, E., Goldberg, M. S., et al. (2002). α-synuclein is phosphorylated in synucleinopathy lesions. *Nat. Cell Biol.* 4, 160–164. doi: 10.1038/ncb748

Fusco, G., Chen, S. W., Williamson, P. T. F., Cascella, R., Perni, M., Jarvis, J. A., et al. (2017). Structural basis of membrane disruption and cellular toxicity by α-synuclein oligomers. *Science* 358, 1440–1443. doi: 10.1126/science.aan6160

Galvagnion, C. (2017). The role of lipids interacting with α-synuclein in the pathogenesis of Parkinson's disease. *J. Parkinsons Dis.* 7, 433–450. doi: 10.3233/JPD-171103

Gao, Q., Binns, D. D., Kinch, L. N., Grishin, N. V., Ortiz, N., Chen, X., et al. (2017). Pet10p is a yeast perilipin that stabilizes lipid droplets and promotes their assembly. *J. Cell Biol.* 216, 3199–3217. doi: 10.1083/jcb.201610013

Garcia, E. J., Vevea, J. D., and Pon, L. A. (2018). Lipid droplet autophagy during energy mobilization, lipid homeostasis and protein quality control. *Front. Biosci.* 23, 1552–1563. doi: 10.2741/4660

Gardai, S. J., Mao, W., Schüle, B., Babcock, M., Schoebel, S., Lorenzana, C., et al. (2013). Elevated alpha-synuclein impairs innate immune cell function and provides a potential peripheral biomarker for Parkinson's disease. *PLoS One* 8:e71634. doi: 10.1371/journal.pone.0071634

Ghio, S., Kamp, F., Cauchi, R., Giese, A., and Vassallo, N. (2016). Interaction of α-synuclein with biomembranes in Parkinson's disease - Role of cardiolipin. *Prog. Lipid Res.* 61, 73–82. doi: 10.1016/j.plipres.2015.10.005

Ghosh, D., Sahay, S., Ranjan, P., Salot, S., Mohite, G. M., Singh, P. K., et al. (2014). The newly discovered Parkinsons disease associated finnish mutation (A53E) attenuates α-synuclein aggregation and membrane binding. *Biochemistry* 53, 6419–6421. doi: 10.1021/bi5010365

Giasson, B. I., Murray, I. V. J., Trojanowski, J. Q., and Lee, V. M. Y. (2001). A hydrophobic stretch of 12 amino acid residues in the middle of α-synuclein is essential for filament assembly. *J. Biol. Chem.* 276, 2380–2386. doi: 10.1074/jbc.M008919200

Giusto, N. M., Salvador, G. A., Castagnet, P. I., Pasquaré, S. J., and Ilincheta de Boschero, M. G. (2002). Age-associated changes in central nervous system glycerolipid composition and metabolism. *Neurochem. Res.* 27, 1513–1523. doi: 10.1023/A:1021604623208

Gluchowski, N. L., Becuwe, M., Walther, T. C., and Farese, R. V. (2017). Lipid droplets and liver disease: from basic biology to clinical implications. *Nat. Rev. Gastroenterol. Hepatol.* 14, 343–355. doi: 10.1038/nrgastro.2017.32

Golovko, M. Y., Barceló-Coblijn, G., Castagnet, P. I., Austin, S., Combs, C. K., and Murphy, E. J. (2009). The role of α-synuclein in brain lipid metabolism: a downstream impact on brain inflammatory response. *Mol. Cell. Biochem.* 326, 55–66. doi: 10.1007/s11010-008-0008-y

Golovko, M. Y., and Murphy, E. J. (2008). Brain prostaglandin formation is increased by α-synuclein gene-ablation during global ischemia. *Neurosci. Lett.* 432, 243–247. doi: 10.1016/j.neulet.2007.12.031

Golovko, M. Y., Rosenberger, T. A., Faergeman, N. J., Feddersen, S., Cole, N. B., Pribill, I., et al. (2006). Acyl-CoA synthetase activity links wild-type but not mutant alpha-synuclein to brain arachidonate metabolism. *Biochemistry* 45, 6956–6966. doi: 10.1021/bi0600289

Golovko, M. Y., Rosenberger, T. A., Feddersen, S., Færgeman, N. J., and Murphy, E. J. (2007). α-Synuclein gene ablation increases docosahexaenoic acid incorporation and turnover in brain phospholipids. *J. Neurochem.* 101, 201–211. doi: 10.1111/j.1471-4159.2006.04357.x

Gorbatyuk, O. S., Li, S., Nha Nguyen, F., Manfredsson, F. P., Kondrikova, G., Sullivan, L. F., et al. (2010). α-synuclein expression in rat substantia nigra suppresses phospholipase D2 toxicity and nigral neurodegeneration. *Mol. Ther.* 18, 1758–1768. doi: 10.1038/mt.2010.137

Guo, J., Shou, C., Meng, L., Jiang, B., Dong, B., Yao, L., et al. (2007). Neuronal protein synuclein γ predicts poor clinical outcome in breast cancer. *Int. J. Cancer* 121, 1296–1305. doi: 10.1002/ijc.22763

Guo, J. T., Chen, A. Q., Kong, Q., Zhu, H., Ma, C. M., and Qin, C. (2008). Inhibition of vesicular monoamine transporter-2 activity in α-synuclein stably transfected SH-SY5Y cells. *Cell. Mol. Neurobiol.* 28, 35–47. doi: 10.1007/s10571-007-9227-0

Guschina, I., Millership, S., O'Donnell, V., Ninkina, N., Harwood, J., and Buchman, V. (2011). Lipid classes and fatty acid patterns are altered in the brain of γ-synuclein null mutant mice. *Lipids* 46, 121–130. doi: 10.1007/s11745-010-3486-0

Hellstrand, E., Grey, M., Ainalem, M. L., Ankner, J., Forsyth, V. T., Fragneto, G., et al. (2013). Adsorption of α-synuclein to supported lipid bilayers: positioning and role of electrostatics. *ACS Chem. Neurosci.* 4, 1339–1351. doi: 10.1021/cn400066t

Hibi, T., Mori, T., Fukuma, M., Yamazaki, K., Hashiguchi, A., Yamada, T., et al. (2009). Synuclein-γ is closely involved in perineural invasion and distant metastasis in mouse models and is a novel prognostic factor in pancreatic cancer. *Clin. Cancer Res.* 15, 2864–2871. doi: 10.1158/1078-0432.CCR-08-2946

Hsiao, J. H. T., Halliday, G. M., and Kim, W. S. (2017). α-Synuclein regulates neuronal cholesterol efflux. *Molecules* 22:E1769. doi: 10.3390/molecules22101769

Hu, R., Diao, J., Li, J., Tang, Z., Li, X., Leitz, J., et al. (2016). Intrinsic and membrane-facilitated α-synuclein oligomerization revealed by label-free detection through solid-state nanopores. *Sci. Rep.* 6:20776. doi: 10.1038/srep20776

Hua, H., Xu, L., Wang, J., Jing, J., Luo, T., and Jiang, Y. (2009). Up-regulation of gamma-synuclein contributes to cancer cell survival under endoplasmic reticulum stress. *J. Pathol.* 217, 507–515. doi: 10.1002/path.2465

Ingelsson, M. (2016). Alpha-synuclein oligomers-neurotoxic molecules in Parkinson's disease and other lewy body disorders. *Front. Neurosci.* 10:408. doi: 10.3389/fnins.2016.00408

Iwai, A., Masliah, E., Yoshimoto, M., Ge, N., Flanagan, L., Rohan de Silva, H. A., et al. (1995). The precursor protein of non-Aβ component of Alzheimer's disease amyloid is a presynaptic protein of the central nervous system. *Neuron* 14, 467–475. doi: 10.1016/0896-6273(95)90302-X

Jakes, R., Spillantini, M. G., and Goedert, M. (1994). Identification of two distinct synucleins from human brain. *FEBS Lett.* 345, 27–32. doi: 10.1016/0014-5793(94)00395-5

Jo, E., Fuller, N., Rand, R. P., St George-Hyslop, P., and Fraser, P. E. (2002). Defective membrane interactions of familial Parkinson's disease mutant A30P α-Synuclein. *J. Mol. Biol.* 315, 799–807. doi: 10.1006/jmbi.2001.5269

Jo, E., McLaurin, J. A., Yip, C. M., St George-Hyslop, and Fraser, P. E. (2000). α-Synuclein membrane interactions and lipid specificity. *J. Biol. Chem.* 275, 34328–34334. doi: 10.1074/jbc.M004345200

Kadamur, G., and Ross, E. M. (2013). Mammalian phospholipase C. *Annu. Rev. Physiol.* 75, 127–154. doi: 10.1146/annurev-physiol-030212-183750

Karube, H., Sakamoto, M., Arawaka, S., Hara, S., Sato, H., Ren, C. H., et al. (2008). N-terminal region of α-synuclein is essential for the fatty acid-induced oligomerization of the molecules. *FEBS Lett.* 582, 3693–3700. doi: 10.1016/j.febslet.2008.10.001

Kory, N., Farese, R. V., and Walther, T. C. (2016). Targeting fat: mechanisms of protein localization to lipid droplets. *Trends Cell Biol.* 26, 535–546. doi: 10.1016/j.tcb.2016.02.007

Krüger, R., Kuhn, W., Müller, T., Woitalla, D., Graeber, M., Kösel, S., et al. (1998). Ala30Pro mutation in the gene encoding α-synuclein in Parkinson's disease. *Nat. Genet.* 18, 106–108. doi: 10.1038/ng0298-106

Kuwahara, T., Tonegawa, R., Ito, G., Mitani, S., and Iwatsubo, T. (2012). Phosphorylation of α-synuclein protein at ser-129 reduces neuronal dysfunction by lowering its membrane binding property in *Caenorhabditis elegans*. *J. Biol. Chem.* 287, 7098–7109. doi: 10.1074/jbc.M111.237131

Lahiri, S., and Futerman, A. H. (2007). The metabolism and function of sphingolipids and glycosphingolipids. *Cell. Mol. Life Sci.* 64, 2270–2284. doi: 10.1007/s00018-007-7076-0

Lashuel, H. A., Overk, C. R., Oueslati, A., and Masliah, E. (2013). The many faces of α-synuclein: from structure and toxicity to therapeutic target. *Nat. Rev. Neurosci.* 14, 38–48. doi: 10.1038/nrn3406

Ledesma, M. D., Martin, M. G., and Dotti, C. G. (2012). Lipid changes in the aged brain: effect on synaptic function and neuronal survival. *Prog. Lipid Res.* 51, 23–35. doi: 10.1016/j.plipres.2011.11.004

Lee, C.-Y. J., Seet, R. C. S., Huang, S. H., Long, L. H., and Halliwell, B. (2009). Different patterns of oxidized lipid products in plasma and urine of dengue fever, stroke, and Parkinson's disease patients: cautions in the use of biomarkers of oxidative stress. *Antioxid. Redox Signal.* 11, 407–420. doi: 10.1089/ars.2008.2179

Li, W. W., Yang, R., Guo, J. C., Ren, H. M., Zha, X. L., Cheng, J. S., et al. (2007). Localization of α-synuclein to mitochondria within midbrain of mice. *Neuroreport* 18, 1543–1546. doi: 10.1097/WNR.0b013e3282f03db4

Liu, L., Zhang, K., Sandoval, H., Yamamoto, S., Jaiswal, M., Sanz, E., et al. (2015). Glial lipid droplets and ROS induced by mitochondrial defects promote neurodegeneration. *Cell* 160, 177–190. doi: 10.1016/j.cell.2014.12.019

López, G. H., Ilincheta de Boschero, M. G., Castagnet, P. I., and Giusto, N. M. (1995). Age-associated changes in the content and fatty acid composition of brain glycerophospholipids. *Comp. Biochem. Physiol. Part B Biochem.* 112, 331–343. doi: 10.1016/0305-0491(95)00079-8

Lou, X., Kim, J., Hawk, B. J., and Shin, Y.-K. (2017). α-Synuclein may cross-bridge v-SNARE and acidic phospholipids to facilitate SNARE-dependent vesicle docking. *Biochem. J.* 474, 2039–2049. doi: 10.1042/BCJ20170200

Luk, K. C., Branch, J. R., Brunden, K. R., Trojanowski, J. Q., O'Brien, P., Lee, V. M.-Y., et al. (2009). Exogenous α-synuclein fibrils seed the formation of Lewy body-like intracellular inclusions in cultured cells. *Proc. Natl. Acad. Sci. U.S.A.* 106, 20051–20056. doi: 10.1073/pnas.0908005106

Lynch, S. M., Zhou, C., and Messer, A. (2008). An scFv intrabody against the nonamyloid component of α-synuclein reduces intracellular aggregation and toxicity. *J. Mol. Biol.* 377, 136–147. doi: 10.1016/j.jmb.2007.11.096

Ma, K. L., Song, L. K., Yuan, Y. H., Zhang, Y., Yang, J. L., Zhu, P., et al. (2014). α-synuclein is prone to interaction with the GC-box-like sequence in vitro. *Cell. Mol. Neurobiol.* 34, 603–609. doi: 10.1007/s10571-014-0046-9

Makwana, P. K., and Sundd, M. (2016). Alpha-synuclein structure, aggregation and modulators. *J. Proteins Proteom.* 7, 83–100.

Marie, G., Dunning, C. J., Gaspar, R., Grey, C., Brundin, P., Sparr, E., et al. (2015). Acceleration of α-synuclein aggregation by exosomes. *J. Biol. Chem.* 290, 2969–2982. doi: 10.1074/jbc.M114.585703

Maroteaux, L., Campanelli, J. T., and Scheller, R. H. (1988). Synuclein: a neuron-specific protein localized to the nucleus and presynaptic nerve terminal. *J. Neurosci.* 8, 2804–2815. doi: 10.1523/JNEUROSCI.08-08-02804.1988

Marquardt, D., Geier, B., and Pabst, G. (2015). Asymmetric lipid membranes: towards more realistic model systems. *Membranes* 5, 180–196. doi: 10.3390/membranes5020180

Martinez-Vicente, M., Talloczy, Z., Wong, E., Tang, G., Koga, H., Kaushik, S., et al. (2010). Cargo recognition failure is responsible for inefficient autophagy in Huntington's disease. *Nat. Neurosci.* 13, 567–576. doi: 10.1038/nn.2528

Martins, M., Rosa, A., Guedes, L. C., Fonseca, B. V., Gotovac, K., Violante, S., et al. (2011). Convergence of miRNA expression profiling, α-synuclein interaction and GWAS in Parkinson's disease. *PLoS One* 6:e25443. doi: 10.1371/journal.pone.0025443

Marwarha, G., and Ghribi, O. (2015). Does the oxysterol 27-hydroxycholesterol underlie Alzheimer's disease-Parkinson's disease overlap? *Exp. Gerontol.* 68, 13–18. doi: 10.1016/j.exger.2014.09.013

Marwarha, G., Rhen, T., Schommer, T., and Ghribi, O. (2011). The oxysterol 27-hydroxycholesterol regulatesα-synuclein and tyrosine hydroxylase expression levels in human neuroblastoma cells through modulation of liver X receptors and estrogen receptors-relevance to Parkinson's disease. *J. Neurochem.* 119, 1119–1136. doi: 10.1111/j.1471-4159.2011.07497.x

Mateos, M. V., Salvador, G. A., and Giusto, N. M. (2010). Selective localization of phosphatidylcholine-derived signaling in detergent-resistant membranes from synaptic endings. *Biochim. Biophys. Acta* 1798, 624–636. doi: 10.1016/j.bbamem.2009.12.008

Miotto, M. C., Rodriguez, E. E., Valiente-Gabioud, A. A., Torres-Monserrat, V., Binolfi, A., Quintanar, L., et al. (2014). Site-specific copper-catalyzed oxidation of α-synuclein: tightening the link between metal binding and protein oxidative damage in Parkinson's disease. *Inorg. Chem.* 53, 4350–4358. doi: 10.1021/ic4031377

Miraglia, F., Ricci, A., Rota, L., and Colla, E. (2018). Subcellular localization of alpha-synuclein aggregates and their interaction with membranes. *Neural Regen. Res.* 13, 1136–1144. doi: 10.4103/1673-5374.235013

Mizuno, S., Sasai, H., Kume, A., Takahashi, D., Satoh, M., Kado, S., et al. (2017). Dioleoyl-phosphatidic acid selectively binds to α-synuclein and strongly induces its aggregation. *FEBS Lett.* 591, 784–791. doi: 10.1002/1873-3468.12592

Mohamed Badawy, S. M., Okada, T., Kajimoto, T., Hirase, M., Matovelo, S. A., Nakamura, S., et al. (2018). Extracellular α-synuclein drives sphingosine 1-phosphate receptor subtype 1 out of lipid rafts, leading to impaired inhibitory G-protein signaling. *J. Biol. Chem.* 293, 8208–8216. doi: 10.1074/jbc.RA118.001986

Muntané, G., Janué, A., Fernandez, N., Odena, M. A., Oliveira, E., Boluda, S., et al. (2010). Modification of brain lipids but not phenotype in α-synucleinopathy transgenic mice by long-term dietary n-3 fatty acids. *Neurochem. Int.* 56, 318–328. doi: 10.1016/j.neuint.2009.10.015

Murphy, E. J. (2013). A lipid neurochemist's siren: docosahexaenoic acid and its elusive function in the central nervous system. *J. Neurochem.* 127, 299–302. doi: 10.1111/jnc.12439

Murray, I. V. J., Giasson, B. I., Quinn, S. M., Koppaka, V., Axelsen, P. H., Ischiropoulos, H., et al. (2003). Role of α-synuclein carboxy-terminus on fibril formation in vitro. *Biochemistry* 22, 8530–8540. doi: 10.1021/bi027363r

Nübling, G. S., Levin, J., Bader, B., Lorenzl, S., Hillmer, A., Högen, T., et al. (2014). Modelling Ser129 phosphorylation inhibits membrane binding of pore-forming alpha-synuclein oligomers. *PLoS One* 9:e98906. doi: 10.1371/journal.pone.0098906

Oaks, A. W., Frankfurt, M., Finkelstein, D. I., and Sidhu, A. (2013). Age-dependent effects of A53T alpha-synuclein on behavior and dopaminergic function. *PLoS One* 8:e60378. doi: 10.1371/journal.pone.0060378

Oertel, W., and Schulz, J. B. (2016). Current and experimental treatments of Parkinson disease: a guide for neuroscientists. *J. Neurochem.* 139(Suppl. 1), 325–337. doi: 10.1111/jnc.13750

Ogawa, K., Hishiki, T., Shimizu, Y., Funami, K., Sugiyama, K., Miyanari, Y., et al. (2009). Hepatitis C virus utilizes lipid droplet for production of infectious virus. *Proc. Jpn. Acad. Ser. B Phys. Biol. Sci.* 85, 217–228. doi: 10.2183/pjab.85.217

O'Leary, E. I., Jiang, Z., Strub, M. P., and Lee, J. C. (2018). Effects of phosphatidylcholine membrane fluidity on the conformation and aggregation of N-terminally acetylated α-Synuclein. *J. Biol. Chem.* 293, 11195–11205. doi: 10.1074/jbc.RA118.002780

O'Leary, E. I., and Lee, J. C. (2018). Interplay between α-synuclein amyloid formation and membrane structure. *Biochim. Biophys. Acta Proteins Proteom.* 1867, 483–491. doi: 10.1016/j.bbapap.2018.09.012

Oueslati, A. (2016). Implication of alpha-synuclein phosphorylation at S129 in synucleinopathies: what have we learned in the last decade? *J. Parkinsons Dis.* 6, 39–51. doi: 10.3233/JPD-160779

Oueslati, A., Fournier, M., and Lashuel, H. A. (2010). Role of post-translational modifications in modulating the structure, function and toxicity of α-synuclein. Implications for Parkinson's disease pathogenesis and therapies. *Prog. Brain Res.* 183, 115–145. doi: 10.1016/S0079-6123(10)83007-9

Outeiro, T. F., and Lindquist, S. (2003). Yeast cells provide insight into alpha-synuclein biology and pathobiology. *Science* 302, 1772–1775. doi: 10.1126/science.1090439

Paleologou, K. E., Oueslati, A., Shakked, G., Rospigliosi, C. C., Kim, H.-Y., Lamberto, G. R., et al. (2010). Phosphorylation at S87 is enhanced in synucleinopathies, inhibits alpha-synuclein oligomerization, and influences synuclein-membrane interactions. *J. Neurosci.* 30, 3184–3198. doi: 10.1523/JNEUROSCI.5922-09.2010

Pan, J., Dalzini, A., Khadka, N. K., Aryal, C. M., and Song, L. (2018). Lipid extraction by α-synuclein generates semi-transmembrane defects and lipoprotein nanoparticles. *ACS Omega* 3, 9586–9597. doi: 10.1021/acsomega.8b01462

Pavlou, M. A. S., Pinho, R., Paiva, I., and Outeiro, T. F. (2017). The yin and yang of α-synuclein-associated epigenetics in Parkinson's disease. *Brain* 140, 878–886. doi: 10.1093/brain/aww227

Peng, X. M. (2005). Alpha-Synuclein activation of protein phosphatase 2A reduces tyrosine hydroxylase phosphorylation in dopaminergic cells. *J. Cell Sci.* 118(Pt 15), 3523–3530. doi: 10.1242/jcs.02481

Periquet, M., Fulga, T., Myllykangas, L., Schlossmacher, M. G., and Feany, M. B. (2007). Aggregated alpha-synuclein mediates dopaminergic neurotoxicity in vivo. *J. Neurosci.* 27, 3338–3346. doi: 10.1523/JNEUROSCI.0285-07.2007

Perrin, R. J., Woods, W. S., Clayton, D. F., and George, J. M. (2000). Interaction of human α-synuclein and Parkinson's disease variants with phospholipids: structural analysis using site-directed mutagenesis. *J. Biol. Chem.* 275, 34393–34398. doi: 10.1074/jbc.M004851200

Perrin, R. J., Woods, W. S., Clayton, D. F., and George, J. M. (2001). Exposure to long chain polyunsaturated fatty acids triggers rapid multimerization of synucleins. *J. Biol. Chem.* 276, 41958–41962. doi: 10.1074/jbc.M105022200

Pineda, A., and Burré, J. (2017). Modulating membrane binding of α-synuclein as a therapeutic strategy. *Proc. Natl. Acad. Sci. U.S.A.* 114, 1223–1225. doi: 10.1073/pnas.1620159114

Pitcairn, C., Wani, W. Y., and Mazzulli, J. R. (2018). Dysregulation of the autophagic-lysosomal pathway in Gaucher and Parkinson's disease. *Neurobiol. Dis.* 122, 72–82. doi: 10.1016/j.nbd.2018.03.008

Polymeropoulos, M. H., Lavedan, C., Leroy, E., Ide, S. E., Dehejia, A., Dutra, A., et al. (1997). Mutation in the α-synuclein gene identified in families with Parkinson's disease. *Science* 276, 2045–2047. doi: 10.1126/science.276.5321.2045

Powers, R., Lei, S., Anandhan, A., Marshall, D. D., Worley, B., Cerny, R. L., et al. (2017). Metabolic investigations of the molecular mechanisms associated with Parkinson's disease. *Metabolites* 7:E22. doi: 10.3390/metabo7020022

Pozo Devoto, V. M., and Falzone, T. L. (2017). Mitochondrial dynamics in Parkinson's disease: a role for α-synuclein? *Dis. Model. Mech.* 10, 1075–1087. doi: 10.1242/dmm.026294

Puspita, L., Chung, S. Y., and Shim, J. W. (2017). Oxidative stress and cellular pathologies in Parkinson's disease. *Mol. Brain* 10:53. doi: 10.1186/s13041-017-0340-9

Qin, Z., Hu, D., Han, S., Reaney, S. H., Di Monte, D. A., and Fink, A. L. (2007). Effect of 4-hydroxy-2-nonenal modification on alpha-synuclein aggregation. *J. Biol. Chem.* 282, 5862–5870. doi: 10.1074/jbc.M608126200

Rappley, I., Gitler, A. D., Selvy, P. E., LaVoie, M. J., Levy, B. D., Brown, H. A., et al. (2009). Evidence that α-synuclein does not inhibit phospholipase D. *Biochemistry* 48, 1077–1083. doi: 10.1021/bi801871h

Reynolds, N. P., Soragni, A., Rabe, M., Verdes, D., Liverani, E., Handschin, S., et al. (2011). Mechanism of membrane interaction and disruption by α-synuclein. *J. Am. Chem. Soc.* 133, 19366–19375. doi: 10.1021/ja2029848

Riedel, M., Goldbaum, O., Wille, M., and Richter-Landsberg, C. (2011). Membrane lipid modification by docosahexaenoic acid (DHA) promotes the formation of alpha-synuclein inclusion bodies immunopositive for SUMO-1 in oligodendroglial cells after oxidative stress. *J. Mol. Neurosci.* 43, 290–302. doi: 10.1007/s12031-010-9439-5

Robotta, M., Cattani, J., Martins, J. C., Subramaniam, V., and Drescher, M. (2017). Alpha-synuclein disease mutations are structurally defective and locally affect membrane binding. *J. Am. Chem. Soc.* 139, 4254–4257. doi: 10.1021/jacs.6b05335

Rodriguez, J. A., Ivanova, M. I., Sawaya, M. R., Cascio, D., Reyes, F. E., Shi, D., et al. (2015). Structure of the toxic core of α-synuclein from invisible crystals. *Nature* 525, 486–490. doi: 10.1038/nature15368

Roy, A., and Pahan, K. (2011). Prospects of statins in Parkinson disease. *Neuroscientist* 17, 244–255. doi: 10.1177/1073858410385006

Ruipérez, V., Darios, F., and Davletov, B. (2010). Alpha-synuclein, lipids and Parkinson's disease. *Prog. Lipid Res.* 49, 420–428. doi: 10.1016/j.plipres.2010.05.004

Salvador, G. A. (2010). Iron in neuronal function and dysfunction. *Biofactors* 36, 103–110. doi: 10.1002/biof.80

Sánchez Campos, S., Alza, N. P., and Salvador, G. A. (2018). Lipid metabolism alterations in the neuronal response to A53T α-synuclein and Fe-induced injury. *Arch. Biochem. Biophys.* 655, 43–54. doi: 10.1016/j.abb.2018.08.007

Sánchez Campos, S., Diez, G. R., Oresti, G. M., and Salvador, G. A. (2015). Dopaminergic neurons respond to iron-induced oxidative stress by modulating lipid acylation and deacylation cycles. *PLoS One* 10:e0130726. doi: 10.1371/journal.pone.0130726

Savage, M. J., Goldberg, D. J., and Schacher, S. (1987). Absolute specificity for retrograde fast axonal transport displayed by lipid droplets originating in the axon of an identified Aplysia neuron in vitro. *Brain Res.* 406, 215–223. doi: 10.1016/0006-8993(87)90785-2

Schneider, S. A., and Bhatia, K. P. (2012). Syndromes of neurodegeneration with brain iron accumulation. *Semin. Pediatr. Neurol.* 19, 57–66. doi: 10.1016/j.spen.2012.03.005

Scott, D., and Roy, S. (2012). α-synuclein inhibits intersynaptic vesicle mobility and maintains recycling-pool homeostasis. *J. Neurosci.* 32, 10129–10135. doi: 10.1523/JNEUROSCI.0535-12.2012

Seet, R. C. S., Lee, C. Y. J., Lim, E. C. H., Tan, J. J. H., Quek, A. M. L., Chong, W. L., et al. (2010). Oxidative damage in Parkinson disease: measurement using accurate biomarkers. *Free Radic. Biol. Med.* 48, 560–566. doi: 10.1016/j.freeradbiomed.2009.11.026

Sere, Y. Y., Regnacq, M., Colas, J., and Berges, T. (2010). A *Saccharomyces cerevisiae* strain unable to store neutral lipids is tolerant to oxidative stress induced by α-synuclein. *Free Radic. Biol. Med.* 49, 1755–1764. doi: 10.1016/j.freeradbiomed.2010.09.007

Serhan, C. N., and Petasis, N. A. (2011). Resolvins and protectins in inflammation resolution. *Chem. Rev.* 111, 5922–5943. doi: 10.1021/cr100396c

Shaltiel-Karyo, R., Frenkel-Pinter, M., Egoz-Matia, N., Frydman-Marom, A., Shalev, D. E., Segal, D., et al. (2010). Inhibiting α-synuclein oligomerization by stable cell-penetrating β-synuclein fragments recovers phenotype of Parkinson's disease model flies. *PLoS One* 5:e13863. doi: 10.1371/journal.pone.0013863

Shamoto-Nagai, M., Hisaka, S., Naoi, M., and Maruyama, W. (2018). Modification of α-synuclein by lipid peroxidation products derived from polyunsaturated fatty acids promotes toxic oligomerization: its relevance to Parkinson disease. *J. Clin. Biochem. Nutr.* 62, 207–212. doi: 10.3164/jcbn.18-25

Sharon, R., Bar-Joseph, I., Frosch, M. P., Walsh, D. M., Hamilton, J. A., Selkoe, D. J., et al. (2003a). The formation of highly soluble oligomers of alpha-synuclein is regulated by fatty acids and enhanced in Parkinson's disease. *Neuron* 37, 583–595. doi: 10.1016/s0896-6273(03)00024-2

Sharon, R., Bar-Joseph, I., Mirick, G. E., Serhan, C. N., and Selkoe, D. J. (2003b). Altered fatty acid composition of dopaminergic neurons expressing α-synuclein and human brains with α-synucleinopathies. *J. Biol. Chem.* 278, 49874–49881. doi: 10.1074/jbc.M309127200

Sharon, R., Goldberg, M. S., Bar-Josef, I., Betensky, R. A., Shen, J., Selkoe, D. J., et al. (2001). α-Synuclein occurs in lipid-rich high molecular weight complexes, binds fatty acids, and shows homology to the fatty acid-binding proteins. *Proc. Natl. Acad. Sci. U.S.A.* 98, 9110–9115. doi: 10.1073/pnas.171300598

Shvadchak, V. V., Falomir-Lockhart, L. J., Yushchenko, D. A., and Jovin, T. M. (2011). Specificity and kinetics of alpha-synuclein binding to model membranes determined with fluorescent excited state intramolecular proton transfer (ESIPT) probe. *J. Biol. Chem.* 286, 13023–13032. doi: 10.1074/jbc.M110.204776

Singleton, A. B., Farrer, M., Johnson, J., Singleton, A., Hague, S., Kachergus, J., et al. (2003). α-synuclein locus triplication causes Parkinson's disease. *Science* 302:841. doi: 10.1126/science.1090278

Stöckl, M., Fischer, P., Wanker, E., and Herrmann, A. (2008). α-synuclein selectively binds to anionic phospholipids embedded in liquid-disordered domains. *J. Mol. Biol.* 375, 1394–1404. doi: 10.1016/j.jmb.2007.11.051

Su, L. J., Auluck, P. K., Outeiro, T. F., Yeger-Lotem, E., Kritzer, J. A., Tardiff, D. F., et al. (2010). Compounds from an unbiased chemical screen reverse both ER-to-Golgi trafficking defects and mitochondrial dysfunction in Parkinson's disease models. *Dis. Model. Mech.* 3, 194–208. doi: 10.1242/dmm.004267

Sumi-Akamaru, H., Beck, G., Shinzawa, K., Kato, S., Riku, Y., Yoshida, M., et al. (2016). High expression of α-synuclein in damaged mitochondria with PLA2G6 dysfunction. *Acta Neuropathol. Commun.* 4:27. doi: 10.1186/s40478-016-0298-3

Surguchev, A. A., and Surguchov, A. (2017). Synucleins and gene expression: ramblers in a crowd or cops regulating traffic? *Front. Mol. Neurosci.* 10:224. doi: 10.3389/fnmol.2017.00224

Surguchov, A., Palazzo, R. E., and Surgucheva, I. (2001). Gamma synuclein: subcellular localization in neuronal and non-neuronal cells and effect on signal transduction. *Cell Motil. Cytoskeleton* 49, 218–228. doi: 10.1002/cm.1035

Swant, J., Goodwin, J. S., North, A., Ali, A. A., Gamble-George, J., Chirwa, S., et al. (2011). α-synuclein stimulates a dopamine transporter-dependent chloride current and modulates the activity of the transporter. *J. Biol. Chem.* 286, 43933–43943. doi: 10.1074/jbc.M111.241232

Sztalryd, C., and Brasaemle, D. L. (2017). The perilipin family of lipid droplet proteins: gatekeepers of intracellular lipolysis. *Biochim. Biophys. Acta Mol. Cell Biol. Lipids* 1862(10 Pt B), 1221–1232. doi: 10.1016/j.bbalip.2017.07.009

Tashiro, M., Kojima, M., Kihara, H., Kasai, K., Kamiyoshihara, T., Uéda, K., et al. (2008). Characterization of fibrillation process of α-synuclein at the initial stage. *Biochem. Biophys. Res. Commun.* 369, 910–914. doi: 10.1016/j.bbrc.2008.02.127

Terakawa, M. S., Lee, Y. H., Kinoshita, M., Lin, Y., Sugiki, T., Fukui, N., et al. (2018). Membrane-induced initial structure of α-synuclein control its amyloidogenesis on model membranes. *Biochim. Biophys. Acta* 1860, 757–766. doi: 10.1016/j.bbamem.2017.12.011

Thiam, A. R., Antonny, B., Wang, J., Delacotte, J., Wilfling, F., Walther, T. C., et al. (2013). COPI buds 60-nm lipid droplets from reconstituted water-phospholipid-triacylglyceride interfaces, suggesting a tension clamp function. *Proc. Natl. Acad. Sci. U.S.A.* 110, 13244–13249. doi: 10.1073/pnas.1307685110

Tirinato, L., Pagliari, F., Limongi, T., Marini, M., Falqui, A., Seco, J., et al. (2017). An overview of lipid droplets in cancer and cancer stem cells. *Stem Cells Int.* 2017:1656053. doi: 10.1155/2017/1656053

Tosatto, L., Andrighetti, A. O., Plotegher, N., Antonini, V., Tessari, I., Ricci, L., et al. (2012). Alpha-synuclein pore forming activity upon membrane association. *Biochim. Biophys. Acta* 1818, 2876–2883. doi: 10.1016/j.bbamem.2012.07.007

Trostchansky, A., Lind, S., Hodara, R., Oe, T., Blair, I. A., Ischiropoulos, H., et al. (2006). Interaction with phospholipids modulates α-synuclein nitration and lipid–protein adduct formation. *Biochem. J.* 393(Pt 1), 343–349. doi: 10.1016/B978-0-12-409547-2.12460-6

Uversky, V. N., and Fink, A. L. (2002). Amino acid determinants of α-synuclein aggregation: putting together pieces of the puzzle. *FEBS Lett.* 522, 9–13. doi: 10.1016/S0014-5793(02)02883-1

van Meer, G., Voelker, D. R., and Feigenson, G. W. (2008). Membrane lipids: where they are and how they behave. *Nat. Rev. Mol. Cell Biol.* 9, 112–124. doi: 10.1038/nrm2330

van Rooijen, B. D., Claessens, M. M., and Subramaniam, V. (2009). Lipid bilayer disruption by oligomeric α-synuclein depends on bilayer charge and accessibility of the hydrophobic core. *Biochim. Biophys. Acta* 1788, 1271–1278. doi: 10.1016/j.bbamem.2009.03.010

Vargas, K. J., Makani, S., Davis, T., Westphal, C. H., Castillo, P. E., and Chandra, S. S. (2014). Synucleins regulate the kinetics of synaptic vesicle endocytosis. *J. Neurosci.* 34, 9364–9376. doi: 10.1523/JNEUROSCI.4787-13.2014

Vasquez, A. M., Mouchlis, V. D., and Dennis, E. A. (2018). Review of four major distinct types of human phospholipase A2. *Adv. Biol. Regul.* 67, 212–218. doi: 10.1016/j.jbior.2017.10.009

Velázquez, A. P., Tatsuta, T., Ghillebert, R., Drescher, I., and Graef, M. (2016). Lipid droplet-mediated ER homeostasis regulates autophagy and cell survival during starvation. *J. Cell Biol.* 212, 621–631. doi: 10.1083/jcb.201508102

Volta, M., Lavdas, A. A., Obergasteiger, J., Überbacher, C., Picard, A., Pramstaller, P. P., et al. (2017). Elevated levels of alpha-synuclein blunt cellular signal transduction downstream of Gq protein-coupled receptors. *Cell. Signal.* 30, 82–91. doi: 10.1016/j.cellsig.2016.11.012

Voshol, P. J., Dennis, R. J., Buchman, V. L., Oort, P. J., Ninkina, N., Guschina, I. A., et al. (2012). Increased lipolysis and altered lipid homeostasis protect γ-synuclein-null mutant mice from diet-induced obesity. *Proc. Natl. Acad. Sci. U.S.A.* 109, 20943–20948. doi: 10.1073/pnas.1210022110

Wakamatsu, M., Ishii, A., Iwata, S., Sakagami, J., Ukai, Y., Ono, M., et al. (2008). Selective loss of nigral dopamine neurons induced by overexpression of truncated human α-synuclein in mice. *Neurobiol. Aging* 29, 574–585. doi: 10.1016/j.neurobiolaging.2006.11.017

Wang, L., Das, U., Scott, D. A., Tang, Y., McLean, P. J., and Roy, S. (2014). α-Synuclein multimers cluster synaptic vesicles and attenuate recycling. *Curr. Biol.* 24, 2319–2326. doi: 10.1016/j.cub.2014.08.027

Wang, W., Perovic, I., Chittuluru, J., Kaganovich, A., Nguyen, L. T. T., Liao, J., et al. (2011). A soluble α-synuclein construct forms a dynamic tetramer. *Proc. Natl. Acad. Sci. U.S.A.* 108, 17797–17802. doi: 10.1073/pnas.1113260108

Watanabe, H., Hongu, T., Yamazaki, M., and Kanaho, Y. (2011). Phospholipase D2 activation by p38 MAP kinase is involved in neurite outgrowth. *Biochem. Biophys. Res. Commun.* 413, 288–293. doi: 10.1016/j.bbrc.2011.08.088

Waxman, E. A., Mazzulli, J. R., and Giasson, B. I. (2009). Characterization of hydrophobic residue requirements for α-synuclein fibrillization. *Biochemistry* 48, 9427–9436. doi: 10.1021/bi900539p

Welte, M. A. (2015). Expanding roles for lipid droplets. *Curr. Biol.* 25, R470–R481. doi: 10.1016/j.cub.2015.04.004

Welte, M. A., and Gould, A. P. (2017). Lipid droplet functions beyond energy storage. *Biochim. Biophys. Acta Mol. Cell Biol. Lipids* 1862(10 Pt B), 1260–1272. doi: 10.1016/j.bbalip.2017.07.006

Wietek, J., Haralampiev, I., Amoussouvi, A., Herrmann, A., and Stöckl, M. (2013). Membrane bound α-synuclein is fully embedded in the lipid bilayer while segments with higher flexibility remain. *FEBS Lett.* 587, 2572–2577. doi: 10.1016/j.febslet.2013.06.034

Wilhelm, B. G., Mandad, S., Truckenbrodt, S., Kröhnert, K., Schäfer, C., Rammner, B., et al. (2014). Composition of isolated synaptic boutons reveals the amounts of vesicle trafficking proteins. *Science* 344, 1023–1028. doi: 10.1126/science.1252884

Winner, B., Jappelli, R., Maji, S. K., Desplats, P. A., Boyer, L., Aigner, S., et al. (2011). In vivo demonstration that α-synuclein oligomers are toxic. *Proc. Natl. Acad. Sci. U.S.A.* 108, 4194–4199. doi: 10.1073/pnas.1100976108

Wood, S. J., Wypych, J., Steavenson, S., Louis, J. C., Citron, M., and Biere, A. L. (1999). α-Synuclein fibrillogenesis is nucleation-dependent. Implications for the pathogenesis of Parkinson's disease. *J. Biol. Chem.* 274, 19509–19512. doi: 10.1074/jbc.274.28.19509

Yakunin, E., Loeb, V., Kisos, H., Biala, Y., Yehuda, S., Yaari, Y., et al. (2012). α-Synuclein neuropathology is controlled by nuclear hormone receptors and enhanced by docosahexaenoic acid in a mouse model for Parkinson's disease. *Brain Pathol.* 22, 280–294. doi: 10.1111/j.1750-3639.2011.00530.x

Yeger-Lotem, E., Riva, L., Su, L. J., Gitler, A. D., Cashikar, A. G., King, O. D., et al. (2009). Bridging high-throughput genetic and transcriptional data reveals cellular responses to alpha-synuclein toxicity. *Nat. Genet.* 41, 316–323. doi: 10.1038/ng.337

Ysselstein, D., Joshi, M., Mishra, V., Griggs, A. M., Asiago, J. M., McCabe, G. P., et al. (2015). Effects of impaired membrane interactions on α-synuclein aggregation and neurotoxicity. *Neurobiol. Dis.* 79, 150–163. doi: 10.1016/j.nbd.2015.04.007

Zaltieri, M., Grigoletto, J., Longhena, F., Navarria, L., Favero, G., Castrezzati, S., et al. (2015). α-synuclein and synapsin III cooperatively regulate synaptic function in dopamine neurons. *J. Cell Sci.* 128, 2231–2243. doi: 10.1242/jcs.157867

Zarranz, J. J., Alegre, J., Gómez-Esteban, J. C., Lezcano, E., Ros, R., Ampuero, I., et al. (2004). The new mutation, E46K, of α-synuclein causes Parkinson and lewy body dementia. *Ann. Neurol.* 55, 164–173. doi: 10.1002/ana.10795

Zhou, Q., Yen, A., Rymarczyk, G., Asai, H., Trengrove, C., Aziz, N., et al. (2016). Impairment of PARK14-dependent Ca2+ signalling is a novel determinant of Parkinson's disease. *Nat. Commun.* 7:10332. doi: 10.1038/ncomms10332

Zhu, M., Li, J., and Fink, A. L. (2003). The association of α-synuclein with membranes affects bilayer structure, stability, and fibril formation. *J. Biol. Chem.* 278, 40186–40197. doi: 10.1074/jbc.M305326200

5

# The *WWOX* Gene Influences Cellular Pathways in the Neuronal Differentiation of Human Neural Progenitor Cells

*Katarzyna Kośla*, Elżbieta Płuciennik, Ewa Styczeń-Binkowska, Magdalena Nowakowska, Magdalena Orzechowska and Andrzej K. Bednarek*

*Department of Molecular Carcinogenesis, Medical University of Łódź, Łódź, Poland*

***Correspondence:**
*Katarzyna Kośla*
*katarzyna.kosla@umed.lodz.pl*

The brain is the most functionally organized structure of all organs. It manages behavior, perception and higher cognitive functions. The *WWOX* gene is non-classical tumor suppressor gene, which has been shown to have an impact on proliferation, apoptosis and migration processes. Moreover, genetic aberrations in *WWOX* induce severe neuropathological phenotypes in humans and rodents. The aim of the present study was to investigate in detail the impact of *WWOX* on human neural progenitor cell (hNPC) maintenance and how depletion of *WWOX* disturbs signaling pathways playing a pivotal role in neuronal differentiation and central nervous system (CNS) organogenesis. hNPC with a silenced *WWOX* gene exhibited lowered mitochondrial redox potential, enhanced adhesion to fibronectin and extracellular matrix protein mixture, downregulation of MMP2/9 expression and impaired 3D growth. Global transcriptome analysis using cap analysis of gene expression (CAGE) found that *WWOX* downregulation significantly changes the expression of multiple genes engaged in cytoskeleton organization, adhesion, cell signaling and chromatin remodeling. The massive changes in gene expression caused by *WWOX* silencing may strongly affect the differentiation and migration of neurons in organogenesis, brain injury, cancerogenesis or neurodifferentiation. *WWOX* gene appears to be an important regulator of neural tissue architecture and function.

**Keywords: *WWOX*, neural progenitor cells, neuronal differentiation, neurodegeneration, WOREE, SCAR, CAGE**

## INTRODUCTION

The *WWOX* gene is an important transcription regulator. It is known to regulate the activity of a number of transcription factors, including Jun, AP2gamma, NFkappaB, ErbB4 (Aqeilan et al., 2004a, 2005; Gaudio et al., 2006; Chen et al., 2013). It has been found to have tumor suppressor activity, and recent studies have investigated its potential new physiological roles in DNA repair and glucose metabolism (Aqeilan et al., 2005; Abu-Remaileh and Aqeilan, 2014; Iatan et al., 2014). In addition to steroid-hormone regulated tissues like those in the testis, ovary and breast, the *WWOX* gene also shows high expression in the brain and cerebellum (Nunez et al., 2006). Loss of correct *WWOX* expression is a common event associated with cancer promotion, progression and resistance to treatment (Płuciennik et al., 2006, 2014; Dias et al., 2007; Donati et al., 2007; Wang et al., 2011; Lan et al., 2012; Sun et al., 2017; Seabra et al., 2018). Unlike classic suppressor genes, the loss of functionality of only one *WWOX* allele is sufficient to increase the chance of cancerogenesis (haploinsufficiency).

WWOX has also been found to play a significant role in glioblastoma (GBM), the most malignant brain tumor. It has been shown that loss of heterozygosity, a relatively frequent occurrence in GBM, along with promoter methylation may decrease the expression of the *WWOX* gene. Our experiment also revealed a correlation between the expression of *WWOX* and that of *Bcl2*, *Ki67*, and *ErbB4* in this type of cancer (Kosla et al., 2011). Further investigations have found *WWOX* expression to modulate the global profile of gene expression in the GBM T98G cell line, and increased *WWOX* expression makes its phenotype less malignant. Cells with ectopically expressed *WWOX* demonstrate significantly different transcription profiles among almost 3000 genes, with WNT, TGFβ, Notch and Hedgehog being the main cellular pathways affected; all of these are involved both in GBM carcinogenesis and neural differentiation. Moreover, the *WWOX*-transfected GBM cells presented greatly altered biological characteristics, lowered proliferation, adhesion and impaired 3D growth (Kośla et al., 2014).

Recent evidence suggests that *WWOX* may play a regulatory role in central nervous system (CNS) development and functioning (Chen et al., 2004; Lo et al., 2008; Suzuki et al., 2009; Tabarki et al., 2015a; Liu et al., 2018; Shaukat et al., 2018; Hussain et al., 2019). Complete loss of WWOX protein function in knock-out mice results in epilepsy and balance disturbances. The animals show progressive susceptibility to spontaneous and audiogenic tonic-clonic epilepsy, which is indicative of a neurodegenerative process (Mallaret et al., 2014). Suzuki et al. (2009) report the presence of a spontaneous homozygous 13-bp deletion in exon 9 of the *WWOX* gene that has also been found in *Ide/Ide* rats. This deletion results in a frameshift in the C-terminus of the WWOX protein and may influence protein stability, since WWOX protein was undetectable in the hippocampus of the *Ide/Ide* rats. In addition to various abnormalities, such as dwarfism, postnatal lethality and male hypogonadism, the animals also display a high incidence of epilepsy, ataxic gait, audiogenic seizures and many vacuoles in the hippocampus and amygdala, indicating the progression of neurodegeneration (Suzuki et al., 2009). There is a strong overlap between the symptoms present in KO *WWOX* rodent models and those observed in humans. The genetic aberrations in the *WWOX* locus has been linked with two human neuropathological phenotypes: Spinocerebellar ataxia, autosomal recessive 12 (SCAR12, MIM 614322) and WWOX-Related Epileptic Encephalopathy/Early Infantile Epileptic Encephalopathy 28 (WOREE/EIEE28, MIM 616211). All known patients suffering from SCAR12 carry a homozygous missense mutation in *WWOX* coding region (139C > A or 1114G > C) that causes a partial loss of gene function, with the resulting substitutions placed in the WW1 protein–protein interaction domain and in the SDR (short-chain dehydrogenase/reductase) domain, respectively. These mutations affect the ability of the protein to bind to its cellular partners and may reduce its catalytic activity. The WOREE patients exhibiting more severe neurological disorders harbor nonsense/frameshift mutations and/or robust deletions of whole exons of *WWOX* gene (Mignot et al., 2015; Tabarki et al., 2015b; Elsaadany et al., 2016; Piard et al., 2018).

Overall, reports describing neural aberrations connected with disruption of *WWOX locus* in humans and animals indicate that germline loss-of-function of *WWOX* leads to serious developmental deficiency in the neural system.

The *WWOX* gene was found to be also involved in neurodegenerative Alzheimer's disease. The level of WWOX protein is much lower in the hippocampal neurons of those suffering from Alzheimer's disease in comparison to healthy individuals (Sze et al., 2004; Teng et al., 2012). Moreover, *in vitro* studies of *WWOX* silencing in neuronal cells have resulted in spontaneous Tau phosphorylation and accumulation of neurofibrillary tangles (NFTs). It has been confirmed that WWOX interacts with GSK3β, ERK and other kinases inhibiting the phosphorylation of Tau and preventing NFTs formation and cell death. The role of WWOX as a Tau phosphorylation regulator is important not only in the context of neurodegeneration, but also neuronal differentiation, where the Tau protein takes part in microtubule assembly and neurite outgrowth. The level of *WWOX* expression was shown to decrease with age and is significantly lower in middle-aged individuals (Sze et al., 2004; Wang et al., 2012).

To date, WWOX has been experimentally shown to act as a regulator of several transcription factors, including p73 (considered as one of the main regulators of CNS organogenesis), ErbB4, Met, c-Jun, Gli1, and AP-2 (Aqeilan et al., 2004a,b, 2005; Gaudio et al., 2006; Matteucci et al., 2009; Xiong et al., 2014). The shared mechanism of regulation is based on partner protein sequestration in the cytoplasm. Upon binding to WWOX, the locked transcription factors are unable to translocate to the nucleus and activate their target genes. A set of 240 proteins thought to be able to bind with WWOX has been given by Abu-Odeh et al. (2014). An analysis of potential WWOX partners shows that the protein can affect pathways critical for neuronal differentiation, such as Notch, Hippo, Wnt, and TGFβ, which are also disturbed in the course of brain cancer.

So far, the molecular mechanism by which WWOX regulates nerve cell functioning is largely unknown. It has been suggested that *WWOX* may influence the CNS by regulating the proteins taking part in neuronal differentiation, through negative regulation of GSK3β, and apoptosis, probably via the mitochondrial pathway by downregulating apoptotic inhibitors Bcl2 and Bcl-xL. WWOX has also been shown to influence the action of such neural pathways as Wnt (Dvl-2), TGFβ (TIAF1, SMAD3, and SMAD7), Hedgehog (Gli1) by interacting with their constituent proteins (Bouteille et al., 2009; Ferguson et al., 2013; Xiong et al., 2014; Chiang et al., 2015; Hsu et al., 2016). A recent study on WWOX KO mice by Hussain et al. (2019) found that lack of the protein leads to a reduction of GABA-ergic hippocampal neurons and a lowered level of GABA synthesis.

The described neuropathological phenotypes arising from genetic aberrations of the *WWOX* locus demonstrates the importance of the gene in CNS development and functioning. Although *WWOX* mutations found in SCAR12 or WOREE are very rare, possibly because of intrauteral lethality, changes in its expression are very common in pathological states like Alzheimer's disease or GBM.

The development of the CNS is a highly organized process consisting of neurogenesis, neuron migration, synaptogenesis and gliogenesis, which is controlled at multiple levels. It is likely that the WWOX protein is involved in at least some of these steps. Briefly, the process of cytoskeleton reorganization requires a complex configuration of intrinsic and extrinsic cues involving the action of membrane and ECM proteins, which triggers specific signaling pathways. Its details are still poorly understood and await further investigation. Our findings indicate that the silencing of WWOX in human neural progenitors results in significant changes in the regulation of genes encoding membrane/ECM, cell signaling, chromatin condensation and cytoskeleton proteins.

The study examines which specific genes and cellular pathways are influenced by WWOX in human neural progenitor cells (hNPC) and how *WWOX* affects their biological properties and differentiation. *WWOX* expression was silenced in the hNPC line, and the cells were tested for their ECM adhesion ability, mitochondrial potential and 3D growth; in addition, a global gene expression analysis was conducted with next generation sequencing (NGS).

## MATERIALS AND METHODS

### Cell Line and Culture Conditions

The human neural stem cells (hNSC, Thermo Fisher Scientific) are derived from H9 embryonic stem cells (hESC). According to manufacturer description they have the potential to differentiate into neurons, astrocytes and oligodendrocytes. The cells were cultured as an adherent culture in vessels coated with ECM protein mixture (Geltrex, Thermo Fisher Scientific). The cells were maintained in KnockOut™ DMEM/F-12 Medium supplemented with 20 ng/ml EGF, FGFb, StemPro Neural Supplement (Thermo Fisher Scientific) and Antibiotic-Antimycotic (Gibco) and handled according to the supplier recommendations.

Spontaneous differentiation of the cells was triggered by culturing in medium without the addition of EGF and FGFb growth factors for 14 days. Although the supplier claims that the cells are able to differentiate into neurons, astrocytes and oligodendrocytes upon growth factor removal, in our conditions all the cells were found to undergo differentiation into neurons, which was confirmed by immunocytochemistry. All differentiated cells were found to be positive for neuronal markers MAP2 and TUJ1 and negative for astrocytes - GFAP or oligodendrocytes - GalC markers (**Supplementary Figure S2**). This suggests that the cells lose their multipotence and instead of being neural stem cells are rather a neural progenitors (hNPC) and were regarded in this study as such.

The 2D differentiation assays were conducted on Geltrex coated vessels, and neuron maturity was assessed by immunocytochemistry with antibodies against neuronal marker MAP2. For a 3D culture assay, 16,000, 25,000, and 35,000 cells were seeded on a solidified 2 mm layer of growth factor-reduced Geltrex basement membrane matrix (Thermo Fisher Scientific).

In every conducted experiment the cells from both experimental variants were in the same, low passage number.

### *WWOX* Gene Silencing

The *WWOX* gene was silenced by a shRNA lentiviral delivery system (Santa Cruz Biotechnology). The control cells were transduced with the same type of vector harboring scrambled shRNA sequence instead of targeting investigated gene. Target cells were seeded at a density of $5 \times 10^4$ cells/cm$^2$, and the next day, were infected with the virus suspension in culturing medium supplemented with polybrene 5 μg/ml (Sigma-Aldrich). After 24 h, the transduction mixture was removed and replaced with regular medium. The stable transductants were selected with 0.4 μg/ml puromycin. The gene silencing efficiency was assessed with Western blot.

### Western Blot

The cellular proteins were extracted with RIPA buffer supplemented with protease inhibitor cocktail, PMSF and Na-orthovanadate (Santa Cruz Biotechnology). Briefly, 60 μg of protein was resolved on SDS-PAGE and transferred to PVDF membrane. After blocking in 5% non-fat milk, membranes were incubated overnight in 4°C with a primary antibody, anti-WWOX (Thermo Fisher Scientific). After 1-h incubation with a suitable secondary antibody conjugated with alkaline phosphatase (Sigma-Aldrich), the membranes were developed with Novex AP Chromogenic Substrate (Thermo Fisher Scientific). The ImageJ software was used for densitometric analysis of protein amount, adjusted to GAPDH as a reference protein.

### Immunocytochemistry

The cells were fixed with ice cold ethanol:acetic acid (95:5) solution for 10 min. After a double wash with DPBS, unspecific antibody binding was blocked with blocking buffer (2% BSA, 1% donkey serum, and 0.1% Triton-X100). Next step was incubation with the primary antibodies (Millipore, Thermo Fisher Scientific) 1:200 solution in 5% donkey serum, 4°C, overnight. After double washing with DPBS, the cells were incubated with secondary antibodies (donkey, Alexa Fluor 488/594 conjugated), diluted 1:1000. The nuclei were counterstained with DAPI and the cells were imagined with FLoid Cell Imaging System (Thermo Fisher Scientific).

### Adhesion Assays

The cells were seeded on 96-well plate coated with Geltrex (Gibco) at a density of 17,500 cells/well. The adhesion to fibronectin was assessed on 48-well fibronectin-coated plate (BD). The cells were seeded at a density of 100,000 cells/well. The cells were incubated for 90 min at 37°C. Next the cells were washed with PBS and adherent cells were stained with Cell Stain Solution (Cell Biolabs, Inc.). The stain was dissolved in Extraction Solution (Cell Biolabs, Inc.) and the absorbance was read with a plate reader (BioTek), $\lambda = 570$ nm.

## Zymography

The level of metalloproteinase 2 and 9 was examined by gelatin zymography. The cells were cultured on a six-well plate for 48 h and the culture medium was collected for protein analysis. Protein concentration was measured with a Qubit Protein Assay with Qubit 2.0 fluorometer (Thermo Fisher Scientific). A total of 2 μg protein extracts was loaded and separated on 10% SDS-PAGE gel prepared with addition of 2 mg/ml gelatin. The gel was washed with Triton X-100 and incubated in a developing buffer (0.5 M Tris–HCl, 2 M NaCl, 50 mM CaCl 2, pH 7.5) at 37°C for 18 h. Next, it was stained with Coomassie Brilliant Blue R-250 and incubated in destaining buffer (methanol: acetic acid: water, 3:1:6) to visualize white bands on a blue background where gelatinolytic metalloproteinases were active. The active or inactive form of MMP2 and 9 was identified according to protein marker separated on the same gel. The amount of the proteins was assessed with ImageJ software, based on the area of the clear band.

## Redox Assay

The mitochondrial metabolic activity was measured using PrestoBlue reagent (resazurin based, Thermo Fisher Scientific). Cells were seeded on 96-well white, clear-bottom 96-well plate at a density of 20,000 cells/well. PrestoBlue was added to fresh medium 18 h post seeding and the cells were incubated in 37°C. The fluorescence of resorufin obtained by reduction of resazurin in mitochondria was measured in intervals for 5 h with Victor X4 plate reader (PerkinElmer), excitation $\lambda = 550$ nm.

## Statistical Analysis of Biological Assays

The results of the adhesion, mitochondrial redox potential and zymography procedures are presented as means. The normality of data distribution was verified with Shapiro–Wilk Normality Test and the statistical relevance was evaluated with unpaired *t*-test. The results are described as significant when $p < 0.05$.

## CAGE Gene Expression Analysis

The gene expression profile of 2D cultured undifferentiated and differentiated cells were analyzed with cap analysis of gene expression (CAGE) technique.

The libraries for sequencing were prepared according to Carnici, described in detail elsewhere (Takahashi et al., 2012). Briefly, polyadenylated and non-polyadenylated RNA was reverse transcribed into cDNA with the use of a random prime-containing *Eco*P15I sequence. The next step was biotinylation of the cap site and the 3′ ends of the hybridized RNAs. Non-hybridized ssRNAs were digested and the 5′ complete cDNAs hybridized to biotin-tagged, cap-containing RNAs were separated on streptavidin-coated magnetic beads. cDNA was released from RNA and a double-stranded 5′ linker with a barcode and *Eco*P15I sequences was ligated. Subsequently, using the biotinylated 2nd SOL primer, a second strand cDNA was synthetized. The digestion with *Eco*P15I allowed 27 bp fragments to be cleaved inside the 5′ end of the cDNA. At the 3′ end of the cDNA, a 3′ linker with 3′ Illumina primer sequence was ligated. Following this, the constructed CAGE tags were amplified and purified. The prepared libraries were sequenced on an Illumina HiSeq System. The data was then analyzed in-house. The raw data from CAGE experiment are deposited in NCBI Gene Expression Omnibus (GEO) Database with accession number GSE126075.

## Data Processing

The obtained CAGE data was processed by the MOIRAI system (Hasegawa et al., 2014), a GUI-based workflow system allowing quality control and further data transformation into multiple file formats for subsequent expression analyses. Briefly, raw input was split by barcode, following which, sequences of low quality (with base N) were removed and processed via BWA to output BAM files. Primarily, the GRCh37/hg19 assembly was used as a reference human genome; however, the data was reprocessed through UCSC liftOver tool (Kuhn et al., 2013) to convert the genomic coordinates of CAGE peaks into current GRCh38/hg38 assembly and make the data meaningful for the recent genome version. Subsequently, CAGE output was analyzed with CAGEr (Haberle et al., 2015), a Bioconductor package enabling preprocessing, identification and normalization of transcription start sites (TSS) and downstream analysis of the promoterome based upon CAGE sequencing with the BSgenome.Hsapiens.UCSC.hg38 package as a referent genome (Pagès, 2018). Analysis was performed according to Haberle and Plessy[1]. In brief, raw CAGE tag counts were normalized with simple TPM method, TSS were clustered into tag clusters corresponding to individual promoters using paraclu clustering algorithm and mapped to known promoters using CAGE peaks identified as true TSS by TSS classifier available at FANTOM5 repository (Lizio et al., 2015) (GRCh38/hg38 assembly).

## Global Biological Differentiation – Gene Set Enrichment Analysis

Global differences between hNPC with silenced *WWOX* expression and controls before and after differentiation were determined in terms of gene ontology (GO), such as biological processes (BP), by applying the gene set enrichment analysis (GSEA) algorithm. Enrichment analysis was performed for 9427 genes between shWWOX and shScrambled, classified as phenotype labels separately for hNPC and neurons through *t*-test with a weighted scoring scheme and a permutation type regarding phenotype. Significance threshold was set as FDR < 0.25.

## Protein–Protein Interaction Analysis

The interaction relationships of the proteins encoded by the differentially expressed genes were searched and visualized with the Search Tool for the Retrieval of Interacting Genes (STRING) Plug-in (version 1.4.0)[2] in Cytoscape software (version 3.6.1)[3]. All the parameters were set as default values, and the confidence (combined score) ≥ 0.4 was used as the cut off criterion.

---

[1] http://bioconductor.org/packages/release/bioc/vignettes/CAGEr/inst/doc/CAGEexp.html

[2] http://www.string-db.org

[3] http://www.cytoscape.org

## Principle Component Analysis

Dimensional grouping investigating hNPC phenotypes according to a set of selected genes was performed using principle component analysis (PCA). The analysis involved 362 genes of several oxidative stress response/antioxidant defense/oxygen species activity connected groups form The Molecular Signatures Database (MSigDB)[4], a collection of annotated gene sets. The PCA was conducted to determine the contribution of particular genes into partitioning of cell genotype across first and second dimensions (dim1 and dim2) with the oxidative gene set as an active variable. All analyses were performed using FactoMineR and Factoextra R packages.

## RESULTS

An analysis of NGS data deposited in the RIKEN Fantom5 Project data repository[5] indicates that the level of *WWOX* expression in the human brain varies according to location (**Figure 1**). The highest levels are observed in the corpus callosum and medulla oblongata, and the lowest in the postcentral and paracentral gyrus. Moreover, adults display greater *WWOX* expression in the brain as a whole than 20–33 weeks fetuses, 17.7 TPM RLE (tags per million, relative log expression) vs. 9.2 TPM RLE.

In the present study, the hNPC cells were transduced with lentiviral shRNA vector. After confirmation of *WWOX* gene silencing by Western blot (**Supplementary Figure S1**) the hNPC/shWWOX cells and control hNPC/shScrambled were cultured either as a 2D monolayer culture using plates coated with a thin layer of diluted Geltrex or as a 3D culture in a thick (2–3 mm) Geltrex scaffold. Next, the cells were used in a number of biological experiments, and global analysis of transcriptome was performed using CAGE.

[4]http://software.broadinstitute.org/gsea/msigdb/index.jsp

[5]http://fantom.gsc.riken.jp/

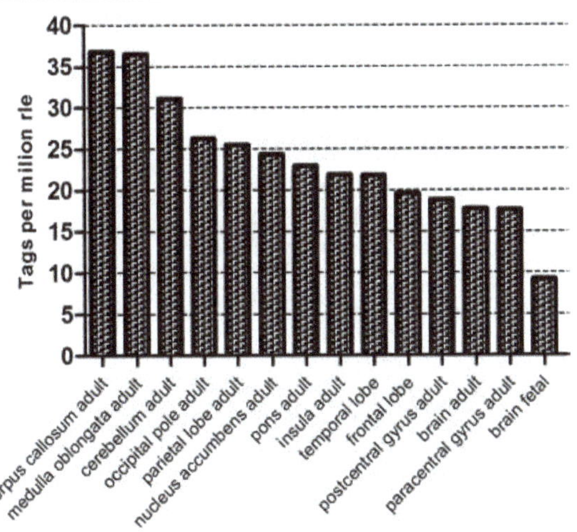


**FIGURE 1 |** The *WWOX* gene expression level in different human brain compartment (Fantom 5, Zenbu, Riken). The counts were normalized as TPM (tags per million) after scaling by normalization factors calculated by RLE (relative log expression) method.

## *WWOX* Depletion Alters the Main Biological Functions of hNPC

A number of biological differences were observed between the hNPC cells with silenced *WWOX* and controls.

*WWOX* silencing reduced the mitochondrial redox activity of the cells (**Figure 2**) and strongly affected their adhesion to ECM proteins. The hNPC cells with silenced *WWOX* demonstrated considerably stronger adhesion to the ECM protein mixture ($p$ = 0.0626) and to fibronectin alone ($p < 0.05$) (**Figure 3**).

It was also found that downregulation of *WWOX* lowered pro-MMP2 and pro-MMP9 metalloproteinase secretion (**Figure 4**).

Most striking was that in 3D culture, the hNPC with silenced *WWOX* remained as isolated, single cells that did not proliferate nor differentiate, while cells with unaltered *WWOX* expression differentiated and exhibited extensive network formation (**Figures 5, 6**). This observation was confirmed in three separate experiments and was not influenced by the seeding density (data not shown). No such phenomenon was observed when the cells were cultured in 2D as a monolayer (**Figure 7**).

## Functional Enrichment Analysis

The global gene expression was assessed in the hNPC with the silenced *WWOX* expression and the control group before and after differentiation by CAGE. Whole transcriptome sequencing revealed global changes in the regulation of a number of pivotal cellular pathways and functions. It was found that 2282 genes were differentially expressed between hNPC/shScrambled and hNPC/sh*WWOX* (log2 FC > ±1, $p < 0.05$) and 7392 differed between differentiated neurons/shScrambled and neurons/sh*WWOX*. To identify global biological changes between cells with different *WWOX* status, enrichment analysis was performed within GO BP using a GSEA algorithm. The top five most altered BP classified according to GO terms are presented in **Table 1** and includes adhesion, neural migration and differentiation. Significantly greater numbers of enriched gene sets was found for undifferentiated cells (44 for hNPC/shScrambled and 109 for hNPC/sh*WWOX*, FDR < 0.25) than for differentiated neurons (no gene sets for neurons/shScrambled and four sets in neurons/sh*WWOX*). The

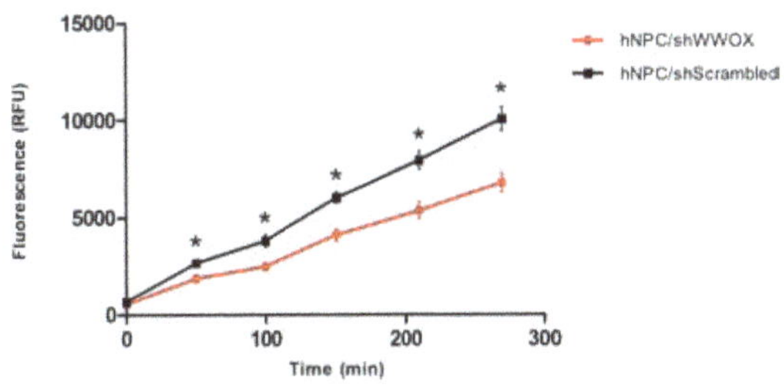


**FIGURE 2 |** Mitochondrial redox activity tested by PrestoBlue® assay based on colorimetric measurement of resofurin, *$p < 0.05$.

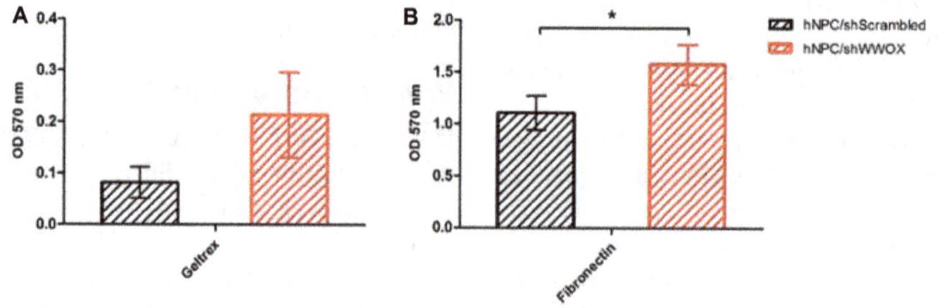


**FIGURE 3 |** Adhesion of *WWOX* silenced hNPC cells to ECM protein mixture (Geltrex, **A**), the tendency not reaching the statistical significance (0.0626) and to fibronectin **(B)**, $*p < 0.05$.

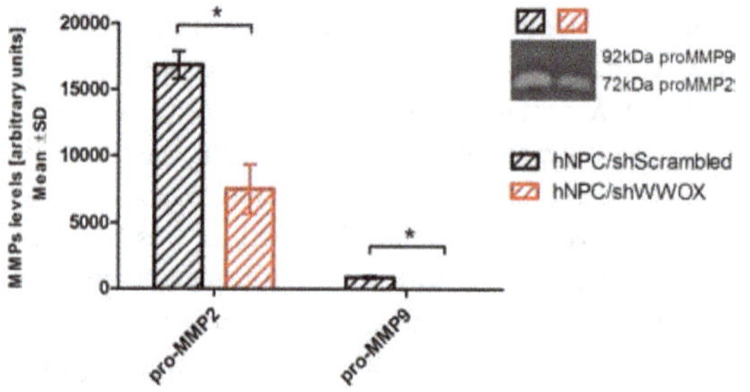


**FIGURE 4 |** Gelatin zymography analysis showing the level of pro-MMP2 (72 kDa) and pro-MMP9 (92 kDa) secreted by control and WWOX-silenced hNPC, $*p < 0.05$.

detailed results are available as **Supplementary Tables S2, S3.** Enrichment plots for selected gene sets are given in **Figure 8**.

The GSEA showed that *WWOX* silencing causes substantial gene expression reorganization. We found dualistic enrichment of GO_Stem_Cell_Differentiation gene set in both phenotypes (**Figure 8B**). In the hNPC/shScrambled the leading edge subset (considered as the most upregulated and promising genes) included LOXL3, JAG1, SOX21, ERBB4, KITLG, GPM6A, EFNB1, FGF10, NRG1, WWTR1, RUNX2, LAMA5, MSI2, SEMA4D, BCHE, FOXC1, SMAD4, SEMA5A, SEMA5B, SEMA6C, SEMA3A, SEMA6A, SEMA3C, GSK3B, BMP7, SFRP1, SEMA4F, and SEMA4B, whereas the hNPC/sh*WWOX* leading edge subset included HHEX, FGFR2, GBX2, SNAI1, GREM1, MSX2, and MSX1.

## Protein–Protein Interaction Network Analysis

Based on information from the STRING database, the protein–protein global interaction network was constructed with Log2 fold change of differentially expressed genes belonging to gene sets related to membrane proteins, cytoskeleton and cell signaling. The selected genes encode proteins that play an important role in the steps of CNS development –

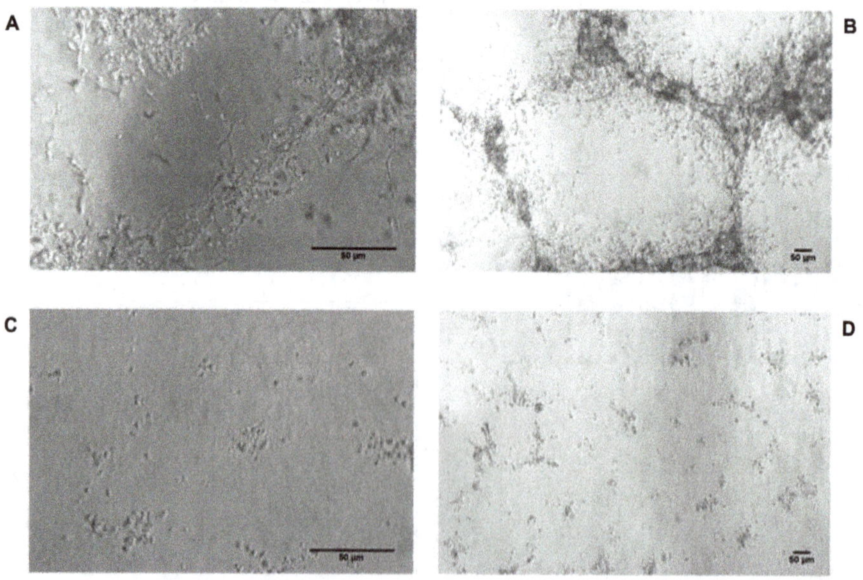


**FIGURE 5 |** hNPC cells cultured for 8 days in thick 3D Geltrex (ECM protein mixture) layer. **(A,B)** hNPC/shScrambled, 200× and 40×, respectively. **(C,D)** hNPC/shWWOX, 200× and 40×, respectively.

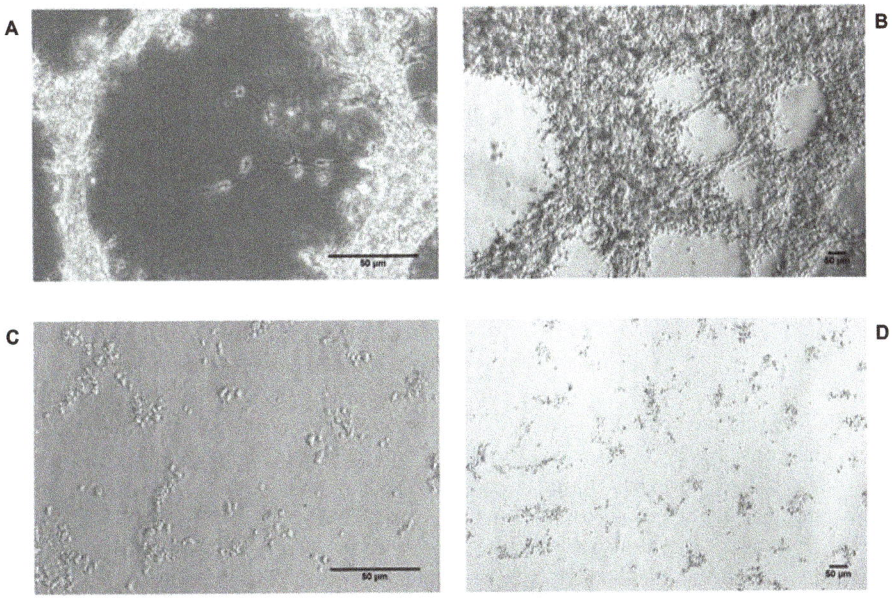

**FIGURE 6 |** hNPC cells cultured for 19 days in thick 3D Geltrex (ECM protein mixture) layer. **(A,B)** hNPC/shScrambled, 200× and 40×, respectively. **(C,D)** hNPC/shWWOX, 200× and 40×, respectively.

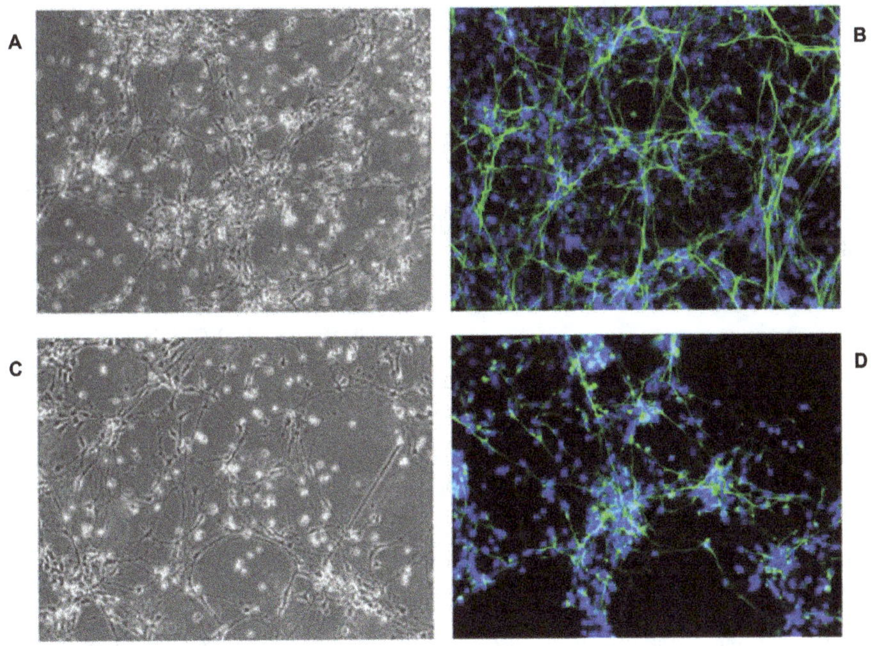

**FIGURE 7 |** hNPC cells cultured for 18 days in 2D ECM protein mixture coated vessels, 200×. **(A,B)** hNPC/shScrambled, **(C,D)** hNPC/shWWOX, green MAP2 neuronal marker, blue DAPI nucleus counterstain.

neurogenesis, neuron migration, and synaptogenesis. The constructed network comprised of 198 nodes and 1113 edges (**Figure 9**; for details see **Supplementary Figure S3**). **Figure 10** presents protein-protein interaction networks of genes which are differentially expressed between undifferentiated hNPC (A) and differentiated neurons (B). In hNPC, the most significantly upregulated genes (Log2 fold change $> \pm 1$, $p < 0.05$) are associated with signaling and chromatin remodeling.

## Principle Component Analysis

Principle component analysis employing the oxidative gene set served to identify genes of the highest contribution to spatial partitioning of the genotypes and selection of

**TABLE 1** | Top gene sets enriched in hNPC with native *WWOX* expression level.

| Gene set name | Gene number | Enrichment score |
|---|---|---|
| GO_neural_crest_cell_differentiation | 33 | 0.622 |
| GO_neural_crest_cell_migration | 21 | 0.677 |
| GO_homophilic_cell_adhesion_via_ plasma_membrane_adhesion_molecules | 53 | 0.511 |
| GO_cell_cell_adhesion_via_plasma _membrane_adhesion_molecules | 69 | 0.428 |
| GO_negative_regulation_of_ axon_extension | 21 | 0.578 |

*FDR q-value < 0.25.*

genes differentiating hNPC/shScrambled, hNPC/shWWOX, neurons/shScrambled and neurons/shWWOX in the most significant manner. As expected, we obviously found clear partitioning of hNPC and neuronal genotypes across the first dimension with a total variance of 77.7%. However, we also observed a clear partitioning across the dim2 with a total variance of 14.6%. The dim2 differentiates shScrambled and shWWOX variants indicating changes in oxidation-related genes induced by *WWOX* depletion (**Figure 11**). PCA analysis showed that among oxidative catabolism and oxidative stress genes that expression differentiates between *WWOX* expressing and *WWOX* depleted hNPC as well as neurons are those important for energy and redox metabolism. Examples of genes mostly involved in such differentiation are: Hexokinase 2 (HK2), Pyruvate Dehydrogenase Kinase 1 (PDK1), Lactate Dehydrogenase A (LDHA), Ferredoxin Reductase (FDXA), Cytochrome C (CYCS), Superoxide Dismutase 1 and 2 (SOD1 and SOD2), and Peroxiredoxin 2 (PRDX2), see **Supplementary Table S1** for all involved genes.

## DISCUSSION

The *WWOX* tumor suppressor gene has been recently recognized as a global modulator of transcription and an important regulator of brain differentiation and maintenance. Aberrations in *WWOX* expression lead to severe developmental neuropathologies as well as metabolic insufficiency and premature death (Shaukat et al., 2018). Public data from the Fantom 5 Project of the Riken Database (Robinson et al., 2010; Lizio et al., 2015) indicate that in human brain, *WWOX* expression is strongly dependent on the brain compartment as well as the age of the organism. In our study, we aimed to clarify the molecular basis of *WWOX* actions in neural tissue by analyzing the changes in phenotype and gene expression in hNPC with silenced *WWOX*.

The process of brain development is highly organized and its precise orchestration is vital to ensure the perfect construction of such a complex organ. Neurons and glial cells must be created in accurate numbers, locations and timing. The differentiation of neural stem cells into neurons, as well as the maintenance of the pool of undifferentiated neural progenitors, is governed by intra and extracellular signaling and involves mainly Notch, Wnt, and Hedgehog signaling pathways (Jiang and Nardelli, 2016). Our analysis of the functional networks of the differentially expressed genes revealed that *WWOX* expression in hNPC is associated with transcription regulation of genes of neural differentiation that take part in such pathways as Notch, PI3K kinase, PDGF, Cadherin, Hedgehog, and Endothelin signaling pathway.

The migration of the newborn neurons to their destination sites requires several major changes in cell polarity and motility. Young neurons leaving the SVZ exhibit multipolarity, and those on their way to target site typically display a bipolar morphology (Marín et al., 2006). This elaborate process is guided by intricate intra and extracellular signals. The pivotal role in migration is played by cytoskeleton components such as actin filaments and microtubules, as well as motor proteins like dyneins and kinesins, which undergo strictly controlled rearrangements to facilitate directional movement (Jiang and Nardelli, 2016). We showed that *WWOX* silencing in neural progenitor cells significantly changed expression of a large set of genes connected to cytoskeleton organization, e.g., MAP2/4/6, DCLK, NEFM, and NEFL that are engaged in microtubule and neurofilament assembly. Spalice et al. (2009) showed that impairment in the function of cytoskeletal genes, such as those associated with tubulins, causes severe disturbances in gyrification and lissencephaly, i.e., lack of brain folds and grooves (Liu, 2011). This emphasize the importance of migration process in cortex development.

During synaptogenesis the targets identification by the protruding ends of the outgrowing axons is mediated by cell adhesion molecules, e.g., NCAMs, N-cadherin and integrins, as well as extracellular matrix proteins (Dickson, 2002). Repulsive or attractive cues triggers signalization leading to reorganization of cytoskeleton facilitating directional movement. A number of cell-adhesion proteins is also involved in pre- and postsynaptic specialization (Li and Sheng, 2003). In our study, the lack of *WWOX* expression resulted in significant changes in cellular adhesion to ECM proteins. The hNPC/sh*WWOX* cells demonstrated increased ability to adhere to fibronectin ($p < 0.05$) and to the ECM protein mixture ($p = 0.0626$). Previous studies conducted on various cancer cell lines also identified a negative correlation between *WWOX* expression level and adherence ability (Zhang et al., 2009; Paige et al., 2010; Kośla et al., 2014). Our data indicates that WWOX is an important regulator of the tissue architecture. The changes in *WWOX* expression influence the levels of a number of pivotal adherence proteins, e.g., CDH2 (expression doubled in hNPC/shScrambled in compare to hNPC/sh*WWOX*) and ITGβ1 (expression lowered twice in hNPC/shScrambled in compare to hNPC/sh*WWOX*). The amount of secreted metalloproteinases (pro-MMP2 and pro-MMP9) was also significantly lowered in *WWOX* depleted cells. Metalloproteinases play a major role in the process of migration for neural progenitor cells and neural crest cells (Wang et al., 2006; Monsonego-Ornan et al., 2012). The interaction between ECM proteins and neural stem/progenitor cells is essential for the process of neurodifferentiation and functional maturation (Li et al., 2014). In addition to differentiation, the biochemical and biomechanical interaction with the extracellular microenvironment is also crucial for neural cell migration during the development of the nervous system, as well as in the case of brain injury (Joo et al., 2015). The precise nature of the effect of

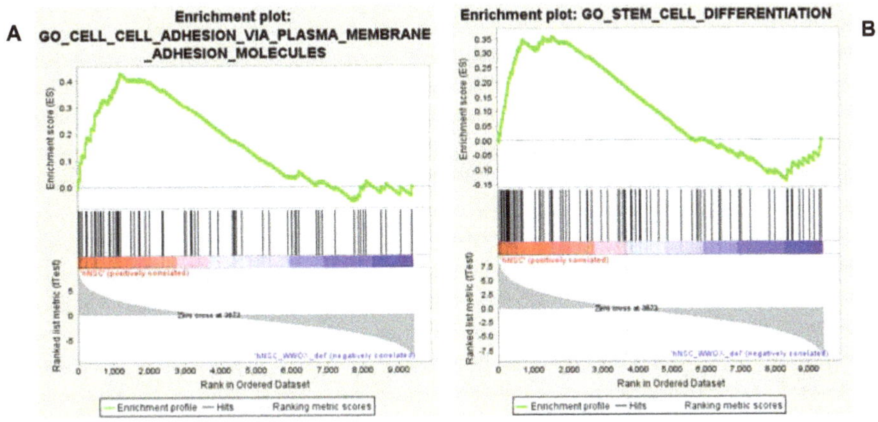


**FIGURE 8 |** GSEA enrichment plots presenting adhesion **(A)** and differentiation **(B)** gene sets enriched in hNPC cells.

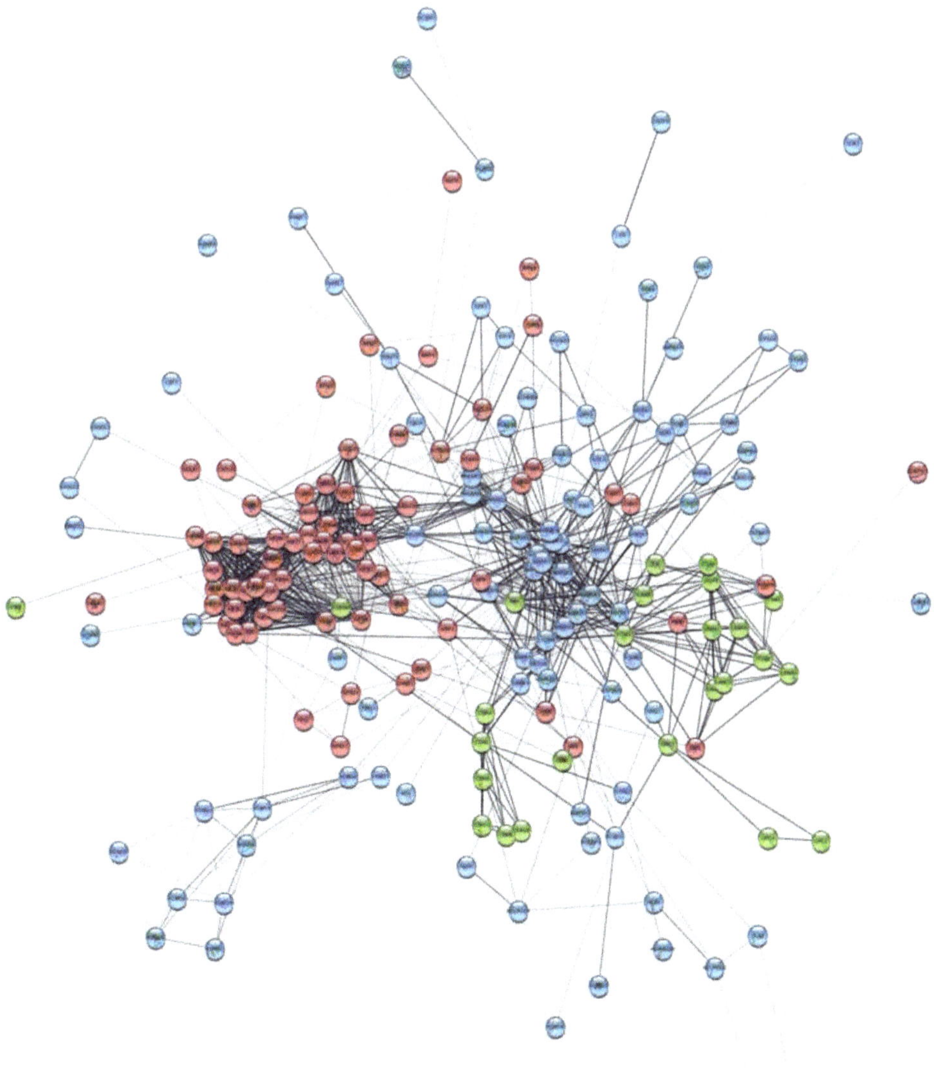

**FIGURE 9 |** Protein–protein interaction network of differentially expressed genes involved in neuron migration. Cytoskeleton and ER are red; membrane and ECM proteins are green; cell signaling and chromatin remodeling are blue. High resolution figure with legible gene names available in **Supplementary Figure S3**.

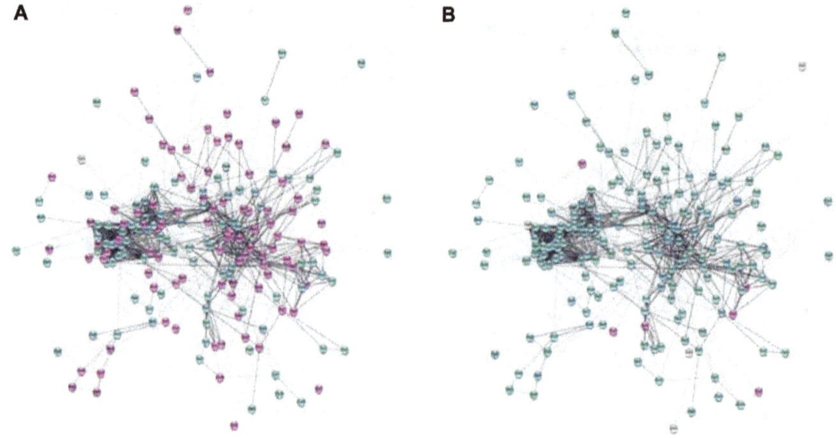


**FIGURE 10 |** Protein–protein interaction network of differentially expressed genes involved in neuron migration. **(A)** Log2 fold change of gene expression in hNPC/shWWOX vs. hNPC/shScrambled. **(B)** Log2 fold change of gene expression in neurons/shWWOX vs. neurons/shScrambled. Significantly upregulated genes are magenta; significantly downregulated genes are turquoise (Log2 fold change > ±1, $p < 0.05$). High resolution figure with legible gene names available in **Supplementary Figures S4, S5**.

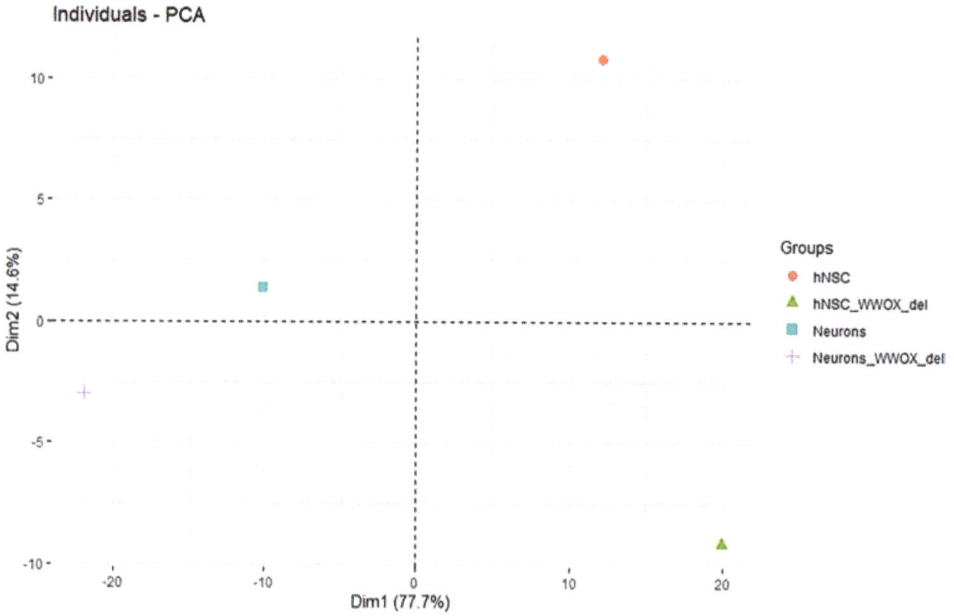


**FIGURE 11 |** The principle component analysis employing the gene set of oxidative gene set for identification of genes of the highest contribution to spatial partitioning of the genotypes and selection of genes differentiating hNPC/shScrambled, hNPC/shWWOX, neurons/shScrambled and neurons/shWWOX in the most significant manner. The partitioning of hNPC and neuron genotypes across the first dimension. The partitioning of shScrambled control and shWWOX genotypes across the second dimension.

WWOX on cell adhesion to ECM proteins remain unclear, but aberrations in WWOX protein level or functionality may disturb this physiologically relevant interactions.

The other main change observed in hNPC phenotype concerned mitochondrial redox potential. A number of papers have presented data suggesting that WWOX is capable of modulating cell metabolism (O'Keefe et al., 2011; Dayan et al., 2013; Abu-Remaileh et al., 2014; Choo et al., 2015). In the presented study, hNPC with silenced *WWOX* exhibit significantly lowered mitochondrial redox potential. Reactive oxygen species levels and mitochondrial metabolic state strongly contribute to neurogenesis and neuron maturation. The balance in this processes is critical for maintaining cellular homeostasis and accurate source, timing and localization of ROS synthesis is crucial for neuron physiology (Beckervordersandforth, 2017; Wilson et al., 2018). In our study, the transcriptome of investigated cells was analyzed to look for a confirmation of the observed decrease of the redox potential in *WWOX* depleted hNPC. A PCA with an oxidative stress response/antioxidant defense gene set was employed. The analysis clearly shows that in the terms of the resultant effect of the considered genes' expression, the control and *WWOX*-depleted genotypes are completely different (**Figure 11**). This is true both for undifferentiated hNPC and differentiated neurons. Amongst the genes with the highest contribution to differentiation between *WWOX* high/low variants are several important players participating in basic metabolism and reactive oxygen species control (**Supplementary Table S1**). Therefore, we conclude that *WWOX* might have considerable impact on neurons through modulation of oxygen metabolism and mitochondria functioning.

The specific mechanisms that underlie the individual stages of brain development process are far from being understood. Even so, our findings suggest that the WWOX protein might be an important regulator of neuronal migration and synaptogenesis. Its expression downregulation is significantly associated with changes in the level of expression of the genes involved in cell motility and adhesion, regulation of chromatin condensation and global cell signaling. The gene expression alternations identified in the CAGE analysis are consistent with phenotypical changes including cell adhesion, motility and ability for 3D growth.

The most striking observation in hNPC phenotype was noted when the cells were cultured in a three dimensional scaffold formed of ECM protein mixture. Under these conditions, the hNPC/sh*WWOX* cells lost their potential for 3D growth. They remained as single cells that did neither proliferate nor differentiate, whereas hNPC/shScrambled controls formed extensive cellular networks. This effect of *WWOX* depletion was observed irrespective of seeding density. This observation, along with changes in cellular adhesion, suggests that *WWOX* deprivation may lead to deficiency in cytoskeleton organization, interactions between cells and extracellular matrix proteins that impair correct tissue formation. In fact, human individuals known to possess dysfunctional *WWOX* variants present physical abnormalities in brain structure, *inter alia* global atrophy and hypoplasia of the corpus callosum (Abdel-Salam et al., 2014; Elsaadany et al., 2016; Johannsen et al., 2018). Similarly, Abdeen et al. (2013) report that silencing *WWOX* expression in MCF-10A normal breast cell line caused impairment of 3D growth and increases levels of fibronectin. In our previous report we demonstrated that differentiation of *WWOX* expression influences the 3D growth of the GBM T98G cell line, with upregulation of its expression disturbing the growth and spread of cancer cells in an ECM matrix (Kośla et al., 2014). This inability to perform 3D growth might by implied by massive gene expression deregulation triggered by *WWOX* depletion.

To identify which specific pathways may be influenced by WWOX protein in hNPC, the transcription profiles of undifferentiated hNPC cells and hNPC differentiated into neurons were compared between *WWOX* high and *WWOX* low variants and analyzed ontologically to match the differentially expressed genes with the BP. The global analysis showed enrichment in 14 gene sets related to neuronal development and differentiation (e.g., neuronal progenitor cell population maintenance, regulation of neuron migration, neural crest cell differentiation) (**Supplementary Table S2**). It was found that the gene sets were enriched in hNPC/shScrambled cells versus hNPC/sh*WWOX*, indicating that WWOX-induced transcription downregulation severely interferes with CNS developmental processes. Our results shows that beside adhesion membrane proteins, *WWOX* expression also influences a significant set of genes engaged in cytoskeleton structure and intracellular signaling. This can directly imply the observed disability for 3D growth and differentiation. *In vivo* the change in cell polarity and morphology is needed to allow migration from neurogenic niches to the final localization, and *WWOX* silencing appears to cause deregulation of the genes crucial for microtubule and neurofilament assembly as well as motor proteins.

The other large functional groups emerging from the ontological analysis were the gene sets connected with cellular adhesion and neurotransmitter management. It was shown recently that in a murine model, *WWOX* knockout may lower GABA synthesis (Hussain et al., 2019).

The multiplicity of molecular changes caused by *WWOX* depletion highlights its importance for the neural differentiation process. Aberration of its expression and/or protein functionality may disturb the delicate balance of this complicated net of connections and consequently lead to severe neuropathological conditions. WWOX has been postulated to act as linker in various protein crosstalk, an important multifunctional node that connects numerous proteins in many pathways, what may nicely explain the versatile effects of its silencing.

## CONCLUSION

Our findings indicate that appropriate *WWOX* expression is required for hNPC maintenance and differentiation. The silencing of *WWOX* expression results in global transcriptional changes, with the upregulation of some group of genes and simultaneous downregulation of others. Hence, it appears that the WWOX protein may be one of the master expression regulators in neural tissue.

## AUTHOR CONTRIBUTIONS

KK planned and performed the experiments, bioinformatic analysis, and wrote the manuscript. EP contributed to the interpretation of the results. ES-B and MN participated in performing the biological experiments. MO performed the statistical and bioinformatic analysis. AB conceived the idea, performed the bioinformatic analysis of CAGE results, and contributed to writing of the manuscript.

## FUNDING

This study was supported by the National Science Centre, Poland, grant no. 2015/17/D/NZ2/01989 and the Medical University of Łódź grant no. 503/0-078-02/503-01-004.

## REFERENCES


Abdeen, S. K., Salah, Z., Khawaled, S., and Aqeilan, R. I. (2013). Characterization of WWOX inactivation in murine mammary gland development. *J. Cell. Physiol.* 228, 1391–1396. doi: 10.1002/jcp.24310

Abdel-Salam, G., Thoenes, M., Afifi, H. H., Körber, F., Swan, D., and Bolz, H. J. (2014). The supposed tumor suppressor gene WWOX is mutated in an early lethal microcephaly syndrome with epilepsy, growth retardation and retinal degeneration. *Orphanet J. Rare Dis.* 9:12. doi: 10.1186/1750-1172-9-12

Abu-Odeh, M., Bar-Mag, T., Huang, H., Kim, T., Salah, Z., Abdeen, S. K., et al. (2014). Characterizing WW domain interactions of tumor suppressor WWOX reveals its association with multiprotein networks. *J. Biol. Chem.* 289, 8865–8880. doi: 10.1074/jbc.M113.506790

Abu-Remaileh, M., and Aqeilan, R. I. (2014). Tumor suppressor WWOX regulates glucose metabolism via HIF1α modulation. *Cell Death Differ.* 21, 1805–1814. doi: 10.1038/cdd.2014.95

Abu-Remaileh, M., Seewaldt, V. L., and Aqeilan, R. I. (2014). WWOX loss activates aerobic glycolysis. *Mol. Cell. Oncol.* 2:e965640. doi: 10.4161/23723548.2014.965640

Aqeilan, R. I., Donati, V., Palamarchuk, A., Trapasso, F., Kaou, M., Pekarsky, Y., et al. (2005). WW domain-containing proteins, WWOX and YAP, compete for interaction with ErbB-4 and modulate its transcriptional function. *Cancer Res.* 65, 6764–6772. doi: 10.1158/0008-5472.CAN-05-1150

Aqeilan, R. I., Palamarchuk, A., Weigel, R. J., Herrero, J. J., Pekarsky, Y., and Croce, C. M. (2004a). Physical and functional interactions between the Wwox tumor suppressor protein and the AP-2gamma transcription factor. *Cancer Res.* 64, 8256–8261. doi: 10.1158/0008-5472.CAN-04-2055

Aqeilan, R. I., Pekarsky, Y., Herrero, J. J., Palamarchuk, A., Letofsky, J., Druck, T., et al. (2004b). Functional association between Wwox tumor suppressor protein and p73, a p53 homolog. *Proc. Natl. Acad. Sci. U.S.A.* 101, 4401–4406. doi: 10.1073/pnas.0400805101

Beckervordersandforth, R. (2017). Mitochondrial metabolism-mediated regulation of adult neurogenesis. *Brain Plast.* 3, 73–87. doi: 10.3233/BPL-170044

Bouteille, N., Driouch, K., Hage, P. E., Sin, S., Formstecher, E., Camonis, J., et al. (2009). Inhibition of the Wnt/beta-catenin pathway by the WWOX tumor suppressor protein. *Oncogene* 28, 2569–2580. doi: 10.1038/onc.2009.120

Chen, S.-J., Huang, S.-S., and Chang, N.-S. (2013). Role of WWOX and NF-kappaB in lung cancer progression. *Transl. Respir. Med.* 1:15. doi: 10.1186/2213-0802-1-15

Chen, S. T., Chuang, J. I., Wang, J. P., Tsai, M. S., Li, H., and Chang, N.-S. (2004). Expression of WW domain-containing oxidoreductase WOX1 in the developing murine nervous system. *Neuroscience* 124, 831–839. doi: 10.1016/j.neuroscience.2003.12.036

Chiang, M.-F., Chen, H.-H., Chi, C.-W., Sze, C.-I., Hsu, M.-L., Shieh, H.-R., et al. (2015). Modulation of sonic hedgehog signaling and WW domain containing oxidoreductase WOX1 expression enhances radiosensitivity of human glioblastoma cells. *Exp. Biol. Med.* 240, 392–399. doi: 10.1177/1535370214565989

Choo, A., O'Keefe, L. V., Lee, C. S., Gregory, S. L., Shaukat, Z., Colella, A., et al. (2015). Tumor suppressor WWOX moderates the mitochondrial respiratory complex. *Genes Chromosomes Cancer* 54, 745–761. doi: 10.1002/gcc.22286

Dayan, S., O'Keefe, L. V., Choo, A., and Richards, R. I. (2013). Common chromosomal fragile site FRA16D tumor suppressor WWOX gene expression and metabolic reprograming in cells. *Genes Chromosomes Cancer* 52, 823–831. doi: 10.1002/gcc.22078

Dias, E. P., Pimenta, F. J., Sarquis, M. S., Dias Filho, M. A., Aldaz, C. M., Fujii, J. B., et al. (2007). Association between decreased WWOX protein expression and thyroid cancer development. *Thyroid* 17, 1055–1059. doi: 10.1089/thy.2007.0232

Dickson, B. J. (2002). Molecular mechanisms of axon guidance. *Science* 298, 1959–1964. doi: 10.1126/science.1072165

Donati, V., Fontanini, G., Dell'Omodarme, M., Prati, M. C., Nuti, S., Lucchi, M., et al. (2007). WWOX expression in different histologic types and subtypes of non-small cell lung cancer. *Clin. Cancer Res.* 13, 884–891. doi: 10.1158/1078-0432.CCR-06-2016

Elsaadany, L., El-Said, M., Ali, R., Kamel, H., and Ben-Omran, T. (2016). W44X mutation in the WWOX gene causes intractable seizures and developmental delay: a case report. *BMC Med. Genet.* 17:53. doi: 10.1186/s12881-016-0317-z

Ferguson, B. W., Gao, X., Zelazowski, M. J., Lee, J., Jeter, C. R., Abba, M. C., et al. (2013). The cancer gene WWOX behaves as an inhibitor of SMAD3 transcriptional activity via direct binding. *BMC Cancer* 13:593. doi: 10.1186/1471-2407-13-593

Gaudio, E., Palamarchuk, A., Palumbo, T., Trapasso, F., Pekarsky, Y., Croce, C. M., et al. (2006). Physical association with WWOX suppresses c-Jun transcriptional activity. *Cancer Res.* 66, 11585–11589. doi: 10.1158/0008-5472.CAN-06-3376

Haberle, V., Forrest, A. R. R., Hayashizaki, Y., Carninci, P., and Lenhard, B. (2015). *CAGEr*: precise TSS data retrieval and high-resolution promoterome mining for integrative analyses. *Nucleic Acids Res.* 43:e51. doi: 10.1093/nar/gkv054

Hasegawa, A., Daub, C., Carninci, P., Hayashizaki, Y., and Lassmann, T. (2014). MOIRAI: a compact workflow system for CAGE analysis. *BMC Bioinformatics* 15:144. doi: 10.1186/1471-2105-15-144

Hsu, L.-J., Chiang, M.-F., Sze, C.-I., Su, W.-P., Yap, Y. V., Lee, I.-T., et al. (2016). HYAL-2-WWOX-SMAD4 signaling in cell death and anticancer response. *Front. Cell Dev. Biol.* 4:141. doi: 10.3389/fcell.2016.00141

Hussain, T., Kil, H., Hattiangady, B., Lee, J., Kodali, M., Shuai, B., et al. (2019). Wwox deletion leads to reduced GABA-ergic inhibitory interneuron numbers and activation of microglia and astrocytes in mouse hippocampus. *Neurobiol. Dis.* 121, 163–176. doi: 10.1016/j.nbd.2018.09.026

Iatan, I., Choi, H. Y., Ruel, I., Reddy, M. V. P. L., Kil, H., Lee, J., et al. (2014). The WWOX gene modulates high-density lipoprotein and lipid metabolism. *Circ. Cardiovasc. Genet.* 7, 491–504. doi: 10.1161/CIRCGENETICS.113.000248

Jiang, X., and Nardelli, J. (2016). Cellular and molecular introduction to brain development. *Neurobiol. Dis.* 92, 3–17. doi: 10.1016/j.nbd.2015.07.007

Johannsen, J., Kortüm, F., Rosenberger, G., Bokelmann, K., Schirmer, M. A., Denecke, J., et al. (2018). ). A novel missense variant in the SDR domain of the WWOX gene leads to complete loss of WWOX protein with early-onset epileptic encephalopathy and severe developmental delay. *Neurogenetics* 19, 151–156. doi: 10.1007/s10048-018-0549-545

Joo, S., Kim, J. Y., Lee, E., Hong, N., Sun, W., and Nam, Y. (2015). Effects of ECM protein micropatterns on the migration and differentiation of adult neural stem cells. *Sci. Rep.* 5:13043. doi: 10.1038/srep13043

Kośla, K., Nowakowska, M., Pospiech, K., and Bednarek, A. K. (2014). WWOX modulates the gene expression profile in the T98G glioblastoma cell line rendering its phenotype less malignant. *Oncol. Rep.* 32, 1362–1368. doi: 10.3892/or.2014.3335

Kosla, K., Pluciennik, E., Kurzyk, A., Jesionek-Kupnicka, D., Kordek, R., Potemski, P., et al. (2011). Molecular analysis of WWOX expression correlation with proliferation and apoptosis in glioblastoma multiforme. *J. Neurooncol.* 101, 207–213. doi: 10.1007/s11060-010-0254-251

Kuhn, R. M., Haussler, D., and Kent, W. J. (2013). The UCSC genome browser and associated tools. *Brief. Bioinform.* 14, 144–161. doi: 10.1093/bib/bbs038

Lan, C., Chenggang, W., Yulan, B., Xiaohui, D., Junhui, Z., and Xiao, W. (2012). Aberrant expression of WWOX protein in epithelial ovarian cancer: a clinicopathologic and immunohistochemical study. *Int. J. Gynecol. Pathol.* 31, 125–132. doi: 10.1097/PGP.0b013e3182297fd2

Li, Y., Liu, M., Yan, Y., and Yang, S.-T. (2014). Neural differentiation from pluripotent stem cells: the role of natural and synthetic extracellular matrix. *World J. Stem Cells* 6, 11–23. doi: 10.4252/wjsc.v6.i1.11

Li, Z., and Sheng, M. (2003). Some assembly required: the development of neuronal synapses. *Nat. Rev. Mol. Cell Biol.* 4, 833–841. doi: 10.1038/nrm1242

Liu, C.-C., Ho, P.-C., Lee, I.-T., Chen, Y.-A., Chu, C.-H., Teng, C.-C., et al. (2018). WWOX phosphorylation, signaling, and role in neurodegeneration. *Front. Neurosci.* 12:563. doi: 10.3389/fnins.2018.00563

Liu, J. S. (2011). Molecular genetics of neuronal migration disorders. *Curr. Neurol. Neurosci. Rep.* 11, 171–178. doi: 10.1007/s11910-010-0176-175

Lizio, M., Harshbarger, J., Shimoji, H., Severin, J., Kasukawa, T., Sahin, S., et al. (2015). Gateways to the FANTOM5 promoter level mammalian expression atlas. *Genome Biol.* 16:22. doi: 10.1186/s13059-014-0560-566

Lo, C.-P., Hsu, L.-J., Li, M.-Y., Hsu, S.-Y., Chuang, J.-I., Tsai, M.-S., et al. (2008). MPP+-induced neuronal death in rats involves tyrosine 33 phosphorylation of WW domain-containing oxidoreductase WOX1. *Eur. J. Neurosci.* 27, 1634–1646. doi: 10.1111/j.1460-9568.2008.06139.x

Mallaret, M., Synofzik, M., Lee, J., Sagum, C. A., Mahajnah, M., Sharkia, R., et al. (2014). The tumour suppressor gene WWOX is mutated in autosomal recessive cerebellar ataxia with epilepsy and mental retardation. *Brain J. Neurol.* 137, 411–419. doi: 10.1093/brain/awt338

Marín, O., Valdeolmillos, M., and Moya, F. (2006). Neurons in motion: same principles for different shapes? *Trends Neurosci.* 29, 655–661. doi: 10.1016/j.tins.2006.10.001

Matteucci, E., Bendinelli, P., and Desiderio, M. A. (2009). Nuclear localization of active HGF receptor met in aggressive MDA-MB231 breast carcinoma cells. *Carcinogenesis* 30, 937–945. doi: 10.1093/carcin/bgp080

Mignot, C., Lambert, L., Pasquier, L., Bienvenu, T., Delahaye-Duriez, A., Keren, B., et al. (2015). WWOX-related encephalopathies: delineation of the phenotypical spectrum and emerging genotype-phenotype correlation. *J. Med. Genet.* 52, 61–70. doi: 10.1136/jmedgenet-2014-102748

Monsonego-Ornan, E., Kosonovsky, J., Bar, A., Roth, L., Fraggi-Rankis, V., Simsa, S., et al. (2012). Matrix metalloproteinase 9/gelatinase B is required for neural crest cell migration. *Dev. Biol.* 364, 162–177. doi: 10.1016/j.ydbio.2012.01.028

Nunez, M. I., Ludes-Meyers, J., and Aldaz, C. M. (2006). WWOX protein expression in normal human tissues. *J. Mol. Histol.* 37, 115–125. doi: 10.1007/s10735-006-9046-9045

O'Keefe, L. V., Colella, A., Dayan, S., Chen, Q., Choo, A., Jacob, R., et al. (2011). Drosophila orthologue of WWOX, the chromosomal fragile site FRA16D tumour suppressor gene, functions in aerobic metabolism and regulates reactive oxygen species. *Hum. Mol. Genet.* 20, 497–509. doi: 10.1093/hmg/ddq495

Pagés, H., (2018). *BSgenome: Software Infrastructure for Efficient Representation of Full Genomes and Their SNPs. R Package Version 1.48.0.* Available at: http://bioconductor.riken.jp/packages/3.7/bioc/html/BSgenome.html

Paige, A. J. W., Zucknick, M., Janczar, S., Paul, J., Mein, C. A., Taylor, K. J., et al. (2010). WWOX tumour suppressor gene polymorphisms and ovarian cancer pathology and prognosis. *Eur. J. Cancer* 46, 818–825. doi: 10.1016/j.ejca.2009.12.021

Piard, J., Hawkes, L., Milh, M., Villard, L., Borgatti, R., Romaniello, R., et al. (2018). The phenotypic spectrum of WWOX-related disorders: 20 additionalcases of WOREE syndrome and review of the literature. *Genet. Med.* 21, 1308–1318. doi: 10.1038/s41436-018-0339-3

Płuciennik, E., Kusińska, R., Potemski, P., Kubiak, R., Kordek, R., and Bednarek, A. K. (2006). WWOX–the FRA16D cancer gene: expression correlation with breast cancer progression and prognosis. *Eur. J. Surg. Oncol.* 32, 153–157. doi: 10.1016/j.ejso.2005.11.002

Płuciennik, E., Nowakowska, M., Stępien, A., Wołkowicz, M., Stawiński, A., Różański, W., et al. (2014). Alternating expression levels of WWOX tumor suppressor and cancer-related genes in patients with bladder cancer. *Oncol. Lett.* 8, 2291–2297. doi: 10.3892/ol.2014.2476

Robinson, M. D., McCarthy, D. J., and Smyth, G. K. (2010). edgeR: a bioconductor package for differential expression analysis of digital gene expression data. *Bioinformatics* 26, 139–140. doi: 10.1093/bioinformatics/btp616

Seabra, M. A. L., Cândido, E. B., Vidigal, P. V. T., Lamaita, R. M., Rodrigues, A. N., and Silva Filho, A. L. D. (2018). Immunohistochemical WWOX expression and association with angiogenesis, p53 expression, cell proliferation and clinicopathological parameters in cervical cancer. *Rev. Bras. Ginecol. Obstet.* 40, 79–85. doi: 10.1055/s-0037-1618597

Shaukat, Q., Hertecant, J., El-Hattab, A. W., Ali, B. R., and Suleiman, J. (2018). West syndrome, developmental and epileptic encephalopathy, and severe CNS disorder associated with WWOX mutations. *Epileptic Disord.* 20, 401–412. doi: 10.1684/epd.2018.1005

Spalice, A., Parisi, P., Nicita, F., Pizzardi, G., Del Balzo, F., and Iannetti, P. (2009). Neuronal migration disorders: clinical, neuroradiologic and genetics aspects. *Acta Paediatr.* 98, 421–433. doi: 10.1111/j.1651-2227.2008.01160.x

Sun, W., Dou, J., Zhang, L., Qiao, L., Shen, N., and Gao, W. (2017). Expression of CD133, E-cadherin and WWOX in colorectal cancer and related analysis. *Pak. J. Med. Sci.* 33, 425–429. doi: 10.12669/pjms.332.11687

Suzuki, H., Katayama, K., Takenaka, M., Amakasu, K., Saito, K., and Suzuki, K. (2009). A spontaneous mutation of the Wwox gene and audiogenic seizures in rats with lethal dwarfism and epilepsy. *Genes Brain Behav.* 8, 650–660. doi: 10.1111/j.1601-183X.2009.00502.x

Sze, C.-I., Su, M., Pugazhenthi, S., Jambal, P., Hsu, L.-J., Heath, J., et al. (2004). Down-regulation of WW domain-containing oxidoreductase induces tau phosphorylation in vitro. A potential role in Alzheimer's disease. *J. Biol. Chem.* 279, 30498–30506. doi: 10.1074/jbc.M401399200

Tabarki, B., Al Mutairi, F., and Al Hashem, A. (2015a). The fragile site WWOX gene and the developing brain. *Exp. Biol. Med.* 240, 400–402. doi: 10.1177/1535370214561952

Tabarki, B., AlHashem, A., AlShahwan, S., Alkuraya, F. S., Gedela, S., and Zuccoli, G. (2015b). Severe CNS involvement in WWOX mutations: description of five new cases. *Am. J. Med. Genet. A.* 167, 3209–3213. doi: 10.1002/ajmg.a.37363

Takahashi, H., Lassmann, T., Murata, M., and Carninci, P. (2012). 5' end-centered expression profiling using cap-analysis gene expression and next-generation sequencing. *Nat. Protoc.* 7, 542–561. doi: 10.1038/nprot.2012.005

Teng, C.-C., Yang, Y.-T., Chen, Y.-C., Kuo, Y.-M., and Sze, C.-I. (2012). Role of WWOX/WOX1 in Alzheimer's disease pathology and in cell death signaling. *Front. Biosci.* 4:1951–1965. doi: 10.2741/e516

Wang, H.-Y., Juo, L.-I., Lin, Y.-T., Hsiao, M., Lin, J.-T., Tsai, C.-H., et al. (2012). WW domain-containing oxidoreductase promotes neuronal differentiation via negative regulation of glycogen synthase kinase 3β. *Cell Death Differ.* 19, 1049–1059. doi: 10.1038/cdd.2011.188

Wang, L., Zhang, Z. G., Zhang, R. L., Gregg, S. R., Hozeska-Solgot, A., LeTourneau, Y., et al. (2006). Matrix metalloproteinase 2 (MMP2) and MMP9 secreted by erythropoietin-activated endothelial cells promote neural progenitor cell migration. *J. Neurosci.* 26, 5996–6003. doi: 10.1523/JNEUROSCI.5380-05.2006

Wang, X., Chao, L., Ma, G., Chen, L., Zang, Y., and Sun, J. (2011). The prognostic significance of WWOX expression in patients with breast cancer and its association with the basal-like phenotype. *J. Cancer Res. Clin. Oncol.* 137, 271–278. doi: 10.1007/s00432-010-0880-881

Wilson, C., Muñoz-Palma, E., and González-Billault, C. (2018). From birth to death: a role for reactive oxygen species in neuronal development. *Semin. Cell Dev. Biol.* 80, 43–49. doi: 10.1016/j.semcdb.2017.09.012

Xiong, A., Wei, L., Ying, M., Wu, H., Hua, J., and Wang, Y. (2014). Wwox suppresses breast cancer cell growth through modulation of the hedgehog-GLI1 signaling pathway. *Biochem. Biophys. Res. Commun.* 443, 1200–1205. doi: 10.1016/j.bbrc.2013.12.133

Zhang, J., Li, L., Song, H., Paige, A., and Gabra, H. (2009). [Effect of WWOX gene on the attachment and adhesion of ovarian cancer cells]. *Zhonghua Fu Chan Ke Za Zhi* 44, 529–532.

6

# Early Developmental Marginal Zinc Deficiency Affects Neurogenesis Decreasing Neuronal Number and Altering Neuronal Specification in the Adult Rat Brain

*Ana M. Adamo*[1†], *Xiuzhen Liu*[2†], *Patricia Mathieu*[1], *Johnathan R. Nuttall*[2], *Suangsuda Supasai*[2,3] and *Patricia I. Oteiza*[2*]

*[1]Department of Biological Chemistry and IQUIFIB (UBA-CONICET), Facultad de Farmacia y Bioquimica, Universidad de Buenos Aires, Buenos Aires, Argentina, [2]Department of Nutrition and Department of Environmental Toxicology, University of California, Davis, Davis, CA, United States, [3]Department of Molecular Tropical Medicine and Genetics, Faculty of Tropical Medicine, Mahidol University, Bangkok, Thailand*

***Correspondence:**
*Patricia I. Oteiza*
*poteiza@ucdavis.edu*

*†These authors have contributed equally to this work*

During pregnancy, a decreased availability of zinc to the fetus can disrupt the development of the central nervous system leading to defects ranging from severe malformations to subtle neurological and cognitive effects. We previously found that marginal zinc deficiency down-regulates the extracellular signal-regulated kinase 1/2 (ERK1/2) signaling pathway and affects neural progenitor cell (NPC) proliferation. This study investigated if marginal zinc deficiency during gestation in rats could disrupt fetal neurogenesis and affect the number and specification of neurons in the adult offspring brain cortex. Rats were fed a marginal zinc deficient or adequate diet throughout gestation and until postnatal day (P) 2, and subsequently the zinc adequate diet until P56. Neurogenesis was evaluated in the offspring at embryonic day (E)14, E19, P2, and P56 measuring parameters of NPC proliferation and differentiation by Western blot and/or immunofluorescence. At E14 and E19, major signals (i.e., ERK1/2, Sox2, and Pax6) that stimulate NPC proliferation and self-renewal were markedly downregulated in the marginal zinc deficient fetal brain. These alterations were associated to a lower number of Ki67 positive cells in the ventricular (VZs) and subventricular zones (SVZs). Following the progression of NPCs into intermediate progenitor cells (IPCs) and into neurons, Pax6, Tbr2 and Tbr1 were affected in the corresponding areas of the brain at E19 and P2. The above signaling alterations led to a lower density of neurons and a selective decrease of glutamatergic neurons in the young adult brain cortex exposed to maternal marginal zinc deficiency from E14 to P2. Current results supports the concept that marginal zinc deficiency during fetal development can disrupt neurogenesis and alter cortical structure potentially leading to irreversible neurobehavioral impairments later in life.

**Keywords: zinc, brain development, ERK1/2, Tbr2, zinc deficiency**

## INTRODUCTION

Prenatal zinc deficiency resulting from insufficient dietary intake, absorption, or transport can compromise development of the central nervous system leading to a spectrum of defects ranging from severe congenital malformations to subtle neurological and cognitive impairments. Severe zinc deficiency during fetal development has been implicated as a mechanism contributing to neural tube defects (NTDs). Severe dietary zinc deficiency in rats during pregnancy leads to NTDs in association with decreased cell proliferation in the ventricular zone (VZ) of the fetal brain (Swenerton et al., 1969). In humans, supplementation with dietary zinc and adequate plasma zinc concentrations are related to a reduced risk of NTDs (Velie et al., 1999; Dey et al., 2010). Although developmental marginal zinc deficiency does not cause gross malformations like NTDs, it is associated with neurological morbidity such as impairments in learning, working memory, and social behavior (Hagmeyer et al., 2015). Similar cognitive defects result from secondary zinc deficiency caused by gestational exposure to infection in rats (Kirsten et al., 2015).

Developmental exposure to a decreased zinc availability could have a long-term and irreversible impact on the offspring's brain leading to neurological and behavioral disorders later in life. In rats, severe postnatal zinc deficiency impairs neurogenesis in the cerebellum (Dvergsten et al., 1983), and decreases the expression of genes related to proliferation and neuronal differentiation in the hippocampus (Gower-Winter et al., 2013). In cultured cells, zinc deficiency impairs human IMR-32 neuroblastoma cell proliferation and induces apoptosis (Adamo et al., 2010), and inhibits retinoic acid-induced neuronal differentiation (Gower-Winter et al., 2013). Furthermore, zinc deficiency alters brain redox regulation and affects signaling pathways involved in neurogenesis (Zago et al., 2005; Aimo et al., 2010a,b; Mackenzie et al., 2011). Thus, we previously observed that gestational marginal zinc deficiency in rats decreases the number of neuronal progenitor cells (NPCs) expressing Ki67 in the VZ at embryonic day (E) 19 (Nuttall et al., 2015). NPCs give rise to all neuronal types present in the brain and play a pivotal role in regulating the balance between cell self-renewal and neurogenesis. Cortical excitatory neurons are directly generated from radial glial progenitors (RGPs) during embryonic neurogenesis or indirectly through intermediate progenitor cells (IPCs) derived from the VZ (Haubensak et al., 2004; Noctor et al., 2004). Radial glia proliferate at the ventricular surface and IPCs divide at a non-surface area in the VZ and subventricular zone (SVZ). The transcription factor cascade involving Pax6, Tbr2 and Tbr1 regulates the different stages of differentiation from NPCs to IPCs to cortical neurons. Tbr1 and Tbr2 are part of the T-box transcription factor subfamily Tbr1, and play key roles in glutamatergic neuron differentiation in the cerebral cortex, olfactory bulbs, hippocampal dentate gyrus, cerebellum and adult SVZ (Mihalas and Hevner, 2017). The extracellular signal-regulated kinase (ERK1/2) pathway is also a key regulator of NPC proliferation and neuronal differentiation (Nuttall and Oteiza, 2012). Marginal zinc deficiency during pregnancy in rats causes a decreased phosphorylation of ERK1/2 in the frontal cortex of the fetal rat brain at E19 (Nuttall et al., 2015) which is associated with a decrease in NPC number. However, it remains unclear if this decrease in NPCs can affect the number of neurons in the adult offspring brain as well as the process of neuronal differentiation and specification.

A complex and tightly regulated cascade of events lead to the differentiation of NPCs into neurons. Our previous results showed impaired NPC proliferation in association with maternal zinc deficiency. Thus, the goal of the present work was to evaluate whether a marginal zinc diet fed throughout gestation and until postnatal day (P) 2 can: (i) affect, in the offspring brain, the transcription factor cascade involved in NPC and IPC proliferation and differentiation into glutamatergic neurons; and (ii) cause long-term effects in the number and specification of cortical neurons in the offspring young adult brain. To such end, the temporal activation/expression of ERK1/2 and transcription factors Sox2, Pax6, Tbr2 and Tbr1 were characterized in the E14, E19 and P2 offspring brain. Alterations in cortical neuronal number and specification to glutamatergic and GABAergic neurons secondary to maternal marginal zinc deficiency were assessed in the adult offspring brain after postnatal repletion of dietary zinc.

## MATERIALS AND METHODS

### Materials

Primary antibodies for β-actin (#12620), phospho (Thr202/Tyr204) ERK (#4370), and ERK (#9102), were from Cell Signaling Technology (Danvers, MA, USA). Antibodies for glutamic acid decarboxylase 65 (GAD65; SC-377154) and Tbr1 (SC-376258; Western blot) were from Santa Cruz Biotechnology (Santa Cruz, CA, USA). Antibodies for Neu-N (MAB377) and Tbr2 (AB15894) were from Millipore (Burlington, MA, USA). The antibody for Ki67 (550609) was obtained from BD Pharmingen (San José, CA, USA). Antibodies for Sox2 (ab97959), Tbr1 (ab31941; immunofluorescence), vGlut1 (ab77822) and Pax6 (ab5790) were from Abcam Inc. (Cambridge, MA, USA). Secondary fluorescent antibodies were obtained from Jackson ImmunoResearch Co. Laboratories (West Grove, PA, USA). Polyvinylidene difluoride (PVDF), membranes and molecular weight standards for Western blot were obtained from BIO-RAD (Hercules, CA, USA). The enhanced chemiluminescence (ECL) Western blotting system was from Thermo Fisher Scientific Inc. (Piscataway, NJ, USA). Zinquin, the antibody for γ amino butyric acid (GABA; A2052), and all other reagents were of the highest quality available and were purchased from Sigma-Aldrich Co. (St. Louis, MO, USA).

### Animals and Animal Care

All procedures were in agreement with standards for the care of laboratory animals as outlined in the National Institutes of Health Guide for the Care and Use of Laboratory Animals. All procedures were administered under the auspices of the Animal Resource Services of the University of California at Davis, which is accredited by the American Association for the Accreditation of Laboratory Animal Care. Experimental protocols were approved before implementation by the University of California at Davis Animal Use and Care Administrative Advisory

Committee and were administered through the Office of the Campus Veterinarian. Adult Sprague-Dawley rats (Charles River, Wilmington, MA, USA; 200–225 g) were housed individually in stainless steel cages in a temperature—(22–23°C) and photoperiod—(12-h light/dark) controlled room. An egg-white protein-based diet with adequate zinc (25 μg zinc/g) was the standard control diet (Keen et al., 1989). Animals were fed the control diet for 1 week before breeding. The overall experimental design is shown in **Figure 1A**. Males and females were caged together overnight and the following morning (E0), after the presence of a sperm plug confirmed a successful breeding, female rats (six animals/group for E14, E19, and P2/P56) were divided into two groups and fed *ad libitum* a control diet (25 μg zinc/g diet, control group) or a diet containing a marginal concentration of zinc (10 μg zinc/g diet; MZD group). Food intake was recorded daily, and body weight was measured at 3-day intervals. On E14 and E19, dams were anesthetized with isoflurane (2 mg/kg body weight) and laparotomies were performed. The gravid uterus was removed and fetuses were weighed. Fetal brains were removed, weighed and immediately either processed for immunohistochemistry, or removed and kept on ice to microdissect regions enriched in cortical tissue (CT), which were then frozen in liquid nitrogen and stored at −80°C. In the E14 offspring, CT included the cortical neuroepithelium with the SVZ and VZ; in E19 offspring, CT included the cortical plate with the SVZ and VZ. At P2, litters were adjusted to eight pups/litter, and brain/brain cortices were dissected from the euthanized pups and processed as described before. Dams from both the control and the MZD groups were subsequently fed the control diet. Pups were weaned at P21 and were all fed the control diet until P56 when euthanized; blood and brain/brain cortex collection was carried out as described before.

With regard to the time of exposure of the offspring to zinc deficiency, it should be considered that milk zinc content does not decrease in conditions of marginal zinc nutrition both in rodents and humans, even when maternal plasma zinc levels are low (Kelleher and Lönnerdal, 2005). Thus, in the current experimental model, it is expected that the offspring would have access to similar amounts of zinc in milk starting at birth in both control and MZD groups.

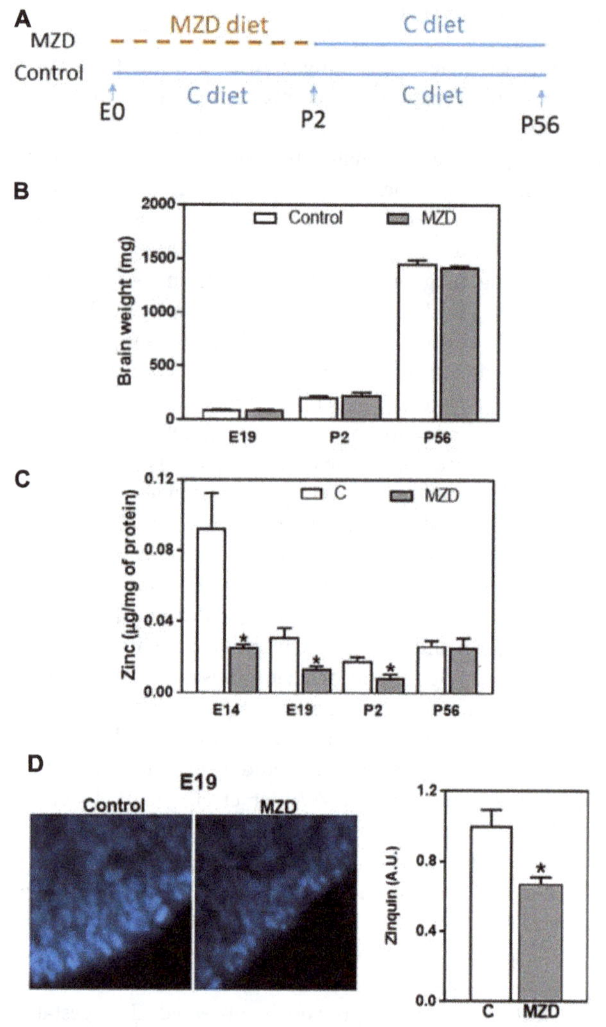


**FIGURE 1** | Fetal/offspring brain weight and zinc concentration after maternal consumption of a control or a marginal zinc diet throughout gestation and until postnatal day (P) 2. **(A)** Experimental design. **(B)** Embryonic day (E) 19–P56 offspring brain weight. **(C)** Zinc concentration in fetal/offspring cortical tissue (CT) and brain cortex 100,000× *g* supernatants were measured by atomic emission spectroscopy (AES). **(D)** Labile zinc was measured in the ventricular zone (VZ) at E19 by zinquin staining (blue fluorescence). Micrographs show the VZ of the dorsomedial frontal cortex at 1,000-fold magnification. Fluorescence was quantified as described in "Materials and Methods" section. **(B–D)** Data are shown as mean ± SEM and are the average of 4–6 litters per group. *Significantly different from the control group at the same developmental stage (*t*-test, $p < 0.05$).

## Determination of Zinc Concentrations

The concentration of zinc in diets and brain supernatants was measured by inductively coupled plasma atomic emission spectroscopy (ICP-AES) as described by Clegg et al. (2005). E14 and E19 brain CT and P2 and P56 cortices were weighed, homogenized in ice-cold PBS (1:10), and centrifuged for 60 min at 100,000× *g* at 4°C. The supernatant was collected and protein concentration was measured using the Bradford assay (Bradford, 1976). Three milliliter of 16 N $HNO_3$ were added to the 100,000× *g* supernatants and diet samples and allowed to digest for 72 h. Samples were dried, and resuspended in ultrapure water. Zinc concentration was determined by inductively coupled plasma atomic emission spectroscopy (ICP-AES; Trace Scan; Thermo Elemental, Franklin, MA, USA). Certified reference solutions (QC 21; Spec CentriPrep, Metuchen, NJ, USA) were used to generate standard curves. A sample of a National Bureau of Standards bovine liver (SRM1577; U.S. Department of Commerce, National Bureau of Standards, Washington, DC, USA) was included with the samples to ensure accuracy and reproducibility.

## Zinquin Staining

Labile zinc was measured in coronal sections from the fetal rat brain at E19. Slides were overlaid with a solution of 25 μM zinquin in Hank's balanced salt solution (HBSS) and incubated at 37°C for 40 min. After washing in HBSS, coverslips were mounted with a solution of 90% glycerol and 10% HBSS and imaged on an Olympus BX50 epifluorescence microscope provided with a Cool-Snap digital camera. Image pro software (Rockville, MD, USA) was used to analyze the resulting micrographs. Three randomly selected fields were measured per animal and experimental condition ($n = 3$).

## Western Blot Analysis

Extraction of total cellular protein from CT and cortex homogenates was done as previously described (Aimo et al., 2010b). Protein concentration was measured using the Bradford assay (Bradford, 1976), and aliquots containing 25–50 μg of protein were separated by reducing 10% (w/v) SDS-PAGE and electroblotted to PVDF membranes. Colored molecular weight standards were run simultaneously. Membranes were blocked for 1 h in 5% (w/v) nonfat milk and incubated overnight with the corresponding primary antibodies (1:1,000–1:5,000) in 1% (w/v) bovine serum albumin in TBST (20 mM Tris, 150 mM NaCl, pH 7.4, 0.1% Tween 20) at 4°C. After incubation for 1 h at room temperature with the corresponding peroxidase-conjugated secondary antibodies (1:10,000–1:30,000), proteins were visualized by chemiluminescence detection, and subsequently quantified, using a Phosphorimager 840 (Amersham, Piscataway, NJ, USA).

## Immunofluorescence

E14, E19, and P2 rat brains were dissected out and fixed in a 4% (w/v) solution of paraformaldehyde in PBS overnight. P56 rats were deeply anesthetized as described above and perfused transcardially with PBS followed by 4% (w/v) solution of paraformaldehyde in PBS, after which brains were collected. In all cases, tissue cryoprotection was subsequently performed in 30% (w/v) sucrose until the tissue sank down, after which, brains were submerged in Cryoplast freezing medium (Biopack, Buenos Aires, Argentina), frozen, cut into 18 μm coronal sections on a Leica CM 1850 cryotome (Leica Microsystems, Nussloch, Germany), and mounted on positively charged microscope slides. Sections were blocked for 45 min in 1% (v/v) donkey serum in 0.1% (v/v) Triton X-100 in PBS, and incubated with the corresponding dilution of primary antibody in blocking solution (1:200 rabbit anti-Sox2, 1:100 rabbit anti-Pax6, 1:200 rabbit anti-Trb1, 1:100 chicken anti-Tbr2, 1:200 mouse anti-NeuN, 1:200 rabbit anti-vGlut1, 1:200 rabbit anti-GABA, 1:100 mouse anti-Ki67) overnight at 4°C. Sections were then washed once in 0.1% (v/v) Triton X-100 in PBS and once in 0.1 M phosphate buffer, pH 7.4, and incubated with the corresponding dilution of secondary antibody (1:500 Cy3-conjugated donkey anti-rabbit, 1:500 Alexa 488 donkey anti-mouse IgG, and 1:500 Alexa 488 donkey anti-chicken) for 2 h at room temperature. After immunostaining, cell nuclei were stained with 1 μg/ml Hoechst 33342 and sections were imaged using an Olympus FV 1000 laser scanning confocal microscope or an Olympus BX50 epifluorescence microscope provided with a Cool-Snap digital camera. Image pro software (Rockville, MD, USA) was used to merge and analyze the resulting micrographs. Marker-positive cells were counted using ImageJ (National Institutes of Health, Bethesda, MD, USA) and results were expressed as the number of positive cells per area. At least 300 cells were counted for each cell marker, analyzed in three independent experiments that were performed in triplicates for four animals per group. Alternatively, fluorescence intensity was measured for vGlut1 and GABA.

## Statistical Analysis

Data for the control and MZD groups at each developmental stage were analyzed by Student's $t$-test using Statview 5.0 (SAS Institute Inc., Cary, NC, USA). The litter was the statistical unit. A $p$ value $< 0.05$ was considered statistically significant. Data are shown as mean ± SE.

# RESULTS

## Animal Outcome

Pregnant dams were fed a marginal zinc or a control diet from E0 until P2. Subsequently all dams until P21, and the

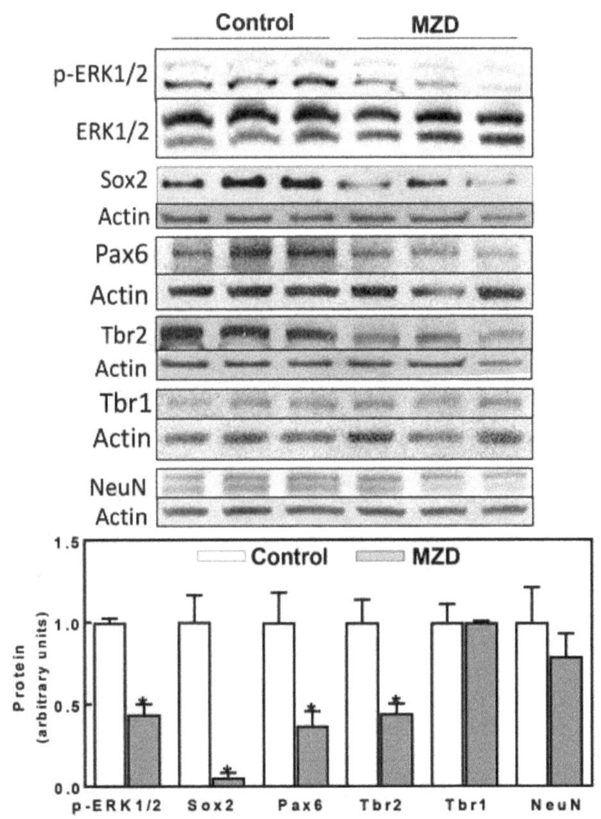


**FIGURE 2** | Maternal marginal zinc deficiency affects parameters of neurogenesis in the E14 rat brain. Phospho extracellular signal-regulated kinase 1/2 (ERK1/2), ERK1/2, Sox2, Pax6, Tbr2, Tbr1 and NeuN protein levels were measured by Western blot in E14 brain CT homogenates. After quantification of bands, phospho-ERK1/2 levels were referred to total ERK1/2 content and the other proteins were referred to β-actin levels. Values (arbitrary units, AUs) were normalized to those of the control group (1) Results are shown as mean ± SE of E14 brain cortices from six litters/group. *Significantly different from the control group ($p < 0.05$, Student's $t$-test).

offspring, until P56, were fed the control diet (**Figure 1A**). As previously described (Aimo et al., 2010b; Nuttall et al., 2015), we observed that a marginal zinc nutrition throughout gestation does not affect overall maternal and fetal outcome (data not shown). Furthermore, consumption of the marginal zinc diet throughout gestational and perinatal period did not affect fetal/offspring brain weight between E19 and P56 (**Figure 1B**). Zinc concentration in E14 and E19 CT and P2 brain cortex 100,000× *g* supernatants was significantly lower (72%, 58% and 56%, respectively) in MZD offspring compared to the control group (**Figure 1C**). Loosely bound zinc in the E19 brain was evaluated by Zinquin staining and subsequent fluorescence microscopy. In the control group, Zinquin fluorescence appeared strongest in the VZ and surrounding blood vessels. In the MZD offspring VZ, the intensity of Zinquin fluorescence was 34% lower than in controls (**Figure 1D**).

## Maternal Marginal Zinc Deficiency Affects Markers of Neurogenesis at E14

Given our previous work showing a decrease in ERK1/2 activation together with a reduction in NPC proliferation, we aimed to investigate the impact of these events on cortical excitatory neurons. Signaling cascades involved in NPC proliferation, self-renewal, and progression to differentiation were evaluated at E14 (**Figure 2**). ERK1/2 phosphorylation was 66%, lower in the MZD E14 brain CT compared to controls (**Figure 2**). Maternal marginal zinc nutrition also affected different markers of NPC proliferation and progression to differentiation as evaluated by Western blot (**Figure 2**). Sox2 is a transcription factor that controls the self-renewal of NPCs throughout development. Maternal marginal zinc deficiency caused a 95% decrease in E14 cortical Sox2 levels compared to controls. Pax6, a transcription factor that is central to the development of the brain cortex, showed 63% lower levels in the E14 cortex from MZD compared to the control group (**Figure 2**). Marginal zinc nutrition also affected the abundance of Tbr2, a transcription factor that regulates the specification of the intermediate neural progenitors (INPs) that will differentiate into excitatory neurons. Tbr2 levels were 55% lower in MZD compared to control E14 CT. Protein levels of Tbr1 and of the marker of post-mitotic mature neurons NeuN were similar between groups.

## Maternal Marginal Zinc Deficiency Affects Markers of Neurogenesis in the Offspring Brain at E19 and P2

At E19, all measured markers of cortical neurogenesis, from NPC proliferation to fully differentiated neurons, were affected in the MZD embryo brain (**Figure 3**). ERK1/2 phosphorylation was lower (36%) in the E19 CT from MZD compared to controls. Sox2, Pax6, Tbr2, Tbr1 and NeuN protein levels were 57, 37, 57, 43 and 42% lower in MZD compared to control embryo CT as measured by Western blot (**Figure 3A**). Immunofluorescence analysis also showed lower levels of total proliferative cells in the E19 SVZ of MZD compared to control

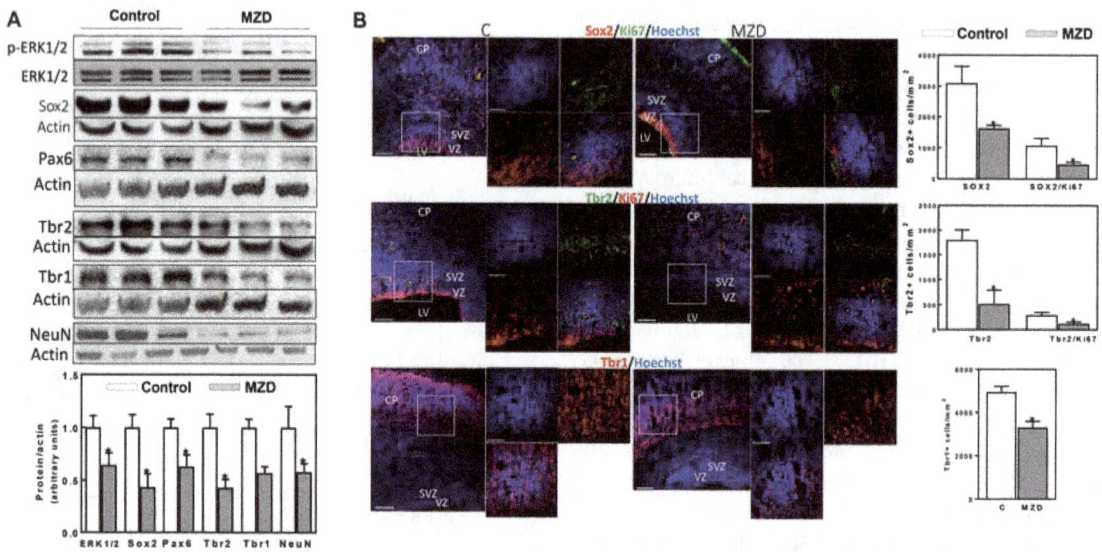


**FIGURE 3** | Maternal marginal zinc deficiency affects parameters of neurogenesis in the E19 rat brain. **(A)** Phospho ERK1/2, ERK1/2, Sox2, Pax6, Tbr2, Tbr1 and NeuN protein levels were measured by Western blot in E19 CT homogenates. After quantification of bands, phospho-ERK1/2 levels were referred to total ERK1/2 content and the other proteins were referred to β-actin levels. Values (AUs) were normalized to those of the control group (1) Results are shown as mean ± SE of fetal brain cortices from six litters/group. *Significantly different from the control group ($p < 0.05$, Student's *t*-test). **(B)** Immunofluorescence for Sox2 (red fluorescence) and Ki67 (green fluorescence); Tbr2 (green fluorescence) and Ki67 (red fluorescence); Tbr1 (red fluorescence) and Ki67 (green fluorescence). Nuclei were visualized with Hoechst staining (blue fluorescence; Scale bar, 100 μm). Images in boxes are shown at a higher magnification (Scale bar, 50 μm). Quantifications were done as described in methods. Results are shown as mean ± SE of E19 brains from four litters/group. *Significantly different from the control group ($p < 0.05$, Student's *t*-test).

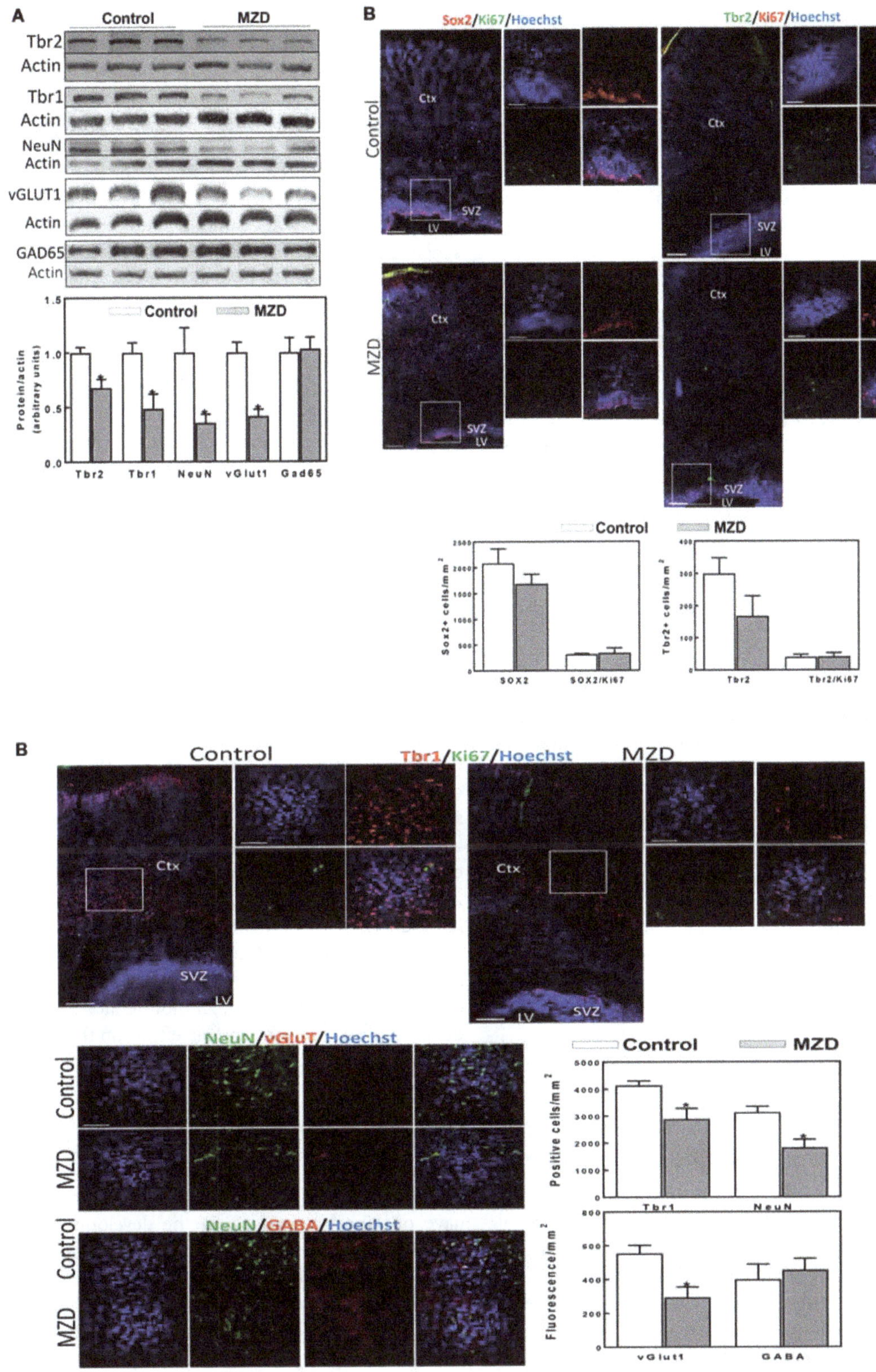


**FIGURE 4 |** Maternal marginal zinc deficiency affects parameters of neurogenesis in the P2 fetal rat brain. **(A)** Tbr2, Tbr1, NeuN, vGlut1 and glutamic acid decarboxylase 65 (GAD65) protein levels were measured by Western blot in P2 brain cortex homogenates. After quantification of bands, values were referred to β-actin levels and values (AUs) were normalized to those of the control group (1) Results are shown as mean ± SE of fetal brain cortices from six litters/group.

*(Continued)*

**FIGURE 4** | Continued
*Significantly different from the control group ($p < 0.05$, Student's $t$-test). **(B)** Immunofluorescence for Sox2 (red fluorescence) and Ki67 (green fluorescence); Tbr2 (green fluorescence) and Ki67 (red fluorescence); Tbr1 (red fluorescence) and Ki67 (green fluorescence); NeuN (green fluorescence) and vGlut1 (red fluorescence); and NeuN (green fluorescence) and $\gamma$ amino butyric acid (GABA; red fluorescence). Nuclei were visualized with Hoechst staining (blue fluorescence; Scale bar, 100 $\mu$m). Images in boxes are shown at a higher magnification (Scale bar, 50 $\mu$m). Quantifications were done as described in methods. Results are shown as mean ± SE of offspring brains from four litters/group. *Significantly different from the control group ($p < 0.05$, Student's $t$-test).

offspring (**Figure 3B**). Thus, NPC Sox2 and IPC Tbr2 positive cells in the SVZ of MZD embryos were 47 and 71%, respectively, compared to controls (**Figure 3B**). The ratio Sox2/Ki67 and Tbr2/Ki67 positive cells were 56 and 59% lower, respectively, in MZD than in control embryo SVZ. The number of Tbr1 positive cells in E19 cortices were 33% lower in MZD compared to controls.

Markers of cortical neurogenesis were measured next at P2 by Western blot (**Figure 4A**). Tbr2 and Tbr1 levels were significantly lower in MZD than in control brain cortices (32 and 51%, respectively). A decrease in mature neurons is supported by a 64% decrease in NeuN levels in MZD compared to controls. Furthermore, alterations in neuronal specification were already evident at P2. Thus, a 58% decrease in vGlut1, a glutamate/proton exchanger indicator of glutamatergic neuron abundance, was observed in MZD offspring brain cortices. On the other hand, the protein abundance of Gad65 an enzyme involved in GABA synthesis, was similar between groups. Immunofluorescence analysis (**Figure 4B**) showed no significant differences between groups for Sox2 and Tbr2. Although values were 44% lower for Tbr2, differences were not significant ($p < 0.15$). The number of Tbr1 positive cells was 30% lower in MZD cortices than in controls. The number of NeuN positive cells and of vGlut1 fluorescence intensity were 42 and 47% lower in MZD compared to control P2 offspring brains, while GABA fluorescence intensity was similar between groups.

### Early Developmental Marginal Zinc Deficiency Disrupted Neurogenesis Leading to a Decreased Neuronal Number and Altered Neuronal Specification in the Adult Brain (P56)

We next investigated if the effects of gestational marginal zinc deficiency on fetal brain development have long lasting repercussions, even following repletion with a diet containing adequate zinc. The total number of mature neurons (NeuN positive cells) in the brain cortex of the P56 offspring was evaluated by immunohistochemistry. Marginal zinc deficiency from E0-P2 resulted in a 29% decrease in the number of cells expressing NeuN in the offspring frontal cortex (**Figure 5**). While no differences in the fluorescence intensity for GABA was observed between groups, 26% lower levels of fluorescence for vGlut1 were observed in the P56 brain cortex from MZD offspring compared to controls (**Figure 5**).

## DISCUSSION

Results from this study demonstrate that a decreased proliferation of NPCs resulting from gestational marginal zinc deficiency leads to the disruption of cortical neurogenesis in the rat offspring brain. This is associated with a decreased number of neurons in the MZD young adult brain cortex, and an altered specification that results in a reduced number of excitatory glutamatergic neurons, not affecting GABAergic neurons.

Severe nutritional zinc deficiency, both due to low zinc content or high content of zinc-binding phytates, during early development causes NTDs and brain/organ teratology (Oteiza et al., 1990; Velie et al., 1999). Also maternal infections, diabetes, and toxicant exposures that stimulate an acute-phase response causes a decreased transport of zinc to the developing fetus (Nuttall et al., 2017), which can lead to increased risk of NTDs (Chua et al., 2006; Uriu-Adams and Keen, 2010). On the other hand, a marginally low dietary zinc intake during pregnancy is associated with decreased fetal heart rate variability, suggesting impaired regulation of the autonomic nervous system (Spann et al., 2015). Accordingly, prenatal zinc supplementation improves the regulation of the autonomic nervous system later in life (Caulfield et al., 2011). Mild developmental zinc deficiency, both in humans and rodents, impairs learning, working memory, and social behavior (Hagmeyer et al., 2015). Similar cognitive defects result from secondary zinc deficiency in a rat model of maternal infection (Kirsten et al., 2015). Importantly, these cognitive defects are consistent with rodent models of autism spectrum disorder, suggesting that disruption of fetal brain development resulting from marginal zinc deficiency could contribute to the risk of developing autism (Grabrucker et al., 2014; Kirsten et al., 2015; Nuttall, 2015). Moreover, reports in humans have established an association between zinc deficiency and Phelan McDermid Syndrome, a genetic disorder characterized by features of autism spectrum disorders (Pfaender et al., 2017). Thus, although not teratogenic, marginal zinc deficiency can have long-lasting effects on the nervous system.

We currently observed that consumption of a marginal zinc deficient diet during pregnancy did not affect the overall pregnancy and fetal/offspring outcome. On the other hand, the concentration of zinc in the offspring brain cytosolic fraction was markedly affected from E14 through P2. This finding stresses the major impact that a mild decrease in zinc availability can have on zinc homeostasis in the developing brain. Cytosolic zinc and Zinquin-reactive zinc largely reflect loosely bound and rapidly available zinc pools, which are highly relevant to the regulation of cell signaling. For example, and stressing the relevance of available zinc pools, both the decrease in ERK1/2 phosphorylation and cell proliferation observed in zinc-deficient IMR-32 cells are rapidly restored upon zinc supplementation and *via* the inhibition of the ERK1/2-directed phosphatase PP2A (Nuttall et al., 2015).

Zinc deficiency affects signaling pathways that can contribute to altered brain development. In this regard, we previously

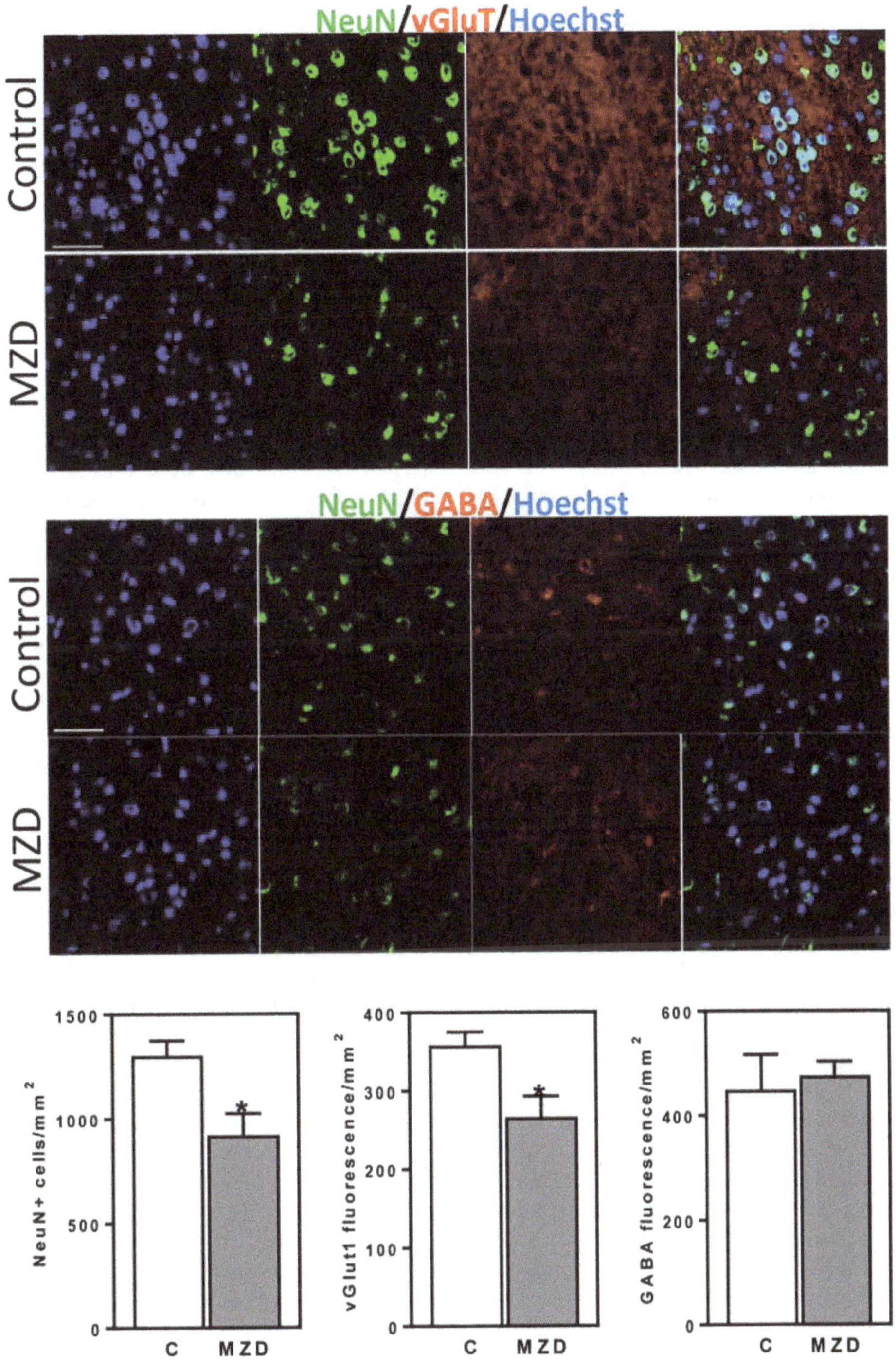


**FIGURE 5** | Maternal marginal zinc deficiency from E0 to P2 affects the number and specification of neurons in the young adult brain. NeuN (green fluorescence), vGlut1 (red fluorescence) and GABA (red fluorescence) were measured by immunofluorescence in the frontal cortex at P56. Nuclei were visualized with Hoechst staining (blue fluorescence; Scale bar, 100 μm). Quantifications were done as described in methods. Results are shown as mean ± SE of offspring brain from four litters/group. *Significantly different from the control group ($p < 0.05$, Student's *t*-test).

observed a downregulation of transcription factors NF-κB and NFAT, the activation of MAPKs p38 and JNK, and a downregulation of ERK1/2 both in zinc deficient IMR-32 cells and E19 fetal rat brain (Zago et al., 2005; Aimo et al., 2010b; Nuttall et al., 2015). In particular, ERK1/2 phosphorylation showed a major decrease in the MZD brain CT at E14 and E19. This can in part explain maternal zinc deficiency-associated decrease in VZ NPC number and proliferation and the observed alterations in neuronal specification. In this regard, ERK1/2 is not only important for NPC proliferation but also for neuronal differentiation (Samuels et al., 2008; Pucilowska et al., 2012). In humans, mutations that disrupt ERK1/2 signaling impair brain development leading to cognitive dysfunction in neuro-cardio-faciocutaneous syndromes and autism spectrum disorders (Samuels et al., 2009; Kalkman, 2012). Mice with a conditional deletion of ERK1/2 in NPCs have decreased NPC proliferation leading to abnormal distribution of neurons in the cortical plate, increased excitability of cortical neurons, increased anxiety-like behavior, reduced memory, and impairments of social behavior (Satoh et al., 2011; Pucilowska et al., 2012). Overall, ERK1/2 can be a key signal underlying the altered neurogenesis and behavior associated with maternal marginal zinc deficiency (Nuttall and Oteiza, 2012).

Transcription factor Sox2 functions by regulating NPC self-renewal in both the developing and mature brain, and inhibiting NPC differentiation (Graham et al., 2003; Favaro et al., 2009). A major decrease of Sox2 was observed in the MZD E14 and E19 embryos, suggesting that Sox2 downregulation can contribute to the observed decrease in NPC proliferation. On the other hand, Sox2 downregulation causes premature neuronal differentiation (Graham et al., 2003), which was not observed in the MZD embryonic brain. Pax6 expression at E14 was also impaired in the MZD group. Pax6, a homeobox and paired domain transcription factor, promotes the expression of Tbr2, inducing the transition of NPC-like RGPs to IPCs (Sansom et al., 2009). Pax6 regulates the proliferation of cortical progenitors being expressed in RGPs at the VZ, but not in IPCs (Manuel et al., 2015). Thus, not only ERK1/2 but also Sox2 and Pax6 downregulation at a period of active progenitor proliferation can contribute to the decrease in the number of fetal brain NPCs as a consequence of maternal marginal zinc deficiency.

We next evaluated the potential disruption of the process of neuronal differentiation and specification that could be associated with an impaired NPC proliferation. Similarly to Sox2 and Pax6, Tbr2 protein levels were markedly low in E14 and E19 MZD brain CT. Tbr2 is expressed in the mouse brain as early as E10.5 in proliferative areas, where neuronal progenitors reside (Kimura et al., 1999). Tbr1 expression is located in the cerebral cortex and other brain areas populated by postmitotic neurons, decreasing the expression postnatally (Bulfone et al., 1995). Tbr2 is a marker of IPCs, being required for the progression of RGPs to IPCs, a process that is in part mediated by the downregulation of Pax6 by Trb2 (Hodge et al., 2012). Most glutamatergic neurons in the brain cortex are originated from a Tbr2 positive lineage (Vasistha et al., 2015). We observed a reduction in the number of Tbr2 positive IPCs in the SVZ and of Tbr1 positive postmitotic neurons in the cortical plate. Thus, while the decrease in NPCs in the MZD embryonic brain may explain a decreased number of neurons, the observed downregulation of Tbr2 during the period of active differentiation suggests that the specification of neurons may also be affected.

As IPCs are necessary to expand the population of cortical glutamatergic neurons, we next analyzed the population of mature NeuN positive neurons and the populations of vGlut1 and GABA positive neurons at P2 and P56. We observed not only a lower number of mature neurons in the MZD mature brain but also, in agreement with alterations in Tbr2 and Tbr1 expression, an impairment in the generation of glutamatergic neurons. Very importantly, even after postnatal zinc repletion, vGlut1 expression in the MZD P56 brain cortex remained markedly affected. The mammalian neocortex has two types of neurons, glutamatergic pyramidal cells and GABAergic non-pyramidal cells (Peters and Jones, 1984; DeFelipe and Fariñas, 1992). Glutamatergic projection neurons give rise from progenitor cells in the VZ of the pallium from where they migrate radially into the neocortex. On the other hand, GABAergic interneurons are born in the subpallium and migrate tangentially into the neocortex (Marin, 2013). They arise from the ventral telencephalon (Anderson et al., 1997), in particular the medial and caudal ganglionic eminences (Wichterle et al., 2001; Wonders and Anderson, 2006; Wonders et al., 2008) from Nkx2.1-expressing progenitors (Butt et al., 2005), in a process modulated by Sonic hedgehog (Hebert and Fishell, 2008). The described diverse origin and regulation of glutamatergic and GABAergic neurons can explain the differential effect of developmental zinc deficiency on these neuronal populations.

The current findings stress the concept that the adverse effects of limited zinc availability during early development can have irreversible consequences in the number and specification of neurons in the mature brain. These results add to previous evidence showing that severe zinc deficiency can disrupt NPC proliferation and neuronal differentiation (Swenerton et al., 1969; Dvergsten et al., 1983; Gower-Winter et al., 2013), but in a condition of marginal zinc availability which can be extrapolated to human populations. The disruption observed in neurogenesis could contribute to the described persistent effects of marginal zinc deficiency on behavior. In this regard, marginal zinc deficiency throughout gestation and lactation decreases working memory in rats after dietary repletion (Halas et al., 1986). In mice, marginal zinc deficiency through gestation leads to increased anxiety-like behavior, abnormal social behavior, and impaired motor learning even after dietary repletion (Grabrucker et al., 2014, 2016). Very relevant to the current results, a dysbalance in excitatory/inhibitory systems has been proposed as a developmental precursor of autism spectrum disorders (Mariani et al., 2015) and a possible target for restoring functional connectivity even in adulthood (Ajram et al., 2017).

In summary, this work demonstrates that gestational marginal zinc deficiency affects neurogenesis in the fetal rat brain leading to a disruption of the cortical excitatory/inhibitory balance that persists into adulthood even after dietary repletion. While earlier studies focused on severely deficient animal models, this is the first study to report disruption of fetal neurogenesis resulting from marginal zinc deficiency that affects the cellularity of the mature brain cortex. These findings stress the relevance of an adequate zinc nutrition during pregnancy to prevent irreversible effects on the offspring cortical structure and ultimately on behavior and cognition.

## AUTHOR CONTRIBUTIONS

PO and AA designed the research. XL, AA, SS, JN and PM performed the research. All authors participated in the analysis and discussion of data. PO, AA and JN wrote the article.

## FUNDING

This work was supported by grants from NIFA-USDA (CA-D*-XXX-7244-H) and the Packer-Wentz Endowment to PO, and grants from Universidad de Buenos Aires (20020160100050BA) and CONICET (PIP 0567), Argentina, to AA. SS, JN and XL were recipients of Jastro Shields awards. XL and JN were supported by a National Institute of Environmental Health Sciences funded training program (T32 ES007058-33 and 2T32ES007059-41). SS was a recipient of a Thai Government Scholarship.

## REFERENCES


Adamo, A. M., Zago, M. P., Mackenzie, G. G., Aimo, L., Keen, C. L., Keenan, A., et al. (2010). The role of zinc in the modulation of neuronal proliferation and apoptosis. *Neurotox. Res.* 17, 1–14. doi: 10.1007/s12640-009-9067-4

Aimo, L., Cherr, G. N., and Oteiza, P. I. (2010a). Low extracellular zinc increases neuronal oxidant production through nadph oxidase and nitric oxide synthase activation. *Free Radic. Biol. Med.* 48, 1577–1587. doi: 10.1016/j.freeradbiomed.2010.02.040

Aimo, L., Mackenzie, G. G., Keenan, A. H., and Oteiza, P. I. (2010b). Gestational zinc deficiency affects the regulation of transcription factors AP-1, NF-kappaB and NFAT in fetal brain. *J. Nutr. Biochem.* 21, 1069–1075. doi: 10.1016/j.jnutbio.2009.09.003

Ajram, L. A., Horder, J., Mendez, M. A., Galanopoulos, A., Brennan, L. P., Wichers, R. H., et al. (2017). Shifting brain inhibitory balance and connectivity of the prefrontal cortex of adults with autism spectrum disorder. *Transl. Psychiatry* 7:e1137. doi: 10.1038/tp.2017.104

Anderson, S. A., Eisenstat, D. D., Shi, L., and Rubenstein, J. L. (1997). Interneuron migration from basal forebrain to neocortex: dependence on *Dlx* genes. *Science* 278, 474–476. doi: 10.1126/science.278.5337.474

Bradford, M. M. (1976). A rapid and sensitive method for the quantitation of microgram quantities of protein utilizing the principle of protein-dye binding. *Anal. Biochem.* 72, 248–254. doi: 10.1006/abio.1976.9999

Bulfone, A., Smiga, S. M., Shimamura, K., Peterson, A., Puelles, L., and Rubenstein, J. L. (1995). T-brain-1: a homolog of Brachyury whose expression defines molecularly distinct domains within the cerebral cortex. *Neuron* 15, 63–78. doi: 10.1016/0896-6273(95)90065-9

Butt, S. J., Fuccillo, M., Nery, S., Noctor, S., Kriegstein, A., Corbin, J. G., et al. (2005). The temporal and spatial origins of cortical interneurons predict their physiological subtype. *Neuron* 48, 591–604. doi: 10.1016/j.neuron.2005.09.034

Caulfield, L. E., Zavaleta, N., Chen, P., Lazarte, F., Albornoz, C., Putnick, D. L., et al. (2011). Maternal zinc supplementation during pregnancy affects autonomic function of Peruvian children assessed at 54 months of age. *J. Nutr.* 141, 327–332. doi: 10.3945/jn.110.128843

Chua, J. S., Rofe, A. M., and Coyle, P. (2006). Dietary zinc supplementation ameliorates LPS-induced teratogenicity in mice. *Pediatr. Res.* 59, 355–358. doi: 10.1203/01.pdr.0000199906.37619.9c

Clegg, M. S., Hanna, L. A., Niles, B. J., Momma, T. Y., and Keen, C. L. (2005). Zinc deficiency-induced cell death. *IUBMB Life* 57, 661–669. doi: 10.1080/15216540500264554

DeFelipe, J., and Fariñas, I. (1992). The pyramidal neuron of the cerebral cortex: morphological and chemical characteristics of the synaptic inputs. *Prog. Neurobiol.* 39, 563–607. doi: 10.1016/0301-0082(92)90015-7

Dey, A. C., Shahidullah, M., Mannan, M. A., Noor, M. K., Saha, L., and Rahman, S. A. (2010). Maternal and neonatal serum zinc level and its relationship with neural tube defects. *J. Health Popul. Nutr.* 28, 343–350. doi: 10.3329/jhpn.v28i4.6040

Dvergsten, C. L., Fosmire, G. J., Ollerich, D. A., and Sandstead, H. H. (1983). Alterations in the postnatal development of the cerebellar cortex due to zinc deficiency. I. Impaired acquisition of granule cells. *Brain Res.* 271, 217–226. doi: 10.1016/0006-8993(83)90284-6

Favaro, R., Valotta, M., Ferri, A. L., Latorre, E., Mariani, J., Giachino, C., et al. (2009). Hippocampal development and neural stem cell maintenance require Sox2-dependent regulation of *Shh. Nat. Neurosci.* 12, 1248–1256. doi: 10.1038/nn.2397

Gower-Winter, S. D., Corniola, R. S., Morgan, T. J. Jr., and Levenson, C. W. (2013). Zinc deficiency regulates hippocampal gene expression and impairs neuronal differentiation. *Nutr. Neurosci.* 16, 174–182. doi: 10.1179/1476830512y.0000000043

Grabrucker, S., Boeckers, T. M., and Grabrucker, A. M. (2016). Gender dependent evaluation of autism like behavior in mice exposed to prenatal zinc deficiency. *Front. Behav. Neurosci.* 3:37. doi: 10.3389/fnbeh.2016.00037

Grabrucker, S., Jannetti, L., Eckert, M., Gaub, S., Chhabra, R., Pfaender, S., et al. (2014). Zinc deficiency dysregulates the synaptic ProSAP/Shank scaffold and might contribute to autism spectrum disorders. *Brain* 137, 137–152. doi: 10.1093/brain/awt303

Graham, V., Khudyakov, J., Ellis, P., and Pevny, L. (2003). SOX2 functions to maintain neural progenitor identity. *Neuron* 39, 749–765. doi: 10.1016/s0896-6273(03)00497-5

Hagmeyer, S., Haderspeck, J. C., and Grabrucker, A. M. (2015). Behavioral impairments in animal models for zinc deficiency. *Front. Behav. Neurosci.* 8:443. doi: 10.3389/fnbeh.2014.00443

Halas, E. S., Hunt, C. D., and Eberhardt, M. J. (1986). Learning and memory disabilities in young adult rats from mildly zinc deficient dams. *Physiol. Behav.* 37, 451–458. doi: 10.1016/0031-9384(86)90205-2

Haubensak, W., Attardo, A., Denk, W., and Huttner, W. B. (2004). Neurons arise in the basal neuroepithelium of the early mammalian telencephalon: a major site of neurogenesis. *Proc. Natl. Acad. Sci. U S A* 101, 3196–3201. doi: 10.1073/pnas.0308600100

Hebert, J. M., and Fishell, G. (2008). The genetics of early telencephalon patterning: some assembly required. *Nat. Rev. Neurosci.* 9, 678–685. doi: 10.1038/nrn2463

Hodge, R. D., Nelson, B. R., Kahoud, R. J., Yang, R., Mussar, K. E., Reiner, S. L., et al. (2012). Tbr2 is essential for hippocampal lineage progression from neural stem cells to intermediate progenitors and neurons. *J. Neurosci.* 32, 6275–6287. doi: 10.1523/JNEUROSCI.0532-12.2012

Kalkman, H. O. (2012). Potential opposite roles of the extracellular signal-regulated kinase (ERK) pathway in autism spectrum and bipolar disorders. *Neurosci. Biobehav. Rev.* 36, 2206–2213. doi: 10.1016/j.neubiorev.2012.07.008

Keen, C. L., Peters, J. M., and Hurley, L. S. (1989). The effect of valproic acid on 65Zn distribution in the pregnant rat. *J. Nutr.* 119, 607–611. doi: 10.1093/jn/119.4.607

Kelleher, S. L., and Lönnerdal, B. (2005). Molecular regulation of milk trace mineral homeostasis. *Mol. Aspects Med.* 26, 328–339. doi: 10.1016/j.mam.2005.07.005

Kimura, N., Nakashima, K., Ueno, M., Kiyama, H., and Taga, T. (1999). A novel mammalian T-box-containing gene, Tbr2, expressed in mouse developing brain. *Dev. Brain Res.* 115, 183–193. doi: 10.1016/s0165-3806(99)00064-4

Kirsten, T. B., Queiroz-Hazarbassanov, N., Bernardi, M. M., and Felicio, L. F. (2015). Prenatal zinc prevents communication impairments and BDNF disturbance in a rat model of autism induced by prenatal lipopolysaccharide exposure. *Life Sci.* 130, 12–17. doi: 10.1016/j.lfs.2015.02.027

Mackenzie, G. G., Salvador, G. A., Romero, C., Keen, C. L., and Oteiza, P. I. (2011). A deficit in zinc availability can cause alterations in tubulin thiol redox status in cultured neurons and in the developing fetal rat brain. *Free Radic. Biol. Med.* 51, 480–489. doi: 10.1016/j.freeradbiomed.2011.04.028

Manuel, M. N., Mi, D., Mason, J. O., and Price, D. J. (2015). Regulation of cerebral cortical neurogenesis by the Pax6 transcription factor. *Front. Cell. Neurosci.* 9:70. doi: 10.3389/fncel.2015.00070

Mariani, J., Coppola, G., Zhang, P., Abyzov, A., Provini, L., Tomasini, L., et al. (2015). FOXG1-dependent dysregulation of GABA/glutamate neuron differentiation in autism spectrum disorders. *Cell* 162, 375–390. doi: 10.1016/j.cell.2015.06.034

Marin, O. (2013). Cellular and molecular mechanisms controlling the migration of neocortical interneurons. *Eur. J. Neurosci.* 38, 2019–2029. doi: 10.1111/ejn.12225

Mihalas, A. B., and Hevner, R. F. (2017). Control of neuronal development by T-box genes in the brain. *Curr. Top. Dev. Biol.* 122, 279–312. doi: 10.1016/bs.ctdb.2016.08.001

Noctor, S. C., Martínez-Cerdeño, V., Ivic, L., and Kriegstein, A. R. (2004). Cortical neurons arise in symmetric and asymmetric division zones and migrate through specific phases. *Nat. Neurosci.* 7, 136–144. doi: 10.1038/nn1172

Nuttall, J. R. (2015). The plausibility of maternal toxicant exposure and nutritional status as contributing factors to the risk of autism spectrum disorders. *Nutr. Neurosci.* 20, 209–218. doi: 10.1080/1028415x.2015.1103437

Nuttall, J. R., Kucera, H. R., Supasai, S., Gaikwad, N. W., and Oteiza, P. I. (2017). Combined effects of gestational phthalate exposure and zinc deficiency on steroid metabolism and growth. *Toxicol. Sci.* 156, 469–479. doi: 10.1093/toxsci/kfx008

Nuttall, J. R., and Oteiza, P. I. (2012). Zinc and the ERK kinases in the developing brain. *Neurotox. Res.* 21, 128–141. doi: 10.1007/s12640-011-9291-6

Nuttall, J. R., Supasai, S., Kha, J., Vaeth, B. M., Mackenzie, G. G., Adamo, A. M., et al. (2015). Gestational marginal zinc deficiency impaired fetal neural progenitor cell proliferation by disrupting the ERK1/2 signaling pathway. *J. Nutr. Biochem.* 26, 1116–1123. doi: 10.1016/j.jnutbio.2015.05.007

Oteiza, P. I., Cuellar, S., Lönnerdal, B., Hurley, L. S., and Keen, C. L. (1990). Influence of maternal dietary zinc intake on *in vitro* tubulin polymerization in fetal rat brain. *Teratology* 41, 97–104. doi: 10.1002/tera.1420410110

Peters, A., and Jones, E. G. (1984). "Classification of cortical neurons," in *Cerebral Cortex, Cellular Components of the Cerebral Cortex*, eds A. Peters and E. G. Jones (New York, NY: Plenum Press), 107–121.

Pfaender, S., Sauer, A. K., Hagmeyer, S., Mangus, K., Linta, L., Liebau, S., et al. (2017). Zinc deficiency and low enterocyte zinc transporter expression in human patients with autism related mutations in SHANK3. *Sci. Rep.* 7:45190. doi: 10.1038/srep45190

Pucilowska, J., Puzerey, P. A., Karlo, J. C., Galán, R. F., and Landreth, G. E. (2012). Disrupted ERK signaling during cortical development leads to abnormal progenitor proliferation, neuronal and network excitability and behavior, modeling human neuro-cardio-facial-cutaneous and related syndromes. *J. Neurosci.* 32, 8663–8677. doi: 10.1523/JNEUROSCI.1107-12.2012

Samuels, I. S., Karlo, J. C., Faruzzi, A. N., Pickering, K., Herrup, K., Sweatt, J. D., et al. (2008). Deletion of ERK2 mitogen-activated protein kinase identifies its key roles in cortical neurogenesis and cognitive function. *J. Neurosci.* 28, 6983–6995. doi: 10.1523/JNEUROSCI.0679-08.2008

Samuels, I. S., Saitta, S. C., and Landreth, G. E. (2009). MAP'ing CNS development and cognition: an ERKsome process. *Neuron* 61, 160–167. doi: 10.1016/j.neuron.2009.01.001

Sansom, S. N., Griffiths, D. S., Faedo, A., Kleinjan, D. J., Ruan, Y., Smith, J., et al. (2009). The level of the transcription factor Pax6 is essential for controlling the balance between neural stem cell self-renewal and neurogenesis. *PLoS Genet.* 5:e1000511. doi: 10.1371/journal.pgen.1000511

Satoh, Y., Endo, S., Nakata, T., Kobayashi, Y., Yamada, K., Ikeda, T., et al. (2011). ERK2 contributes to the control of social behaviors in mice. *J. Neurosci.* 31, 11953–11967. doi: 10.1523/JNEUROSCI.2349-11.2011

Spann, M. N., Smerling, J., Gustafsson, H., Foss, S., Altemus, M., and Monk, C. (2015). Deficient maternal zinc intake-but not folate-is associated with lower fetal heart rate variability. *Early Hum. Dev.* 91, 169–172. doi: 10.1016/j.earlhumdev.2015.01.007

Swenerton, H., Shrader, R., and Hurley, L. S. (1969). Zinc-deficient embryos: reduced thymidine incorporation. *Science* 166, 1014–1015. doi: 10.1126/science.166.3908.1014

Uriu-Adams, J. Y., and Keen, C. L. (2010). Zinc and reproduction: effects of zinc deficiency on prenatal and early postnatal development. *Birth Defects Res. B Dev. Reprod. Toxicol.* 89, 313–325. doi: 10.1002/bdrb.20264

Vasistha, N. A., García-Moreno, F., Arora, S., Cheung, A. F., Arnold, S. J., Robertson, E. J., et al. (2015). Cortical and clonal contribution of Tbr2 expressing progenitors in the developing mouse brain. *Cereb. Cortex* 25, 3290–3302. doi: 10.1093/cercor/bhu125

Velie, E. M., Block, G., Shaw, G. M., Samuels, S. J., Schaffer, D. M., and Kulldorff, M. (1999). Maternal supplemental and dietary zinc intake and the occurrence of neural tube defects in California. *Am. J. Epidemiol.* 150, 605–616. doi: 10.1093/oxfordjournals.aje.a010059

Wichterle, H., Turnbull, D. H., Nery, S., Fishell, G., and Alvarez-Buylla, A. (2001). *In utero* fate mapping reveals distinct migratory pathways and fates of neurons born in the mammalian basal forebrain. *Development* 128, 3759–3771.

Wonders, C. P., and Anderson, S. A. (2006). The origin and specification of cortical interneurons. *Nat. Rev. Neurosci.* 7, 687–696. doi: 10.1038/nrn1954

Wonders, C. P., Taylor, L., Welagen, J., Mbata, I. C., Xiang, J. Z., and Anderson, S. A. (2008). A spatial bias for the origins of interneuron subgroups within the medial ganglionic eminence. *Dev. Biol.* 314, 127–136. doi: 10.1016/j.ydbio.2007.11.018

Zago, M. P., Mackenzie, G. G., Adamo, A. M., Keen, C. L., and Oteiza, P. I. (2005). Differential modulation of MAP kinases by zinc deficiency in IMR-32 cells: role of $H_2O_2$. *Antioxid. Redox Signal.* 7, 1773–1782. doi: 10.1089/ars.2005.7.1773

# 7

# Neuroprotection: Pro-Survival and Anti-Neurotoxic Mechanisms as Therapeutic Strategies in Neurodegeneration

*Horacio Uri Saragovi[1,2,3]*, Alba Galan[1,2] and Leonard A. Levin[3,4,5]*

*[1] Lady Davis Institute, Montreal, QC, Canada, [2] Jewish General Hospital, Montreal, QC, Canada, [3] Department of Ophthalmology and Visual Sciences, McGill University, Montreal, QC, Canada, [4] McGill University Health Centre, Montreal, QC, Canada, [5] Montreal Neurological Institute, Mcgill University, Montreal, QC, Canada*

***Correspondence:***
*Horacio Uri Saragovi*
*uri.saragovi@mcgill.ca*

Neurotrophins (NTs) are a subset of the neurotrophic factor family. These growth factors were originally named based on the nerve growth functional assays used to identify them. NTs act as paracrine or autocrine factors for cells expressing NT receptors. The receptors and their function have been studied primarily in cells of the nervous system, but are also present in the cardiovascular, endocrine, and immune systems, as well as in many neoplastic cells. The signals activated by NTs can be varied, depending on cellular stage and context, healthy or disease states, and depending on whether the specific NTs and their receptors are expressed in the relevant cells. In the healthy central and peripheral adult nervous systems, NTs drive neuronal survival, phenotype, synaptic maintenance, and function. Deficiencies of the NT/NT receptor axis are causally associated with disease onset or disease progression. Paradoxically, NTs can also drive synaptic loss and neuronal death. In the embryonic stage this activity is essential for proper developmental pruning of the nervous system, but in the adult it can be associated with neurodegenerative disease. Given their key role in neuronal survival and death, NTs and NT receptors have long been considered therapeutic targets to achieve neuroprotection. The first neuroprotective approaches consisted of enhancing neuronal survival signals using NTs. Later strategies selectively targeted receptors to induce survival signals specifically, while avoiding activation of death signals. Recently, the concept of selectively targeting receptors to reduce neuronal death signals has emerged. Here, we review the rationale of each neuroprotective strategy with respect to the complex cell biology and pharmacology of each target receptor.

**Keywords: small molecule, mimetic, antibody, growth factor, neurotrophin, receptor, neurodegeneration, therapy**

## INTRODUCTION

Neurotrophins (NTs) are a family of growth factors that include nerve growth factor (NGF), brain-derived neurotrophic factor (BDNF), neurotrophin-3 (NT-3), and neurotrophin 4/5 (NT-4/5). Neurotrophin mRNAs are translated into larger precursors named pro-NTs, which are then processed into mature NTs by enzymatic cleavage. The pro-NTs and the mature NTs activate different and sometimes opposing signals and physiological pathways, acting through different receptors (Teng , and Hempstead, 2004).

Mature NTs preferentially activate Trk receptors, which are generally associated with survival signals, whereas pro-NTs activate p75 receptors, which are generally associated with death signals (Chao et al., 2006). Neurodegenerative diseases often exhibit imbalances either in NT (e.g., poor processing of pro-NTs to the mature state or poor transport of NTs to the site, where they are needed) or imbalances in NT receptors (e.g., decreases in pro-survival Trks and increases in pro-death p75). This summary is a simplification, and there are additional issues, such as positive and negative functional cross-regulation of Trks and p75, when these receptors are co-expressed. In certain cellular contexts the receptors may also have altered functions, for example in neoplasia.

Clinical trials using NTs as drugs to promote neuroprotection have consistently failed, in large part due to poor receptor selectivity (e.g., binding to Trks and p75), their pleiotropic pro-survival and pro-death activities, short half-lives, poor pharmacokinetics and bioavailability (Yuen and Mobley, 1996; Thoenen and Sendtner, 2002), or because pro-death p75 receptors may be up-regulated in disease (Rudzinski et al., 2004; Ibanez and Simi, 2012), thus negating the full benefit of Trk activation (Josephy-Hernandez et al., 2017). In addition, in some cases Trk receptors can also promote neuronal death (Tauszig-Delamasure et al., 2007), resulting in a confusing pattern of *in vivo* physiology and hard-to-predict pharmacology.

Many excellent reviews of the NT field discuss the biology and physiology of each factor and receptor (Ibanez and Simi, 2012; Bothwell, 2016), and postulate reasons to explain clinical failures (Yuen and Mobley, 1996; Thoenen and Sendtner, 2002). Other comprehensive reviews describe compounds reported to activate/inactivate Trks and p75 receptors, some of which were used as proof-of-concept therapeutics [reviewed in (Longo and Massa, 2004; Josephy-Hernandez et al., 2017)].

Here, we present a reassessment of neuroprotection strategies and their challenges, focusing on the paradoxes of receptor pharmacology and signals. We distinguish strategies that promote survival and strategies that reduce neurotoxicity, as separate but complementary approaches. Each strategy faces challenges which must be addressed for successful translation into clinically effective neuroprotective therapies.

## NEUROTROPHIN RECEPTORS AND ROLES IN DISEASE

Neurotrophins (NTs) act through two distinct receptor families: three receptor tyrosine kinases named TrkA TrkB and TrkC, and a receptor named p75. NGF binds TrkA, BDNF and NT-4 bind TrkB, and NT-3 prefers TrkC but also can bind TrkA and TrkB (**Figure 1**).

Ligands binding to Trks drive the activation of the receptor tyrosine kinase enzymatic activity and the tyrosine phosphorylation of intracellular proteins (e.g., PLCγ, PI3K, Ras and Raf/MEK/Erk1) to initiate signaling pathways (Saragovi and Gehring, 2000; Miller and Kaplan, 2001). These intracellular signaling pathways are usually associated with neuronal survival, maintenance and function in the peripheral and central nervous systems (CNS), and the survival of stressed neurons (Huang and Reichardt, 2003). Therefore, activation of Trks or their signaling cascades has been sought as a mechanism to thwart neuronal degeneration (Saragovi and Gehring, 2000; Saragovi et al., 2009).

All NTs, including the pro-NTs, also bind to p75, a member of the Tumor Necrosis Factor-α (TNFα) receptor superfamily. NTs binding to p75 lead to the activation of complex cascades that are stage- or tissue-specific. Generally, p75 is believed to signal neuronal atrophy, synaptic loss, loss of function, and cell death (Zaccaro et al., 2001; Hempstead, 2002, 2006; Saragovi and Zaccaro, 2002; Ivanisevic et al., 2003; Chao et al., 2006; Saragovi et al., 2009), and is commonly upregulated in neurodegenerative diseases. In pathological states (**Table 1**), pro-NTs binding to p75 promotes the production of inflammatory cytokines TNFα and α2 Macroglobulin (α2M) by glial cells, and increase levels of pro-NGF itself, thus perpetuating the deleterious activation of p75. All of these factors are neurotoxic at increased levels, and result in a vicious cycle of neurotoxic events (Barcelona and Saragovi, 2015).

Adding another layer of complexity to this signaling axis, the biological function of p75 depends on several factors. The p75 receptor cooperates with other proteins, such as the sortilin family of receptors, which are integral to p75 signaling (Vaegter et al., 2011; Skeldal et al., 2012). Additionally, co-expression of Trks can influence p75 biology, as can the type of cell and its stage of maturation/differentiation. As mentioned above, the p75 receptor also has multiple ligands (all NTs as well as all pro-NTs) (Dechant and Barde, 2002; Nykjaer et al., 2005; Al-Shawi et al., 2007), and co-expression of p75 and Trks regulates ligand binding and affinity (Hempstead and Chao, 1997), as well as functional signaling (Zaccaro et al., 2001; Saragovi and Zaccaro, 2002) in a positive or negative manner (**Figure 1**). Due to the complexity of the signaling pathways, the consequences of pharmacological modulation of p75 *in vivo* are difficult to predict.

Yet another level of complexity in Trk receptor signaling emerges from the presence of Trk receptor isoforms. Trks can be expressed as full-length Trk tyrosine kinase receptors (Trk-FL) or as truncated isoforms without a kinase domain. The truncated isoforms are generated by alternative mRNA splicing, gaining a new and distinct intracellular sequence while lacking intrinsic tyrosine kinase activity (Brahimi et al., 2016). Both truncated TrkB.T1 and TrkC.T1 are able to mediate signals, either by inhibiting full-length tyrosine kinase as a dominant-negative mechanism (Valenzuela et al., 1993; Palko et al., 1999; Das et al., 2000) or by being activated in a ligand-dependent manner (Baxter et al., 1997; Esteban et al., 2006). Pathological upregulation of TrkC.T1 induces neuronal cell death through activation of Rac1 GTPase and pERK signaling pathways, with subsequent increase of TNFα production to toxic levels (Esteban et al., 2006; Galán et al., 2017b). Expression of TrkB.T1 and TrkC.T1 receptors increases in many neurodegenerative diseases (**Table 1**; Bai et al., 2010b; Yanpallewar et al., 2012; Galán et al., 2017b).

**TABLE 1** | Experimental (and in some cases clinical) validation of the indicated receptor targets as "proof-of-concept" in neurodegenerative diseases affecting the CNS.

| | TrkC | TrkC.T1 | p75 | TrkA | TrkB | TrkB.T1 | RET |
|---|---|---|---|---|---|---|---|
| **Brain / Spinal Cord** | | | | | | | |
| Alzheimer's/memory | | | Antag. | Agonist | Agonist | Prevent splicing* | |
| Parkinson's | | | ? | | Agonist | | Agonist |
| ALS | Agonist | Antag. or prevent splicing* | Antag. | | Agonist | Prevent splicing* | Agonist |
| Huntington's | | | Antag. | | Agonist | | Agonist |
| **Cochlea** | | | | | | | |
| Hearing loss | Agonist | Antag. or prevent splicing* | ? | | Agonist | | Agonist |
| **Retina** | | | | | | | |
| Retinitis pigmentosa | | Antag. | Antag. | | | | Agonist |
| Glaucoma | | Antag. or prevent splicing* | Antag. | Agonist | Agonist | | Agonist |
| Diabetic retinopathy | | | Antag. | | | | |
| Optic nerve injury | | | Antag. | Agonist | Agonist | | Agonist |
| Retinal angiogenesis | | Antag. | Antag. | | | | |

*Antag = antagonist. ALS = amyotrophic lateral sclerosis. *Prevention of TrkB or TrkC mRNA splicing to their truncated isoforms was achieved by an engineered mutation of the splicing site in transgenic mice. ? = unclear or contradictory data.*

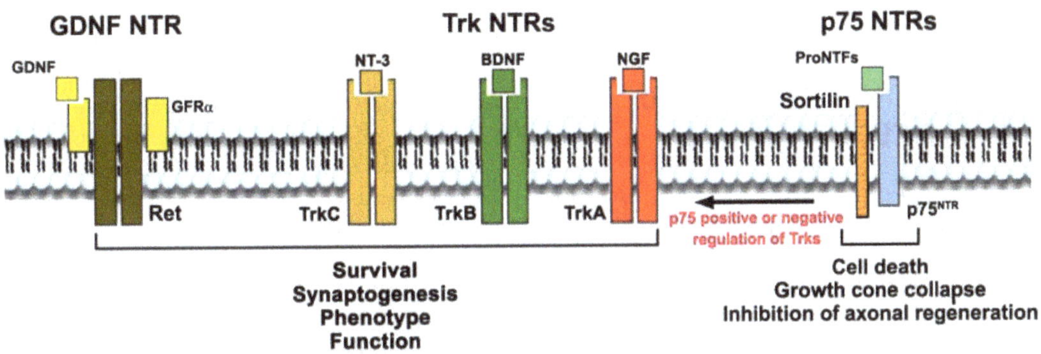


**FIGURE 1** | Neurotrophic Factors, their receptors (NTRs) and functions. NTs activate signaling receptors TrkA, TrkB, TrkC, and p75$^{NTR}$. Each NT receptor (NTR) can act alone, and all Trks can also cooperate positively or negatively with p75$^{NTR}$. GDNF acts through RET but binds the glycosyl-phosphatidylinositol-anchored co-receptor (GFRα1–4) subunits. Mature NTs (NGF, BDNF, NT-3) bind, respectively, TrkA, TrkB and TrkC with some selectivity. All NTs and the precursor pro-neurotrophin proteins bind to p75$^{NTR}$. Growth factor activation of Trks or RET promote survival, growth, differentiation and synaptogenesis. Trk receptors may be present in truncated forms that are not protective (not shown). Growth factor activation of p75$^{NTR}$/sortilin complex in neurons leads to apoptosis, growth cone collapse, and inhibition of axonal regeneration; and in glia, activation of p75$^{NTR}$ leads to production of pro-inflammatory and neurotoxic factors. p75$^{NTR}$ can also regulate the action of Trk receptors positively or negatively, depending on its binding partners and other factors.

Given that truncated isoforms are increased in disease and can be activated by NTs to cause toxicity, it would seem counterintuitive to use NTs as therapeutic agents in these conditions.

## NEUROTROPHIC FACTORS IN CLINICAL DEVELOPMENT

Neurotrophins (NTs) are part of a larger family of neurotrophic factors (NTFs). Among the NTFs, glial-derived neurotrophic factor (GDNF), ciliary-derived neurotrophic factor (CNTF), and insulin-like growth factor-1 (IGF-1) are key determinants of neuronal health (Sakowski et al., 2009; Pasquin et al., 2015) and were tested for clinical efficacy (Yuen and Mobley, 1996; Thoenen and Sendtner, 2002).

Glial-derived neurotrophic factor (GDNF) signals by binding to a co-receptor known as GFRα1, leading to the activation of the tyrosine kinase Ret. Similarly to its counterparts in the Trk family, Ret induces survival through the PI3K/Akt, Ras/Erk, Src and PLCγ signaling pathways (Ibanez, 2013). The absolute requirement of GFRα co-receptors for GDNF activation of Ret limits the number of neurons targeted by GDNF.

## THE EVOLUTION OF THE CONCEPT OF NT-BASED NEUROPROTECTION

The translational potential of NTs as drugs and NT receptors as targets for neuroprotection has long been recognized, and several clinical trials were carried out in the 1990's, none resulting in regulatory approval, the main problems attributed to lack of specific targeting, not achieving an effective dose, and failure to avoid side effects (Thoenen and Sendtner, 2002). The failure of these trials to achieve their endpoints led to a re-evaluation of the validity and druggability of these targets in disease, and particularly the scrutiny of the physiological basis for their pharmacology.

Below we present evolving concepts of NT receptor biology and receptor physiology relevant to their roles in disease. We discuss 4 generations of neuroprotection strategies. Neuroprotection strategy 1.0 refers to the use of NTs or NT-inducing agents regardless of receptor selectivity, pharmacokinetics, or receptor expression patterns. Neuroprotection strategy 2.0 refers to the selective activation of Trk receptors without p75 binding and activation, particularly in diseases, where p75 is upregulated. Neuroprotection strategy 3.0 refers to inhibition of p75-mediated signals, which are pro-inflammatory and neurotoxic. Neuroprotection strategy 4.0 refers to improved Trk-activation in a selective manner, not only circumventing p75 activation but also the activation of truncated Trk isoforms that mediate neurotoxicity (**Figure 2**). Conceivably, these 4 strategies may be combined to achieve synergy, given that they have different mechanisms of action.

## NEUROPROTECTION STRATEGY 1.0: ACTIVATING NT RECEPTORS

Neurotrophins (NTs) normally drive neuronal survival, maintenance of phenotype and synapses, and function. Ligand-dependent activation of the Trk receptors is associated with those survival signals (Sendtner et al., 1996; Bechade et al., 2002; Wan et al., 2014; Brahimi et al., 2016). As mentioned earlier, deficits in the activation of Trk receptor tyrosine kinases (for instance, impaired cellular transport, decreased receptor expression, or agonist deficiency) are linked to early stages of neurodegeneration, and precede neuronal death and symptoms. These data supported the rationale that Trk-agonism may be therapeutic, and NTs were evaluated in multiple experimental models with the expectation that they would solely act as Trk agonists.

Nerve growth factor (NGF) was studied therapeutically to activate TrkA in models of Alzheimer disease (AD) (Schindowski et al., 2008; Cuello et al., 2010), and ageing (Mufson et al., 2000; Bruno et al., 2004; Saragovi, 2005), or Down syndrome (Sendera et al., 2000; Dorsey et al., 2006), models with cholinergic deficits and memory impairment. BDNF and GDNF were studied therapeutically in models of Parkinson disease (PD) (Rangasamy et al., 2010) and Huntington disease (HD) (Alberch et al., 2004), with loss of neurons that express TrkB and RET. NT-3 was studied therapeutically in models of amyotrophic lateral sclerosis (ALS) with loss of spinal cord motor neurons that express TrkC (Ekestern, 2004). Ophthalmic neurodegenerative diseases such as glaucoma (Rudzinski et al., 2004; Nafissi and Foldvari, 2016), retinitis pigmentosa (RP) (Thanos and Emerich, 2005), and diabetic retinopathy (DR) (Bikbova et al., 2014) were studied using NTs as therapeutic agents. In most of these diseases, growth factors other than NTs were explored, including GDNF, CNTF, and IGF-1 (Kaspar et al., 2003; Dupraz et al., 2013; Bassil et al., 2014; Ma et al., 2015; Agostinone et al., 2018) [reviewed in (Gould and Oppenheim, 2011)].

Clinical trials using exogenous delivery of these factors or cells secreting these factors, designed to agonize Trk or RET or IGF-1 receptors, have been consistently unsuccessful. Reasons include the poor pharmacokinetics and pharmacodynamics of NTs, short half-lives, undesirable high potency and pleiotropic effects, inability to penetrate tissue barriers, and difficulty in delivery of these large proteins across the BBB, requiring increasingly sophisticated and risky methods of administration (Weissmiller and Wu, 2012; Rafii et al., 2018), with consequent limitations in reaching the relatively high doses required for efficacy in experimental studies.

Notably, the reasons thought to be responsible for failure are not exclusive to NTs: they generally affect most protein-based therapies, and the issues are resolvable. But there are problems specific to NTs. These include poor receptor selectivity and unpredictable *in vivo* pharmacology, particularly off-target effects on unintended activation of p75 or truncated Trk receptors (Saragovi and Gehring, 2000; Josephy-Hernandez et al., 2017). The expression and activity of these receptors are increased in neurodegenerative states, and given that they are neurotoxic, they invalidate the benefit of Trk activation, decrease the therapeutic effect, and create a poor risk/benefit ratio (**Figure 2A**; Peleshok and Saragovi, 2006; Josephy-Hernandez et al., 2017).

## NEUROPROTECTION STRATEGY 2.0: TARGETING FULL LENGTH Trk RECEPTORS AND AVOIDING p75 ACTIVATION

Based on the many failures of neuroprotection strategy 1.0, we hypothesized that selective Trk-activating agents which circumvent p75 binding and activation would be neuroprotective. To test this idea, we produced a wide range of TrkA-, TrkB-, and TrkC-selective agonists and tested them in different neurodegenerative pathologies (**Figure 2B**). GDNF agonists are also briefly summarized.

### TrkA-, TrkB-, or TrkC-Selective Agonists

We generated small molecule mimetics of NTs (LeSauteur et al., 1995, 1996a; Debeir et al., 1999; Maliartchouk et al., 2000a,b; Pattarawarapan et al., 2002; Zaccaro et al., 2005; Chen et al., 2009), agonistic mAbs (LeSauteur et al., 1996b, Saragovi et al., 1998; Bai et al., 2010c; Guillemard et al., 2010), small molecule mimetics of the mAbs (Brahimi et al., 2009, 2010, 2014; Chen et al., 2009), and mutant NTs (Saragovi et al., 1998; Ivanisevic et al., 2007; Bai et al., 2010a; Aboulkassim et al., 2011). We then tested them in animal models of neurodegenerative disease, demonstrating effectiveness *in vivo*.

For instance, a TrkA-selective NGF mutant that does not activate p75 (Bai et al., 2010a) and the selective small molecule

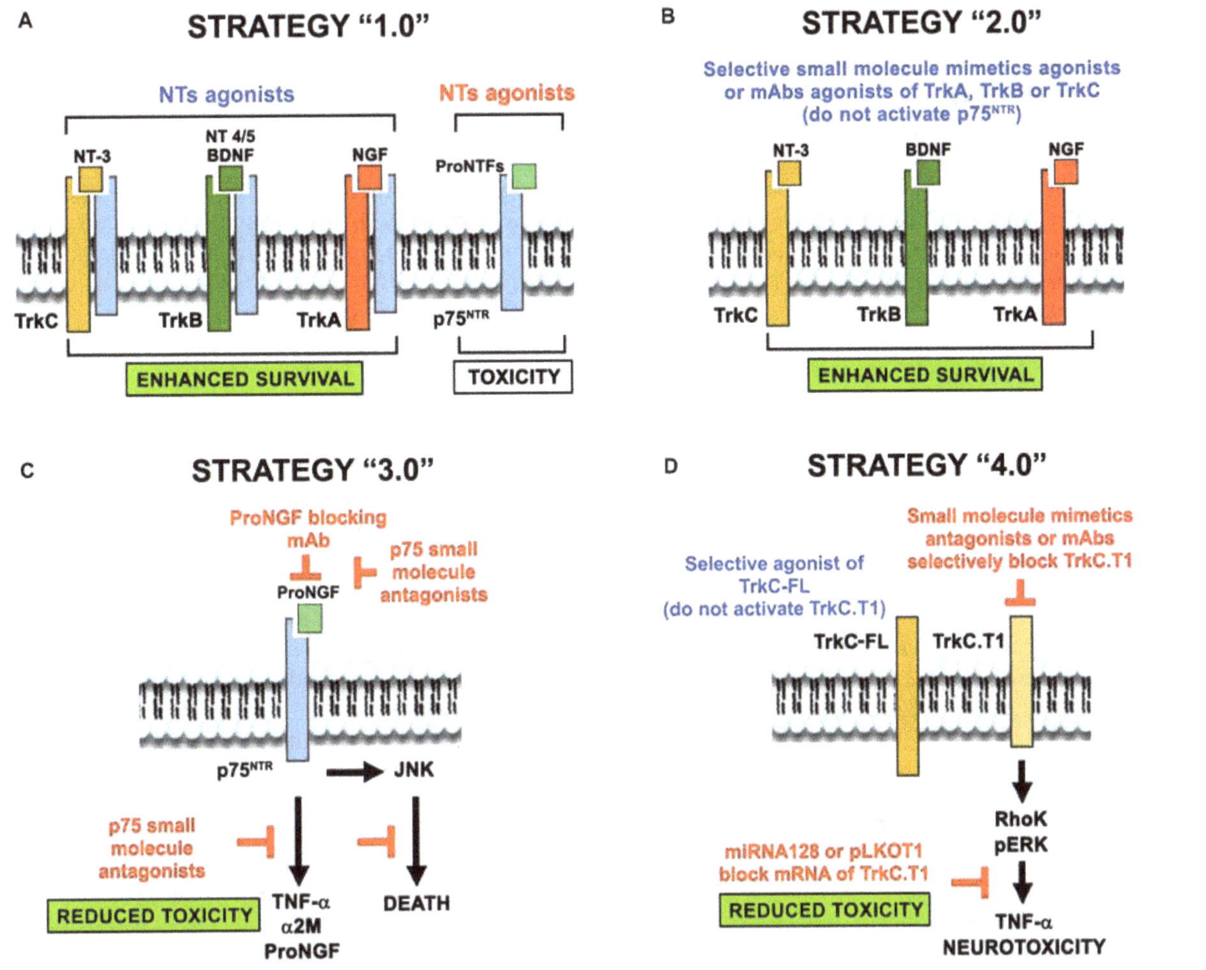


**FIGURE 2 |** The evolution of the concept of NT-based neuroprotection. Four neuroprotective strategies evolved from the use of NTs-based therapies in neurodegenerative diseases. **(A)** Neuroprotection strategy 1.0 was the original use of NTs regardless of receptor selectivity, causing unintended signaling through p75$^{NTR}$ or truncated Trk isoforms that are up-regulated in neurodegenerative pathologies. **(B)** Neuroprotection strategy 2.0 overcomes some of the drawbacks by using selective agonists of Trk receptors (small molecules, mAbs, and mutant NTs that do not bind p75), circumventing p75$^{NTR}$ activation. **(C)** Neuroprotection strategy 3.0 addresses p75$^{NTR}$ neurotoxicity using selective blocking antibodies and small molecules antagonists. **(D)** Neuroprotection strategy 4.0 addresses the toxic function of truncated Trk isoforms by using selective Trk full-length agonists (that do not activate the truncated forms) or selective antagonists of truncated isoforms (small molecules, mAbs, miRNAs and shRNA vectors). Co-expression of p75 and TrkC.T1 in glia may exacerbate neurotoxicity. We predict that combinations of these strategies (e.g., strategy 2 + strategy 3) may be synergistic because of their complementary mechanisms of action.

TrkA agonist D3 (Shi et al., 2007) rescued retinal ganglion cells (RGCs) in glaucoma and optic nerve axotomy models. A selective agonistic mAb that binds TrkB delayed RGC death and preserved the structure of retinal layers from degenerating in optic nerve axotomy and glaucoma (Bai et al., 2010c). A mutant NT-3 selective for TrkC, and an agonistic mAb that activates TrkC (Guillemard et al., 2010) selectively protected motor neurons in an ALS model (Enomoto et al., 2013; Brahimi et al., 2016). None of these ligands bind or activate p75. Many of these agents were very effective *in vivo* in disease states and paradigms, where the native NTs were ineffective unless p75 was concomitantly silenced or neutralized (Bruno et al., 2004; Shi et al., 2007; Lebrun-Julien et al., 2009b, 2010).

Later, other groups validated the concept by generating TrkB small molecule agonists and TrkB and TrkC agonistic mAbs that were protective in the MPTP neurotoxicity mouse model of PD (Berezov et al., 2002; Jang et al., 2010; Devi and Ohno, 2012; Bollen et al., 2013; Coles et al., 2014; Chitranshi et al., 2015; Nie et al., 2015), HD (Jiang et al., 2013; Simmons et al., 2013), and ALS. These agents were effective in experimental paradigms, where the wild type NTs were ineffective, whether endogenously produced or added as therapeutic agents. Yet the wild type NTs became effective when p75 expression was concomitantly silenced or inhibited [reviewed in Josephy-Hernandez et al. (2017)].

With respect to translation to clinical use, one of our TrkA-selective small molecule agonists is currently in Phase 3 clinical trials for an ophthalmic indication, a TrkC-selective mAb agonist is in pre-clinical studies for ALS, and Trk-selective agonistic mAbs and NT mutants are under investigation for neurosensory hearing loss. Other translational efforts with Trk-selective agonists are in progress in PD, ALS, AD, and HD.

### GDNF/Ret Agonists

The GDNF/Ret/GFRα1 axis plays an important neuroprotective role in the retina and other anatomical sites. GDNF causes upregulation of the glutamate aspartate transporter in glial cells, and therefore counteracts the excitotoxic environment in the degenerating retina (Delyfer et al., 2005). GDNF also stimulates the secretion of osteopontin and basic fibroblast growth factor (bFGF), which have been shown to prolong rod survival (Hauck et al., 2006; Del Rio et al., 2011). Following the initial evaluation of GDNF therapies (Strategy 1.0), new efforts have led to the generation of small-molecule agonists with GDNF-like activity or Ret modulatory activity (Sidorova et al., 2017).

Norgestrel is a small molecule related to progesterone that has been demonstrated to be neuroprotective in the rd10 model of RP (Doonan et al., 2011), possibly through the upregulation of bFGF. XIB4035t is a small molecule with effects on GFRα1/Ret signaling. Originally, it was inappropriately characterized as a GFRα1 agonist (Tokugawa et al., 2003), but is nowadays considered to be a GFRα1 modulator, able to potentiate signaling in the presence of GDNF (Hedstrom et al., 2014; Sidorova et al., 2017; Ivanova et al., 2018).

## NEUROPROTECTION STRATEGY 3.0: INHIBITING p75 RECEPTORS

In the adult, the p75 receptor is expressed at low levels in healthy states (Tomellini et al., 2014), but is upregulated in disease. This injury-induced expression recapitulates the role of p75 in development (Ibanez and Simi, 2012), where p75 is expressed at high levels and modulates synaptic pruning and the death of unwanted neurons (Lebrun-Julien et al., 2009b; Bai et al., 2010b). The upregulated p75 receptor is generally associated with neuronal death and is activated primarily by proNGF (**Figure 2C**; Teng et al., 2005).

In neurons, activation of p75 by proNGF triggers apoptotic death, decreases synaptic function (Jansen et al., 2007), and reduces the neuroprotective effect associated with agonists of full-length Trk receptors (Zaccaro et al., 2001; Saragovi and Zaccaro, 2002; Ivanisevic et al., 2003; Saragovi et al., 2009).

In the vasculature, p75 activation causes pericyte dysfunction (Siao et al., 2013; Barcelona et al., 2016) and breakdown of blood–tissue barriers, causing vascular permeability and edema, and leading to vascular endothelial cell death and hypoxia (Shanab et al., 2015). Consequent vaso-obliteration and hypoxia induce VEGF, angiogenic remodeling, and pathological neovascularization (Siao et al., 2013; Barcelona et al., 2016). Thus, p75 on pericytes is relevant to deficits after cardiac hypoxia associated with cardiac injury, retinal neovascularization in DR, and choroidal neovascularization in the wet form of age-related macular degeneration.

In glia, p75 enhances production of the inflammatory mediators TNFα (Srinivasan et al., 2004; Nakazawa et al., 2006; Lebrun-Julien et al., 2009a, Lebrun-Julien et al., 2010; Bai et al., 2010b; Barcelona et al., 2016; Galan et al., 2017a; Platon-Corchado et al., 2017), proNGF (Srinivasan et al., 2004; Lim et al., 2008; Lebrun-Julien et al., 2009b, 2010; Xu et al., 2009; Barcelona et al., 2016), and α2M (Shi et al., 2008; Bai et al., 2010a,b; Barcelona et al., 2016; Galan et al., 2017a; Platon-Corchado et al., 2017). Each of these factors is neurotoxic, and they cooperate to synergistically worsen pathology (Mysona et al., 2013; Barcelona and Saragovi, 2015). Mechanistically, α2M extends the half-lives of TNFα and proNGF (Barcelona and Saragovi, 2015), and p75-driven production of proNGF generates an autocrine loop, resulting in its persistent activation.

Notably, TNFα, proNGF, and α2M are each validated therapeutic targets. Inhibition of TNFα (Nakazawa et al., 2006; Roh et al., 2012), proNGF (Barcelona et al., 2013; Barcelona and Saragovi, 2015), or α2M (Shi et al., 2008; Bai et al., 2010a,b) as monotherapy affords moderate efficacy in retinal neurodegeneration, and other pathologies. Thus, p75 overexpression in disease creates an unfavorable environment by driving at least three neurotoxic proteins, which then feeds back in an autocrine-mediated vicious cycle. Expression and activity of p75 in disease disrupts neuro-glia-vascular homeostasis, with progressive pathology, whereby inflammation causes neuronal death, and neuronal death causes more inflammation and vascular pathology.

These observations in animal models are relevant to human neurodegenerative and vascular diseases because increased levels of p75, TNFα, proNGF, and α2M, alone or in combination, have been documented in ALS, cardiac hypoxia, RP, DR, and others. Inhibition of p75 should also prevent direct neuronal death, vascular deficits, acute inflammation, and chronic production of TNFα, proNGF, and α2M.

We developed a family of drug-like agents that selectively inhibit p75 activity (Bai et al., 2010a; Josephy-Hernandez et al., 2017). These p75 antagonists were therapeutic in models of glaucoma and optic nerve injury (Bai et al., 2010a), RP (Galán et al., 2017b; Platon-Corchado et al., 2017), and neovascularization in DR (Barcelona et al., 2016; Galan et al., 2017a), even when applied as monotherapy after disease onset. Other small p75 ligands reduced tau-related pathology in AD (Massa et al., 2002; Nguyen et al., 2014) and p75-induced motor neuron cell death in ALS (Pehar et al., 2006).

## NEUROPROTECTION STRATEGY 4.0: INHIBITING TRUNCATED Trk RECEPTORS

As described above, the full length Trk receptors have a tyrosine kinase intracellular domain that phosphorylates and activates survival signals such as Akt or PLCγ pathways in a ligand-dependent manner. The "full length" (FL) receptor activity is critical to the survival and function of neurons, where they are expressed. For instance, TrkC-FL is necessary for the physiology of motor neurons and cochlear neurons (Sendtner et al., 1996; Bechade et al., 2002; Mellado Lagarde et al., 2014; Wan et al., 2014; Wan and Corfas, 2015; Brahimi et al., 2016;

Suzuki et al., 2016), whereas TrkB-FL is necessary for brain dopaminergic neurons (Nie et al., 2015).

However, there are truncated Trk receptors which arise from alternative mRNA splicing of Trk-FL mRNAs. The resulting truncated isoforms lack the kinase domain, and signal differently. The most common truncated TrkC and TrkB isoforms in humans and rodents are TrkC.T1 (Tessarollo, 1998; Palko et al., 1999) and TrkB.T1, respectively, (**Figure 2D**; Yanpallewar et al., 2012).

## Truncated TrkC Isoform (TrkC.T1)

TrkC.T1 arises from alternative mRNA splicing of TrkC-FL mRNA, resulting in deletion of the kinase domain, and gain of a new intracellular domain with a unique sequence from a spliced-in exon. For this reason, the TrkC-FL and TrkC.T1 isoforms only differ at the intracellular domain primary sequences, but retain the same extracellular primary sequence. Both TrkC-FL and TrkC.T1 bind NT-3 equally well and both signal in an NT-3–dependent manner (Esteban et al., 2006).

TrkC.T1 acts by activation of Rho kinase-Erk pathways (Esteban et al., 2006; Galán et al., 2017b), and via tamalin (Esteban et al., 2006). One physiological consequence of TrkC.T1 activity is an NT-3–dependent increase in TNFα, which is neurotoxic (Bai et al., 2010b; Brahimi et al., 2016; Galán et al., 2017b). Hence there must be a balance of TrkC-FL and TrkC.T1 signals in health and disease. In healthy adult tissue TrkC.T1 is low or undetectable, but it is significantly upregulated shortly after injury, but before degeneration and detectable symptoms, in neurodegenerative diseases such as glaucoma, RP, and ALS (Bai et al., 2010b; Brahimi et al., 2016; Galán et al., 2017b), as well as in noise-induced hearing loss (Saragovi, unpublished).

TrkC.T1 mRNA is produced constitutively and is immediately degraded by miRNA128. miRNA128 is reduced and TrkC.T1 mRNA is increased in neurodegenerative diseases (Brahimi et al., 2016). Hence, at the onset of neurodegenerative diseases TrkC.T1 protein is upregulated, but without a decrease in TrkC-FL until very late in disease, when neurons die (Bai et al., 2010b; Brahimi et al., 2016; Galán et al., 2017b).

TrkC-FL is present mainly in neurons, whereas in disease states TrkC.T1 is mainly in glia and astrocytes. Hence the TrkC.FL/TrkC.T1 ratio is reduced in diseased tissues with a difference in cellular distribution that is relevant to the mechanisms of action. In glia, TrkC.T1 activity promotes TNFα production in a pErk–dependent manner, and *in vivo* all TrkC.T1 mRNA co-localizes in cells expressing TNFα mRNA (Brahimi et al., 2016; Galan et al., 2017a; Galán et al., 2017b). The TrkC.T1–dependent increase in TNFα is neurotoxic and neurodegenerative, and relevant to the etiology of glaucoma and RP (Bai et al., 2010b; Galán et al., 2017b).

NT-3 binds TrkC-FL and TrkC.T1, and therefore paradoxically activates both neuroprotective and neurodegenerative signals. In this context, we postulated that NT-3 would be therapeutically useful if administered before disease onset (e.g., before TrkC.T1 upregulation), whereas neurotoxicity would predominate when NT-3 was applied after disease onset (e.g., after TrkC.T1 upregulation) (Corse et al., 1999; Park et al., 2009; Wyatt et al., 2011; Suzuki et al., 2016). Indeed, this paradox has been reported in motor neuron degeneration (such as SOD1 mutant rodent models of ALS) (Brahimi et al., 2016), in the death of retinal ganglion cell neurons in a model of RP (Galán et al., 2017b), and may be germane to the death of spiral ganglion neurons in a noise-induced hearing loss model (NIHL).

To directly test the hypothesis that the therapeutic failure of NT-3 is due in part to the unintended activation of TrkC.T1, we developed selective agonists of TrkC-FL. These agents activate TrkC-FL but do not bind or activate TrkC.T1, and therefore do not stimulate TNFα production (Guillemard et al., 2010; Brahimi et al., 2016). In an animal model of ALS these selective TrkC-FL agonists protect motor neuron health and significantly prolong life-span, even when injected after disease onset (Brahimi et al., 2016).

Additionally, we validated this concept by showing that in disease models of neurodegeneration (glaucoma causing RGC neuronal death (Bai et al., 2010b) and a genetically driven model of RP causing photoreceptor neuronal death (Galán et al., 2017b), reduced TrkC.T1 expression had significantly reduced disease progression. reduced levels of TNFα, lower activation of pErk in glia, and reduced neuronal death and neurodegeneration.

With respect to pharmacological inhibition, we have also developed highly selective inhibitors of TrkC.T1 expression (miRNA128 and shRNA vectors) which silence or inhibit TrkC.T1 and prevent induction of TNFα by NT-3 *in vitro* (Brahimi et al., 2016) and *ex vivo* in organotypic cultures (Galán et al., 2017b). Published small molecule inhibitors of TrkC (Brahimi et al., 2010, Brahimi et al., 2014, 2016; Liu et al., 2010) are non-selective between TrkC-FL and TrkC.T1, but significantly decrease TNFα levels and neuronal cell death in a mouse model of glaucoma (Bai et al., 2010b). The non-selective TrkC antagonists used in glaucoma were useful because virtually all the TrkC in the glaucomatous retina is TrkC.T1. However, selective TrkC.T1 inhibitors would be preferable, and we have developed and evaluated such agents (Brahimi et al., 2009, Brahimi et al., 2016).

## Truncated TrkB Isoform (TrkB.T1)

TrkB.T1 (T1) is the main TrkB isoform in the mature brain (Dorsey et al., 2006) and its function was studied *in vivo* (Ferrer et al., 1999). Similar to TrkC.T1, TrkB.T1 inhibits TrkB.FL signaling acting as a dominant-negative receptor, thereby decreasing the effects of BDNF on neuronal survival, differentiation, and plasticity. TrkB.T1 also has BDNF-independent functions and regulates Rho GTPase activity (Ohira et al., 2006) and may stimulate PLCγ and MAPK signaling (Ohira et al., 2007).

TrkB.T1 is upregulated in neurodegenerative diseases such as AD (Ferrer et al., 1999) and ALS (Yanpallewar et al., 2012). Genetic deletion of TrkB.T1 in the SOD mouse model of ALS significantly delayed the onset of motor neuron degeneration (Yanpallewar et al., 2012) and restored cognitive abnormalities (Quarta et al., 2018).

In summary, TrkC.T1 (along with p75, TNFα, proNGF, and α2M) and TrkB.T1 are upregulated in animal and in human diseases (Sanchez et al., 2007; Bai et al., 2011; Roh et al., 2012; Yanpallewar et al., 2012; Siao et al., 2013; Shepheard et al., 2014) and are relevant to pathophysiology, making them excellent therapeutic targets.

## CONCLUSION

It has been 25 years since the first clinical trials of NTs in CNS neurodegenerative disorders. These and subsequent studies failed, due not only to poor pharmacokinetics, short half-lives and/or poor bioavailability of the drugs, but also due to the complex biology of NTs and their receptors. Our understanding of the finely tuned physiology of NT receptors is critical to developing strategies for selectively restoring the balance between neuroprotective and neurotoxic signals. Over the years, we have learned that failures of NTs (neuroprotection strategy 1.0) were related to their pleiotropic effects, poor selectivity and off-target effects on unintended p75 or truncated Trk isoforms. More specific and successful strategies were developed using specific Trk-activating agents that circumvented p75 (neuroprotection strategy 2.0) and therefore potentiated neuroprotection, or by specifically inhibiting p75 receptors (neuroprotection strategy 3.0) or truncated Trk isoforms (neuroprotection strategy 4.0), both signaling neurotoxicity.

NT-based neuroprotection is still an evolving concept, and we can expect the development of even more focused strategies in coming years, which should deal with the complex nature of NT receptor physiology. We envision a future neuroprotection strategy 5.0 based on combining strategies, for example a synergistic neuroprotective and anti-neurotoxic combination, which might finally provide successful translation for treatment of chronic neurodegenerative diseases.

## AUTHOR CONTRIBUTIONS

All authors listed have made a substantial, direct and intellectual contribution to the work, and approved it for publication.

## FUNDING

This work was supported by grants from the Canadian Institutes of Health Research (HS and LL), NIH (LL), and Canada Research Chairs (LL). HS has licensed products for neuroprotection, and is a consultant to Otonomy Inc. LL is a consultant to Aerie, Eyevensys, Galimedix, Prilenia, Quark, and Regenera on neuroprotection.

## REFERENCES

Aboulkassim, T., Tong, X. K., Chung Tse, Y., Wong, T. P., Woo, S. B., Neet, K. E., et al. (2011). Ligand-dependent TrkA activity in brain differentially affects spatial learning and long-term memory. *Mol. Pharmacol.* 80, 498–508. doi: 10.1124/mol.111.071332

Agostinone, J., Alarcon-Martinez, L., Gamlin, C., Yu, W. Q., Wong, R. O. L., and Di Polo, A. (2018). Insulin signalling promotes dendrite and synapse regeneration and restores circuit function after axonal injury. *Brain* 141, 1963–1980. doi: 10.1093/brain/awy142

Alberch, J., Perez-Navarro, E, and Canals, J. M. (2004). Neurotrophic factors in Huntington's disease. *Prog. Brain Res.* 146, 195–229.

Al-Shawi, R., Hafner, A., Chun, S., Raza, S., Crutcher, K., Thrasivoulou, C., et al. (2007). ProNGF, sortilin, and age-related neurodegeneration. *Ann. N. Y. Acad. Sci.* 1119, 208–215. doi: 10.1196/annals.1404.024

Bai, Y., Dergham, P., Nedev, H., Xu, J., Galan, A., Rivera, J. C., et al. (2010a). Chronic and acute models of retinal neurodegeneration TrkA activity are neuroprotective whereas p75NTR activity is neurotoxic through a paracrine mechanism. *J. Biol. Chem.* 285, 39392–39400. doi: 10.1074/jbc.M110.147801

Bai, Y., Shi, Z., Zhuo, Y., Liu, J., Malakhov, A., Ko, E., et al. (2010b). In glaucoma the upregulated truncated TrkC.T1 receptor isoform in glia causes increased TNF-alpha production, leading to retinal ganglion cell death. *Invest. Ophthalmol. Vis. Sci.* 51, 6639–6651. doi: 10.1167/iovs.10-5431

Bai, Y., Sivori, D., Woo, S. B., Neet, K. E., Lerner, S. F., Saragovi, H. U. et al. (2011). During glaucoma, alpha2-macroglobulin accumulates in aqueous humor and binds to nerve growth factor, neutralizing neuroprotection. *Invest. Ophthalmol. Vis. Sci.* 52, 5260–5265. doi: 10.1167/iovs.10-6691

Bai, Y., Xu, J., Brahimi, F., Zhuo, Y., Marinko Sarunic, V., and Saragovi, H. U. et al. (2010c). An agonistic anti-TrkB mAb, but not BDNF, causes sustained TrkB activation, delays RGC death, and protects the retinal structure in optic nerve axotomy and in glaucoma. *Invest. Ophthalmol. Vis. Sci.* 51, 4722–4731.

Barcelona, P. F., Ortiz, S. G., Chiabrando, G. A., and Sanchez, M. C. (2013). alpha2-Macroglobulin induces glial fibrillary acidic protein expression mediated by low-density lipoprotein receptor-related protein 1 in Muller cells. *Invest. Ophthalmol. Vis. Sci.* 52, 778–786. doi: 10.1167/iovs.10-5759

Barcelona, P. F., Sitaras, N., Galan, A., Esquiva, G., Jmaeff, S., Jian, Y., et al. (2016). p75NTR and its ligand ProNGF activate paracrine mechanisms etiological to the vascular, inflammatory, and neurodegenerative pathologies of diabetic retinopathy. *J. Neurosci.* 36, 8826–8841. doi: 10.1523/JNEUROSCI.4278-15.2016

Barcelona, P. F and Saragovi, H. U. (2015). A pro-nerve growth factor (proNGF) and NGF binding protein, alpha2-macroglobulin, differentially regulates p75 and TrkA receptors and is relevant to neurodegeneration *ex vivo* and *in vivo*. *Mol. Cell. Biol.* 35, 3396–3408. doi: 10.1128/mcb.00544-15

Bassil, F., Fernagut, P. O., Bezard, E., and Meissner, W. G. (2014). Insulin, IGF-1 and GLP-1 signaling in neurodegenerative disorders: targets for disease modification? *Prog. Neurobiol.* 118, 1–18. doi: 10.1016/j.pneurobio.2014.02.005

Baxter, G. T., Radeke, M. J., Kuo, R. C., Makrides, V., Hinkle, B., Hoang, R., et al. (1997). Signal transduction mediated by the truncated trkB receptor isoforms, trkB.T1 and trkB.T2. *J. Neurosci.* 17, 2683–2690. doi: 10.1523/jneurosci.17-08-02683.1997

Bechade, C., Mallecourt, C., Sedel, F., Vyas, S., and Triller, A. (2002). Motoneuron-derived neurotrophin-3 is a survival factor for PAX2-expressing spinal interneurons. *J. Neurosci.* 22, 8779–8784. doi: 10.1523/jneurosci.22-20-08779.2002

Berezov, A., Chen, J., Liu, Q., Zhang, H. T., Greene, M. I., Murali, R. et al. (2002). Disabling receptor ensembles with rationally designed interface peptidomimetics. *J. Biol. Chem.* 277, 28330–28339. doi: 10.1074/jbc.m202880200

Bikbova, G., Oshitari, T., Baba, T., and Yamamoto, S. (2014). Neurotrophic factors for retinal ganglion cell neuropathy - with a special reference to diabetic neuropathy in the retina. *Curr. Diabetes Rev.* 10, 166–176. doi: 10.2174/1573399810666140508121927

Bollen, E., Vanmierlo, T., Akkerman, S., Wouters, C., Steinbusch, H. M., Prickaerts, J. et al. (2013). 7,8-Dihydroxyflavone improves memory consolidation processes in rats and mice. *Behav. Brain Res.* 257, 8–12. doi: 10.1016/j.bbr.2013.09.029

Bothwell, M. (2016). Recent advances in understanding neurotrophin signaling. *F1000Res.* 5:F1000 Faculty Rev-1885.

Brahimi, F., Ko, E., Malakhov, A., Burgess, K., and Saragovi, H. U. (2014). Combinatorial assembly of small molecules into bivalent antagonists of TrkC or TrkA receptors. *PLoS One* 9:e89617. doi: 10.1371/journal.pone.0089617

Brahimi, F., Liu, J., Malakhov, A., Chowdhury, S., Purisima, E. O., Ivanisevic, L., et al. (2010). A monovalent agonist of TrkA tyrosine kinase receptors can be converted into a bivalent antagonist. *Biochim. Biophys. Acta* 1800, 1018–1026. doi: 10.1016/j.bbagen.2010.06.007

Brahimi, F., Maira, M., Barcelona, P. F., Galan, A., Aboulkassim, T., Teske, K., et al. (2016). The Paradoxical Signals of Two TrkC Receptor Isoforms Supports a Rationale for Novel Therapeutic Strategies in ALS. *PLoS One* 11:e0162307. doi: 10.1371/journal.pone.0162307

Brahimi, F., Malakhov, A., Lee, H. B., Pattarawarapan, M., Ivanisevic, L., Burgess, K., et al. (2009). A peptidomimetic of NT-3 acts as a TrkC antagonist. *Peptides* 30, 1833–1839. doi: 10.1016/j.peptides.2009.07.015

Bruno, M. A., Clarke, P. B., Seltzer, A., Quirion, R., Burgess, K., Cuello, A. C., et al. (2004). Long-lasting rescue of age-associated deficits in cognition and the CNS cholinergic phenotype by a partial agonist peptidomimetic ligand of TrkA. *J. Neurosci.* 24, 8009–8018. doi: 10.1523/jneurosci.1508-04.2004

Chao, M. V., Rajagopal, R., and Lee, F. S. (2006). Neurotrophin signalling in health and disease. *Clin. Sci.* 110, 167–173. doi: 10.1042/cs20050163

Chen, D., Brahimi, F., Angell, Y., Li, Y. C., Moscowicz, J., Saragovi, H. U., et al. (2009). Bivalent peptidomimetic ligands of TrkC are biased agonists and selectively induce neuritogenesis or potentiate neurotrophin-3 trophic signals. *ACS Chem. Biol.* 4, 769–781. doi: 10.1021/cb9001415

Chitranshi, N., Gupta, V., Kumar, S., and Graham, S. L. (2015). Exploring the molecular interactions of 7,8-dihydroxyflavone and its derivatives with TrkB and VEGFR2 proteins. *Int. J. Mol. Sci.* 16, 21087–21108. doi: 10.3390/ijms160921087

Coles, C. H., Mitakidis, N., Zhang, P., Elegheert, J., Lu, W., Stoker, A. W., et al. (2014). Structural basis for extracellular cis and trans RPTPsigma signal competition in synaptogenesis. *Nat. Commun.* 5:5209. doi: 10.1038/ncomms6209

Corse, A. M., Bilak, M. M., Bilak, S. R., Lehar, M., Rothstein, J. D., Kuncl, R. W. et al. (1999). Preclinical testing of neuroprotective neurotrophic factors in a model of chronic motor neuron degeneration. *Neurobiol. Dis.* 6, 335–346. doi: 10.1006/nbdi.1999.0253

Cuello, A. C., Bruno, M. A., Allard, S., Leon, W., and Iulita, M. F. (2010). Cholinergic involvement in Alzheimer's disease. A link with NGF maturation and degradation. *J. Mol. Neurosci.* 40, 230–235. doi: 10.1007/s12031-009-9 238-z

Das, I., Sparrow, J. R., Lin, M. I., Shih, E., Mikawa, T., Hempstead BL. (2000). Trk C signaling is required for retinal progenitor cell proliferation [published erratum appears. *J. Neurosci.* 20, 2887–2895. doi: 10.1523/jneurosci.20-08-02887.2000

Debeir, T., Saragovi, H. U., and Cuello, A. C. (1999). A nerve growth factor mimetic TrkA antagonist causes withdrawal of cortical cholinergic boutons in the adult rat. *Proc. Natl. Acad. Sci. U.S.A.* 96, 4067–4072. doi: 10.1073/pnas.96.7.4067

Dechant, G., and Barde, Y. A. (2002). The neurotrophin receptor p75(NTR): novel functions and implications for diseases of the nervous system. *Nat. Neurosci.*refvol5, 1131–1136. doi: 10.1038/nn1102-1131

Del Rio, P., Irmler, M., Arango-Gonzalez, B., Favor, J., Bobe, C., Bartsch, U., et al. (2011). GDNF-induced osteopontin from Muller glial cells promotes photoreceptor survival in the Pde6brd1 mouse model of retinal degeneration. *Glia* 59, 821–832. doi: 10.1002/glia.21155

Delyfer, M. N., Forster, V., Neveux, N., Picaud, S., Leveillard, T., Sahel, J. A. et al. (2005). Evidence for glutamate-mediated excitotoxic mechanisms during photoreceptor degeneration in the rd1 mouse retina. *Mol. Vis.* 11, 688–696.

Devi, L, and Ohno, M. (2012). 7,8-dihydroxyflavone, a small-molecule TrkB agonist, reverses memory deficits and BACE1 elevation in a mouse model of Alzheimer's disease. *Neuropsychopharmacology* 37, 434–444. doi: 10.1038/npp.2011.191

Doonan, F., O'Driscoll, C., Kenna, P., and Cotter, T. G. (2011). Enhancing survival of photoreceptor cells in vivo using the synthetic progestin Norgestrel. *J. Neurochem.* 118, 915–927. doi: 10.1111/j.1471-4159.2011.07354.x

Dorsey, S. G., Renn, C. L., Carim-Todd, L. Barrick, C. A., Bambrick, L., Krueger, B. K., et al. (2006). In vivo restoration of physiological levels of truncated TrkB.T1 receptor rescues neuronal cell death in a trisomic mouse model. *Neuron* 51, 21–28. doi: 10.1016/j.neuron.2006.06.009

Dupraz, S., Grassi, D., Karnas, D., Nieto, A. F., Guil, D., Hicks, D et al. (2013). The insulin-like growth factor 1 receptor is essential for axonal regeneration in adult central nervous system neurons. *PLoS One* 8:e54462. doi: 10.1371/journal.pone.0054462

Ekestern, E. (2004). Neurotrophic factors and amyotrophic lateral sclerosis. *Neurodegener. Dis.* 1, 88–100. doi: 10.1159/000080049

Enomoto, M., Bunge, M. B., and Tsoulfas, P. (2013). A multifunctional neurotrophin with reduced affinity to p75NTR enhances transplanted Schwann cell survival and axon growth after spinal cord injury. *Exp. Neurol.* 248, 170–182. doi: 10.1016/j.expneurol.2013.06.013

Esteban, P. F., Yoon, H. Y., Becker, J., Dorsey, S. G., Caprari, P., Palko, M. E., et al. (2006). A kinase-deficient TrkC receptor isoform activates Arf6-Rac1 signaling through the scaffold protein tamalin. *J. Cell Biol.* 173, 291–299. doi: 10.1083/jcb.200512013

Ferrer, I., Marin, C., Rey, M. J., Ribalta, T., Goutan, E., Blanco, R., et al. (1999). BDNF and full-length and truncated TrkB expression in Alzheimer disease. Implications in therapeutic strategies. *J. Neuropathol. Exp. Neurol.* 58, 729–739. doi: 10.1097/00005072-199907000-00007

Galan, A., Barcelona, P. F., Nedev, H., Sarunic, M. V., Jian, Y., Saragovi, H. U., et al. (2017a). Subconjunctival delivery of p75NTR antagonists reduces the inflammatory, vascular, and neurodegenerative pathologies of diabetic retinopathy. *Invest. Ophthalmol. Vis. Sci.* 58, 2852–2862. doi: 10.1167/iovs.16-20988

Galán, A., Jmaeff, S., Barcelona, P. F., Brahimi, F., Sarunic, M. V., and Saragovi, H. U. (2017b). In retinitis pigmentosa TrkC.T1-dependent vectorial Erk activity upregulates glial TNF-alpha, causing selective neuronal death. *Cell Death Dis.* 8, 3222. doi: 10.1038/s41419-017-0074-8

Gould, T. W, and Oppenheim, R. W. (2011). Motor neuron trophic factors: therapeutic use in ALS? *Brain Res. Rev.* 67, 1–39. doi: 10.1016/j.brainresrev.2010.10.003

Guillemard, V., Ivanisevic, L., Garcia, A. G., Scholten, V., Lazo, O. M., Bronfman, F. C., et al. (2010). An agonistic mAb directed to the TrkC receptor juxtamembrane region defines a trophic hot spot and interactions with p75 coreceptors. *Dev. Neurobiol.* 70, 150–164. doi: 10.1002/dneu.20776

Hauck, S. M., Kinkl, N., Deeg, C. A., Swiatek-de Lange, M., Schoffmann, S., and Ueffing, M. (2006). GDNF family ligands trigger indirect neuroprotective signaling in retinal glial cells. *Mol. Cell. Biol.* 26, 2746–2757. doi: 10.1128/mcb.26.7.2746-2757.2006

Hedstrom, K. L., Murtie, J. C., Albers, K., Calcutt, N. A., and Corfas, G. (2014). Treating small fiber neuropathy by topical application of a small molecule modulator of ligand-induced GFRalpha/RET receptor signaling. *Proc. Natl. Acad. Sci. U.S.A.* 111, 2325–2330. doi: 10.1073/pnas.1308889111

Hempstead, B. L. (2002). The many faces of p75NTR. *Curr. Opin. Neurobiol.* 12, 260–267. doi: 10.1016/s0959-4388(02)00321-5

Hempstead, B. L. (2006). Dissecting the diverse actions of pro- and mature neurotrophins. *Curr. Alzheimer Res.* 3, 19–24. doi: 10.2174/156720506775697061

Hempstead, B. L, and Chao, M. V. (1997). Entering the domain of neurotrophin binding. *Nat. Biotechnol.* 15, 623–624. doi: 10.1038/nbt0797-623

Huang, E. J, and Reichardt, L. F. (2003). Trk receptors: roles in neuronal signal transduction. *Annu. Rev. Biochem.* 72, 609–642. doi: 10.1146/annurev.biochem.72.121801.161629

Ibanez, C. F. (2013). Structure and physiology of the RET receptor tyrosine kinase. *Cold Spring Harb. Perspect. Biol.* 5:a009134. doi: 10.1101/cshperspect.a009134

Ibanez, C. F, and Simi, A. (2012). p75 neurotrophin receptor signaling in nervous system injury and degeneration: paradox and opportunity. *Trends Neurosci.* 35, 431–440. doi: 10.1016/j.tins.2012.03.007

Ivanisevic, L., Banerjee, K., and Saragovi, H. U. (2003). Differential cross-regulation of TrkA and TrkC tyrosine kinase receptors with p75. *Oncogene* 22, 5677–5685. doi: 10.1038/sj.onc.1206864

Ivanisevic, L., Zheng, W., Woo, S. B., Neet, K. E., Saragovi, H. U. (2007). TrkA receptor hot spots for binding of NT-3 as a heterologous ligand. *J. Biol. Chem.* 282, 16754–16763. doi: 10.1074/jbc.m701996200

Ivanova, L., Tammiku-Taul, J., Garcia-Sosa, A. T., Sidorova, Y., Saarma, M., and Karelson, M. (2018). Molecular Dynamics Simulations of the Interactions between Glial Cell Line-Derived Neurotrophic Factor Family Receptor GFRalpha1 and Small-Molecule Ligands. *ACS Omega* 3, 11407–11414. doi: 10.1021/acsomega.8b01524

Jang, S. W., Liu, X., Yepes, M., Shepherd, K. R., Miller, G. W., Liu, Y., et al. (2010). A selective TrkB agonist with potent neurotrophic activities by 7,8-dihydroxyflavone. *Proc. Natl. Acad. Sci. U.S.A.* 107, 2687–2692. doi: 10.1073/pnas.0913572107

Jansen, P., Giehl, K., Nyengaard, J. R., Teng, K., Lioubinski, O., Sjoegaard, S. S., et al. (2007). Roles for the pro-neurotrophin receptor sortilin in neuronal development, aging and brain injury. *Nat. Neurosci.* 10, 1449–1457. doi: 10.1038/nn2000

Jiang, M., Peng, Q., Liu, X., Jin, J., Hou, Z., Zhang, J., et al. (2013). Small-molecule TrkB receptor agonists improve motor function and extend survival in a mouse model of Huntington's disease. *Hum. Mol. Genet.* 22, 2462–2470. doi: 10.1093/hmg/ddt098

Josephy-Hernandez, S., Jmaeff, S., Pirvulescu, I., Aboulkassim, T., and Saragovi, H. U. (2017). Neurotrophin receptor agonists and antagonists as therapeutic agents: an evolving paradigm. *Neurobiol. Dis.* 97(Pt. B), 139–155. doi: 10.1016/j.nbd.2016.08.004

Kaspar, B. K., Llado, J., Sherkat, N., Rothstein, J. D., and Gage, F. H. (2003). Retrograde viral delivery of IGF-1 prolongs survival in a mouse ALS model. *Science* 301, 839–842. doi: 10.1126/science.1086137

Lebrun-Julien, F., Bertrand, M. J., De Backer, O., Stellwagen, D., Morales, C. R., Di Polo, A, and Barker, P. A. (2010). ProNGF induces TNFalpha-dependent death of retinal ganglion cells through a p75NTR non-cell-autonomous signaling pathway. *Proc. Natl. Acad. Sci. U.S.A.* 107, 3817–3822. doi: 10.1073/pnas.0909276107

Lebrun-Julien, F., Duplan, L., Pernet, V., Osswald, I., Sapieha, P., Bourgeois, P., et al. (2009a). Excitotoxic death of retinal neurons in vivo occurs via a non-cell-autonomous mechanism. *J. Neurosci.* 29, 5536–5545. doi: 10.1523/JNEUROSCI.0831-09.2009

Lebrun-Julien, F., Morquette, B., Douillette, A., Saragovi, H. U., and Di Polo, A. (2009b). Inhibition of p75(NTR) in glia potentiates TrkA-mediated survival of injured retinal ganglion cells. *Mol. Cell. Neurosci.* 40, 410–420. doi: 10.1016/j.mcn.2008.12.005

LeSauteur, L., Cheung, N. K., Lisbona, R., and Saragovi, H. U. (1996a). Small molecule nerve growth factor analogs image receptors *in vivo*. *Nat. Biotechnol.* 14, 1120–1122.

LeSauteur, L., Maliartchouk, S., Le Jeune, H., Quirion, R., and Saragovi, H. U. (1996b). Potent human p140-TrkA agonists derived from an anti-receptor monoclonal antibody. *J. Neurosci.* 16, 1308–1316. doi: 10.1523/jneurosci.16-04-01308.1996

LeSauteur, L., Wei, L., Gibbs, B. F., and Saragovi, H. U. (1995). Small peptide mimics of nerve growth factor bind TrkA receptors and affect biological responses. *J. Biol. Chem.* 270, 6564–6569. doi: 10.1074/jbc.270.12.6564

Lim, Y. S., McLaughlin, T., Sung, T. C., Santiago, A., Lee, K. F., and O'Leary, D. D. (2008). p75(NTR) mediates ephrin-A reverse signaling required for axon repulsion and mapping. *Neuron* 59, 746–758. doi: 10.1016/j.neuron.2008.07.032

Liu, J., Brahimi, F., Saragovi, H. U., and Burgess, K. (2010). Bivalent diketopiperazine-based tropomysin receptor kinase C (TrkC) antagonists. *J. Med. Chem.* 53, 5044–5048. doi: 10.1021/jm100148d

Longo, F. M, and Massa, S. M. (2004). Neurotrophin-based strategies for neuroprotection. *J. Alzheimers Dis.* 6:S13–S17.

Ma, J., Guo, C., Guo, C., Sun, Y., Liao, T., Beattie, U., et al. (2015). Transplantation of human neural progenitor cells expressing IGF-1 enhances retinal ganglion cell survival. *PLoS One* 10:e0125695. doi: 10.1371/journal.pone.0125695

Maliartchouk, S., Debeir, T., Beglova, N., Cuello, A. C., Gehring, K., and Saragovi, H. U. (2000a). Genuine monovalent ligands of TrkA nerve growth factor receptors reveal a novel pharmacological mechanism of action. *J. Biol. Chem.* 275, 9946–9956. doi: 10.1074/jbc.275.14.9946

Maliartchouk, S., Feng, Y., Ivanisevic, L., Debeir, T., Cuello, A. C., Burgess, K., et al. (2000b). A designed peptidomimetic agonistic ligand of TrkA nerve growth factor receptors. *Mol. Pharmacol.* 57, 385–391.

Massa, S. M., Xie, Y., and Longo, F. M. (2002). Alzheimer's therapeutics: neurotrophin small molecule mimetics. *J. Mol. Neurosci.* 19, 107–111. doi: 10.1007/s12031-002-0019-1

Mellado Lagarde, M. M., Wan, G., Zhang, L., Gigliello, A. R., McInnis, J. J., Zhang, Y., et al. (2014). Spontaneous regeneration of cochlear supporting cells after neonatal ablation ensures hearing in the adult mouse. *Proc. Natl. Acad. Sci. U.S.A.* 111, 16919–16924. doi: 10.1073/pnas.1408064111

Miller, F. D, and Kaplan, D. R. (2001). Neurotrophin signalling pathways regulating neuronal apoptosis. *Cell. Mol. Life Sci.* 58, 1045–1053. doi: 10.1007/pl00000919

Mufson, E. J., Ma, S. Y., Cochran, E. J., Bennett, D. A., Beckett, L. A., Jaffar, S., et al. (2000). Loss of nucleus basalis neurons containing trkA immunoreactivity in individuals with mild cognitive impairment and early Alzheimer's disease. *J. Comp. Neurol.* 427, 19–30. doi: 10.1002/1096-9861(20001106)427:1<19::aid-cne2>3.0.co;2-a

Mysona, B. A., Al-Gayyar, M. M., Matragoon, S., Abdelsaid, M. A., El-Azab, M. F., Saragovi, H. U., et al. (2013). Modulation of p75(NTR) prevents diabetes- and proNGF-induced retinal inflammation and blood-retina barrier breakdown in mice and rats. *Diabetologia* 56, 2329–2339. doi: 10.1007/s00125-013-2998-6

Nafissi, N., and Foldvari, M. (2016). Neurotrophin signalling pathways regulating neuronal apoptosis. *Wiley Interdiscip. Rev. Nanomed. Nanobiotechnol.* 8, 240–254.

Nakazawa, T., Nakazawa, C., Matsubara, A., Noda, K., Hisatomi, T., She, H., et al. (2006). Tumor necrosis factor-alpha mediates oligodendrocyte death and delayed retinal ganglion cell loss in a mouse model of glaucoma. *J. Neurosci.* 26, 12633–12641. doi: 10.1523/jneurosci.2801-06.2006

Nguyen, T. V., Shen, L., Vander Griend, L., Quach, L. N., Belichenko, N. P., Saw, N., et al. (2014). Small molecule $p75^{NTR}$ ligands reduce pathological phosphorylation and misfolding of tau, inflammatory changes, cholinergic degeneration, and cognitive deficits in $AbetaPP^{L/S}$ transgenic mice. *J. Alzheimers Dis.* 42, 459–483. doi: 10.3233/JAD-140036

Nie, S., Xu, Y., Chen, G., Ma, K., Han, C., Guo, Z., et al. (2015). Small molecule TrkB agonist deoxygedunin protects nigrostriatal dopaminergic neurons from 6-OHDA and MPTP induced neurotoxicity in rodents. *Neuropharmacology* 99, 448–458. doi: 10.1016/j.neuropharm.2015.08.016

Nykjaer, A., Willnow, T. E., and Petersen, C. M. (2005). p75NTR–live or let die. *Curr. Opin. Neurobiol.* 15, 49–57. doi: 10.1016/j.conb.2005.01.004

Ohira, K., Funatsu, N., Homma, K. J., Sahara, Y., Hayashi, M., Kaneko, T., et al. (2007). Truncated TrkB-T1 regulates the morphology of neocortical layer I astrocytes in adult rat brain slices. *Eur. J. Neurosci.* 25, 406–416. doi: 10.1111/j.1460-9568.2007.05282.x

Ohira, K., Homma, K. J., Hirai, H., Nakamura, S., and Hayashi, M. (2006). TrkB-T1 regulates the RhoA signaling and actin cytoskeleton in glioma cells. *Biochem. Biophys. Res. Commun.* 342, 867–874. doi: 10.1016/j.bbrc.2006.02.033

Palko, M. E., Coppola, V., and Tessarollo, L. (1999). Evidence for a role of truncated trkC receptor isoforms in mouse development. *Neurosci. J.* 19, 775–782. doi: 10.1523/jneurosci.19-02-00775.1999

Park, S., Kim, H. T., Yun, S., Kim, I. S., Lee, J., Lee, I. S., et al. (2009). Growth factor-expressing human neural progenitor cell grafts protect motor neurons but do not ameliorate motor performance and survival in ALS mice. *Exp. Mol. Med.* 41, 487–500. doi: 10.3858/emm.2009.41.7.054

Pasquin, S., Sharma, M., and Gauchat, J. F. (2015). Ciliary neurotrophic factor (CNTF): new facets of an old molecule for treating neurodegenerative and metabolic syndrome pathologies. *Cytokine Growth Factor Rev.* 26, 507–515. doi: 10.1016/j.cytogfr.2015.07.007

Pattarawarapan, M., Zaccaro, M. C., Saragovi, U. H., and Burgess, K. (2002). New templates for syntheses of ring-fused, C(10) beta-turn peptidomimetics leading to the first reported small-molecule mimic of neurotrophin-3. *J. Med. Chem.* 45, 4387–4390. doi: 10.1021/jm0255421

Pehar, M., Cassina, P., Vargas, M. R., Xie, Y., Beckman, J. S., Massa, S. M., et al. (2006). Modulation of p75-dependent motor neuron death by a small non-peptidyl mimetic of the neurotrophin loop 1 domain. *Eur. J. Neurosci.* 24, 1575–1580. doi: 10.1111/j.1460-9568.2006.05040.x

Peleshok, J., and Saragovi, H. U. (2006). Functional mimetics of neurotrophins and their receptors. *Biochem. Soc. Trans.* 34(Pt. 4), 612–617. doi: 10.1042/bst0340612

Platon-Corchado, M., Barcelona, P. F., Jmaeff, S., Marchena, M., Hernandez-Pinto, A. M., Hernandez- Sanchez, C., et al. (2017). p75NTR antagonists attenuate photoreceptor cell loss in murine models of retinitis pigmentosa. *Cell Death Dis.* 8:e2922. doi: 10.1038/cddis.2017.306

Quarta, E., Fulgenzi, G., Bravi, R., Cohen, E. J., Yanpallewar, S., Tessarollo, L., et al. (2018). Deletion of the endogenous TrkB.T1 receptor isoform restores the number of hippocampal CA1 parvalbumin-positive neurons and rescues long-term potentiation in pre-symptomatic mSOD1(G93A) ALS mice. *Mol. Cell. Neurosci.* 89, 33–41. doi: 10.1016/j.mcn.2018.03.010

Rafii, M. S., Tuszynski, M. H., Thomas, R. G., Barba, D., Brewer, J. B., Rissman, R. A., et al. (2018). Adeno-associated viral vector (Serotype 2)-nerve growth factor for patients with Alzheimer disease: a randomized clinical trial. *JAMA Neurol.* 75, 834–841. doi: 10.1001/jamaneurol.2018.0233

Rangasamy, S. B., Soderstrom, K., Bakay, R. A., and Kordower, J. H. (2010). Neurotrophic factor therapy for Parkinson's disease. *Prog. Brain Res.* 184, 237–264. doi: 10.1016/S0079-6123(10)84013-0

Roh, M., Zhang, Y., Murakami, Y., Thanos, A., Lee, S. C., Vavvas, D. G., et al. (2012). Etanercept, a widely used inhibitor of tumor necrosis factor-alpha (TNF-alpha), prevents retinal ganglion cell loss in a rat model of glaucoma. *PLoS One* 7:e40065. doi: 10.1371/journal.pone.0040065

Rudzinski, M., Wong, T. P., and Saragovi, H. U. (2004). Changes in retinal expression of neurotrophins and neurotrophin receptors induced by ocular hypertension. *J. Neurobiol.* 58, 341–354. doi: 10.1002/neu.10293

Sakowski, S. A., Schuyler, A. D., and Feldman, E. L. (2009). Insulin-like growth factor-I for the treatment of amyotrophic lateral sclerosis. *Amyotroph. Lateral Scler.* 10, 63–73. doi: 10.1080/17482960802160370

Sanchez, M. C., Luna, J. D., Barcelona, P. F., Gramajo, A. L., Juarez, P. C., Riera, C. M., et al. (2007). Effect of retinal laser photocoagulation on the activity of metalloproteinases and the alpha(2)-macroglobulin proteolytic state in the vitreous of eyes with proliferative diabetic retinopathy. *Exp. Eye Res.* 85, 644–650. doi: 10.1016/j.exer.2007.07.018

Saragovi, H. U. (2005). Progression of age-associated cognitive impairment correlates with quantitative and qualitative loss of TrkA receptor protein in nucleus basalis and cortex. *J. Neurochem.* 95, 1472–1480. doi: 10.1111/j.1471-4159.2005.03479.x

Saragovi, H. U., Hamel, E., and Di Polo A. (2009). A neurotrophic rationale for the therapy of neurodegenerative disorders. *Curr. Alzheimer Res.* 6, 419–423. doi: 10.2174/156720509789207912

Saragovi, H. U., Zheng, W., Maliartchouk, S., DiGugliemo, G. M., Mawal, Y. R., Kamen, A., et al. (1998). A TrkA-selective, fast internalizing nerve growth factor-antibody complex induces trophic but not neuritogenic signals. *Biol. J. Chem.* 273, 34933–34940. doi: 10.1074/jbc.273.52.34933

Saragovi, H. U, and Zaccaro, M. C. (2002). Small molecule peptidomimetic ligands of neurotrophin receptors, identifying binding sites, activation sites and regulatory sites. *Curr. Pharm. Des.* 8, 2201–2216. doi: 10.2174/1381612023393215

Saragovi, H. U., and Gehring, K. (2000). Development of pharmacological agents for targeting neurotrophins and their receptors. *Trends Pharmacol. Sci.*refvol 21, 93–98. doi: 10.1016/s0165-6147(99)01444-3

Schindowski, K., Belarbi, K., and Buee, L. (2008). Neurotrophic factors in Alzheimer's disease: role of axonal transport. *Genes Brain Behav.* 7, 43–56. doi: 10.1111/j.1601-183X.2007.00378.x

Sendera, T. J., Ma, S. Y., Jaffar, S., Kozlowski, P. B., Kordower, J. H., Mawal, Y., et al. (2000). Reduction in TrkA-immunoreactive neurons is not associated with an overexpression of galaninergic fibers within the nucleus basalis in Down's syndrome. *Neurochem. J.* 74, 1185–1196. doi: 10.1046/j.1471-4159.2000.741185.x

Sendtner, M., Holtmann, B., and Hughes, R. A. (1996). The response of motoneurons to neurotrophins. *Neurochem. Res.* 21, 831–841. doi: 10.1007/bf02532307

Shanab, A. Y., Mysona, B. A., Matragoon, S., and El-Remessy, A. B. (2015). Silencing p75(NTR) prevents proNGF-induced endothelial cell death and development of acellular capillaries in rat retina. *Mol. Ther. Methods Clin. Dev.* 2:15013. doi: 10.1038/mtm.2015.13

Shepheard, S. R., Chataway, T., Schultz, D. W., Rush, R. A., and Rogers, M. L. (2014). The extracellular domain of neurotrophin receptor p75 as a candidate biomarker for amyotrophic lateral sclerosis. *PLoS One* 9:e87398. doi: 10.1371/journal.pone.0087398

Shi, Z., Birman, E., and Saragovi, H. U. (2007). Neurotrophic rationale in glaucoma: a TrkA agonist, but not NGF or a p75 antagonist, protects retinal ganglion cells in vivo. *Dev. Neurobiol.* 67, 884–894. doi: 10.1002/dneu.20360

Shi, Z., Rudzinski, M., Meerovitch, K., Lebrun-Julien, F., Birman, E., Di, A., et al. (2008). Alpha2-macroglobulin is a mediator of retinal ganglion cell death in glaucoma. *J. Biol. Chem.* 283, 29156–29165. doi: 10.1074/jbc.M802365200

Siao, C. J., Lorentz, C. U., Kermani, P., Marinic, T., Carter, J., McGrath, K., et al. (2013). ProNGF, a cytokine induced after myocardial infarction in humans, targets pericytes to promote microvascular damage and activation. *J. Exp. Med.* 209, 2291–2305. doi: 10.1084/jem.20111749

Sidorova, Y. A., Bespalov, M. M., Wong, A. W., Kambur, O., Jokinen, V., Lilius, T. O., et al. (2017). A novel small molecule GDNF receptor RET agonist, BT13, promotes neurite growth from sensory neurons *in vitro* and attenuates experimental neuropathy in the rat. *Front. Pharmacol.* 8:365. doi: 10.3389/fphar.2017.00365

Simmons, D. A., Belichenko, N. P., Yang, T., Condon, C., Monbureau, M., Shamloo, M., et al. (2013). A small molecule TrkB ligand reduces motor impairment and neuropathology in R6/2 and BACHD mouse models of Huntington's disease. *J. Neurosci.* 33, 18712–18727. doi: 10.1523/JNEUROSCI.1310-13.2013

Skeldal, S., Sykes, A. M., Glerup, S., Matusica, D., Palstra, N., Autio, H., et al. (2012). Mapping of the interaction site between sortilin and the p75 neurotrophin receptor reveals a regulatory role for the sortilin intracellular domain in p75 neurotrophin receptor shedding and apoptosis. *J. Biol. Chem.* 287, 43798–43809. doi: 10.1074/jbc.M112.374710

Srinivasan, B., Roque, C. H., Hempstead, B. L., Al-Ubaidi, M. R., and Roque, R. S. (2004). Microglia-derived pronerve growth factor promotes photoreceptor cell death via p75 neurotrophin receptor. *J. Biol. Chem.*refvol 279, 41839–41845. doi: 10.1074/jbc.m402872200

Suzuki, J., Corfas, G., and Liberman, M. C. (2016). Round-window delivery of neurotrophin 3 regenerates cochlear synapses after acoustic overexposure. *Sci. Rep.* 6:24907. doi: 10.1038/srep24907

Tauszig-Delamasure, S., Yu, L. Y., Cabrera, J. R., Bouzas-Rodriguez, J., Mermet-Bouvier, C., Guix, C., et al. (2007). The TrkC receptor induces apoptosis when the dependence receptor notion meets the neurotrophin paradigm. *Proc. Natl. Acad. Sci. U.S.A.* 104, 13361–13366. doi: 10.1073/pnas.0701243104

Teng, H. K., Teng, K. K., Lee, R., Wright, S., Tevar, S., Almeida, R. D., et al. (2005). ProBDNF induces neuronal apoptosis via activation of a receptor complex of p75NTR and sortilin. *J. Neurosci.* 25, 5455–5463. doi: 10.1523/jneurosci.5123-04.2005

Teng K. K., and Hempstead, B. L. (2004). Neurotrophins and their receptors: signaling trios in complex biological systems. *Cel Mol. Life Sci.* 61, 35–48. doi: 10.1007/s00018-003-3099-3

Tessarollo, L. (1998). Pleiotropic functions of neurotrophins in development. *Cytokine Growth Factor Rev.* 9, 125–137. doi: 10.1016/s1359-6101(98)00003-3

Thanos C. and Emerich, D. (2005). Delivery of neurotrophic factors and therapeutic proteins for retinal diseases. *Expert Opin. Biol. Ther.*refvol 5, 1443–1452. doi: 10.1517/14712598.5.11.1443

Thoenen H. and Sendtner, M. (2002). Neurotrophins: from enthusiastic expectations through sobering experiences to rational therapeutic approaches. *Nat. Neurosci.*refvol 5 1046–1050. doi: 10.1038/nn938

Tokugawa, K., Yamamoto, K., Nishiguchi, M., Sekine, T., Sakai, M., Ueki, T., et al. (2003). XIB4035, a novel nonpeptidyl small molecule agonist for GFRalpha-1. *Neurochem. Int.* 42, 81–86. doi: 10.1016/s0197-0186(02)00053-0

Tomellini, E., Lagadec, C., Polakowska, R., and Le Bourhis, X. (2014). Role of p75 neurotrophin receptor in stem cell biology: more than just a marker. *Cell. Mol. Life Sci.* 71, 2467–2481. doi: 10.1007/s00018-014-1564-9

Vaegter, C. B., Jansen, P., Fjorback, A. W., Glerup, S., Skeldal, S., Kjolby, M., et al. (2011). Sortilin associates with Trk receptors to enhance anterograde transport and neurotrophin signaling. *Nat. Neurosci.* 14, 54–61. doi: 10.1038/nn.2689

Valenzuela, D. M., Maisonpierre, P. C., Glass, D. J., Rojas, E., Nunez, L., Kong, Y., et al. (1993). Alternative forms of rat TrkC with different functional capabilities. *Neuron* 10, 963–974. doi: 10.1016/0896-6273(93)90211-9

Wan, G., and Corfas, G. (2015). No longer falling on deaf ears: mechanisms of degeneration and regeneration of cochlear ribbon synapses. *Hear. Res.* 329, 1–10. doi: 10.1016/j.heares.2015.04.008

Wan, G., Gomez-Casati, M. E., Gigliello, A. R., Liberman, M. C., and Corfas, G. (2014). Neurotrophin-3 regulates ribbon synapse density in the cochlea and induces synapse regeneration after acoustic trauma. *eLife* 3:e03564.

Weissmiller, A. M, and Wu, C. (2012). Current advances in using neurotrophic factors to treat neurodegenerative disorders. *Transl. Neurodegener.* 1:14. doi: 10.1186/2047-9158-1-14

Wyatt, T. J., Rossi, S. L., Siegenthaler, M. M., Frame, J., Robles, R., Nistor, G., et al. (2011). Human motor neuron progenitor transplantation leads to endogenous neuronal sparing in 3 models of motor neuron loss. *Stem Cells Int.* 2011:207230. doi: 10.4061/2011/207230

Xu, F., Wei, Y., Lu, Q., Zheng, D., Zhang, F., Gao, E., et al. (2009). Immunohistochemical localization of sortilin and p75(NTR) in normal and ischemic rat retina. *Neurosci. Lett.* 454, 81–85. doi: 10.1016/j.neulet.2009.02.036

Yanpallewar, S. U., Barrick, C. A., Buckley, H., Becker, J., and Tessarollo, L. (2012). Deletion of the BDNF truncated receptor TrkB.T1 delays disease onset in a mouse model of amyotrophic lateral sclerosis. *PLoS One* 7:e39946. doi: 10.1371/journal.pone.0039946

Yuen, E. C, and Mobley, W. C. (1996). Therapeutic potential of neurotrophic factors for neurological disorders. *Ann. Neurol.* 40, 346–354. doi: 10.1002/ana.410400304

Zaccaro, M. C., Ivanisevic, L., Perez, P., Meakin, S. O., and Saragovi, H. U. (2001). p75 Co-receptors regulate ligand-dependent and ligand-independent Trk receptor activation, in part by altering Trk docking subdomains. *J. Biol. Chem.* 276, 31023–31029. doi: 10.1074/jbc.m104630200

Zaccaro, M. C., Lee, H. B., Pattarawarapan, M., Xia, Z., Caron, A., L'Heureux, P. J., et al. (2005). Selective small molecule peptidomimetic ligands of TrkC and TrkA receptors afford discrete or complete neurotrophic activities. *Chem. Biol.* 12, 1015–1028. doi: 10.1016/j.chembiol.2005.06.015

# 8

# Effect of Autophagy Modulators on Vascular, Glial and Neuronal Alterations in the Oxygen-Induced Retinopathy Mouse Model

*Paula V. Subirada[1,2], María C. Paz[1,2], Magali E. Ridano[1,2], Valeria E. Lorenc[3], Claudio M. Fader[4,5], Gustavo A. Chiabrando[1,2] and María C. Sánchez[1,2]**

*[1] Departamento de Bioquímica Clínica, Facultad de Ciencias Químicas, Universidad Nacional de Córdoba, Córdoba, Argentina, [2] Consejo Nacional de Investigaciones Científicas y Técnicas (CONICET), Centro de Investigaciones en Bioquímica Clínica e Inmunología (CIBICI), Córdoba, Argentina, [3] Nanomedicine and Vision Group, Facultad de Ciencias Biomédicas, Instituto de Investigaciones en Medicina Traslacional, Universidad Austral, Consejo Nacional de Investigaciones en Ciencia y Tecnología (CONICET), Pilar, Argentina, [4] Facultad de Odontología Mendoza, Universidad Nacional de Cuyo, Mendoza, Argentina, [5] Instituto de Histología y Embriología (IHEM), Facultad de Ciencias Médicas, Universidad Nacional de Cuyo, Consejo Nacional de Investigaciones Científicas y Técnicas (CONICET), Mendoza, Argentina*

***Correspondence:**
*María C. Sánchez*
*csanchez@fcq.unc.edu.ar*

Hypoxia is one of the main insults in proliferative retinopathies, leading to neovascularization and neurodegeneration. To maintain homeostasis, neurons require efficient degradation and recycling systems. Autophagy participates in retinal cell death, but it is also a cell survival mechanism. Here, we analyzed the role of autophagy at the three characteristic time periods in the oxygen-induced retinopathy (OIR) mouse model and determined if its modulation can improve vascular and non-vascular alterations. Experiments were performed with chloroquine (CQ) in order to monitor autophagosome accumulation by lysosomal blockade. Post natal day (P)17 OIR mouse retinas showed a significant increase in autophagy flux. In particular, an intense LC3B and p62 staining was observed in inner layers of the retina, mainly proliferating endothelial cells. After a single intraocular injection of Rapamycin at P12 OIR, a decreased neovascular area and vascular endothelial growth factor (VEGF) protein expression were observed at P17 OIR. In addition, whereas the increased expression of glial fibrillary acidic protein (GFAP) was reversed at P26 OIR, the functional alterations persisted. Using a similar therapeutic schedule, we analyzed the effect of anti-VEGF therapy on autophagy flux. Like Rapamycin, VEGF inhibitor treatment not only reduced the amount of neovascular tufts, but also activated autophagy flux at P17 OIR, mainly in ganglion cell layer and inner nuclear layer. Finally, the effects of the disruption of autophagy by Spautin-1, were evaluated at vascular, glial, and neuronal levels. After a single dose of Spautin-1, Western blot analysis showed a significant decrease in LC3B II and p62 protein expression at P13 OIR, returning both autophagy markers to OIR control levels at P17. In addition, neither gliosis nor functional alterations were attenuated. In line with these results, TUNEL staining showed a slight increase in the number of positive cells in the outer nuclear layer at P17 OIR. Overall, our results demonstrate that all treatments of induction or inhibition of the autophagic flux reduced neovascular area but were unable to completely reverse the neuronal damage. Besides, compared to current treatments, rapamycin provides a more promising therapeutic strategy as it reduces both neovascular tufts and persistent gliosis.

**Keywords: autophagy, hypoxia, proliferative retinopathies, vascular endothelial growth factor, retinal functionality, gliosis, neurodegeneration**

## INTRODUCTION

Retinal neovascular pathologies are still leading causes of blindness worldwide in middle age (DR) and pediatric [retinopathy of prematurity (ROP)] population (Campochiaro, 2015; Rubio and Adamis, 2016). Currently, there is a wide spectrum of treatments available for these diseases including laser photocoagulation and, more recently the intraocular injections of anti-VEGF agents (Evans et al., 2014; Diabetic Retinopathy Clinical Research Network et al., 2015; Tah et al., 2015). Independently of the etiology, retinal neovascular pathologies are characterized by an increase in cytoplasmic HIF-1α levels, a subsequent dimerization with HIF-1β and translocation to the nucleus (Semenza, 2012). Vascular endothelial growth factor is one of the most critical target genes of HIF, and a well-known key player in neovascularization (NV) (Nagy et al., 2008). This trophic factor has pleiotropic functions over neurons and ECs in health and disease (Saint-Geniez et al., 2008; Zhang et al., 2009). In hypoxic environment VEGF levels largely increase and is the main responsible of ECs survival, migration, and proliferation (Gerhardt, 2008). Nowadays, anti-VEGF therapies are the most recommended treatment for retinal NV as they have proved high efficacy in animal models and clinical trials (Tah et al., 2015). Although anti-VEGF treatment has shown better outcomes than alternative treatments, ophthalmologists have detected unequal response of patients to the same administration scheme. Moreover, they have observed that some patients lost visual acuity after the chronic treatment (Osaadon et al., 2014; Yang et al., 2016). There are two main explanations that shed light on these events. On one hand, other proteins involved in NV, inflammation, vascular tone and metabolism have critical roles, whereby, VEGF inhibition would result insufficient to restore retinal homeostasis and regresses NV in the hypoxic milieu. On the other hand, VEGF is also a neuroprotective factor and its further depletion has deleterious effects over neuronal survival.

Consequently, many researchers have designed new pharmacological strategies to cope with NV through the modulation of different proteins or molecular pathways. Based on multiple studies carried out in the field of cancer angiogenesis, recently, it has been proposed that autophagy flux would have an important role as a potential therapeutic tool in clinical medicine (Mizushima and Komatsu, 2011). Autophagy is a catabolic intracellular mechanism that provides recycling of its components through the engulfment of damaged proteins and organelles in a double membrane vesicle (Levine et al., 2015). As it participates in retinal cell death but it is also a cell survival mechanism, its modulation may be either beneficial or deleterious depending on the retinal cell type involved or the disease context (Boya et al., 2016; Chai et al., 2016; Rosa et al., 2016; Amato et al., 2018). In this work, we intend to unravel the role of autophagy on retinal pathological NV and neurodegeneration in mice with oxygen-induced retinopathy (OIR), an animal model of proliferative ischemic retinopathy, and determine if its modulation can improve retinal functionality, gliosis, and avoid neuronal cell death.

**Abbreviations:** CQ, chloroquine; DR, diabetic retinopathy; ECs, endothelial cells; ERG, electroretinogram; GCL, ganglion cell layer; GFAP, glial fibrilar acid protein; GS, glutamine synthase; HIF, hypoxia inducible factor; ILM, inner limitant membrane; INL, inner nuclear layer; LAMP1, lysosomal-associated membrane protein 1; LC3B, microtubule-associated proteins 1A/1B light chain 3B; MGCs, Muller glial cells; NG-2, neuron-glial 2; NV, neovascularization; OIR, oxygen induced retinopathy; ONL, outer nuclear layer; P, post natal day; RA, room air; ROP, retinopathy of prematurity; VEGF, vascular endothelial growth factor; VO, vaso-obliteration.

## MATERIALS AND METHODS

C57BL/6J mice were handled according to guidelines of the ARVO Statement for the Use of Animals in Ophthalmic and Vision Research. Experimental procedures were designed and approved by the Institutional Animal Care and Use Committee (CICUAL) of the Faculty of Chemical Sciences, National University of Córdoba (Res. HCD 1216/18). All efforts were made to reduce the number of animals used.

### Oxygen-Induced Retinopathy (OIR) Mouse Model

In the OIR mouse model (Smith et al., 1994), litters of mice pups and their mothers were exposed to high oxygen concentration (75 ± 2%) from P7 to P12 (hyperoxic period) in an incubator chamber. Oxygen was checked twice daily with an oxygen analyzer (Teledyne Analytical Instruments, Industry, CA, United States). Then, mice were brought to room air (RA) for additional 5 or 14 days. Age-matched control C57BL/6 mice were kept continuously at RA. Animals were maintained in clear plastic cages with standard light cycles (12 h light/12 h dark). At P12, OIR mice were intravitreally injected with a 1.0 μl of solution containing a specific treatment: (a) Rapamycin: 0.5 μg/ml (R0395 Sigma Aldrich, St. Louis, MO, United States); (b) Anti-VEGF mAb: 1.25 μg anti-VEGF diluted 1/20 with phosphate buffered saline (PBS) (Bevacizumab; Genentech, San Francisco, CA, United States) as previously reported (Ridano et al., 2017); (c) Spautin-1 200 μM (SML0440, Sigma Aldrich, St. Louis, MO, United States). Vehicle (DMSO/PBS or PBS)/-injected mice were used as controls. Rapamycin and Spautin-1 concentrations were selected according to *in vitro* assays

(Chen et al., 2014; Russo et al., 2018) and concentrations 10 folds higher than in cell cultures were used (taking in account the dilution of the drug in the vitreous cavity). Briefly, pups were locally anesthetized with one drop of proparacaine hydrochloride 0.5% (Anestalcon, Alcon), exophthalmia was induced with one drop of tropicamide 1% (Midril, Alcon, Buenos Aires, Argentina) and eyes were injected at the upper nasal limbus as described previously (Barcelona et al., 2011). Some mice were sacrificed at three typical times in the OIR mouse model: P12 (maximum vaso-obliteration, VO), P17 (maximum NV) and P26 (vascular alteration resolution) (Smith et al., 1994). To evaluate the effect of Rapamycin or Spautin-1 mice were sacrificed 24 h after the injection (P13). In order to analyze the autophagy flux, some mice received an intraperitoneal (i.p.) injection of chloroquine (CQ) 60 mg/kg (Sigma Aldrich, St. Louis, MO, United States) diluted in sterile PBS 4 h before sacrifice. Eyes or retinas of sacrificed mice with CQ pre-treatment were collected and processed for Western blot and immunofluorescence assays and without CQ pre-treatment for quantitative real-time PCR (qRT-PCR), immunohistochemistry, or flat-mount assays. At least six mice per group were used for each condition at each survival time examined. Data were collected from both males and females as there were no apparent sex differences. All mice were sacrificed at the same time of day in order to avoid the circadian effects and to reduce the mouse-to-mouse variability in autophagy markers and flux. Lysosomal analyses were carried out with intraocular injection of 1 μl of red DQ-BSA (1 mg/ml dissolved in PBS pH 7.2; D12051, Invitrogen). The reagent is taken up by every cell and then the red dye is detected in acidic compartments, where DQ is hydrolyzed from albumin. Mice were sacrificed 4 h after DQ injection (without CQ pre-treatment), fixed with 4% paraformaldehyde (PFA) and dehydrated by sucrose gradient for further cryosection.

## Electroretinography (ERG)

Electroretinographic activity was assessed as previously described (Ridano et al., 2017). Briefly, after overnight (ON) dark adaptation and under dim red illumination, mice were anesthetized via i.p. injections with a solution containing ketamine (90 mg/kg)/xilacine (8 mg/kg). The pupils were dilated with 1% tropicamide and the cornea was lubricated with gel drops of 0.4% polyethyleneglycol 400 and 0.3% propylene glycol (Systane, Alcon, Buenos Aires, Argentina) to prevent damage. Mice were exposed to stimuli at a distance of 20 cm. A reference electrode was inserted on the back in the neck, a grounding electrode was attached to the tail, and a gold electrode was placed in contact with the central cornea. Electroretinograms were simultaneously recorded from both eyes and 10 responses to flashes of unattenuated white light (5 cd.s/m$^2$, 0.2 Hz) from a photic stimulator (light-emitting diodes) set at maximum brightness were amplified, filtered (1.5-Hz low-pass filter, 1000 high-pass filter, notch activated) and averaged (Akonic BIO-PC, Argentina). The a-wave was measured as the difference in amplitude between the recording at onset and trough of the negative deflection, and the b-wave amplitude was measured from the trough of the a-wave to the peak of the b-wave. The latencies of the a- and b-waves were measured from the time of flash presentation to the trough of the a-wave or the peak of the b-wave, respectively. Responses were averaged across the two eyes for each mouse.

## Labeling of Flat-Mount Retinas

Mice were euthanized at P17 and eyes were enucleated and fixed with freshly prepared 4% PFA for 1–2 h at room temperature (RT). Corneas were removed with scissors along the limbus and the whole retinas were dissected. Then, they were blocked and permeabilized in Tris-buffered saline (TBS) containing 5% Bovine Serum Albumin (BSA) and 0.1% Triton-X-100 during6 h at 4°C. After that, retinas were incubated ON with 0.01 μg/μl of Isolectin IB4 Alexa fluor-488 conjugate (GSA-IB4) from Molecular Probes, Inc. (Eugene, OR, United States) and anti-GFAP (1/200; Dako, Carpinteria, CA, United States) or anti-microtubule-associated protein-1 light-chain 3 (LC3) B (1:100; L7543, Sigma). Retinas were then washed with TBS containing 0.1% Triton-X-100, stored in PBS at 4°C and examined by confocal laser-scanning microscopy (Olympus FluoView FV1200; Olympus, Corp., New York, NY, United States).

## Retinal Cryosection, Protein Extract, and RNA Sample Preparation

For cryosection, enucleated eyes were fixed during 2 h with 4% PFA at RT, and incubated ON in 10, 20, and 30% of sucrose in PBS at 4°C. Then, they were embedded in optimum cutting temperature (OCT) (Tissue-TEK, Sakura) compound, and 10 μm-thick radial sections were obtained by using a cryostat, as described (Sanchez et al., 2006). Retinal cryosections were stored at −20°C under dry conditions until immunohistochemical analysis.

Neural retinas were dissected from RPE/choroid layers for Western blot and qRT-PCR analysis. Protein extracts were obtained from retinas after homogenization with a lysis buffer containing 20 mM Tris-HCl pH 7.5, 137 mM NaCl, 2 mM EDTA pH 8, 1% Nonidet P40, 1 mM phenylmethylsulfonyl fluoride (PMSF), 2 mM sodium ortovanadate and protease inhibitor cocktail (Sigma Aldrich, St. Louis, MO, United States) (Sanchez et al., 2006), and were sonicated during 20 s at 40% amplitude. In addition, some neural retinas were disrupted in 500 μL Trizol (Invitrogen) and were stored at −80°C until RNA extraction. All the assays were performed in triplicate and results are representative of at least three independent experiments (animals in each group).

## Immunofluorescence

Immunostaining was performed as described previously (Ridano et al., 2017). Briefly, mouse cryosections were washed in PBS, blocked with 2% of BSA in PBS containing 0.1% Tween-20, for 1 h and then incubated ON at 4°C with the following primary antibodies, respectively: rabbit polyclonal anti-LC3B (1/100; L7543, Sigma Aldrich), mouse monoclonal anti-p62 (1/100; ab56416, Abcam), rabbit polyclonal anti- GS (1/100; ab16802, Abcam), rat monoclonal anti- LAMP1 (1/350; ab25245, Abcam), mouse monoclonal anti- GS (1/100; MAB 302, Millipore), mouse monoclonal anti-CD31 (1/50; Abcam, Inc., Cambridge, MA,

United States) and rabbit polyclonal anti-NG-2 (1/100; AB5320, Millipore). Then, sections were washed with TBS 0.1% Triton-X-100 and incubated with secondary antibodies including goat against rabbit or mouse IgG conjugated with Alexa Fluor 488 and 594 (1/250; Molecular Probes, Eugene, OR, United States) and goat anti rat IgG conjugated with Alexa Fluor 594 (1/200; ab150160, Abcam), during 1 h at RT. The sections were also counterstained with Hoechst 33258 (1:3000; Molecular Probes) for 7 min. After a thorough rinse, the sections were mounted with Fluor Save (Calbiochem, La Jolla, CA, United States) and cover slipped. The labeling was visualized using a confocal laser-scanning microscope (Olympus Fluvial FV300 or FV1200; Olympus, Corp., New York, NY, United States). Finally, images were processed with Image J 2 software (National Institutes of Health, Bethesda, MD, United States), including spatial deconvolution, vesicle quantification and colocalization. Negative controls without incubation with primary antibody were carried out to detect unspecific staining (data not shown).

## Western Blot

Protein concentration of retinal extracts were determined by a BCA kit (Pierce, Buenos Aires, Argentina) and 10–20 μg of proteins were electrophoresed in 15% SDS-PAGE. After electrophoresis, proteins were transferred to nitrocellulose membranes (Amersham Hybond ECL; GE Healthcare Bio-Sciences AB, Uppsala, Sweden). To prevent non-specific binding, membranes were blocked with 5% milk in TBS containing 0.1% Tween-20 (TBST) during at least 1 h at RT. Then, blots were incubated with primary antibodies diluted in TBST or 5% BSA in TBST for 1 h at RT or overnight at 4°C, according to the antibody. The following antibodies were used: rabbit polyclonal anti-LC3 (1/1000; L7543, Sigma Aldrich), mouse monoclonal anti p62 (1/1000; ab56416, Abcam) mouse monoclonal anti- VEGF (1/500; R&D system), rabbit polyclonal anti-GFAP (1/1000; Dako, Carpinteria, CA, United States), mouse monoclonal anti-GS (1/500; MAB 302, Millipore Corporation MA, United States), rabbit polyclonal anti-caspase 3 (1/300; HPA 002643, Sigma Aldrich) and mouse monoclonal anti-β-actin (1/2000; ab8226, Abcam). Blots were incubated with IRDye 800 CW donkey anti-rabbit Ig, or IRDye 800 CW donkey anti-mouse IgG antibodies (1/15000 in TBS with 5% BSA) for 1 h, protected from light. After washing with TBST, membranes were visualized and quantified using the Odyssey Infrared Imaging System (LI-COR, Inc., Lincoln, NE, United States).

## Quantitative Real-Time Polymerase Chain Reaction

Total RNA was extracted from neural retinas using Trizol (Invitrogen), according to the manufacturer's instructions and was processed as previously reported (Ridano et al., 2017). Briefly, 1 μg of total RNA was reverse-transcribed in a total volume of 20 μl using random primers (Invitrogen, Buenos Aires, Argentina) and 50 U of M-MLV reverse transcriptase (Promega, Corp.). Then, cDNA was mixed with 1x SYBR Green PCR Master Mix (Applied Biosystems) and forward and reverse primers: Beclin1 forward: ATGGAGGGGTCTAAGGCGTC/ Beclin 1 reverse: TGGGCTGTGGTAAGTAATGGA; ATG5 forward: TGTGCTTCGAGATGTGTGGTT/ ATG5 reverse: GTCAAATAGCTGACTCTTGGCAA; MAPLC3 forward: CGCTTGCAGCTCAATGCTAAC/ MAPLC3 reverse: TCG TACACTTCGGAGATGGG; P62 forward: TGTGGAACAT GGAGGGAAGAG/ P62 reverse: TGTGCCTGTGCTGGAA CTTTC. qPCR were carried out on an Applied Biosystems 7500 Real-Time PCR System with Sequence Detection Software v1.4. The cycling conditions included a hot start at 95°C for 10 min, followed by 40 cycles at 95°C for 15 s and 60°C for 1 min. Specificity was verified by melting curve analysis. Results were normalized to β-actin (Forward: GGCTGTATTCCCCTCCATCG/ Reverse: CCAGTTGGTAACAATGCCATGT). Relative gene expression was calculated according to the 2-ΔΔCt method. Each sample was analyzed in triplicate. No amplification was observed in PCRs using as template water during the cDNA synthesis (data not shown).

## TUNEL Assay

Cell death was examined by terminal deoxynucleotidyltransferase biotin dUTP nick end labeling (TUNEL) assay (Roche, Mannheim, Germany), which contain an anti-dUTP antibody labeled with peroxidase (POD), according to manufacturer's instructions. Slides were counterstained with methyl green to visualize total nuclei and then mounted with DPX Mounting Media (Sigma Aldrich, St. Louis, MO, United States). Negative controls without enzyme were processed in order to avoid false positive results (data not shown). Images were obtained under a light microscope (Nikon Eclipse TE2000-E, United States).

## Statistical Analysis

Statistical analysis was performed using the GraphPad Prism 5.0 software. A $p$-value < 0.05 was considered statistically significant. Parametric or non-parametric tests were used according to variance homogeneity evaluated by F or Barlett's tests. Two-tailed unpaired t or Mann–Whitney tests were used in analysis of two groups. One-way analysis of variance (ANOVA) followed by Dunnett´s multiple comparison post-test or Kruskal–Wallis followed by Dunn's multiple comparison post-test were used to determine statistical significance among more than two different groups. Two-way ANOVA followed by Bonferroni post-test was used in comparisons between groups when two variables were affecting the dependent variable. Mean ± standard error (SEM) are shown in graphs analyzed with parametric tests and median with interquartile range are shown when data were analyzed with non-parametric test.

# RESULTS

## Hypoxia Induced Autophagy During Neovascular Stage in the OIR Mouse Model

Autophagy is a strictly regulated process that plays a vital role in cell growth, transition, and death (Kimura et al., 2017). In the nervous system it is a matter of intense investigation as these pathways are often missregulated during neovascular and neurodegenerative conditions (Harris and Rubinsztein, 2011; Du et al., 2012; Liu et al., 2016). In this regard, the mouse model of OIR offers an opportunity to examine the role of hypoxia in the pathogenesis of retinal NV, neuroinflammation, oxidative stress, and neurovascular cross-talk (Kim et al., 2016). Thus, in order to study autophagy flux, we determined the expression of classical autophagy markers at the three relevant time points in the OIR mouse model (**Figure 1A**). As we expected, GSA-IB4 lectin-labeled blood vessels in flat-mount retinas showed, at P17 OIR, a central zone of VO in addition to the characteristic vitreoretinal neovascular tufts, which were not observed in P17 RA controls (**Figure 1B**). Post-mitotic cells, especially neurons, are highly dependent on intracellular degradation systems because they provide adequate waste products elimination. The retina is known to have a fast autophagy flux due to the constant exposure to light and increased production of reactive oxygen species (Trachsel-Moncho et al., 2018). Therefore, we decided to block the autophagosome fusion with lysosomes and degradation with an i.p. injection of CQ to evaluate the accumulation of autophagosomes. Retinal levels for LC3B and p62 protein expression, at each temporal point, were measured in both RA and OIR mice by Western blot assays (**Figure 1C**). Quantitative analysis revealed a slight increase in LC3B II protein expression level at P12 in OIR mice, which was markedly upregulated in P17, returning to baseline levels at P26. In our experimental conditions, upregulation of LC3B II in retinal extracts at P17 OIR was associated with an increase, although not statistically significant, in p62 protein expression (**Figure 1D**). To gain more insight into autophagy regulation at the time point where most changes have been observed (P17), additional Western blot assays in mice injected with vehicle or CQ were performed (**Figure 1E**). Quantitative analysis showed an increase, although not statistically significant, in both LC3B II and p62 levels at P17 OIR compared to RA mice retinas injected with vehicle, which were further enhanced after CQ treatment (**Figure 1F**). Our data showed that the augmentation of LC3B II by hypoxic injury is due to the enhancement of autophagic flux rather than impaired clearance of autophagosomes.

Next, we examined the transcript expression of molecules involved in nucleation (Beclin-1), elongation (ATG-5), and structure (LC3) of the autophagosome (Yin et al., 2016), and also the autophagy substrate p62 at the peak of NV. Beclin-1, ATG-5 and LC3 mRNA levels did not showed changes at P17, whereas expression of p62 mRNA was increased $\sim$1.8–fold at this time point (**Figure 1G**).

By immunostaining of retinal cryosections we confirmed the increase in LC3B and p62 protein expression at P17 OIR (**Figure 1H**). Given that there is a tissue gradient of hypoxia in OIR retinas (Rodrigues et al., 2013), we decided to evaluate whether variations in autophagy flux were similar in every retinal layer. The analysis revealed an intense LC3B and p62 signal in the inner limiting membrane (ILM) at P17 OIR (**Figure 1I**). As neurons in the INL and GCL are severely affected by hypoxia (Ridano et al., 2017), quantification evidenced an increase in LC3B puncta mainly in these areas. At the same time, no modification in the autophagy marker puncta was observed in the ONL (**Figures 1I,J**).

Finally, we explored in more detail the presence of autophagosomes in the ILM, a region where vascular and macroglial cells actively interact. In cryosections, we identified Müller glial cells (MGCs) and vascular cells by staining with GS and CD31 respectively, whereas in retinal flat-mounts ECs were isolectin IB4$^{+}$ cells (**Figure 2**, upper panel). Both macroglial and ECs showed, at P17 OIR, a slight increase in LC3B vesicles within the cells (**Figures 2A,B**). However, in neovascular tufts, ECs showed the great number of autophagic vesicles (**Figure 2C**).

In order to determine if the degradative pathway is activated at P17 OIR, we performed immunofluorescence assays using a combination of LC3B antibody along with the late endosomal compartments and lysosomes marker LAMP1 antibody (**Figure 2D**). Fusion of LC3B and LAMP1 positive vesicles was observed in ILM, GCL, and INL in OIR and RA neural retinas (**Figure 2E**). Our statistical analysis did not found differences in colocalization quantification in absence of CQ, probably due to the fast flux in the retina (**Figure 2F**). Through the injection of CQ, we could detect an increase of LAMP-1 vesicles, suggesting that lysosomes and late endosomes are following the degradation pathway properly (**Figures 2G,H**). To further examine the lysosomal activity, mice were intravitreally injected with bovine serum albumin derivate DQ-BSA (Frost et al., 2017). Confocal images showed an increased DQ-BSA staining in ECs at the time when the NV peaks in the OIR mice, compared to RA control retinas (**Figure 2I**), correlating with the observed in **Figure 2E**. However, this increase was not observed in the retinal layers where death was increased (**Figure 2I**). Collectively, our results showed an increase in autophagy flux mainly in proliferating ECs, and inner layers of the retina whereas neurons from the ONL did not showed modifications in autophagic flux at P17 OIR.

## Rapamycin Promoted Autophagy, Prevented NV and Improved Gliosis in the OIR Mice Model

Rapamycin is a potent inhibitor of the complex mTORC1. One of the functions of this multi-protein complex is to prevent the formation of new autophagosomes by phosphorylation of ATG13. In this sense, Rapamycin acts as an autophagy inductor and its different pharmacological formulations (everolimus, sirolimus, among others) have shown beneficial effects in cancer therapies (Li et al., 2014). On the other hand, mTORC1 phosphorylation increase VEGF synthesis, a trophic factor required for vessel survival, proliferation and migration (Wei et al., 2016). New insights in retinal neurodegeneration pointed Rapamycin as a promising therapy as it could both activate autophagy and decrease angiogenesis (Zhu and Du, 2018). Hence, we decided to evaluate neovascular and neurodegenerative processes in the OIR mouse model after Rapamycin treatment (**Figure 3A**). After a single intraocular injection at P12 OIR, we verified the increase in the autophagy flux 24 h later by Western blot assay (**Figure 3B**). In addition, as Yagasaki et al. (2014) demonstrated previously, Rapamycin decreased the NV in P17 OIR retinas. Quantitative analysis

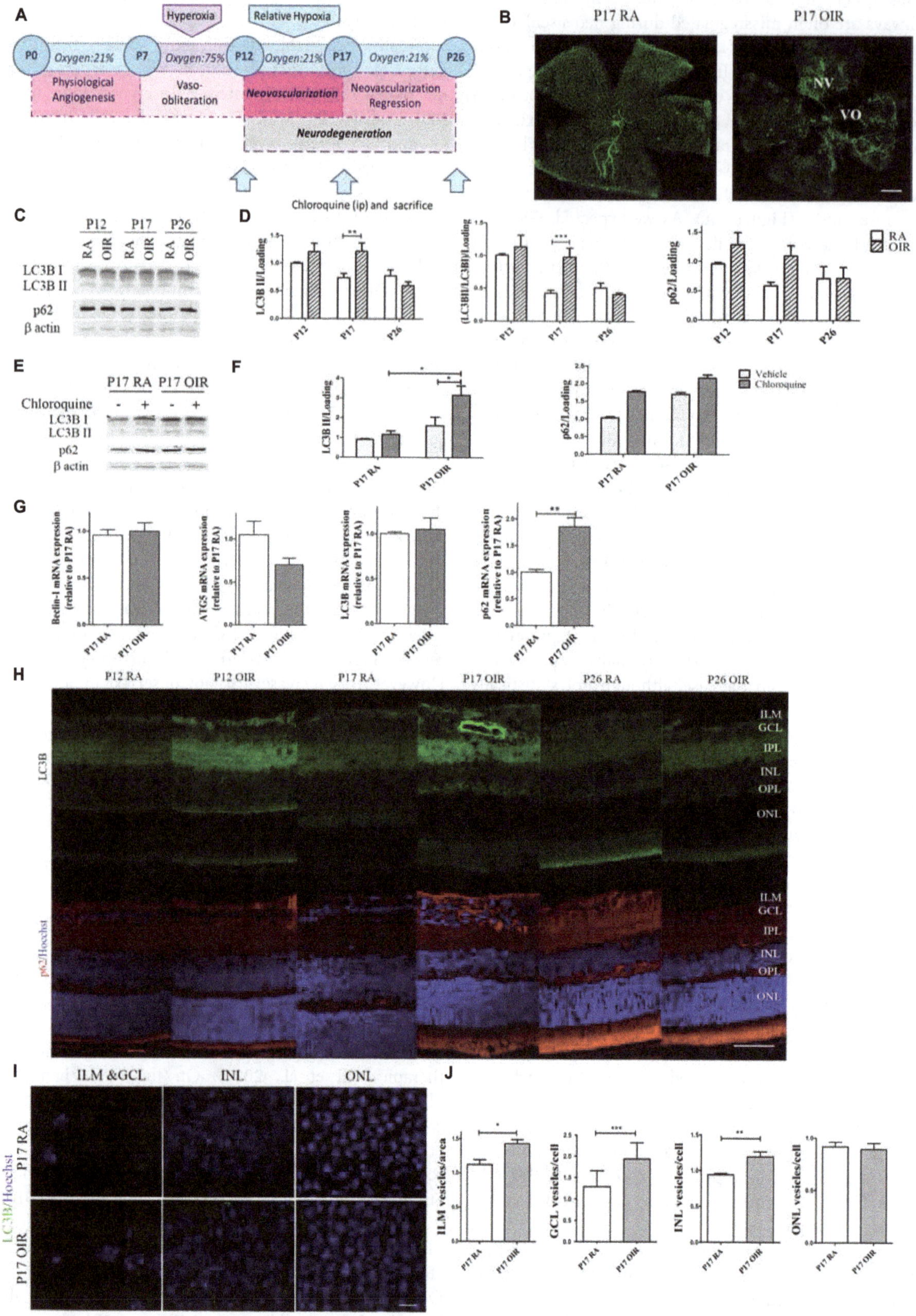


**FIGURE 1** | Continued

**FIGURE 1 |** Effect of hypoxia on the autophagic flux during NV and neurodegeneration in OIR mouse retinas. **(A)** Scheme representing the OIR mouse model with hallmark time points during experimental disease development. Neonatal mice and their nursing mother are kept in room air from birth to P7. At P7, they are exposed to 75% oxygen, which inhibits retinal vessel growth and causes significant VO. Mice are returned to RA at P12; the avascular retina becomes hypoxic, eliciting both normal vessel regrowth and pathological neovascular response. NV reaches its maximum at P17. Shortly thereafter, it spontaneously regresses and the vascular alterations resolve by P25. **(B)** Representative images of flat-mount retinas at P17 showing GSA-IB4 vascular staining in RA and OIR mice. Areas with VO and NV are indicated. Scale bar: 500 μm. **(C,D)** Representative Western blot and quantification data of autophagy markers LC3B II and p62 from neural retinal extracts of RA and OIR at P12, P17, and P26. Mice were injected i.p. with CQ 4 h before sacrifice. β-Actin is shown as a loading control. Graph shows results of three independent experiments. **(E,F)** Representative Western blot and quantification data of autophagy markers, LC3B II and p62, from neural retinal samples of RA and OIR mice injected with vehicle or CQ at P17, and evaluated 4 h after administration. β-Actin is shown as a loading control. Graph shows results of three independent experiments. **(G)** Beclin-1, ATG5, LC3, and p62 mRNA levels were quantified by qRT-PCR in neurosensory retinas of P17 OIR and RA mice. Results were normalized to β-actin and expressed according to the 2-ΔΔCt method using as calibrator the mRNA level obtained from P17 RA mouse retinas. **(H)** Representative immunofluorescence analysis of LC3B (green) and p62 (red) in cryosections of RA and OIR mice injected with CQ at P12, P17, or P26 and evaluated 4 h after administration. Cell nuclei were counterstained with Hoechst 33258 (blue). **(I)** Representative labeling of LC3B (green) in cryosections of RA and OIR mouse retinas at P17, 4 h after CQ administration. Images were taken with oil 60X objective in the best confocal resolution condition. Cell nuclei were counterstained with Hoechst 33258 (blue) Scale bar: 5 μm. **(J)** Quantification of LC3B puncta per area or cell with ImageJ analyze particles software. ILM, inner limiting membrane; GCL, ganglion cell layer; IPL, inner plexiform layer; INL, inner nuclear layer; OPL, outer plexiform layer; ONL, outer nuclear layer. Data are presented as mean ± SEM. $*p < 0.05$, $**p < 0.01$, $***p < 0.001$.

revealed a decrease of more than 75% of retinal NV area. However, the treatment was not able to attenuate other vascular alterations as avascular area, vessel dilatation and tortuosity (**Figures 3C,D**). In line with these observations, our next goal was to determine the protein expression levels of VEGF after Rapamycin treatment. Our results demonstrate that Rapamycin injection at P12 OIR significantly reduced VEGF protein expression in P17, respect to vehicle-injected OIR mouse samples (**Figure 3E**). Pericytes are mesenchymal cells that make important contributions to the microvascular tree in both normal and pathologic tissues (Gerhardt and Betsholtz, 2003). To determine the effect of Rapamycin on pericytes, retinal cryosections at P17 OIR were analyzed by immunofluorescence assay. Confocal microscopy analysis revealed no significant changes in NG-2 (a pericyte marker) staining after Rapamycin injection at P12 among both conditions (**Figure 3F**).

Persistent glial activation is considered a bad prognosis sign, as macroglial reactive cells frequently secrete cytokines and chemokines, contributing to the proinflammatory environment and mediating neuronal death (Subirada et al., 2018). Recently, we have demonstrated that P17 OIR mouse retinas showed the highest neovascular profile and exhibited neuro-glial injury as well as retinal functional loss, which persisted until P26 OIR (Ridano et al., 2017). Herein, we further analyzed if the inhibition of mTORC1 improved gliosis. By Western blot assays we observed comparable protein expression of GFAP in Rapamycin and vehicle-injected P17 OIR retinas (**Figures 4A,B**), which was corroborated by confocal microscopy analysis of flat mounts retinas (**Figure 4C**). However, the quantification at P26 evidenced a significant decrease of the GFAP protein expression after Rapamycin injection at P12. At the same time, we evaluated glial ability to prevent excitotoxicity by analyzing GS protein expression. Quantification of protein levels of the detoxifying enzyme indicated that it was not modified after Rapamycin treatment neither at P17 nor at P26 (**Figures 4A,B**), although a slight increase in the inner layers was detected by immunofluorescence staining (**Figure 4D**).

In retinal neovascular pathologies there is a direct relationship between vascular changes and neuronal dysfunction (Kern, 2014). Thus, we performed ERG studies in both OIR groups (vehicle and Rapamycin) and recorded the intensity (amplitude) and the speed (latency) of the neuronal response after light stimuli. Results demonstrated that neurodegeneration associated to NV was not prevented by the injection at P12 of Rapamycin as ERG signals at P17 and P26 did not show differences after treatment (**Figure 4E**). In line with this result, TUNEL assay (**Figure 4F**) and Western blot quantification of total caspase-3, in retinal extracts of OIR mice (**Figures 4G,H**), were similar in Rapamycin-injected respect to vehicle-injected OIR mouse samples.

We also evaluated changes in autophagy flux at P17 and P26 OIR after Rapamycin treatment. As shown in **Figures 4G,H**, increased levels of LC3B II and p62 expression persisted up to P17. Immunofluorescence assays (**Figure 4I**), were consistent with the Western blot results demonstrating LC3B and p62 staining mainly at GCL and INL. Together, these results indicate that a single injection of Rapamycin was able to prevent the formation of neovessels at P17 OIR by decreasing VEGF protein expression and ameliorate gliosis at P26. By contrast, other vascular and neuronal abnormalities were not reverted.

## Anti-VEGF Treatment Increased the Autophagy Flux in OIR Mouse Retinas

In recent years, several studies have shown that VEGF inhibitors can lead to the activation of autophagy, including ranibizumab, bevacizumab, and several other vascular inhibitors (Liang et al., 2015; Lytvynchuk et al., 2015; Liu et al., 2016). Thus, we decided to determine whether the classical anti-angiogenic treatment was able to modulate the autophagic flux. For this purpose, using a similar treatment schedule (**Figure 5A**), we verified the anti-VEGF effect on vascular alteration in flat-mount retinas, where a significant reduction in neovascular and avascular areas was observed (**Figure 5B**). In addition, as expected, the administration of anti-VEGF mAb at P12 significantly reduced VEGF protein expression in P17 respect to vehicle-injected OIR mouse samples (**Figures 5C,D**).

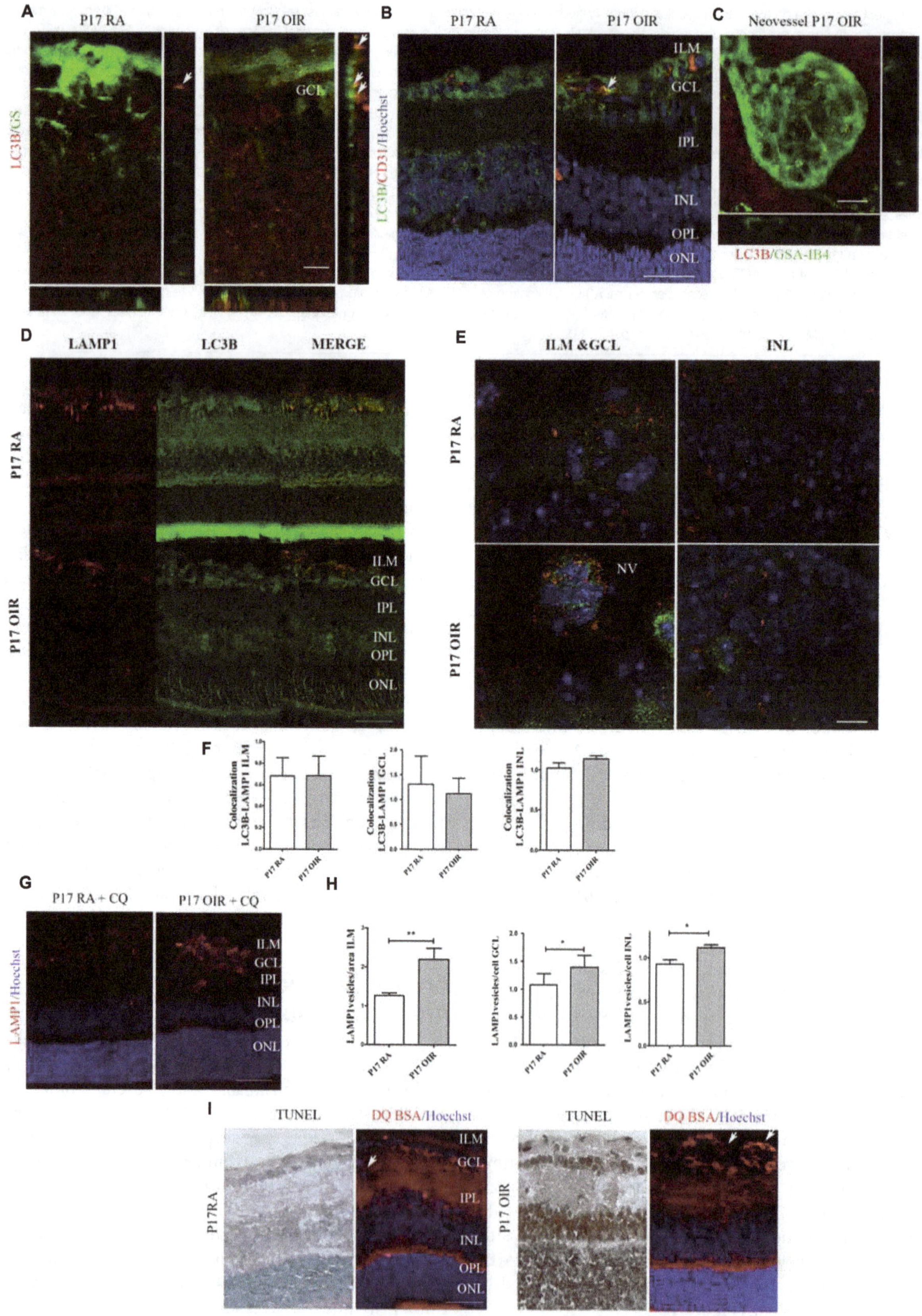


**FIGURE 2** | Continued

**FIGURE 2 |** Effect of hypoxia on LC3B expression and distribution in P17 mouse retinas. Double labeling using: **(A)** a mouse monoclonal antibody for LC3B (red) and a MGC marker, anti-GS (green). Representative merged fluorescence confocal images of entire z-stack (XY) with orthogonal views, XZ and YZ of a mouse retina. Arrows are indicating autophagosomes in MGCs. Scale bar: 5 μm; **(B)** a mouse monoclonal antibody for LC3B (green) and an EC-specific marker, anti-CD31 (red). Cell nuclei were counterstained with Hoechst 33258 (blue). Arrows are indicating autophagosomes in ECs. Scale bar: 50 μm. **(C)** High magnification confocal micrograph of the representative P17 OIR retina showing a typical neovascular tuft (GSA-IB4, green) staining with LC3B (red). Images were taken with oil 60X objective in the best confocal resolution condition. Representative merged fluorescence confocal images of entire z-stack (XY) with orthogonal views, XZ and YZ. Scale bar: 15 μm **(D)** Representative immunofluorescence analysis of LAMP1 (red) and LC3B (green) in cryosections of P17 RA and OIR mice. Scale bar: 50 μm. **(E)** Representative immunofluorescence analysis of LAMP1 (red) and LC3B (green) in cryosections of P17 RA and OIR mice. Images were taken with oil 60X objective and zoom 5x in the best confocal resolution condition. Cell nuclei were counterstained with Hoechst 33258 (blue) Scale bar: 5 μm. **(F)** Quantification of LC3B/LAMP1 vesicles per area (ILM) or cell (GCL and INL) with ImageJ JACoP software. Pearson values were compared statistically. Statistical *t*-test was performed. **(G)** Representative immunofluorescence analysis of LAMP1 (red) in cryosections of RA and OIR mice injected with CQ at P17, and evaluated 4 h after administration. Scale bar: 50 μm. **(H)** Quantification of LAMP1 puncta per area or cell with ImageJ analyze particles software. Data are presented as mean ± SEM. $^{*}p < 0.05$, $^{**}p < 0.01$. **(I)** Representative TUNEL-labeled cryosections of P17 RA and OIR mice and cryosections of mice intravitreally injected with bovine serum albumin derivate DQ-BSA and co stained with anti-LC3B (green). Arrows are indicating DQ-BSA staining in ECs. Scale bar: 50 μm. ILM, inner limiting membrane; GCL, ganglion cell layer; IPL, inner plexiform layer; INL, inner nuclear layer; OPL, outer plexiform layer; ONL, outer nuclear layer; NV, neovascularization.

To determine the effect of anti-VEGF treatment on the autophagic process in the OIR mouse model we first examined the classical autophagy markers by Western blot assays. Quantitative analysis revealed a slight but significantly increase in LC3B II levels at P17 OIR (**Figures 5E,F**). This increase was corroborated by immunofluorescence assays where LC3B was detected mainly in GCL and INL (**Figure 5G**). These findings demonstrated that targeting VEGF prevented vascular alterations and also increased the autophagic flux in P17 OIR retinas.

## Spautin-1 Inhibited Autophagy, Reduced NV but Did Not Prevented Neurodegeneration in the OIR Mouse Model

As autophagy seemed a key feature during NV, we next decided to decrease the autophagy flux by a single administration of Spautin-1 at P12 and to evaluate vascular, neuronal, and glial parameters at P17 and P26, respectively (**Figure 6A**). Western blot analysis showed a significant decrease in LC3B II expression at P13 (**Figure 6B**). Quantitative analysis of flat-mounts labeled with GSA-IB4 lectin showed a significant reduction of more than 70% in neovascular area after Spautin-1 treatment. However, other vascular alterations did not improved in OIR Spautin-1 mice, suggesting that autophagy is important for NV and that the activation in the OIR mouse is not mediating physiological revascularization (**Figures 6C,D**). In addition, a slight decrease in NG-2 staining was observed in Spautin-1 mice at P17 OIR (**Figure 6E**).

After Spautin-1 or vehicle treatment, no changes in GFAP levels were detected by Western blot of neural retinas samples (**Figures 7A,B**) or in flat-mount of retinas (**Figure 7C**). Similarly, no statistically differences in the expression of GS protein were found by Western blot (**Figures 7A,B**) or immunofluorescence (**Figure 7D**) after Spautin-1 treatment neither at P17 nor at P26.

In regard to neuronal functionality, the amplitude of the a-wave showed a tendency to decrease in OIR Spautin-1 mice at P17. In accordance, a later response (increased latency) was detected in photoreceptors as well as in inner neurons after autophagy inhibition (**Figure 7E**). Quantitative analysis of a-wave and b-wave amplitudes and latencies evidence no significant changes in neuronal functionality at P26. In line with these results, TUNEL staining showed a slight increase in the number of positive cells in the ONL after Spautin-1 treatment at P17 OIR (**Figure 7F**). Activation of apoptosis, measured by a reduction in total caspase 3 protein levels was not significantly different at both time points evaluated (**Figures 7G,H**). Finally, we evaluated protein expression of LC3B and p62 5 days (P17) or 14 days (P26) after Spautin-1 treatment. Quantitative analysis of Western blot assays (**Figures 7G,H**) and confocal microscopy images (**Figure 7I**) evidenced that both autophagy markers returned to OIR levels. These results showed that the inhibition of autophagy by Spautin-1 was harmful for the functionality and survival of photoreceptors in P17 OIR retinas.

# DISCUSSION

Preretinal NV is a common feature in many diseases, including ROP, DR and Sickle cell retinopathy. Even though their pathophysiology is different, this family of retinopathies is characterized by the decrease in oxygen tension at a certain stage. The immediate response is the increase in VEGF synthesis, a trophic factor responsible of the proliferation of ECs that originate fragile and immature vascular tufts (Campochiaro, 2015; Rubio and Adamis, 2016). Simultaneously, other events take place in the retina as gliosis and neurodegeneration, which can be developed by the hypoxic stimulus or another primary injury (Ridano et al., 2017). Coincidentally, proliferative retinopathies treatments are palliative and aim to manage NV. However, ongoing inflammation, neuronal death, and impaired oxygen supply frequently lead to neovascular recurrence. Thus, previous studies indicated that a more appropriate therapy should encompass the normalization of both vascular and non-vascular alterations in proliferative retinopathies (Liang et al., 2012).

Modulation of autophagy flux results an attractive target, as this intracellular process occurs in every cell and has proven relationship with neurodegeneration, angiogenesis, and inflammation (Boya et al., 2016). Several research studies have demonstrated that inhibition or stimulation of the autophagic flux is able to reverse the alterations of multiple chronic or acute pathologies, including visual disturbances (Mitter et al., 2012; Russo et al., 2013; Chinskey et al., 2014;

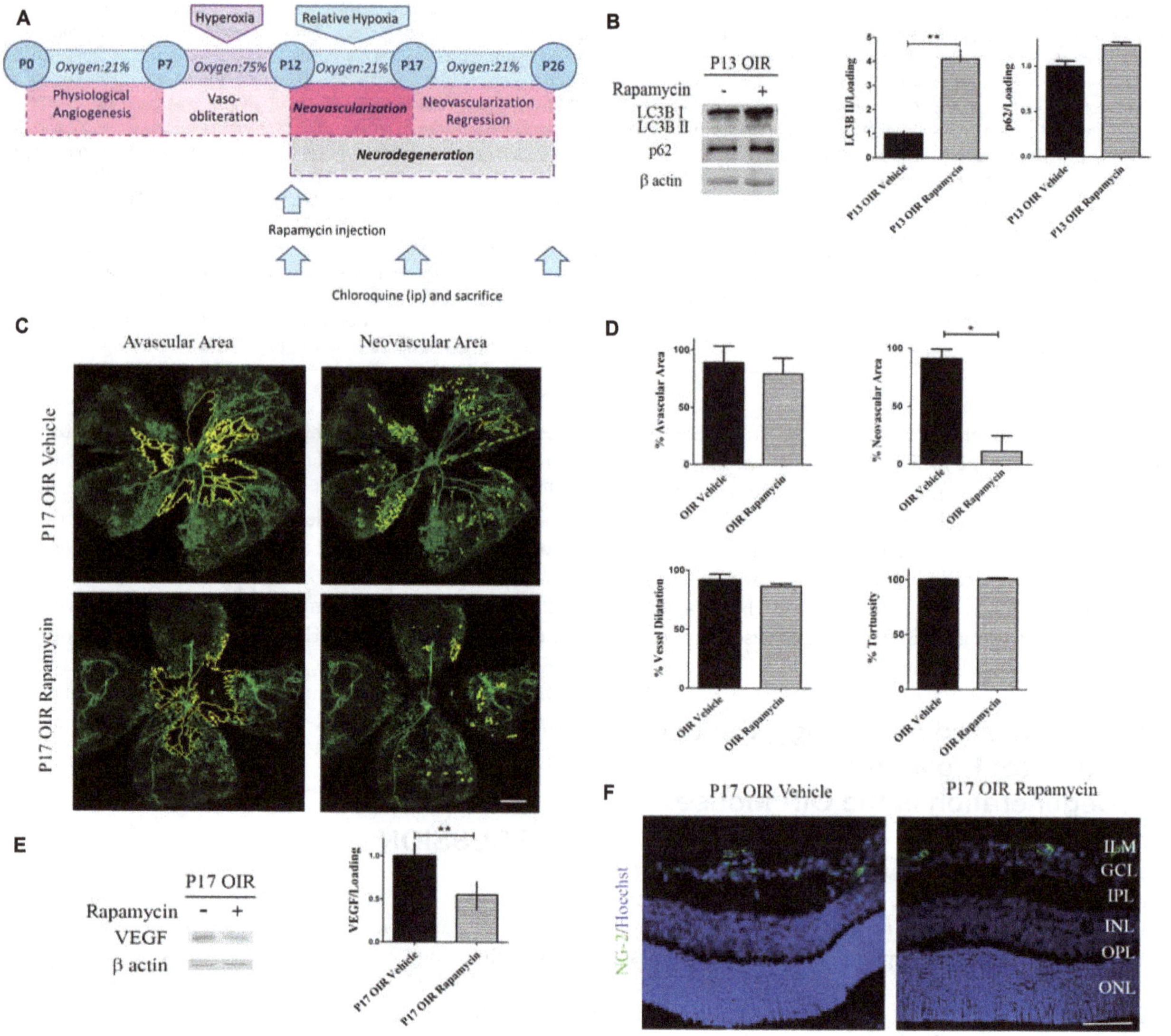


**FIGURE 3 |** Effect of Rapamycin on the vascular alterations in the OIR mouse retinas. **(A)** Rapamycin treatment schedule. Rapamycin (0,5 μg/ml) or vehicle was intravitreally injected at P12 and evaluated at P13, P17, or P26 after 4 h of CQ administration. **(B)** Representative Western blot and quantification data of autophagy markers, LC3B II and p62, from neural retinal extracts of OIR mice intravitreally injected with vehicle or Rapamycin at P12 and evaluated at P13, 4 h after CQ administration. β-Actin is shown as a loading control. Graph shows results of three independent experiments. **(C)** Representative images of flat-mount retinas at P17 showing GSA-IB4 vascular staining in OIR-vehicle and OIR-Rapamycin mice. Areas with VO and NV are indicated. Scale bar: 500 μm. **(D)** The VO (%) was quantified as the ratio of central avascular area to whole retinal area, the NV (%) was quantified as a percentage of whole retinal area. In mayor vessels of the retina, diameter was quantified by tracing a transversal line to the vessel. The tortuosity was obtained by drawing a line along the vessel and comparing it to a straight line traced from the optic nerve to the first branching point. **(E)** Representative Western blot and quantification data of VEGF from neural retinal extracts in OIR mice intravitreally injected with vehicle or Rapamycin at P12 and evaluated at P17, 4 h after CQ administration. β-Actin is shown as a loading control. Graph shows results of three independent experiments. **(F)** Representative immunofluorescence analysis of NG-2 (green) in cryosections of OIR mice intravitreally injected with vehicle or Rapamycin at P12 and evaluated at P17, 4 h after CQ administration. Scale bar: 50 μm. ILM, inner limiting membrane; GCL, ganglion cell layer; IPL, inner plexiform layer; INL, inner nuclear layer; OPL, outer plexiform layer; ONL, outer nuclear layer. Data are presented as mean ± SEM. *$p < 0.05$, **$p < 0.01$.

Frost et al., 2014; Chai et al., 2016; Rosa et al., 2016; Amato et al., 2018). Rapamycin, rapalogs and CQ are the most habitual choice for experimental design as they have been approved by FDA for a specific treatment (Nalbandian et al., 2015; Kezic et al., 2018) and it would be easier to execute clinical trials for second uses of these drugs.

Therefore, we initially explored changes in the autophagy flux in the OIR mouse model. To note, OIR model very closely recapitulates the pathologic events occurring in ROP and some aspects of proliferative DR (Smith et al., 1994). Treatments were carried out at different postnatal days when pups were still in developmental phase, where autophagy plays a crucial role (Boya et al., 2016). Indeed, Western blot assays in RA showed a decrease of LC3B II and p62 protein levels from P12 to P26, indicating a high autophagy flux early after birth. In contrast, OIR mice showed an increase in LC3B II and p62 protein levels

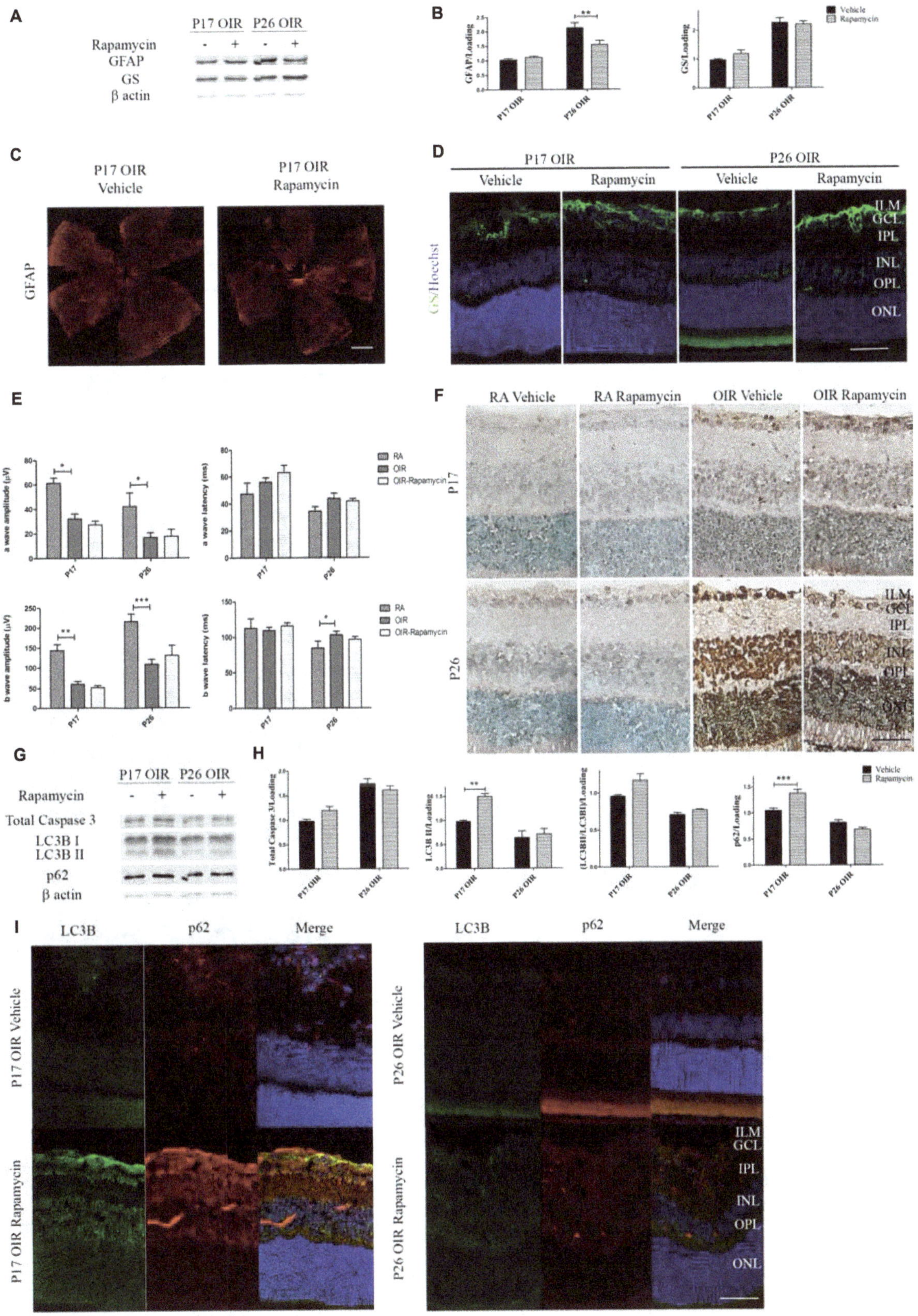


**FIGURE 4** | Continued

**FIGURE 4 |** Effect of Rapamycin on the glial reactivity, neuronal functionality, and autophagy markers in OIR mouse retinas. **(A)** Representative Western blot of GS and GFAP from neural retina extracts of OIR mice intravitreally injected with vehicle or Rapamycin at P12 and evaluated at P17, 4 h after CQ administration. β-Actin is shown as a loading control. **(B)** Levels of GS and GFAP were quantified by densitometry and normalized to β-actin. Graph shows results of three independent experiments. **(C)** Representative images of flat-mount retinas at P17 showing GFAP staining in OIR-vehicle and OIR-Rapamycin mice. Scale bar: 500 μm. **(D)** Representative immunofluorescence analysis of GS (green) in cryosections of OIR mice intravitreally injected with vehicle or Rapamycin at P12 and evaluated at P17, 4 h after CQ administration. Scale bar: 50 μm. **(E)** Amplitudes and latencies of a- and b-waves from scotopic ERG were recorded at P17 and P26 in RA and OIR mice injected at P12 with vehicle or Rapamycin. Data show the average of responses of both eyes with eight mice per condition. **(F)** Representative TUNEL-labeled cryosections of RA and OIR mice injected with vehicle or Rapamycin at P12 and evaluated at P17 and P26. Scale bar: 50 μm. **(G,H)** Representative Western blot and quantification data of total caspase-3, LC3B II and p62 from neural retina samples of OIR mice intravitreally injected with vehicle or Rapamycin at P12 and evaluated at P17 and P26, 4 h after CQ administration. β-Actin is shown as a loading control. Graph shows results of three independent experiments. **(I)** Representative immunofluorescence analysis of LC3B (green) and p62 (red) in cryosections of OIR mice intravitreally injected with vehicle or Rapamycin at P12 and evaluated at P17 and P26, 4 h after CQ administration. Cell nuclei were counterstained with Hoechst 33258 (blue). Scale bar: 50 μm. ILM, inner limiting membrane; GCL, ganglion cell layer; IPL, inner plexiform layer; INL, inner nuclear layer; OPL, outer plexiform layer; ONL, outer nuclear layer. Data are presented as mean ± SEM. $^{*}p < 0.05$, $^{**}p < 0.01$, $^{***}p < 0.001$.

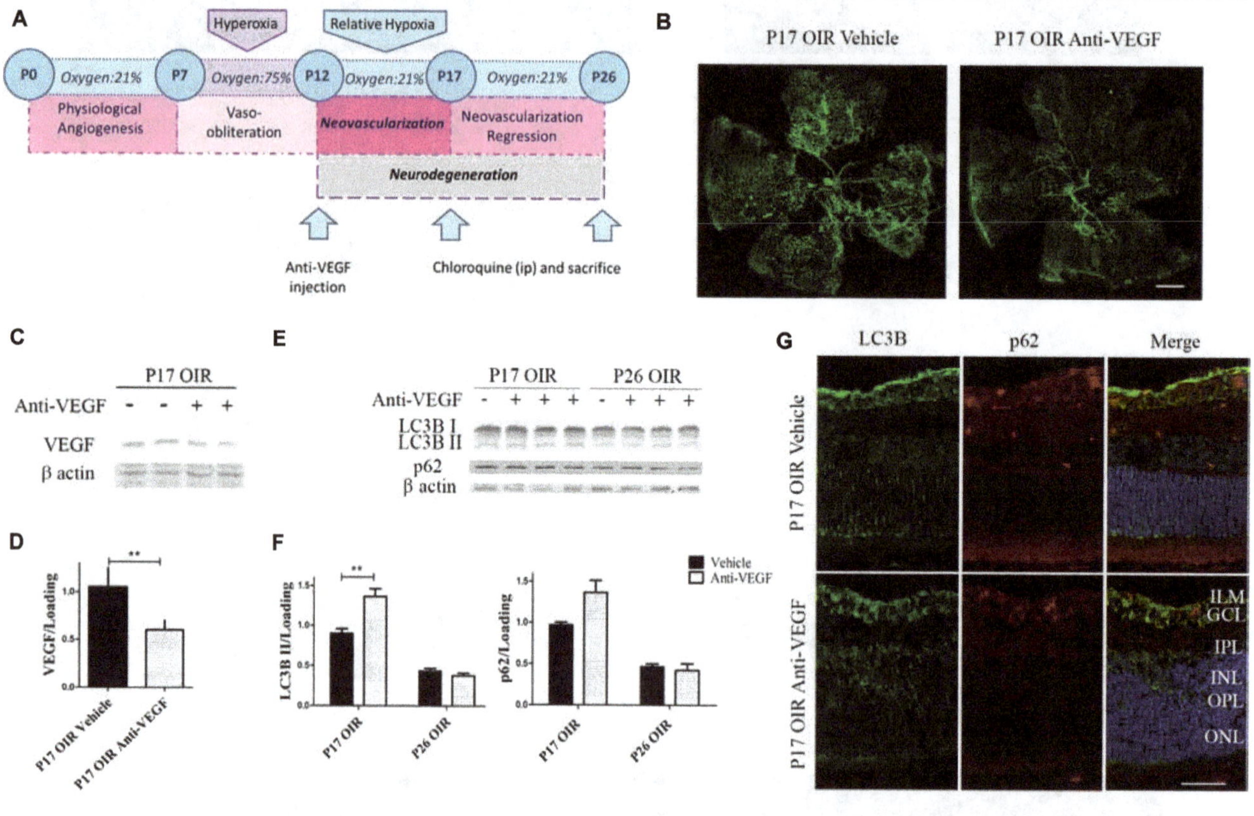


**FIGURE 5 |** Effect of Anti-VEGF treatment on autophagy markers in the OIR mouse retinas. **(A)** Anti-VEGF mAb treatment schedule. Anti-VEGF mAb (1.25 μg) or vehicle was intravitreally injected at P12 and evaluated a P17 or P26, 4 h after CQ administration. **(B)** Representative images of flat-mount retinas at P17 OIR showing GSA-IB4 vascular staining in vehicle or anti-VEGF-injected eyes. Areas with VO and NV are indicated. Scale bar: 500 μm. **(C)** Representative Western blot of VEGF from P17 neural retinal extracts of OIR mice injected at P12 with vehicle or anti-VEGF mAb. β-Actin is shown as a loading control. **(D)** Levels of VEGF were quantified by densitometry and normalized to β-actin. Graph shows results of three independent experiments. **(E)** Representative Western blot of LC3B II and p62 from neural retina extracts of OIR mice intravitreally injected with vehicle or anti-VEGF mAb at P12 and evaluated at P17 and P26, 4 h after CQ administration. β-Actin is shown as a loading control. **(F)** Levels of LC3B II and p62 were quantified by densitometry and normalized to β-actin. Graph shows results of four independent experiments. **(G)** Representative immunofluorescence analysis of LC3B (green) and p62 (red) in cryosections of OIR mice intravitreally injected with vehicle or anti-VEGF mAb at P12 and evaluated at P17, 4 h after CQ administration. Cell nuclei were counterstained with Hoechst 33258 (blue). Scale bar: 50 μm. ILM, inner limiting membrane; GCL, ganglion cell layer; IPL, inner plexiform layer; INL, inner nuclear layer; OPL, outer plexiform layer; ONL, outer nuclear layer. Data are presented as mean ± SEM. $^{**}p < 0.01$.

at P17 OIR, compared to RA controls demonstrating a rise in autophagosomes in the cytosol of retinal cells. Transcriptional activity of autophagy proteins revealed a significant increase in p62 mRNA levels at P17OIR. Upon induction of the flux, p62 is degraded into the autophagosome and it would be necessary to synthesize more protein. This result would indicate that the increase in p62 protein levels at this time point is a consequence of the increased protein synthesis but not of its accumulation.

Physiological vascularization of the retina completes at P21 in mice, when the provisional hyaloid vasculature is replaced

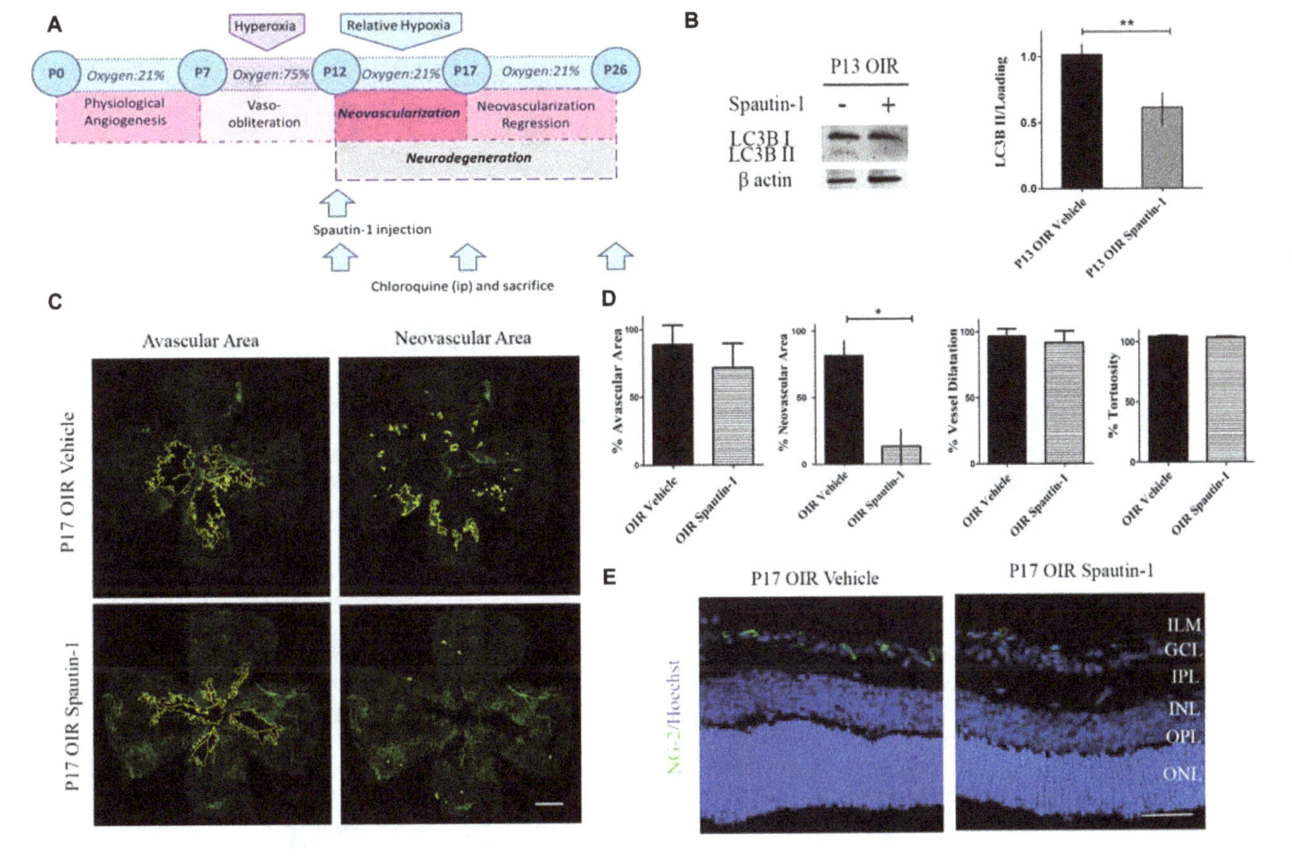


**FIGURE 6 |** Effect of the Spautin-1 on the NV in OIR mouse retinas. **(A)** Spautin-1 treatment schedule. Spautin-1 (200 $\mu$M) or vehicle was intravitreally injected at P12 and evaluated at P17 or P26, 4 h after of CQ administration. **(B)** Representative Western blot and quantification data of autophagy marker LC3B II from neural retinal extracts of OIR mice intravitreally injected with Spautin-1 or vehicle at P12 and evaluated at P13, 4 h after CQ administration. β-Actin is shown as a loading control. Graph shows results of three independent experiments. **(C)** Representative images of flat-mount retinas at P17 showing GSA-IB4 vascular staining in OIR-vehicle and OIR-Spautin-1 mice. Areas with VO and NV are indicated. Scale bar: 500 $\mu$m. **(D)** The VO (%) was quantified as the ratio of central avascular area to whole retinal area, the NV (%) was quantified as a percentage of whole retinal area. In mayor vessels of the retina, diameter was quantified by tracing a transversal line to the vessel. The tortuosity was obtained by drawing a line along the vessel and comparing it to a straight line traced from the optic nerve to the first branching point. **(E)** Representative immunofluorescence analysis of NG-2 (green) in cryosections of OIR mice intravitreally injected with vehicle or Spautin-1 at P12 and evaluated at P17, 4 h after CQ administration. Scale bar: 50 $\mu$m. ILM, inner limiting membrane; GCL, ganglion cell layer; IPL, inner plexiform layer; INL, inner nuclear layer; OPL, outer plexiform layer; ONL, outer nuclear layer. Data are presented as mean ± SEM. $^{*}p < 0.05$, $^{**}p < 0.01$.

by the definite one following a hypoxic gradient. Firstly, the superficial plexus is formed by the radial sprouting of vessels from the optic nerve. Later, the deep plexus is formed by transversal outgrowth of superficial vessels and the retinal vasculature achieves completion with the formation of the intermediate plexus (Stahl et al., 2010). Due to the fact that there is an irregular oxygen supply in the different layers of the retina, the sensing of the hypoxic stimulus could vary along the neural retina and therefore the cellular response (Rodrigues et al., 2013). Confocal images showed that areas near the vascular plexus, GCs and neurons residing in the INL increased LC3B protein expression in P17 OIR mice, whereas autophagy markers were not modified in ONL neurons. Unchanged autophagic flux in photoreceptors could be explained by the provision of oxygen by the choroid vasculature to rods and cones, preventing severe hypoxia in this layer. Although photoreceptors are damaged in OIR model, a reduced cell death rate is observed (Ridano et al., 2017). Nearby to the ILM, both MGCs and ECs showed an increase in LC3B staining. Interestingly, at P17 OIR, LC3B-positive vesicles were found inside ECs in neovascular tufts, suggesting an increased autophagic flux in proliferating cells.

We further confirmed the activation in autophagy flux at P17 OIR by observing a greater number of LC3B/LAMP1 double labeled vesicles, indicating an increase in amphisomes in the inner layers of the retina compared to control mice. An increase in LAMP1 structures was observed after blockade of the flux with CQ, mainly in the ILM, evidencing that the degradation pathway is activated. In addition, neovessels in the ILM hydrolyzed DQ-BSA in lysosomes in great proportion. By TUNEL assay, we demonstrate that cell viability is reduced in INL and GCL. Indeed, neurons undergoing cell death or high hypoxic stress could activate autophagy flux as a survival mechanism.

Next we wonder if the administration of Rapamycin at P12 could improve vascular, glial, or neuronal alterations in OIR mice. We took into account that mTORC1 inhibition increases autophagy flux, but also modulates multiple intracellular

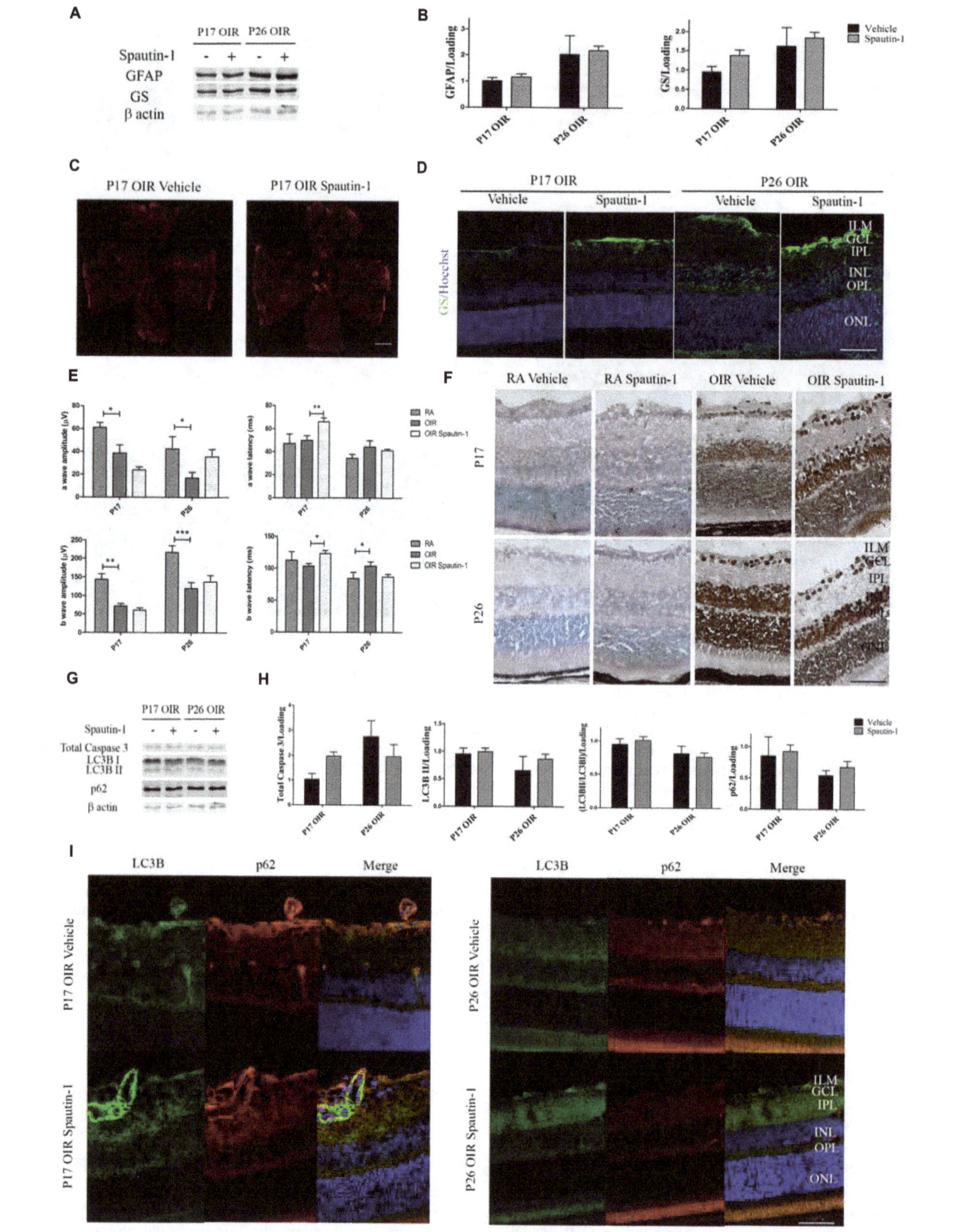


**FIGURE 7** | Continued

**FIGURE 7 | (A)** Effect of Spautin-1 on the glial reactivity, neuronal functionality and autophagy markers in OIR mouse retinas. Representative Western blot of GFAP and GS from neural retina extracts of OIR mice intravitreally injected with Spautin-1 or vehicle at P12 and evaluated at P17, 4 h after CQ treatment. β-Actin is shown as a loading control. **(B)** Levels of GFAP and GS were quantified by densitometry and normalized to β-actin. Graph shows results of four independent experiments. **(C)** Representative images of flat-mount retinas at P17 showing GFAP staining in OIR-vehicle and OIR-Spautin-1 mice. Scale bar: 500 μm. **(D)** Representative immunofluorescence analysis of GS (green) in cryosections of OIR mice intravitreally injected with vehicle or Spautin-1 at P12 and evaluated at P17, 4 h after CQ administration. Scale bar: 50 μm. **(E)** Amplitudes and latencies of a- and b-waves from scotopic ERG were recorded at P17 and P26 in RA and OIR mice injected at P12 with vehicle or Spautin-1. Data show the average of responses in both eyes with eight mice per condition. **(F)** Representative TUNEL-labeled cryosections of RA and OIR mice injected with vehicle or Spautin-1 at P12 and evaluated at P17 and P26. Scale bar: 50 μm. **(G,H)** Representative Western blot and quantification data of total caspase-3, LC3B II and p62 from neural retina samples of OIR mice intravitreally injected with vehicle or Spautin-1 at P12 and evaluated at P17 and P26, 4 h after CQ administration. β-Actin is shown as a loading control. Graph shows results of three independent experiments. **(I)** Representative immunofluorescence analysis of LC3B (green) and p62 (red) in cryosections of OIR mice intravitreally injected with vehicle or Spautin-1 at P12 and evaluated at P17 and P26, 4 h after CQ administration. Cell nuclei were counterstained with Hoechst 33258 (blue). Scale bar: 50 μm. ILM, inner limiting membrane; GCL, ganglion cell layer; IPL, inner plexiform layer; INL, inner nuclear layer; OPL, outer plexiform layer; ONL, outer nuclear layer. Data are presented as mean ± SEM. ns, non-significant, $^{*}p < 0.05$, $^{**}p < 0.01$, $^{***}p < 0.001$.

pathways related to inflammation, angiogenesis and metabolism. A single intraocular injection of Rapamycin decreased the area occupied by neovessels, however the treatment did not promote physiological revascularization (evaluated by avascular area, vessel dilatation, and tortuosity). The normalization of the vascular plexus is essential for the proper irrigation of the retinal tissue and prevents future alterations derived from the turbulence in the blood flow or stasis of blood cells (Liang et al., 2012). The reduction in NV area was supported by the decrease in VEGF levels. It has been described that inhibition of mTORC1 decreases the synthesis of the transcription factor HIF-1α and consequently downregulates the expression of its target genes (Liu et al., 2015). Notably, in the retina VEGF is produced mainly in MGCs, astrocytes, GCs, retinal pigmented epithelium and ECs in a minor proportion (Wang et al., 2010). Then, it is possible that the modulation of the neovascular process is due to the direct effect of Rapamycin on other cells rather than endothelium. In fact, Rapamycin could be a more successful therapeutic strategy because it decreases the synthesis of VEGF, providing an adequate level of the trophic factor. The excessive inhibition of VEGF signaling would be detrimental for neurons. Under certain pathological conditions, increased autophagy flux can also induce cell death (Hirt et al., 2018). In our model, Rapamycin did not alter pericytes viability, one of the most susceptive cells in the vasculature. Persistence of mural cells is a good marker of vascular maturation, indicating that final stage of vasculogenesis is not altered and the newly formed vessels are functional.

Related to gliosis, Rapamycin markedly reduced GFAP expression at P26 OIR, indicating a decrease in the glial response during the neovascular regression stage. This would contribute to the reduction in the persistent pro-inflammatory response that promotes damage in the retinal tissue. Unfortunately, a single dose of Rapamycin was insufficient to increase neuronal functionality. Further studies would be necessary to evaluate if a prolonged administration schedule improves visual function.

Previously, it has been reported that high dose of Rapamycin increases the avascular area (Yagasaki et al., 2014) which could be a result of reduced proliferation or increased cell death of ECs. Here, the induction in autophagy flux did not resulted in an increase of apoptosis, measured by total caspase 3, suggesting that the crosstalk between both pathways is not the responsible of the caspase mediated cell death. Our results showed that the increase in autophagy flux continue up to P17 OIR, indicating that Rapamycin has a relatively long half-life in the vitreous, as previously reported (Nguyen et al., 2018).

In a comparative experiment, we analyzed the effect of the anti-VEGF therapy on the autophagy flux. Western blot analysis revealed a slight induction of the flux at P17 OIR. As confocal images showed an increase in the autophagy proteins, LC3B and p62, in GCL and INL, we consider that the deprivation of the trophic factor VEGF can activate survival mechanisms as autophagy. Previously, we reported that intravitreal administration of anti-VEGF does not improve neuronal functionality and gliosis (Ridano et al., 2017). Thereby, Rapamycin benefits over anti-VEGF therapy rely on the multiplicity of events modulated through the inhibition of mTORC1. Although both treatments reduced NV and activated autophagy, neither of them prevented neurodegeneration in our experimental conditions.

To unravel the role of autophagy in the OIR mouse model, we injected at P12 a single dose of Spautin-1, an inhibitor of the ubiquitin-specific peptidases USP10 and USP13, which target the Beclin-1 subunit of Vps34 complexes (Liu et al., 2011). Remarkably, vascular effects were similar to those observed with Rapamycin. Spautin-1 decreased the neovascular area without modifying other vascular parameters. In this sense, confocal images of neovessels shed light on this result demonstrating that proliferating ECs, highly metabolic cells, showed a fast autophagy flux. Thus, the inhibition of this process would lead to vascular death or a decreased proliferation rate. The interaction between ECs and pericytes is critical for the formation of a structurally sound microvasculature. In this study, we found a reduced NG-2 staining in OIR mice retinas after Spautin-1 treatment indicating an apparent decrease in pericyte density, which may exacerbate vascular alterations.

In regard to non-vascular cells, glial response remained unchanged as no modifications in GS and GFAP levels were detected after Spautin-1 treatment. Electroretinographic recording showed that photoreceptors functionality tend to decrease at P17 OIR in Spautin-1 treated mice. This result reinforces the idea that retinal layers with high autophagy flux at the neovascular peak activate this pathway as a survival mechanism. In this sense, the importance of the autophagic flow became more evident in the photoreceptors because it is the layer less affected in the OIR. Correlatively, an increase in TUNEL positive staining was observed in the ONL when autophagy was inhibited. Five days after Spautin-1 injection, LC3B II and p62 protein levels returned to OIR control levels, indicating a reduced half-life of the drug in the eye.

Presumably, all retinal cells are intended to activate autophagy flux in hypoxic conditions. However, the ability to respond will depend on the status of the cell as well as the intensity and duration of the stimuli (Boya et al., 2016). Prior to the hypoxic stage in the OIR model, the hyperoxic phase induces several alterations in retinal cells originated by apoptotic events at P12 (Sennlaub et al., 2002; Vecino et al., 2004; Narayanan et al., 2011). Recently, it has been demonstrated that retinas of OIR mice are characterized by increased apoptosis and decreased autophagy from P13 to P15 (Cammalleri et al., 2017). Here, using the same *in vivo* model, we completed the analysis including, in addition to P12 and P17, the vascular regression stage (P26). Overall, our results demonstrate that all treatments of induction or inhibition of the autophagic flux reduced neovascular area but were unable to completely reverse the neuronal damage. Besides, compared to current treatments, rapamycin provides a more promising therapeutic strategy as it reduces both neovascular tufts and persistent gliosis.

## AUTHOR CONTRIBUTIONS

PS and MS designed the experiments. PS, MP, MR, and VL conducted the experiments. PS, MP, MR, VL, and MS interpreted the data. GC and CF contributed new reagents, analytic tools, and analyzed and discussed the available data. PS and MS wrote and edited the manuscript.

## FUNDING

This study was funded by the Secretaría de Ciencia y Tecnología, Universidad Nacional de Córdoba (SECyT-UNC) No. 366/16 and the Fondo para la Investigación Científica y Tecnológica (FONCyT), Préstamo BID 2015 PICT No. 1314 (all to MS).

## ACKNOWLEDGMENTS

We thank Gustavo Bonacci for advice and Pablo Barcelona for technical assistance. We also thank Carlos Mas, María Pilar Crespo, and Cecilia Sampedro for assistance in confocal microscopy and Soledad Miró and Victoria Blanco for dedicated animal care.

## REFERENCES


Amato, R., Catalani, E., Dal Monte, M., Cammalleri, M., Di Renzo, I., Perrotta, C., et al. (2018). Autophagy-mediated neuroprotection induced by octreotide in an ex vivo model of early diabetic retinopathy. *Pharmacol. Res.* 128, 167–178. doi: 10.1016/j.phrs.2017.09.022

Barcelona, P. F., Ortiz, S. G., Chiabrando, G. A., and Sanchez, M. C. (2011). Alpha2-macroglobulin induces glial fibrillary acidic protein expression mediated by low-density lipoprotein receptor-related protein 1 in muller cells. *Invest. Ophthalmol. Vis. Sci.* 52, 778–786. doi: 10.1167/iovs.10-5759

Boya, P., Esteban-Martinez, L., Serrano-Puebla, A., Gomez-Sintes, R., and Villarejo-Zori, B. (2016). Autophagy in the eye: development, degeneration, and aging. *Prog. Retin. Eye Res.* 55, 206–245. doi: 10.1016/j.preteyeres.2016.08.001

Cammalleri, M., Locri, F., Catalani, E., Filippi, L., Cervia, D., Dal Monte, M., et al. (2017). The beta adrenergic receptor blocker propranolol counteracts retinal dysfunction in a mouse model of oxygen induced retinopathy: restoring the balance between apoptosis and autophagy. *Front. Cell. Neurosci.* 11:395. doi: 10.3389/fncel.2017.00395

Campochiaro, P. A. (2015). Molecular pathogenesis of retinal and choroidal vascular diseases. *Prog. Retin. Eye Res.* 49, 67–81. doi: 10.1016/j.preteyeres.2015.06.002

Chai, P., Ni, H., Zhang, H., and Fan, X. (2016). The evolving functions of autophagy in ocular health: a double-edged sword. *Int. J. Biol. Sci.* 12, 1332–1340. doi: 10.7150/ijbs.16245

Chen, S., Zhou, L., Zhang, Y., Leng, Y., Pei, X. Y., Lin, H., et al. (2014). Targeting SQSTM1/p62 induces cargo loading failure and converts autophagy to apoptosis via NBK/Bik. *Mol. Cell. Biol.* 34, 3435–3449. doi: 10.1128/MCB.01383-13

Chinskey, N. D., Besirli, C. G., and Zacks, D. N. (2014). Retinal cell death and current strategies in retinal neuroprotection. *Curr. Opin. Ophthalmol.* 25, 228–233. doi: 10.1097/ICU.0000000000000043

Diabetic Retinopathy Clinical Research Network, Wells, J. A., Glassman, A. R., Ayala, A. R., Jampol, L. M., Aiello, L. P., et al. (2015). Aflibercept, bevacizumab, or ranibizumab for diabetic macular edema. *N. Engl. J. Med.* 372, 1193–1203. doi: 10.1056/NEJMoa1414264

Du, J., Teng, R. J., Guan, T., Eis, A., Kaul, S., Konduri, G. G., et al. (2012). Role of autophagy in angiogenesis in aortic endothelial cells. *Am. J. Physiol. Cell Physiol.* 302, C383–C391. doi: 10.1152/ajpcell.00164.2011

Evans, J. R., Michelessi, M., and Virgili, G. (2014). Laser photocoagulation for proliferative diabetic retinopathy. *Cochrane Database Syst. Rev.* 11, CD011234. doi: 10.1002/14651858.CD011234.pub2

Frost, L. S., Dhingra, A., Reyes-Reveles, J., and Boesze-Battaglia, K. (2017). The use of DQ-BSA to monitor the turnover of autophagy-associated cargo. *Methods Enzymol.* 587, 43–54. doi: 10.1016/bs.mie.2016.09.052

Frost, L. S., Mitchell, C. H., and Boesze-Battaglia, K. (2014). Autophagy in the eye: implications for ocular cell health. *Exp. Eye Res.* 124, 56–66. doi: 10.1016/j.exer.2014.04.010

Gerhardt, H. (2008). VEGF and endothelial guidance in angiogenic sprouting. *Organogenesis* 4, 241–246. doi: 10.4161/org.4.4.7414

Gerhardt, H., and Betsholtz, C. (2003). Endothelial-pericyte interactions in angiogenesis. *Cell Tissue Res.* 314, 15–23. doi: 10.1007/s00441-003-0745-x

Harris, H., and Rubinsztein, D. C. (2011). Control of autophagy as a therapy for neurodegenerative disease. *Nat. Rev. Neurol.* 8, 108–117. doi: 10.1038/nrneurol.2011.200

Hirt, J., Porter, K., Dixon, A., McKinnon, S., and Liton, P. B. (2018). Contribution of autophagy to ocular hypertension and neurodegeneration in the DBA/2J spontaneous glaucoma mouse model. *Cell. Death Discov.* 4:14. doi: 10.1038/s41420-018-0077-y

Kern, T. S. (2014). Interrelationships between the retinal neuroglia and vasculature in diabetes. *Diabetes Metab. J.* 38, 163–170. doi: 10.4093/dmj.2014.38.3.163

Kezic, A., Popovic, L., and Lalic, K. (2018). mTOR Inhibitor therapy and metabolic consequences: where do we stand? *Oxid. Med. Cell Longev.* 2018:2640342. doi: 10.1155/2018/2640342

Kim, C. B., D'Amore, P. A., and Connor, K. M. (2016). Revisiting the mouse model of oxygen-induced retinopathy. *Eye Brain* 8, 67–79. doi: 10.2147/EB.S94447

Kimura, T., Jia, J., Claude-Taupin, A., Kumar, S., Choi, S. W., Gu, Y., et al. (2017). Cellular and molecular mechanism for secretory autophagy. *Autophagy* 13, 1084–1085. doi: 10.1080/15548627.2017.1307486

Levine, B., Packer, M., and Codogno, P. (2015). Development of autophagy inducers in clinical medicine. *J. Clin. Invest.* 125, 14–24. doi: 10.1172/JCI73938

Li, J., Kim, S. G., and Blenis, J. (2014). Rapamycin: one drug, many effects. *Cell Metab.* 19, 373–379. doi: 10.1016/j.cmet.2014.01.001

Liang, J., Piao, Y., Henry, V., Tiao, N., and de Groot, J. F. (2015). Interferon-regulatory factor-1 (IRF1) regulates bevacizumab induced autophagy. *Oncotarget* 6, 31479–31492. doi: 10.18632/oncotarget.5491

Liang, X., Zhou, H., Ding, Y., Li, J., Yang, C., Luo, Y., et al. (2012). TMP prevents retinal neovascularization and imparts neuroprotection in an oxygen-induced retinopathy model. *Invest. Ophthalmol. Vis. Sci.* 53, 2157–2169. doi: 10.1167/iovs.11-9315

Liu, J., Fan, L., Wang, H., and Sun, G. (2016). Autophagy, a double-edged sword in anti-angiogenesis therapy. *Med. Oncol.* 33, 10. doi: 10.1007/s12032-015-0721-9

Liu, J., Xia, H., Kim, M., Xu, L., Li, Y., Zhang, L., et al. (2011). Beclin1 controls the levels of p53 by regulating the deubiquitination activity of USP10 and USP13. *Cell* 147, 223–234. doi: 10.1016/j.cell.2011.08.037

Liu, N. N., Zhao, N., and Cai, N. (2015). Suppression of the proliferation of hypoxia-Induced retinal pigment epithelial cell by rapamycin through the /mTOR/HIF-1alpha/VEGF/ signaling. *IUBMB Life* 67, 446–452. doi: 10.1002/iub.1382

Lytvynchuk, L., Sergienko, A., Lavrenchuk, G., and Petrovski, G. (2015). Antiproliferative, apoptotic, and autophagic activity of ranibizumab, bevacizumab, pegaptanib, and aflibercept on fibroblasts: implication for choroidal neovascularization. *J. Ophthalmol.* 2015:934963. doi: 10.1155/2015/934963

Mitter, S. K., Rao, H. V., Qi, X., Cai, J., Sugrue, A., Dunn, W. A., et al. (2012). Autophagy in the retina: a potential role in age-related macular degeneration. *Adv. Exp. Med. Biol.* 723, 83–90. doi: 10.1007/978-1-4614-0631-0_12

Mizushima, N., and Komatsu, M. (2011). Autophagy: renovation of cells and tissues. *Cell* 147, 728–741. doi: 10.1016/j.cell.2011.10.026

Nagy, J. A., Benjamin, L., Zeng, H., Dvorak, A. M., and Dvorak, H. F. (2008). Vascular permeability, vascular hyperpermeability and angiogenesis. *Angiogenesis* 11, 109–119. doi: 10.1007/s10456-008-9099-z

Nalbandian, A., Llewellyn, K. J., Nguyen, C., Yazdi, P. G., and Kimonis, V. E. (2015). Rapamycin and chloroquine: the in vitro and in vivo effects of autophagy-modifying drugs show promising results in valosin containing protein multisystem proteinopathy. *PLoS One* 10:e0122888. doi: 10.1371/journal.pone.0122888

Narayanan, S. P., Suwanpradid, J., Saul, A., Xu, Z., Still, A., Caldwell, R. W., et al. (2011). Arginase 2 deletion reduces neuro-glial injury and improves retinal function in a model of retinopathy of prematurity. *PLoS One* 6:e22460. doi: 10.1371/journal.pone.0022460

Nguyen, Q. D., Merrill, P. T., Sepah, Y. J., Ibrahim, M. A., Banker, A., Leonardi, A., et al. (2018). Intravitreal sirolimus for the treatment of noninfectious uveitis: evolution through preclinical and clinical studies. *Ophthalmology* 125, 1984–1993. doi: 10.1016/j.ophtha.2018.06.015

Osaadon, P., Fagan, X. J., Lifshitz, T., and Levy, J. (2014). A review of anti-VEGF agents for proliferative diabetic retinopathy. *Eye* 28, 510–520. doi: 10.1038/eye.2014.13

Ridano, M. E., Subirada, P. V., Paz, M. C., Lorenc, V. E., Stupirski, J. C., Gramajo, A. L., et al. (2017). Galectin-1 expression imprints a neurovascular phenotype in proliferative retinopathies and delineates responses to anti-VEGF. *Oncotarget* 8, 32505–32522. doi: 10.18632/oncotarget.17129

Rodrigues, M., Xin, X., Jee, K., Babapoor-Farrokhran, S., Kashiwabuchi, F., Ma, T., et al. (2013). VEGF secreted by hypoxic Muller cells induces MMP-2 expression and activity in endothelial cells to promote retinal neovascularization in proliferative diabetic retinopathy. *Diabetes* 62, 3863–3873. doi: 10.2337/db13-0014

Rosa, M. D., Distefano, G., Gagliano, C., Rusciano, D., and Malaguarnera, L. (2016). Autophagy in diabetic retinopathy. *Curr. Neuropharmacol.* 14, 810–825. doi: 10.2174/1570159x14666160321122900

Rubio, R. G., and Adamis, A. P. (2016). Ocular Angiogenesis: vascular endothelial growth factor and other factors. *Dev. Ophthalmol.* 55, 28–37. doi: 10.1159/000431129

Russo, R., Berliocchi, L., Adornetto, A., Amantea, D., Nucci, C., Tassorelli, C., et al. (2013). In search of new targets for retinal neuroprotection: is there a role for autophagy? *Curr. Opin. Pharmacol.* 13, 72–77. doi: 10.1016/j.coph.2012.09.004

Russo, R., Varano, G. P., Adornetto, A., Nazio, F., Tettamanti, G., Girardello, R., et al. (2018). Rapamycin and fasting sustain autophagy response activated by ischemia/reperfusion injury and promote retinal ganglion cell survival. *Cell Death Dis.* 9:981. doi: 10.1038/s41419-018-1044-5

Saint-Geniez, M., Maharaj, A. S., Walshe, T. E., Tucker, B. A., Sekiyama, E., Kurihara, T., et al. (2008). Endogenous VEGF is required for visual function: evidence for a survival role on muller cells and photoreceptors. *PLoS One* 3:e3554. doi: 10.1371/journal.pone.0003554

Sanchez, M. C., Barcelona, P. F., Luna, J. D., Ortiz, S. G., Juarez, P. C., Riera, C. M., et al. (2006). Low-density lipoprotein receptor-related protein-1 (LRP-1) expression in a rat model of oxygen-induced retinal neovascularization. *Exp. Eye Res.* 83, 1378–1385. doi: 10.1016/j.exer.2006.07.016

Semenza, G. L. (2012). Hypoxia-inducible factors in physiology and medicine. *Cell* 148, 399–408. doi: 10.1016/j.cell.2012.01.021

Sennlaub, F., Courtois, Y., and Goureau, O. (2002). Inducible nitric oxide synthase mediates retinal apoptosis in ischemic proliferative retinopathy. *J. Neurosci.* 22, 3987–3993. doi: 10.1523/jneurosci.22-10-03987.2002

Smith, L. E., Wesolowski, E., McLellan, A., Kostyk, S. K., D'Amato, R., Sullivan, R., et al. (1994). Oxygen-induced retinopathy in the mouse. *Invest. Ophthalmol. Vis. Sci.* 35, 101–111.

Stahl, A., Connor, K. M., Sapieha, P., Chen, J., Dennison, R. J., Krah, N. M., et al. (2010). The mouse retina as an angiogenesis model. *Invest. Ophthalmol. Vis. Sci.* 51, 2813–2826. doi: 10.1167/iovs.10-5176

Subirada, P. V., Paz, M. C., Ridano, M. E., Lorenc, V. E., Vaglienti, M. V., Barcelona, P. F., et al. (2018). A journey into the retina: muller glia commanding survival and death. *Eur. J. Neurosci.* 47, 1429–1443. doi: 10.1111/ejn.13965

Tah, V., Orlans, H. O., Hyer, J., Casswell, E., Din, N., Sri Shanmuganathan, V., et al. (2015). Anti-VEGF therapy and the retina: an update. *J. Ophthalmol.* 2015:627674. doi: 10.1155/2015/627674

Trachsel-Moncho, L., Benlloch-Navarro, S., Fernandez-Carbonell, A., Ramirez-Lamelas, D. T., Olivar, T., Silvestre, D., et al. (2018). Oxidative stress and autophagy-related changes during retinal degeneration and development. *Cell. Death Dis.* 9:812. doi: 10.1038/s41419-018-0855-8

Vecino, E., Hernandez, M., and Garcia, M. (2004). Cell death in the developing vertebrate retina. *Int. J. Dev. Biol.* 48, 965–974. doi: 10.1387/ijdb.041891ev

Wang, J., Xu, X., Elliott, M. H., Zhu, M., and Le, Y. Z. (2010). Muller cell-derived VEGF is essential for diabetes-induced retinal inflammation and vascular leakage. *Diabetes* 59, 2297–2305. doi: 10.2337/db09-1420

Wei, J., Jiang, H., Gao, H., and Wang, G. (2016). Blocking mammalian target of rapamycin (mtor) attenuates hif-1alpha pathways engaged-vascular endothelial growth factor (vegf) in diabetic Retinopathy. *Cell Physiol. Biochem.* 40, 1570–1577. doi: 10.1159/000453207

Yagasaki, R., Nakahara, T., Ushikubo, H., Mori, A., Sakamoto, K., and Ishii, K. (2014). Anti-angiogenic effects of mammalian target of rapamycin inhibitors in a mouse model of oxygen-induced retinopathy. *Biol. Pharm. Bull.* 37, 1838–1842. doi: 10.1248/bpb.b14-00487

Yang, S., Zhao, J., and Sun, X. (2016). Resistance to anti-VEGF therapy in neovascular age-related macular degeneration: a comprehensive review. *Drug Des. Devel. Ther.* 10, 1857–1867. doi: 10.2147/DDDT.S97653

Yin, Z., Pascual, C., and Klionsky, D. J. (2016). Autophagy: machinery and regulation. *Microb. Cell* 3, 588–596. doi: 10.15698/mic2016.12.546

Zhang, X., Bao, S., Hambly, B. D., and Gillies, M. C. (2009). Vascular endothelial growth factor-A: a multifunctional molecular player in diabetic retinopathy. *Int. J. Biochem. Cell Biol.* 41, 2368–2371. doi: 10.1016/j.biocel.2009.07.011

Zhu, X. R., and Du, J. H. (2018). Autophagy: a potential target for the treatment of intraocular neovascularization. *Int. J. Ophthalmol.* 11, 695–698. doi: 10.18240/ijo.2018.04.26

# 9

# Lipopolysaccharide-Induced Autophagy Mediates Retinal Pigment Epithelium Cells Survival: Modulation by the Phospholipase D Pathway

*Vicente Bermúdez* [1,2], *Paula Estefanía Tenconi* [1,2], *Norma María Giusto* [1,2] *and Melina Valeria Mateos* [1,2]*

[1] *Instituto de Investigaciones Bioquímicas de Bahía Blanca (INIBIBB), Consejo Nacional de Investigaciones Científicas y Técnicas (CONICET), Bahía Blanca, Argentina,* [2] *Departamento de Biología, Bioquímica y Farmacia (DBByF), Universidad Nacional del Sur (UNS), Bahía Blanca, Argentina*

***Correspondence:**
*Melina Valeria Mateos*
*mvmateos@inibibb-conicet.gob.ar;*
*melinavaleriamateos@gmail.com*

Inflammation and oxidative stress are common factors involved in the pathogenesis of retinal diseases, such as aged-related macular degeneration (AMD) and diabetic retinopathy (DR). Autophagy is a catabolic process essential to cell survival in response to stress. This process is highly active in retinal pigment epithelium (RPE) cells. Our previous findings demonstrated that lipopolysaccharide (LPS) induces an inflammatory response of RPE cells that implies classical phospholipases D (PLD1 and 2) activation, cyclooxygenase-2 (COX-2) expression, prostaglandin $E_2$ ($PGE_2$) production and reduced cell viability. In this work, we studied the autophagic process and its modulation by the PLD pathway in D407 and ARPE-19 RPE cells exposed to LPS. LPS (10 μg/ml or 25 μg/ml) exposure for 24 h increased light chain 3B-II (LC3B-II) content (an autophagy marker) and LC3B-positive punctate structures in both RPE cell lines studied. Next, the drug bafilomycin $A_1$ (BAF, 50 nM) was used to block the autophagic flux. In cells pre-incubated with BAF, LC3B-II and sequestosome 1 (SQSTM1/p62) levels and autophagosome-like structures were increased by LPS, demonstrating that the inflammatory injury increases the autophagic process in RPE cells. To study the role of the PLD pathway, cells were pre-incubated for 1 h with selective PLD1 (VU0359595) or PLD2 (VU0285655-1) inhibitors prior to LPS addition. Under control condition, LC3B-positive punctate structures were increased in cells pre-incubated with PLD2 inhibitor while with PLD1 inhibitor were increased in cells exposed to LPS. MTT reduction assays showed that early autophagy inhibitors, 3-methyladenin (3-MA) or LY294002, enhanced the loss in cell viability induced by LPS exposure for 48 h. On the contrary, the inhibition of PLD1 and PLD2 prevented the loss in cell viability induced by LPS. In conclusion, our results show that even though LPS treatment promotes

**Abbreviations:** 3-MA, 3-methyladenine; BAF, bafilomycin $A_1$; BECN1, beclin1; COX-2, cyclooxygenase-2; DAG, diacylglycerol; ERK, extracellular signal-regulated kinase; HRP, horseradish peroxidase; LC3, microtubule-associated protein 1 light chain 3; LPS, lipopolysaccharide; LPPs, lipid phosphate phosphatases; mTOR, mammalian target of rapamycin; NFκB, nuclear factor kappa B; RAP, rapamycin; SQSTM1/p62, sequestosome 1; PA, phosphatidic acid; PC, phosphatidylcholine; PGs, prostaglandins; PKC, protein kinase C; PKD, protein kinases D; PLD, phospholipase D; POS, photoreceptor outer segments; PR, photoreceptor; PVDF, polyvinylidene fluoride; RasGRP, Ras guanine-releasing protein; RPE, retinal pigment epithelium; WB, western blot.

an inflammatory response in RPE cells, it also triggers the activation of the autophagic process which in turn may serve as a protective mechanism for the cells. In addition, we demonstrate that the PLD pathway modulates the autophagic process in RPE cells. Our findings contribute to the knowledge of the molecular basis of retinal inflammatory and degenerative diseases and open new avenues for potential therapeutic exploration.

**Keywords: retinal pigment epithelium, lipopolysaccharide, autophagy, inflammation, phospholipase D**

## INTRODUCTION

The retinal pigment epithelium (RPE) is a monolayer of pigmented epithelial cells located between the retina and the vascular choroid, constituting the outer blood-retinal barrier (BRB). These epithelial cells play various critical roles for the correct function of the neural retina and photoreceptor (PR) survival, such as the secretion of several growth factors and cytokines and the transport of nutrients and water to the retina. Also, they protect against photo-oxidation and mediate the re-isomerization of all-trans-retinal and the renewal of photoreceptor outer segments (POS) by phagocytosis (Strauss, 2005; Strauß, 2016; Carr et al., 2009). Being a fundamental part in the BRB, RPE cells contribute to establishing the immunological privilege of the eye (Simó et al., 2010; Perez et al., 2013; Pavan et al., 2014). Likewise, RPE mediates in the immune response of the retina, by secreting pro- and anti-inflammatory cytokines, chemoattractants proteins, adhesion molecules and complement factors (Strauss, 2005; Strauß, 2016; Simó et al., 2010; Viringipurampeer et al., 2013).

Inflammation is a key factor in the pathogenesis of several retinal diseases such as age-related macular degeneration (AMD), diabetic retinopathy (DR), retinitis pigmentosa and uveitis, ultimately leading to varying degrees of vision loss (Shen et al., 2000; Rodrigues, 2007; Leung et al., 2009; Kauppinen et al., 2016). The inflammatory response is characterized by a series of reactions, including vasodilation and recruitment of immune cells and plasma proteins to the site of infection or tissue injury (Medzhitov, 2008; Ahmed, 2011; Liu et al., 2017). Inflammation can be both a protective and adaptive response while its deregulation can cause excessive or long-lasting tissue damages, contributing to the development of chronic inflammatory diseases (Medzhitov, 2008; Ahmed, 2011; Whitcup et al., 2013; Liu et al., 2017). It has been demonstrated that RPE cells can participate in the inflammatory response observed in several retinal degenerative diseases through the modification of its secretome (Arjamaa et al., 2017; Datta et al., 2017; Willermain et al., 2018). In view of the essential role of the RPE in PR viability and in visual function, elucidating the molecular mechanisms elicited by inflammation in this tissue could provide new insights for the treatment of retinal diseases.

Previous work from our laboratory demonstrated that the human RPE cell line ARPE-19 expresses both classical phospholipase D isoforms (PLD1 and PLD2) and that lipopolysaccharide (LPS) stimulates PLD activity (Mateos et al., 2014). Classical PLDs hydrolyze phosphatidylcholine (PC) to generate the lipid second messenger phosphatidic acid (PA) and choline (Exton, 2002; Foster and Xu, 2003; Peng and Frohman, 2012; Frohman, 2015). PA can be further dephosphorylated by lipid phosphate phosphatases (LPPs) in order to generate diacylglycerol (DAG), another lipid messenger (Brindley, 2004; Brindley et al., 2009). DAG and PA, as bioactive lipids, can modulate the activity of various proteins involved in cell signaling events, such as protein kinases C (PKC), protein kinase D (PKD), and the mammalian target of rapamycin (mTOR) complex, among others (Wang, 2006; Carrasco and Mérida, 2007; Newton, 2010; Foster et al., 2014). Through the modulation of these signaling proteins, DAG and PA participate in various cellular processes, such as vesicular trafficking, endo and exocytosis and cell survival.

Our previous study constituted the first evidence of classical PLDs participation in the LPS-induced inflammatory response of RPE cells through extracellular signal-regulated kinase (ERK1/2) activation and cyclooxygenase-2 (COX-2) expression (Mateos et al., 2014). Furthermore, we showed that PLD1 plays a dual role in LPS-exposed RPE cells, on the one hand by promoting cell damage through COX-2 induction and on the other by preventing LPS-induced apoptotic signals through PKCε modulation (Tenconi et al., 2016).

Autophagy is a conserved lysosomal self-digestion process ubiquitous in eukaryotic cells that respond to stress conditions, allowing them to adapt to environmental and developmental changes (Klionsky, 2007). Autophagy is initiated by the formation of double membrane-bound vesicles, called autophagosomes, which sequester cytoplasmic material. Finally, the fusion of autophagosomes with lysosomes allows the degradation of autophagic cargo and the subsequent recycling of nutrients and membranes (Yang and Klionsky, 2010). Autophagy is highly active in RPE and PR, being responsible for the lysosomal degradation and recycling of proteins and organelles (Wang et al., 2009). As a recycling process, autophagy has been described as a cellular pro-survival process, although other evidence indicates that under certain circumstances it may conduct to programmed cell death (Ferrington et al., 2016; Montagna et al., 2016; Deretic and Klionsky, 2018). Recently, evidences relating autophagy and inflammation have been described that may lead to therapeutic targeting (Netea-Maier et al., 2016), also in the RPE (Liu et al., 2016). Within the kinases that regulate the onset of autophagy, mTOR is the most important since the active mTORC1 complex prevents the formation of autophagosomes (Saxton and Sabatini, 2017).

Taking into account: (i) the participation of classical PLDs in the LPS-induced inflammatory process in RPE cells through ERK1/2 activation; (ii) the role the latter performs in mTOR regulation (Wang et al., 2017); and (iii) the role of PA and DAG signaling in autophagy (Dall'Armi et al., 2013), PLD possible participation in the regulation of the autophagic process in RPE cells exposed to an inflammatory context was further explored in the present work.

In view of the above, this study aims at arriving at a better understanding of the role of PA- and DAG-mediated signaling pathways in RPE cells exposed to inflammatory conditions.

# MATERIALS AND METHODS

## Reagents

Triton X-100 (octyl phenoxy polyethoxyethanol), dimethyl sulfoxide (DMSO), LPS from *Klebsiella pneumoniae* (LPS, L4268), LY294002 (2-(4-Morpholinyl)-8-phenyl-1(4H)-benzopyran-4-one hydrochloride) and MTT (3-(4,5-dimethylthiazol-2-yl)-2, 5-diphenyltetrazolium bromide) were from Sigma-Aldrich (St. Louis, MO, USA). VU0359595 (PLD1i) and VU0285655-1 (PLD2i) were from Avanti Polar Lipids, Inc. (Alabaster, AL, USA). 4′,6-diamidino-2-phenylindole dihydrochloride (DAPI) was from Life Technologies Corporation (Grand Island, NY, USA). 3-methyladenine (3-MA), rapamycin (RAP) and bafilomycin $A_1$ (BAF) were from Santa Cruz Biotechnology, Inc. (Santa Cruz, CA, USA). 5(6)-carboxy-2′7′-dichlorodihydrofluorescein diacetate (DCDCDHF), TO-PRO$^{TM}$-3 Iodide and DAPI were from Molecular Probes (Eugene, OR, USA). All other chemicals were of the highest purity available.

## Antibodies

Rabbit polyclonal antibody anti-light chain 3B (anti-LC3B; #2775) was from Cell Signaling (Beverly, MA, USA). Mouse monoclonal anti-SQSTM1/p62 (sc-28359) and rabbit polyclonal anti-nuclear factor kappa B (anti-NFκB) p65 (sc-109) antibody were purchased from Santa Cruz Biotechnology, Inc. (Santa Cruz, CA, USA). Mouse monoclonal anti-α Tubulin (DM1-A; CP06) was from EMD/Biosciences-Calbiochem (San Diego, CA, USA). Polyclonal horse radish peroxidase (HRP)-conjugated sheep anti-mouse IgG (NA931V) and polyclonal HRP-conjugated donkey anti-rabbit IgG (NA934V) were purchased from GE Healthcare (Malborough, MA, USA). Alexa Fluor$^{®488}$ goat anti-rabbit (A11008) and Alexa Fluor$^{®488}$ goat anti-mouse (A11001) were from Life Technologies Corporation (Grand Island, NY, USA).

## Retinal-Pigmented Epithelium Cell Cultures and Treatments

Two human retinal-pigmented epithelium cell lines (ARPE-19 and D407) were used in this work. ARPE-19 cells from the American Type Culture Collection (ATCC, Manassas, VA, USA) were generously donated by Dr. E. Politi and Dr. N. Rotstein (INIBIBB, Bahía Blanca, Argentina). D407 cells were a generous gift from Dr E. Rodriguez-Bouland (Weill Medical College of Cornell University, New York, NY, USA). ARPE-19 cells were maintained in Dulbecco's Modified Eagle's Medium (DMEM) supplemented with 10% fetal bovine serum (FBS, Natocor, Córdoba, Argentina) and antibiotic-antimycotic (Anti-Anti 100×, Gibco by Life Technologies) at 37°C under 5% $CO_2$. D407 cells were maintained in 5% FBS DMEM. For western blot (WB) assays, cells were grown to 100% confluence on plastic 35 mm diameter culture dishes. Cell cultures were serum-starved for 30 min prior to LPS treatment with different concentrations (10 or 25 μg/ml) in serum-free DMEM or the same volume of sterile ultra pure water (control condition), for 24 or 48 h. LPS stock (4 mg/ml) was prepared in sterile ultra-pure water. Cells were pre-incubated with different concentrations (0.5 or 5 μM) of VU0359595 (PLD1i) to inhibit PLD1 activity or with different concentrations (0.5 or 5 μM) of VU0285655-1 (PLD2i) to inhibit PLD2 activity for 30 min at 37°C prior to cell stimulation with LPS. To inhibit the autophagic process cells were pre-incubated with 3-MA (5 mM) or with LY294002 (10 μM) for 30 min prior to LPS treatment. To block autophagosome fusion with lysosomes cells were pre-incubated with BAF (50 nM) for 30 min at 37°C prior to LPS treatment. As a positive control, cells were treated with the mammalian target of rapamycin complex 1 (mTORC1) inhibitor rapamycin (RAP, 1 μM) for 24 h in order to induce autophagy. DMSO (vehicle of the inhibitors) was added to all conditions to achieve a final concentration of 0.05%.

## MTT Reduction Assay

Cell viability was measured in terms of mitochondrial function. D407 cells ($1.5 \times 10^4$ cells/well) were seeded in 96-well plates. Cells were pre-incubated with different inhibitors as described above and after a 48 h LPS treatment, mitochondrial function was assessed by MTT reduction assay. MTT is reduced by mitochondrial dehydrogenases of metabolically viable cells to a colored, water-insoluble formazan salt. MTT (5 mg/ml) was prepared in phosphate buffer saline (PBS) and was added to the cell culture medium at a final concentration of 0.5 mg/ml. The culture plates were incubated for 1 h at 37°C in a 5% $CO_2$ atmosphere, cells were then washed twice with PBS and lysed with 100 μl of a buffer containing 10% Triton X-100 and 0.1N HCl in isopropanol. The extent of MTT reduction was measured spectrophotometrically (570 nm absorbance–650 nm absorbance) using a Multiskan$^{TM}$ 60 microplate spectrophotometer (Thermo Fisher Scientific, Waltham, MA, USA). Results are expressed as arbitrary units (AUs) with respect to the control condition.

## Western Blot (WB)

WB assays were performed as previously described (Mateos et al., 2014). Briefly, after experimental treatment the medium was removed from confluent 35 mm dishes, cells were washed with PBS and scraped off with 80 μl ice-cold RIPA lysis buffer [10 mM Tris-HCl (pH 7.4), 15 mM NaCl, 1% Triton X-100, 5 mM NaF, 1 mM $Na_2VO_4$ and the complete protease inhibitor cocktail]. Protein content of total cell lysates was determined by the Bradford method (Bradford, 1976; Bio-Rad Life Science group, Hercules, CA, USA, #500-0006) and samples were denatured with Laemmli sample buffer at

100°C for 5 min (Laemmli, 1970). Thirty micrograms protein were separated by sodium dodecylsulfate polyacrylamide gel electrophoresis (SDS-PAGE) on 10% or 16% polyacrylamide gels and transferred to polyvinylidene fluoride (PVDF) membranes (Millipore, Bedford, MA, USA). Membranes were blocked with 10% bovine serum albumin (BSA) in TTBS buffer [20 mM Tris–HCl (pH 7.4), 100 mM NaCl and 0.1% (w/v) Tween 20] at room temperature for 2 h and subsequently incubated with primary antibodies overnight at 4°C. After three washes with TTBS, membranes were exposed to the appropriate HRP-conjugated secondary antibody for 2 h at room temperature. Immunoreactive bands were detected by enhanced chemiluminescence (Pierce®ECL Western Blotting Substrate, #32209, Thermo scientific) using UltraCruz# Autoradiography Film, Santa Cruz Biotechnology, Inc. (Santa Cruz, CA, USA). Densitometry values of the immunoreactive bands were determined using ImageJ 1.46 software (NIH). The molecular weight of bands was determined using the spectra multicolor broad range protein ladder (26634, Thermo Scientific).

### Measurement of Reactive Oxygen Species (ROS) Production

Reactive oxygen species (ROS) production was measured using the probe DCDCDHF (Molecular Probes, Eugene, OR, USA). This probe can cross the membrane and, after oxidation, it is converted into a fluorescent compound. $6 \times 10^4$ D407 cells were seeded onto 12 mm coverslips and exposed to LPS (10 μg/ml) or to control condition for 24 h. After the experimental treatment, the cell culture medium was removed and replaced by medium containing 10 μM DCDCDHF and cells were incubated for 30 min at 37°C. Cells were subsequently washed three times with PBS and coverslips were mounted for examination with a Nikon Eclipse TE2000-S microscope coupled to a Nikon DS-Qi2 camera (1,608 × 1,608 pixels) and a 60× Plan Apo (1.4 N.A.) oil-immersion objective. Fluorescence intensity values were determined using ImageJ 1.46 software.

### Immunocytochemistry and Fluorescence Microscopy

For immunocytochemistry assays, $6 \times 10^4$ cells were seeded onto 12 mm coverslips on 24-well plates. After LPS treatment (10 or 25 μg/ml) for 24 h cells were washed twice with ice-cold PBS and fixed with methanol for 15 min at −20°C. Cells were then blocked with 2% BSA in PBS for 15 min and exposed to primary anti-LC3B antibody (1:200 in blocking solution), anti-p62 (1:100 in blocking solution) or anti-NFκB p65 (1:100 in blocking solution). Cells were then exposed to the appropriate Alexa Fluor®488-conjugated secondary antibodies (1:500 in blocking solution). Finally, nuclei were stained with DAPI or TO-PRO-3 for 10 min at room temperature. The whole immunocytochemical method was performed at room temperature and three washes with ice-cold PBS were performed between each step of the procedure and after nuclear staining. Coverslips were mounted for examination with a Nikon Eclipse TE2000-S microscope coupled to a Nikon DS-Qi2 camera (1,608 × 1,608 pixels) and a 60× Plan Apo (1.4 N.A.) oil-immersion objective or with a TCS-SP2 confocal microscope (Leica Mikrosysteme Vertrieb GmbH, Wetzlar, Germany) equipped with an acousto optical beam splitter using a 63× (1.2 N.A.) objective. Fluorescence intensity values were determined using ImageJ 1.46 software.

### Data Quantification and Statistical Analysis

In immunocytochemistry images, the percentage of cells with LC3B- or p62- positive punctate structures was manually scored by a blinded operator. With this aim, at least 100 cells of each condition were counted. Data shown in bar graphs represent the percentage mean value ± SD of four independent experiments ($n$ = 4). Fluorescence intensity values from immunocytochemistry images and densitometry values of the WB immunoreactive bands were determined using ImageJ 1.46 software. WBs shown are representative images of samples from four independent experiments ($n$ = 4).

Statistical analysis of the data was performed using ANOVA followed by Tuckey's test to compare means or Student's $t$-test when only two conditions were compared. $p$-values lower than 0.05 were considered statistically significant.

## RESULTS

### LPS Induces NFκB Nuclear Translocation, ROS Generation and Reduces Cell Viability in D407 RPE Cells

Our previous results demonstrated that the exposure of ARPE-19 cells to LPS induces an inflammatory response that engages NO production, PLD activation, COX-2 expression, prostaglandin E2 ($PGE_2$) secretion and reduced cell viability (Mateos et al., 2014). To further characterize the inflammatory response of RPE cells induced by LPS, immunocytochemistry assays were performed in order to evaluate NFκB translocation to the nucleus. In addition, ROS generation was evaluated by using the probe DCDCDHF.

In D407 cells exposed to LPS (10 μg/ml) for 24 h epifluorescence microscope images show an increment in NFκB (p65) nuclear translocation (by 60%) and ROS generation (by 220%) with respect to control condition (**Figures 1A,B**). Similar results were obtained when p65 nuclear translocation was observed by confocal microscopy (**Supplementary Figure S1**). Our previous findings in ARPE-19 cells showed that cell viability was affected only after a 48 h exposure to LPS (Mateos et al., 2014). Similar results were obtained in D407 RPE cells, in which cell viability was reduced by 15% and by 27% in cells exposed to 10 and 25 μg/ml for 48 h, respectively (**Figure 1C**). These results together with our previous findings demonstrate that LPS treatment induces a typical inflammatory response of RPE cells. Taking all these data into account, we next used both RPE cell lines (D407 and ARPE-19) to study the role of the autophagic process in the LPS-induced RPE inflammatory response.

### LPS Exposure Induces an Increment in LC3-II Content in RPE Cells

To study the effect of LPS on the autophagic process of RPE cells, D407 cells were exposed to LPS (10 or 25 μg/ml) for 24 or

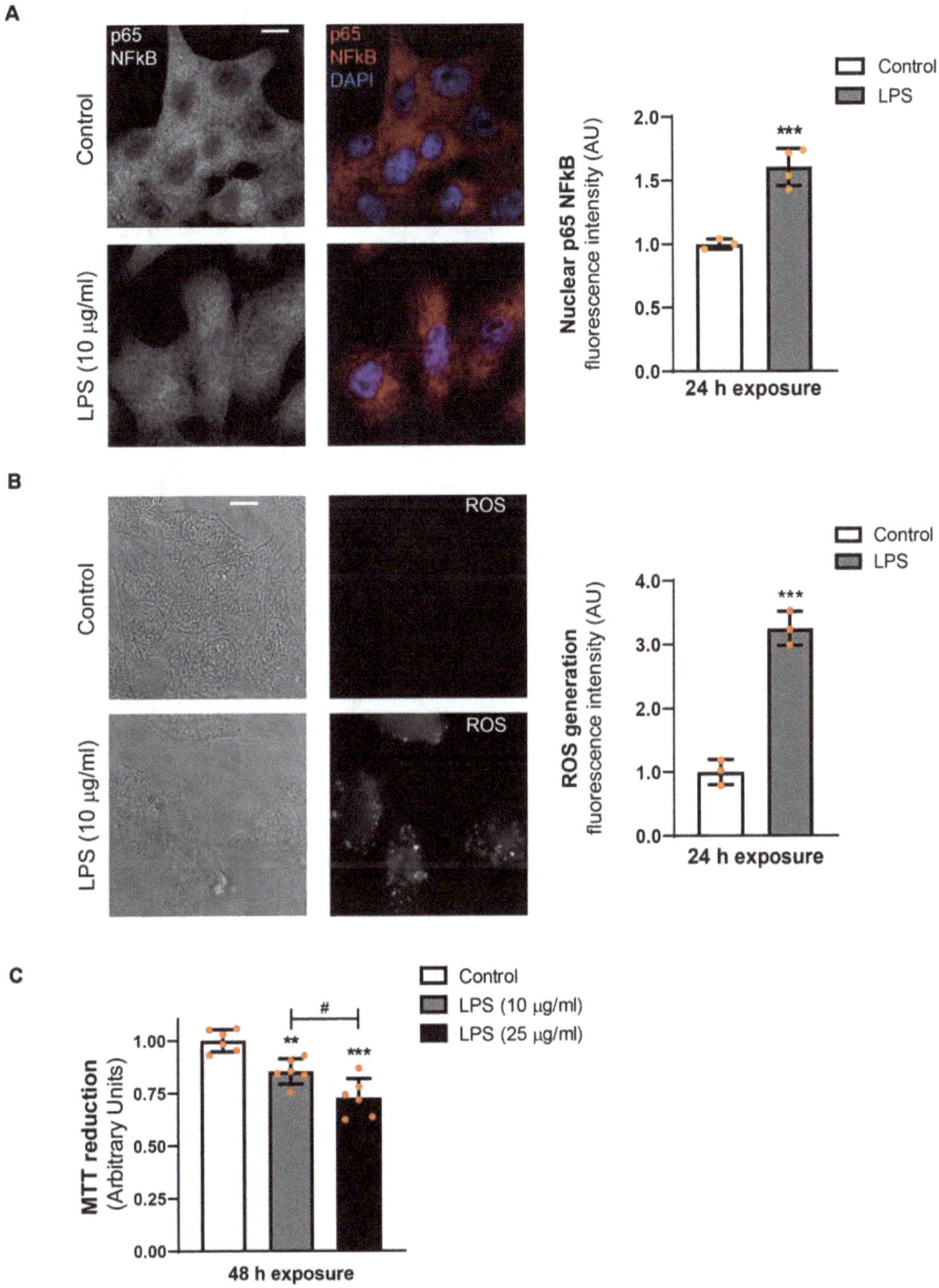


**FIGURE 1** | Lipopolysaccharide (LPS) inflammatory model in D407 cells. **(A)** Immunofluorescence assays for analysis of nuclear factor kappa B (NFκB; p65) subcellular distribution were performed as described in "Materials and Methods" section in D407 cells exposed to LPS (10 μg/ml) or to control condition (ultrapure water) for 24 h. Results are expressed as arbitrary units (AU). **(B)** Reactive oxygen species (ROS) generation was analyzed in D407 cells treated with LPS (10 μg/ml) or under control condition (ultrapure water) for 24 h as detailed in "Materials and Methods" section. Left panel show light microscopy images of the cells. For **(A,B)**, bar graph shows fluorescence intensity expressed as arbitrary units with respect to control conditions (mean ± SD). Dots indicate individual values of different experiments ($n \geq 3$). Asterisks (*) indicate significant differences with respect to control condition (***$p < 0.0001$). Scale bar = 10 μm. **(C)** Cell viability was evaluated using the MTT reduction assay in D407 cells treated with LPS (10 or 25 μg/ml) or ultrapure water (control condition) for 48 h. Results are expressed as arbitrary units. Dots indicate individual values from six different experiments ($n = 6$). Asterisks (*) indicate significant differences with respect to control condition (**$p < 0.001$; ***$p < 0.0001$). Number signs (#) indicate significant differences between LPS conditions ($^{\#}p < 0.05$).

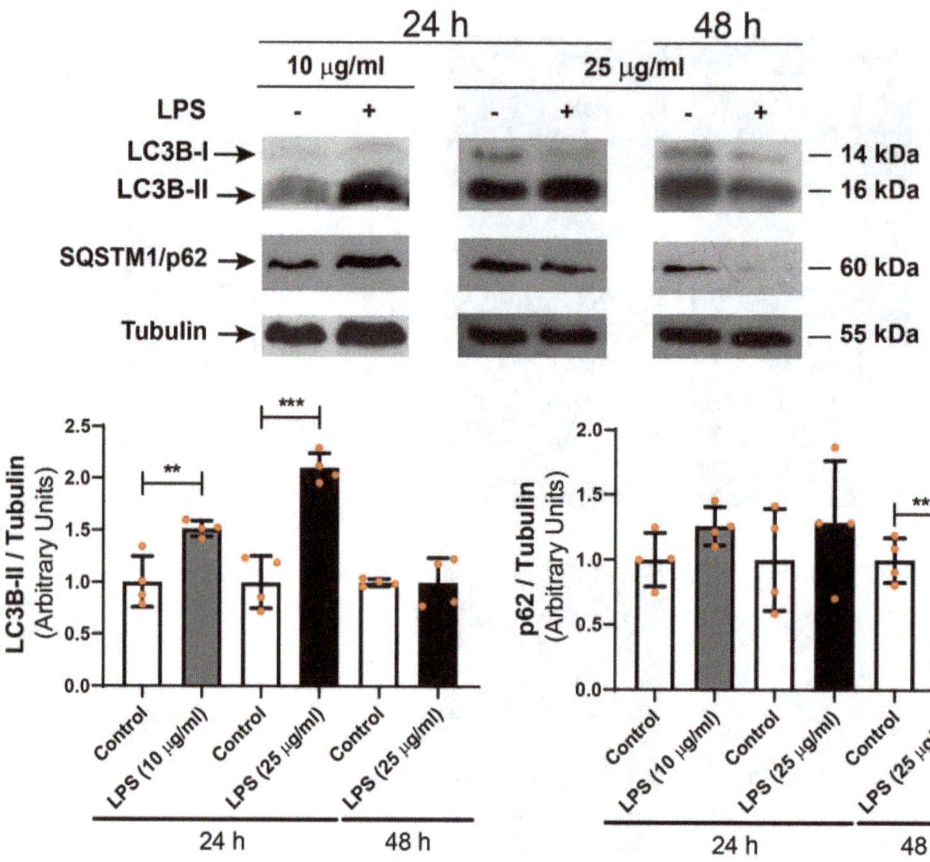


**FIGURE 2 |** Western blot (WB) assays were performed in order to determine light chain 3B-II (LC3B-II) and p62 levels in D407 cells exposed to LPS (10 or 25 μg/ml) or to control condition (ultrapure water), for 24 or 48 h. Numbers to the right indicate molecular weights designated by standard markers. Bar graphs show the densitometry values of LC3B-II/α-Tubulin or p62/α-Tubulin. Results are expressed as arbitrary units. Dots indicate individual values from four independent experiments ($n = 4$). Asterisks (*) indicate significant differences with respect to each control condition (**$p < 0.01$; ***$p < 0.0001$).

48 h and WB assays were performed in order to determine microtubule-associated protein 1 light chain 3B-II (LC3B-II) and sequestosome 1 (SQSTM1/p62) levels. WB showed that 10 and 25 μg/ml LPS increased LC3B-II content by 51% and by 100% with respect to control condition after 24 h treatment, respectively (**Figure 2**). No changes in LC3B-II content were detected after a 48 h exposure to LPS (25 μg/ml; **Figure 2**). SQSTM1/p62 content was not significantly changed after 24 h treatment with both LPS concentrations but was reduced by 70% after a 48 h LPS exposure (**Figure 2**).

In order to study the subcellular distribution of autophagy markers LC3B and p62, immunocytochemistry assays were performed as described in "Materials and Methods" section. **Figure 3** shows that LPS (10 or 25 μg/ml) treatment for 24 h increased LC3B-positive punctate structures in D407 cells (**Figure 3A**) and similar results were observed in ARPE-19 cells exposed to 25 μg/ml LPS for 24 h (**Supplementary Figure S2**). Under control condition, 22% of D407 cells presented LC3B-positive punctate structures and this percentage raised to 58% in cells treated with 10 μg/ml LPS and to 73% in cells treated with 25 μg/ml LPS (**Figure 3A**). The mTORC1 inhibitor rapamycin (RAP, 1 μM) was used as positive control (**Figure 3A**) and no significant differences were detected in LC3B-punctate structure formation between cells incubated with or without FBS (data not shown). Furthermore, larger LC3B-punctate structures were observed in D407 cells exposed to 25 μg/ml LPS with respect to cells exposed to 10 μg/ml LPS (**Figure 3A**). Although WB assays showed no significant changes in p62 content after a 24 h exposure to LPS (**Figure 2**), immunocytochemistry assays showed that a 24 h LPS (10 μg/ml) treatment increases significantly the percentage of D407 cells with p62-positive punctate structures (**Figure 3B**). These results demonstrate that LPS enhances autophagosome-like structures formation in RPE cells.

In view of our results, most of the following experiments were performed with 10 μg/ml LPS since this concentration induced an inflammatory-like response in RPE cells and increased LC3B-II content and autophagosome-like structures formation with fewer effects on cell metabolic state and viability.

To discern whether LPS treatment induces the autophagic process or blocks the autophagic flux, D407 cells were pre-incubated with BAF (50 nM) in order to block autophagosome fusion with lysosomes and thus, autolysosome formation, prior to LPS (10 μg/ml) treatment for 24 h.

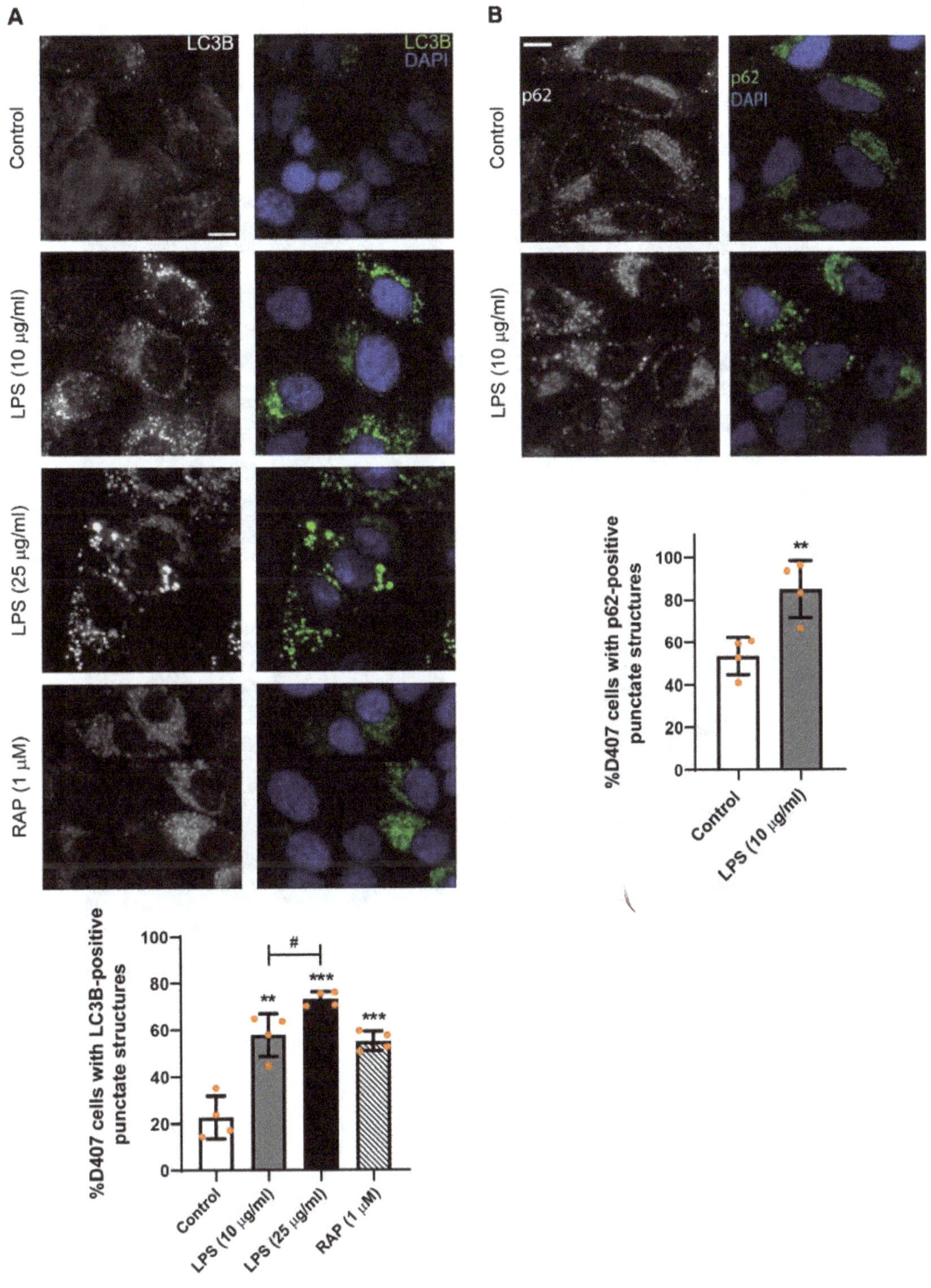


**FIGURE 3 |** Immunofluorescence assays of D407 cells were performed as described in "Materials and Methods" section. **(A)** LC3B-positive punctate structures were analyzed in D407 cells exposed to LPS (10 or 25 μg/ml) or to control condition (vehicle). The mTORC1 inhibitor rapamycin (RAP, 1 μM) was used as positive control. Bar graph shows the percentage of cells presenting LC3B-positive punctate structures in each condition. Cells showing punctate structures similar or bigger to those observed in RAP condition were considered positives. Graph shows the mean percentage ± SD. Dots indicate individual values from four independent experiments ($n = 4$). **(B)** p62-positive punctate structures were analyzed in D407 cells exposed to LPS (10 μg/ml) or to control condition (ultrapure water) for 24 h. Bar graph shows the % of cells presenting p62-positive punctate structures in each condition. Graph shows the mean percentage ± SD. Dots indicate individual values from four independent experiments ($n = 4$). For **(A,B)**, cells were stained with DAPI to visualize the nuclear structure. Scale bar = 10 μm. Asterisks (*) indicate significant differences with respect to control condition ($^{**}p < 0.01$; $^{***}p < 0.001$). Number signs (#) indicate significant differences between LPS conditions ($^{\#}p < 0.05$).

In D407 cells, the blockage of the autophagic flux with BAF increased to 86 the percentage of cells with LC3B-positive punctate structures (**Figures 4A,C**) and to 98 the percentage of cells with p62-positive punctate structures under control condition (**Figures 4B,C**). 100% of the cells pre-incubated with BAF and exposed to LPS for 24 h presented LC3B-positive punctae and p62-positive punctae (**Figures 4A–C**). In addition, WBs showed that pre-incubation with BAF induces an increment

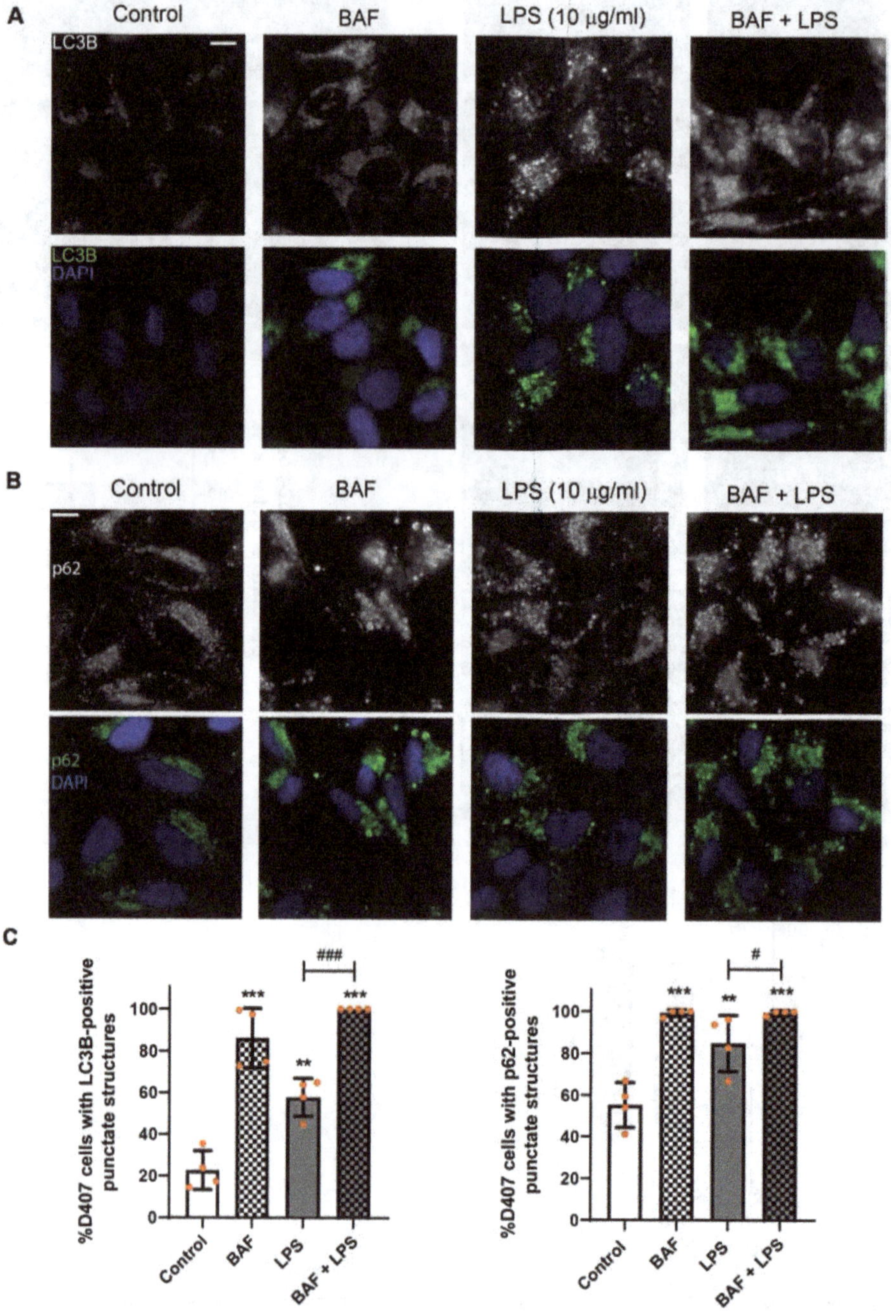


**FIGURE 4 |** Evaluation of autophagic flux in LPS treated retinal pigment epithelium (RPE) cells. RPE cells were pre-incubated with bafilomycin $A_1$ (BAF, 50 nM) or with vehicle dimethyl sulfoxide (DMSO) prior to incubation with LPS (10 µg/ml) or under control condition for 24 h. **(A,B)** Immunofluorescence assays were performed in D407 cells as described in "Materials and Methods" section to determine LC3B-positive **(A)** and p62-positive **(B)** punctate structures. Cells were stained with 4′,6-diamidino-2-phenylindole (DAPI) to visualize the nuclear structure. Scale bar = 10 µm. **(C)** Bar graphs show the percentage of cells presenting LC3B- or p62-positive punctate structures in each condition. Graphs show the mean percentage ± SD. Dots indicate individual values from four independent experiments ($n = 4$). Asterisks (*) indicate significant differences with respect to control condition ($^{**}p < 0.01$; $^{***}p < 0.001$). Number signs (#) indicate significant differences between indicated conditions ($^{\#}p < 0.05$; $^{\#\#\#}p < 0.001$).

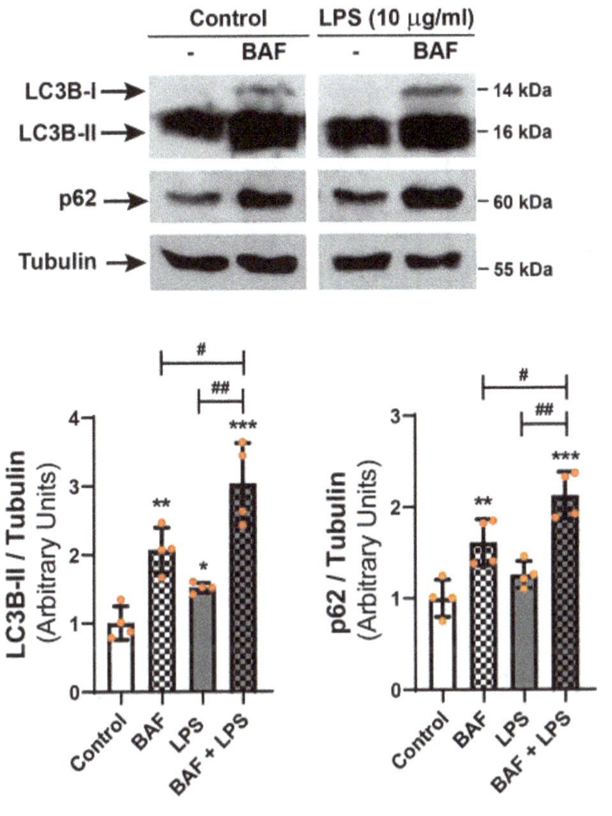


**FIGURE 5 |** D407 cells were pre-incubated with BAF (50 nM) or with vehicle (DMSO) prior to incubation with LPS (10 μg/ml) or under control condition for 24 h. WBs were performed and analyzed as described in "Materials and Methods" section in order to determine LC3B-II and p62 levels. Numbers to the right indicate molecular weights designated by standard markers. Bar graphs show the densitometry values of LC3B-II/α-Tubulin or p62/α-Tubulin. Dots indicate individual values from four independent experiments ($n = 4$). Results are expressed as arbitrary units. Asterisks (*) indicate significant differences with respect to each control condition ($^{*}p < 0.05$; $^{**}p < 0.01$; $^{***}p < 0.001$). Number signs (#) indicate significant differences between indicated conditions ($^{\#}p < 0.05$; $^{\#\#}p < 0.01$).

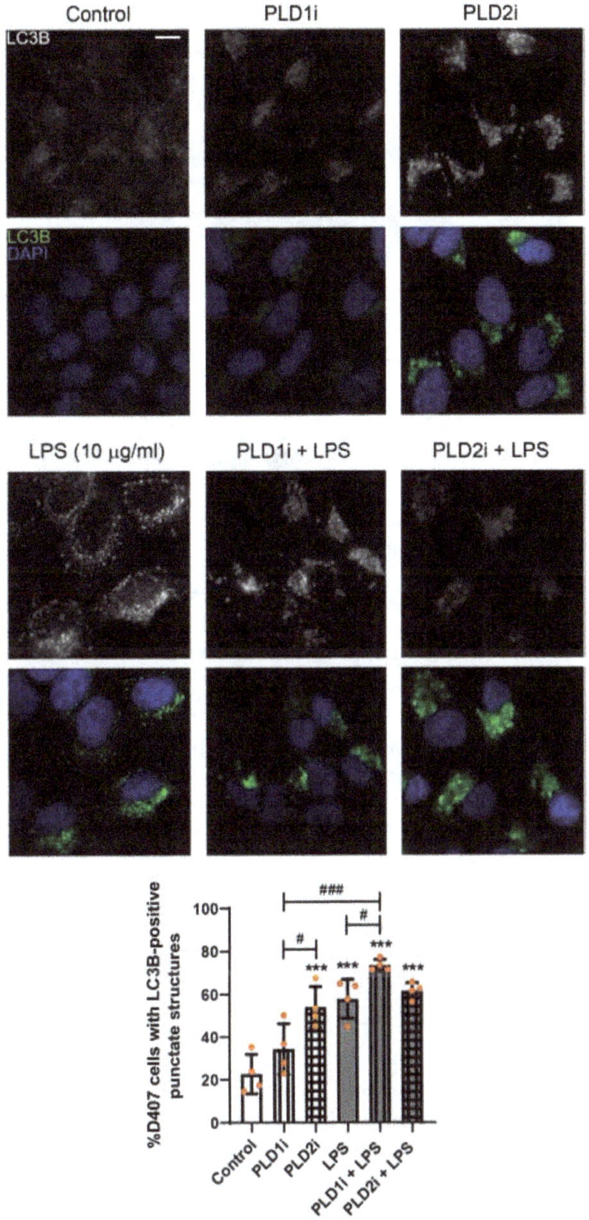


**FIGURE 6 |** Role of phospholipase D (PLD) isoforms 1 and 2 in the autophagic process of RPE cells. D407 cells were pre-incubated with PLD1 or PLD2 selective inhibitors (PLD1i and PLD2i, 5 μM) or vehicle (DMSO) prior to incubation with LPS (10 μg/ml) or under control condition for 24 h. Immunofluorescence assays were performed to determine LC3B-positive punctate structures. Cells were stained with DAPI to visualize the nuclear structure. Scale bar = 10 μm. Bar graph shows the percentage of cells presenting LC3B-positive punctate structures in each condition. Graph shows the mean percentage ± SD. Dots indicate individual values from four independent experiments ($n = 4$). Asterisks (*) indicate significant differences with respect to control condition ($^{***}p < 0.001$). Number signs (#) indicate significant differences between indicated conditions ($^{\#}p < 0.05$; $^{\#\#\#}p < 0.001$).

in LC3B-II and p62 content under control condition and this increment was higher in cells pre-incubated with BAF and exposed to LPS for 24 h (**Figure 5**). Same results were observed in ARPE-19 cells (Data not shown). These results demonstrate that LPS treatment is not blocking the autophagic flux but is inducing the autophagic process in RPE cells.

## PLD1 and PLD2 Inhibition Modulates the Autophagic Process of RPE Cells

As stated above, our previous findings demonstrated the participation of classical PLDs in the LPS-induced inflammatory response of RPE cells (Mateos et al., 2014). To study the role of PLD1 and PLD2 in the LPS-induced autophagic process, D407 cells were pre-incubated with PLD1 or PLD2 selective inhibitors (PLD1i and PLD2i, 5 μM) prior to LPS treatment for 24 h, as described in "Materials and Methods" section. Immunofluorescence assays showed that under control condition the percentage of D407 cells with LC3B-positive punctate structures was increased significantly (to 53%) in cells pre-incubated with PLD2i while PLD1i increased this percentage (to 73%) only in cells exposed to LPS (**Figure 6**). To further support these results, WBs assays show that PLD1 and

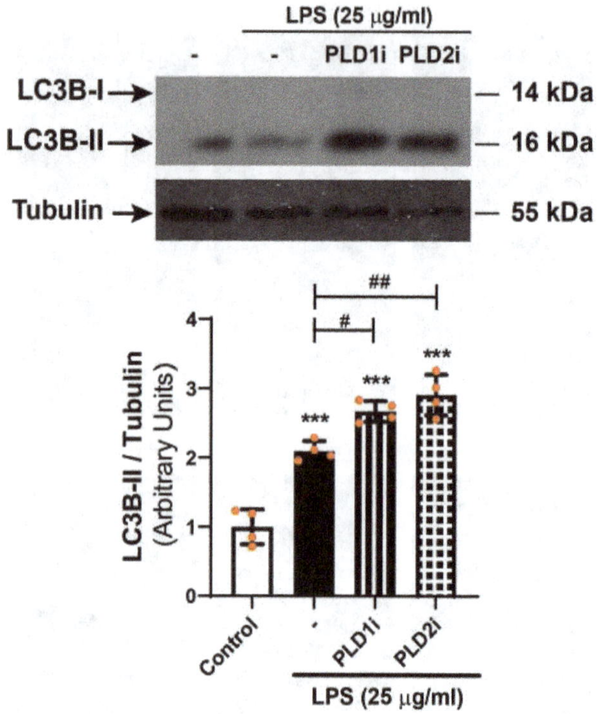


**FIGURE 7 |** WBs were performed and analyzed as described in "Materials and Methods" section in order to determine LC3B-II levels in D407 cells pre-incubated with PLD1i (0.5 μM), PLD2i (0.5 μM) or vehicle (DMSO) prior to incubation with LPS (25 μg/ml) or under control condition for 24 h. The bar graph shows the densitometry values of LC3B-II/α-Tubulin. Dots indicate individual values from four independent experiments ($n$ = 4). Results are expressed as arbitrary units. Asterisks (*) indicate significant differences with respect to control condition ($^{***}p < 0.001$). Number signs (#) indicate significant differences with respect to LPS control condition ($^{\#}p < 0.05$; $^{\#\#}p < 0.01$).

PLD2 inhibition (with lower inhibitor concentrations than those used for immunofluorescence assays, 0,5 μM) also increased LC3B-II content in D407 cells exposed to a higher LPS concentration (25 μg/ml) for 24 h (**Figure 7**). These results suggest that PLD2 modulates basal autophagy under control condition while both PLDs modulate the autophagic process under LPS-induced inflammatory conditions.

## The Activation of the Autophagic Process Protects RPE Cells From the Inflammatory Injury

To assess the role of the autophagic process in LPS-induced cell damage, D407 cells were pre-incubated with autophagy inhibitors 3-MA and LY294002 prior to LPS exposure for 48 h since, as stated above, we previously demonstrated that RPE cell viability is not affected after shorter exposures to LPS (Mateos et al., 2014). These inhibitors block autophagy at an early stage by inhibiting class III phosphatidylinositol 3-kinase (PI3K; Klionsky et al., 2016). **Figure 8A** shows that under control condition 3-MA (5 mM) and LY294002 (10 μM) reduced D407 cell viability by 32% and by 39%, respectively. Furthermore, both inhibitors enhanced the cell viability loss

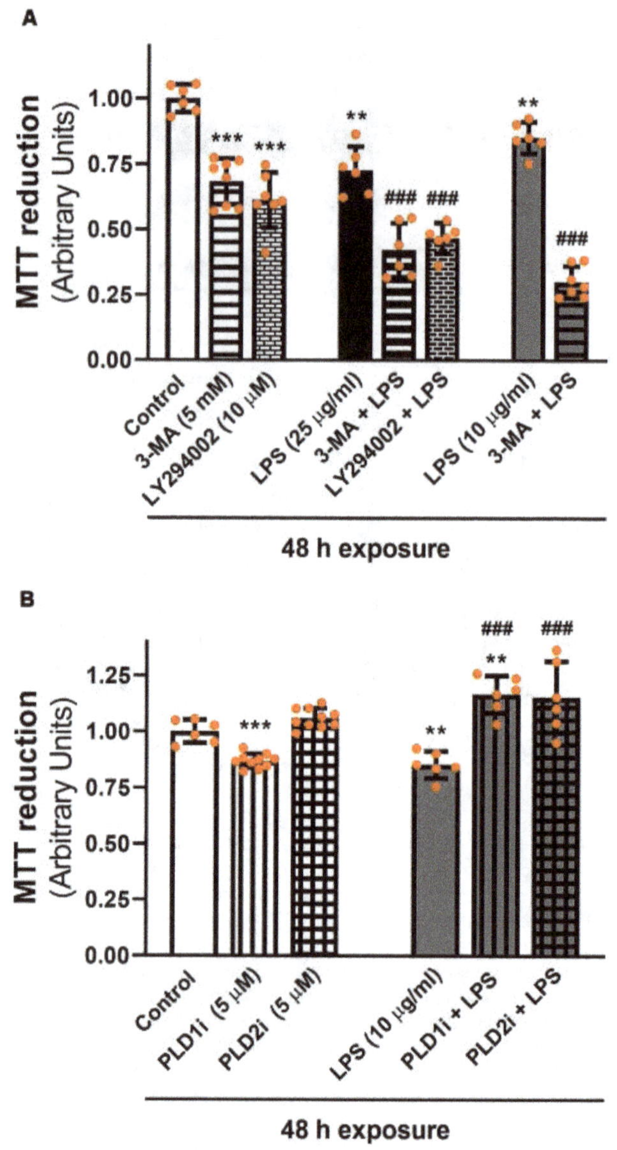


**FIGURE 8 |** **(A)** Effect of autophagy inhibitors on cell viability. D407 cells were pre-incubated with autophagy inhibitor 3-methyladenine (3-MA), LY294002 or vehicle (DMSO) prior to LPS (10 or 25 μg/ml) or control condition exposure for 48 h. **(B)** Effect of PLD inhibitors on cell viability. D407 cells were pre-incubated with PLD1i (5 μM), PLD2i (5 μM) or vehicle (DMSO) prior to LPS (10 μg/ml) or control condition exposure for 48 h. For **(A,B)**, cell viability was evaluated using the MTT reduction assay, as described in "Materials and Methods" section expressed as arbitrary units. Dots indicate individual values from different experiments ($n \geq 6$). Asterisks (*) indicate significant differences with respect to control condition (vehicle; $^{**}p < 0.01$; $^{***}p < 0.0001$). Number signs (#) indicate significant differences with respect to each LPS (vehicle) condition ($^{\#\#\#}p < 0.0001$).

induced by LPS since MTT reduction was reduced by 58% and by 54% in cells pre-incubated with 3-MA and LY294002 and exposed to LPS (25 μg/ml) for 48 h, respectively. Cell viability loss was also enhanced by 70% in cells pre-incubated with 3-MA and exposed to a lower LPS concentration (10 μg/ml) for 48 h (**Figure 8A**). On the contrary, the inhibition of PLD1 and PLD2 with 5 μM PLD1i or PLD2i prevented the loss in cell viability induced by LPS (10 μg/ml) in D407 cells (**Figure 8B**). Lower concentrations (0.5 μM) of PLD1i and PLD2i did not prevent the LPS-induced viability loss of D407 cells (Data not shown). Our results show that the autophagic process is a protective mechanism triggered under LPS-induced inflammation in RPE cells.

## DISCUSSION

LPS can reach and directly stimulate RPE cells in situations of acute ocular inflammation, such as bacterial endophthalmitis (posterior segment eye infection) and uveitis (Leung et al., 2009; Pollreisz et al., 2012). Endophthalmitis can arise after an eye surgery, intravitreal injections, trauma and sepsis (endogenous endophthalmitis), the latter mostly seen in immunocompromised patients (Pollreisz et al., 2012; Haddock et al., 2014; Holland et al., 2014). Although bacterial endophthalmitis is an unusual pathology, it is a vital ocular emergency since it usually ends up in vision loss (Haddock et al., 2014; Holland et al., 2014). Additionally, LPS is often used to induce an inflammatory response in cell cultures. In line with this, our previous findings demonstrated that the exposure of ARPE-19 cells to LPS induces a typical inflammatory response which involves PLD and ERK1/2 activation, COX-2 expression, $PGE_2$ secretion, reduced cell viability and increased caspase-3 cleavage (Mateos et al., 2014; Tenconi et al., 2016). In the present work, we demonstrate that the LPS-induced inflammatory response of RPE cells also involves NFκB nuclear translocation and ROS generation.

Autophagy is a very active catabolic process in RPE cells. It is essential for cell survival in response to stress (Frost et al., 2014; Sinha et al., 2016). Different studies reported that autophagy is selectively dysregulated in the RPE from AMD patients and that downregulation of the autophagic pathway renders the RPE more susceptible to oxidative stress while increased autophagic flux protected the RPE from oxidative damage (Mitter et al., 2014; Golestaneh et al., 2017). In this work, we demonstrate that LPS increases autophagy in RPE cells mediating cell survival. Furthermore, our results show that the PLD pathway can modulate the autophagic process.

Once autophagy is initiated the cytosolic form of LC3 (LC3-I) is processed and transformed by the addition of a group of phosphatidylethanolamine to form LC3-II. This lipidation reaction permits the recruitment of the protein to autophagosome membranes. There are three human isoforms of LC3, LC3A, LC3B, and LC3C. Among the three isoforms, LC3B has been the most studied and has become one of the most reliable markers for characterization of the autophagic process (Klionsky et al., 2016). Similarly, SQSTM1/p62 by interaction with LC3 is associated with the autophagosomal membrane to facilitate the degradation of ubiquitinated protein aggregates (Rubinsztein et al., 2009; Ferrington et al., 2016; Rosa et al., 2016). Finally, p62 is degraded together with ubiquitinated protein in the autolysosome (Rubinsztein et al., 2009; Ferrington et al., 2016; Rosa et al., 2016). Thus, an increase in LC3B-II content and decreased p62 levels are associated with autophagic activation, although p62 changes can be cell type, time and context specific (Klionsky et al., 2016).

The increase in LC3B-II content and in the percentage of cells with LC3B- and p62-positive punctate structures demonstrates that a 24 h LPS exposure induces autophagy in RPE cells. Furthermore, the reduced p62 content observed after a 48 h LPS exposure and the results obtained in the presence of BAF confirm that LPS treatment is inducing the autophagic process in RPE cells rather than blocking its flux. In agreement with our results, Wang and collaborators reported that in ARPE-19 cells LPS plus tetrachlorodibenzo-*p*-dioxin induces the formation of autophagosome-like structures observed by transmission electron microscopy (Wang et al., 2016). The inhibition of autophagy with 3-MA and LY294002, which target early events in the autophagy cycle through irreversible inhibition of class III PI3K, worsened LPS-induced viability loss demonstrating that autophagy is a protective mechanism elicited under LPS condition in RPE cells. Moreover, early autophagy inhibition reduced RPE cell viability in our control condition suggesting that autophagy in a basal context is important for RPE cell maintenance.

The PLD pathway has been postulated both as a positive as well as a negative autophagy modulator (Gomez-Cambronero and Kantonen, 2014). It has been demonstrated that PLD-generated PA induces membrane curvatures necessary for phagocytosis as well as for the formation of the initial autophagosome (Dall'Armi et al., 2010; Holland et al., 2016). On the contrary, PLD-generated PA activates mTORC1, the main inhibitor of the autophagy initiation machinery (Sun and Chen, 2008; Foster et al., 2014; Munson and Ganley, 2015). Moreover, the PLD-mediated autophagic regulation has been proposed as a potential target for cancer therapy (Jang et al., 2014). PA was also shown to bind and activate the mTOR effector S6 kinase (S6K) independently of mTOR (Lehman et al., 2007). An interrelation between PLD2 and mTOR/S6K has been demonstrated in HL-6 leukemia cells, where PLD2 was shown to mediate IL-8-induced mTOR/S6K mRNA up-regulation and, in reverse direction, mTOR and S6K were shown to down-regulate PLD2 activity and gene expression (Tabatabaian et al., 2010). Furthermore, inhibition and genetic knockdown of PLD2 significantly induced autophagy in HT29 and HCT116 colorectal cancer cells (Hwang et al., 2014). However, the role of the PLD pathway in RPE cells autophagic process was a complete unstudied research field. The novelty of our findings is that we show that under control (basal) condition autophagosome-like structures were increased in cells pre-incubated with PLD2i while PLD1i increased autophagosome-like structures in cells exposed to LPS. Our results constitute the first evidence that the PLD pathway is a negative autophagy modulator in RPE cells, possibly through PLD-mediated PA generation and mTORC1 activation. Whereas PLD2 modulates basal autophagy under control condition, both PLDs inhibit the autophagic process under LPS conditions. The PLD2-modulation of basal autophagy in RPE cells is in agreement with the fact that, of both classical PLD isoforms, PLD2 presents higher basal activity.

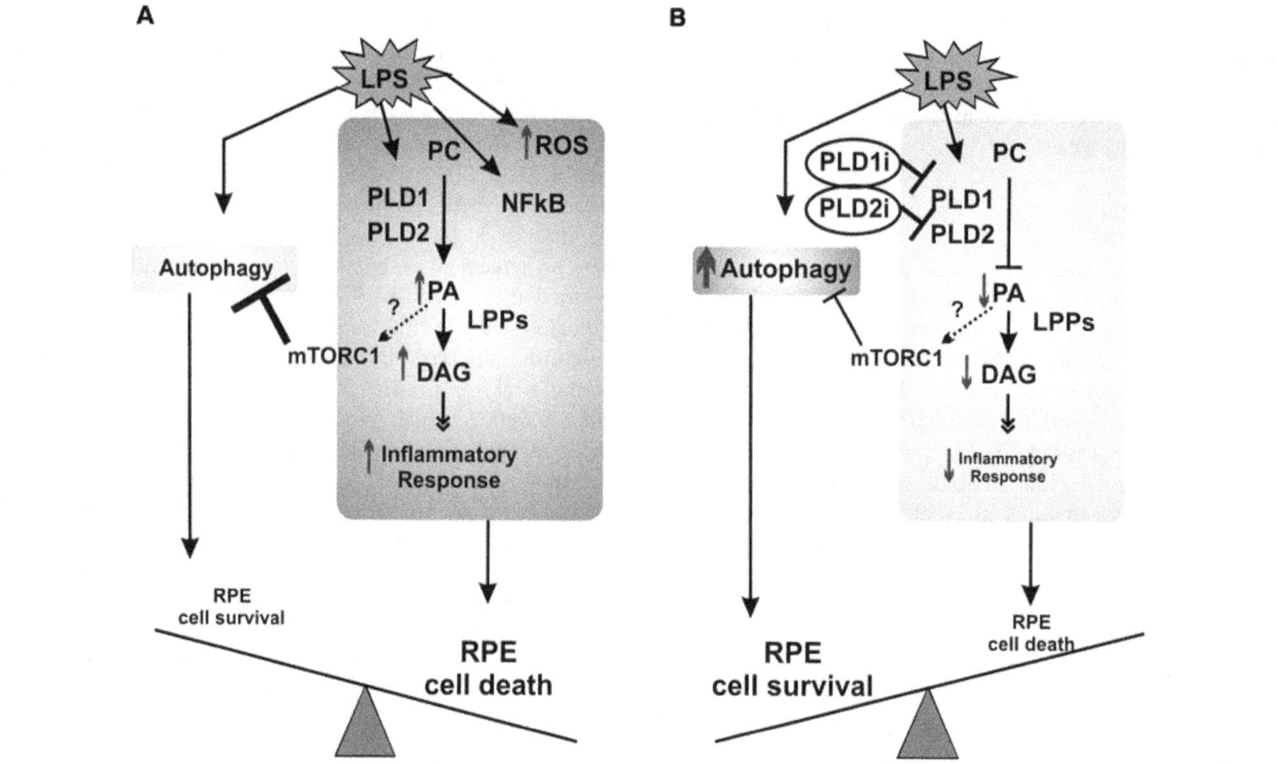


**FIGURE 9 |** Schematic view of signaling events elicited by LPS in RPE cells. **(A)** PLD activation, ROS generation and NFκB nuclear translocation are part of the inflammatory signaling cascade induced in RPE cells exposed to LPS that ultimately leads to cell viability loss. RPE cells answer to LPS also involves the induction of the autophagic process which mediates cells survival. **(B)** When PLD1 and PLD2 are inhibited, the inflammatory response of RPE cells is reduced and autophagy is enhanced, possibly through a reduced phosphatidic acid (PA)-dependent mTORC1 activation, leading to RPE cell survival. Dashed arrows and question marks indicate possible but unstudied mechanisms.

In agreement with results obtained in RPE cells incubated with early autophagy inhibitors (which worsen cell viability loss), PLD inhibitors (which increase autophagy) prevented LPS-induced viability loss in D407 RPE cells. Together, our findings demonstrate that autophagy is a protective mechanism elicited under the LPS-induced inflammatory response of RPE cells. Certainly, the protective effect of PLD inhibitors does not reside only in the modulation of autophagy since our previous findings demonstrated that the pharmacological inhibition of classical PLDs prevents LPS-induced COX-2 expression and $PGE_2$ production in ARPE-19 cells (Mateos et al., 2014). To sum up, our previous work and the findings reported herein demonstrate that in RPE cells LPS induces an inflammatory-like response that involves PLD activation, ROS generation and NFκB nuclear translocation, leading to cell viability loss. Furthermore, LPS induces RPE autophagic process which mediates cells survival (**Figure 9A**). The inhibition of the PLD pathway not only reduces the inflammatory response but also enhances autophagy in RPE cells, possibly through a reduced PA-dependent mTORC1 activation, leading to RPE cell survival (**Figure 9B**).

It is well-recognized the role of NFκB in the regulation of inflammatory responses, by mediating the induction of various pro-inflammatory genes, the activation and differentiation of inflammatory T cells and the activation of inflammasomes (Liu et al., 2017). Furthermore, several studies have linked NFκB signaling with autophagy. It has been reported that NFκB is involved in advanced glycation end-products (AGE)-induced autophagy in diverse cell lines (Verma and Manna, 2016, 2017) and in the autophagic process observed in lung tissues from rats with induced pulmonary arterial hypertension (Zhai et al., 2018). Moreover, in several cell lines NFκB (p65) was shown to induce the expression of beclin1 (BECN1), a central protein that assembles the class III PI3K complex to trigger macroautophagy (Copetti et al., 2009; Han et al., 2018). In LPS-primed macrophages, NFκB was shown to upregulate p62 expression (Zhong et al., 2016) and in head and neck squamous cell carcinoma cells the expression of BECN1 and LC3 was also demonstrated to be modulated by NFκB (p65; He et al., 2017). However, the link between NFκB activation and the expression of autophagy-related proteins in the RPE has not been studied yet. Our results demonstrate that in RPE cells NFκB nuclear translocation and autophagy flux are triggered by LPS at the same time frame, opening interesting questions about the role of this transcription factor in RPE autophagic process.

In conclusion, our results showed that LPS treatment enhances autophagy in RPE cells as a protective mechanism triggered under inflammatory conditions. Furthermore, we demonstrated that the PLD pathway modulates the autophagic process in RPE cells. Further experiments are certainly needed to fully elucidate the mechanisms by which classical PLDs modulates autophagy in RPE cells exposed to inflammatory injury. Our findings contribute to the knowledge of the molecular basis of retinal inflammatory and degenerative diseases, such as AMD, DR and endophthalmitis and open possible avenues of therapeutic exploration.

## AUTHOR CONTRIBUTIONS

VB and PT performed the experiments. VB and MM designed the experiments and wrote the manuscript. MM supervised the study. NG provided equipment and reagents and revised the manuscript.

## FUNDING

This work was supported by grants from Agencia Nacional de Promoción Científica y Tecnológica (ANPCYT; PICTs 2013-2317, 2014-3352 and 2017-0350). MM and NG are research members of CONICET. VB is a postdoctoral fellow. PT is a doctoral fellow from CONICET.

## ACKNOWLEDGMENTS

We want to thank Dr. Ana Sofía Vallés (INIBIBB-UNS-CONICET, Bahía Blanca, Argentina) for the critical reading of the manuscript.

## SUPPLEMENTARY MATERIAL

**FIGURE S1** | Confocal images showing NFκB (p65) subcellular distribution in D407 cells exposed to LPS (10 μg/ml) or to control condition (vehicle) for 24 h. Cells were stained with TO-PRO-3 to visualize the nuclear structure. Scale bar = 10 μm.

**FIGURE S2** | Immunofluorescence assays of ARPE-19 cells. LC3B-positive punctate structures were analyzed by wide-field fluorescence microscopy in ARPE-19 cells exposed for 24 h to 25 μg/ml LPS or control condition (vehicle), with or without FBS. Cells were stained with DAPI to visualize the nuclear structure. Scale bar = 10 μm.

## REFERENCES


Ahmed, A. (2011). An overview of inflammation: mechanism and consequences. *Front. Biol.* 6, 274–281. doi: 10.1007/s11515-011-1123-9

Arjamaa, O., Aaltonen, V., Piippo, N., Csont, T., Petrovski, G., Kaarniranta, K., et al. (2017). Hypoxia and inflammation in the release of VEGF and interleukins from human retinal pigment epithelial cells. *Graefes Arch. Clin. Exp. Ophthalmol.* 255, 1757–1762. doi: 10.1007/s00417-017-3711-0

Bradford, M. M. (1976). A rapid and sensitive method for the quantitation of microgram quantities of protein utilizing the principle of protein-dye binding. *Anal. Biochem.* 72, 248–254. doi: 10.1016/0003-2697(76) 90527-3

Brindley, D. N. (2004). Lipid phosphate phosphatases and related proteins: signaling functions in development, cell division and cancer. *J. Cell. Biochem.* 92, 900–912. doi: 10.1002/jcb.20126

Brindley, D. N., Pilquil, C., Sariahmetoglu, M., and Reue, K. (2009). Phosphatidate degradation: phosphatidate phosphatases (lipins) and lipid phosphate phosphatases. *Biochim. Biophys. Acta* 1791, 956–961. doi: 10.1016/j.bbalip.2009.02.007

Carr, A. J., Vugler, A., Lawrence, J., Chen, L. L., Ahmado, A., Chen, F. K., et al. (2009). Molecular characterization and functional analysis of phagocytosis by human embryonic stem cell-derived RPE cells using a novel human retinal assay. *Mol. Vis.* 15, 283–295.

Carrasco, S., and Mérida, I. (2007). Diacylglycerol, when simplicity becomes complex. *Trends Biochem. Sci.* 32, 27–36. doi: 10.1016/j.tibs.2006.11.004

Copetti, T., Bertoli, C., Dalla, E., Demarchi, F., and Schneider, C. (2009). p65/RelA modulates BECN1 transcription and autophagy. *Mol. Cell. Biol.* 29, 2594–2608. doi: 10.1128/MCB.01396-08

Dall'Armi, C., Devereaux, K. A., and Di, P. G. (2013). The role of lipids in the control of autophagy. *Curr. Biol.* 23, R33–R45. doi: 10.1016/j.cub.2012.10.041

Dall'Armi, C., Hurtado-Lorenzo, A., Tian, H., Morel, E., Nezu, A., Chan, R. B., et al. (2010). The phospholipase D1 pathway modulates macroautophagy. *Nat. Commun.* 1:142. doi: 10.1038/ncomms1144

Datta, S., Cano, M., Ebrahimi, K., Wang, L., and Handa, J. T. (2017). The impact of oxidative stress and inflammation on RPE degeneration in non-neovascular AMD. *Prog. Retin. Eye Res.* 60, 201–218. doi: 10.1016/j.preteyeres.2017.03.002

Deretic, V., and Klionsky, D. J. (2018). Autophagy and inflammation: a special review issue. *Autophagy* 14, 179–180. doi: 10.1080/15548627.2017.1412229

Exton, J. H. (2002). Regulation of phospholipase D. *FEBS Lett.* 531, 58–61. doi: 10.1016/S0014-5793(02)03405-1

Ferrington, D. A., Sinha, D., and Kaarniranta, K. (2016). Defects in retinal pigment epithelial cell proteolysis and the pathology associated with age-related macular degeneration. *Prog. Retin. Eye Res.* 51, 69–89. doi: 10.1016/j.preteyeres.2015.09.002

Foster, D. A., Salloum, D., Menon, D., and Frias, M. A. (2014). Phospholipase D and the maintenance of phosphatidic acid levels for regulation of mammalian target of rapamycin (mTOR). *J. Biol. Chem.* 289, 22583–22588. doi: 10.1074/jbc.r114.566091

Foster, D. A., and Xu, L. (2003). Phospholipase D in cell proliferation and cancer. *Mol. Cancer Res.* 1, 789–800.

Frohman, M. A. (2015). The phospholipase D superfamily as therapeutic targets. *Trends Pharmacol. Sci.* 36, 137–144. doi: 10.1016/j.tips.2015.01.001

Frost, L. S., Mitchell, C. H., and Boesze-Battaglia, K. (2014). Autophagy in the eye: implications for ocular cell health. *Exp. Eye Res.* 124, 56–66. doi: 10.1016/j.exer.2014.04.010

Golestaneh, N., Chu, Y., Xiao, Y. Y., Stoleru, G. L., and Theos, A. C. (2017). Dysfunctional autophagy in RPE, a contributing factor in age-related macular degeneration. *Cell Death Dis.* 8:e2537. doi: 10.1038/cddis.2016.453

Gomez-Cambronero, J., and Kantonen, S. (2014). A river runs through it: how autophagy, senescence and phagocytosis could be linked to phospholipase D by Wnt signaling. *J. Leukoc. Biol.* 96, 779–784. doi: 10.1189/jlb.2vmr0214-120RR

Haddock, L. J., Ramsey, D. J., and Young, L. H. (2014). Complications of subspecialty ophthalmic care: endophthalmitis after intravitreal injections of anti-vascular endothelial growth factor medications. *Semin. Ophthalmol.* 29, 257–262. doi: 10.3109/08820538.2014.959616

Han, T., Guo, M., Gan, M., Yu, B., Tian, X., and Wang, J. B. (2018). TRIM59 regulates autophagy through modulating both the transcription and the ubiquitination of BECN1. *Autophagy* 14, 2035–2048. doi: 10.1080/15548627.2018.1491493

He, Z. J., Zhu, F. Y., Li, S. S., Zhong, L., Tan, H. Y., and Wang, K. (2017). Inhibiting ROS-NF-κB-dependent autophagy enhanced brazilin-induced apoptosis in head and neck squamous cell carcinoma. *Food Chem. Toxicol.* 101, 55–66. doi: 10.1016/j.fct.2017.01.002

Holland, P., Knaevelsrud, H., Søreng, K., Mathai, B. J., Lystad, A. H., Pankiv, S., et al. (2016). HS1BP3 negatively regulates autophagy by modulation of phosphatidic acid levels. *Nat. Commun.* 7:13889. doi: 10.1038/ncomms 13889

Holland, E. J., McDonald, M. B., Parekh, J. G., and Sheppard, J. D. (2014). Antibiotic resistance in acute postoperative endophthalmitis. *Ophthalmology* 121, S1–S9. doi: 10.1016/j.ophtha.2014.06.049

Hwang, W. C., Kim, M. K., Song, J. H., Choi, K. Y., and Min, D. S. (2014). Inhibition of phospholipase D2 induces autophagy in colorectal cancer cells. *Exp. Mol. Med.* 46:e124. doi: 10.1038/emm.2014.74

Jang, Y. H., Choi, K. Y., and Min, D. S. (2014). Phospholipase D-mediated autophagic regulation is a potential target for cancer therapy. *Cell Death Differ.* 21, 533–546. doi: 10.1038/cdd.2013.174

Kauppinen, A., Paterno, J. J., Blasiak, J., Salminen, A., and Kaarniranta, K. (2016). Inflammation and its role in age-related macular degeneration. *Cell. Mol. Life Sci.* 73, 1765–1786. doi: 10.1007/s00018-016-2147-8

Klionsky, D. J. (2007). Autophagy: from phenomenology to molecular understanding in less than a decade. *Nat. Rev. Mol. Cell Biol.* 8, 931–937. doi: 10.1038/nrm2245

Klionsky, D. J., Abdelmohsen, K., Abe, A., Abedin, M. J., Abeliovich, H., Acevedo, A. A., et al. (2016). Guidelines for the use and interpretation of assays for monitoring autophagy (3rd edition). *Autophagy* 12, 1–222. doi: 10.1080/15548627.2015.1100356

Laemmli, U. K. (1970). Cleavage of structural proteins during the assembly of the head of bacteriophage T4. *Nature* 227, 680–685. doi: 10.1038/227680a0

Lehman, N., Ledford, B., Di, F. M., Frondorf, K., McPhail, L. C., and Gomez-Cambronero, J. (2007). Phospholipase D2-derived phosphatidic acid binds to and activates ribosomal p70 S6 kinase independently of mTOR. *FASEB J.* 21, 1075–1087. doi: 10.1096/fj.06-6652com

Leung, K. W., Barnstable, C. J., and Tombran-Tink, J. (2009). Bacterial endotoxin activates retinal pigment epithelial cells and induces their degeneration through IL-6 and IL-8 autocrine signaling. *Mol. Immunol.* 46, 1374–1386. doi: 10.1016/j.molimm.2008.12.001

Liu, J., Copland, D. A., Theodoropoulou, S., Chiu, H. A., Barba, M. D., Mak, K. W., et al. (2016). Impairing autophagy in retinal pigment epithelium leads to inflammasome activation and enhanced macrophage-mediated angiogenesis. *Sci. Rep.* 6:20639. doi: 10.1038/srep20639

Liu, T., Zhang, L., Joo, D., and Sun, S.-C. (2017). NF-κB signaling in inflammation. *Signal Transduct. Target. Ther.* 2:e17023. doi: 10.1038/sigtrans.2017.23

Mateos, M. V., Kamerbeek, C. B., Giusto, N. M., and Salvador, G. A. (2014). The phospholipase D pathway mediates the inflammatory response of the retinal pigment epithelium. *Int. J. Biochem. Cell Biol.* 55, 119–128. doi: 10.1016/j.biocel.2014.08.016

Medzhitov, R. (2008). Origin and physiological roles of inflammation. *Nature* 454, 428–435. doi: 10.1038/nature07201

Mitter, S. K., Song, C., Qi, X., Mao, H., Rao, H., Akin, D., et al. (2014). Dysregulated autophagy in the RPE is associated with increased susceptibility to oxidative stress and AMD. *Autophagy* 10, 1989–2005. doi: 10.4161/auto.36184

Montagna, C., Rizza, S., Maiani, E., Piredda, L., Filomeni, G., and Cecconi, F. (2016). To eat, or NOt to eat: S-nitrosylation signaling in autophagy. *FEBS J.* 283, 3857–3869. doi: 10.1111/febs.13736

Munson, M. J., and Ganley, I. G. (2015). MTOR, PIK3C3 and autophagy: signaling the beginning from the end. *Autophagy* 11, 2375–2376. doi: 10.1080/15548627.2015.1106668

Netea-Maier, R. T., Plantinga, T. S., van de Veerdonk, F. L., Smit, J. W., and Netea, M. G. (2016). Modulation of inflammation by autophagy: consequences for human disease. *Autophagy* 12, 245–260. doi: 10.1080/15548627.2015.1071759

Newton, A. C. (2010). Protein kinase C: poised to signal. *Am. J. Physiol. Endocrinol. Metab.* 298, E395–E402. doi: 10.1152/ajpendo.00477.2009

Pavan, B., Capuzzo, A., and Forlani, G. (2014). High glucose-induced barrier impairment of human retinal pigment epithelium is ameliorated by treatment with Goji berry extracts through modulation of cAMP levels. *Exp. Eye Res.* 120, 50–54. doi: 10.1016/j.exer.2013.12.006

Peng, X., and Frohman, M. A. (2012). Mammalian phospholipase D physiological and pathological roles. *Acta Physiol.* 204, 219–226. doi: 10.1111/j.1748-1716.2011.02298.x

Perez, V. L., Saeed, A. M., Tan, Y., Urbieta, M., and Cruz-Guilloty, F. (2013). The eye: a window to the soul of the immune system. *J. Autoimmun.* 45, 7–14. doi: 10.1016/j.jaut.2013.06.011

Pollreisz, A., Rafferty, B., Kozarov, E., and Lalla, E. (2012). Klebsiella pneumoniae induces an inflammatory response in human retinal-pigmented epithelial cells. *Biochem. Biophys. Res. Commun.* 418, 33–37. doi: 10.1016/j.bbrc.2011.12.102

Rodrigues, E. B. (2007). Inflammation in dry age-related macular degeneration. *Ophthalmologica* 221, 143–152. doi: 10.1159/000099293

Rosa, M. D., Distefano, G., Gagliano, C., Rusciano, D., and Malaguarnera, L. (2016). Autophagy in diabetic retinopathy. *Curr. Neuropharmacol.* 14, 810–825. doi: 10.2174/1570159x14666160321122900

Rubinsztein, D. C., Cuervo, A. M., Ravikumar, B., Sarkar, S., Korolchuk, V., Kaushik, S., et al. (2009). In search of an "autophagomometer". *Autophagy* 5, 585–589. doi: 10.4161/auto.5.5.8823

Saxton, R. A., and Sabatini, D. M. (2017). mTOR signaling in growth, metabolism and disease. *Cell* 168, 960–976. doi: 10.1016/j.cell.2017.02.004

Shen, D. F., Chang, M. A., Matteson, D. M., Buggage, R., Kozhich, A. T., and Chan, C. C. (2000). Biphasic ocular inflammatory response to endotoxin-induced uveitis in the mouse. *Arch. Ophthalmol.* 118, 521–527. doi: 10.1001/archopht.118.4.521

Simó, R., Villarroel, M., Corraliza, L., Hernandez, C., and Garcia-Ramirez, M. (2010). The retinal pigment epithelium: something more than a constituent of the blood-retinal barrier–implications for the pathogenesis of diabetic retinopathy. *J. Biomed. Biotechnol.* 2010:190724. doi: 10.1155/2010/190724

Sinha, D., Valapala, M., Shang, P., Hose, S., Grebe, R., Lutty, G. A., et al. (2016). Lysosomes: regulators of autophagy in the retinal pigmented epithelium. *Exp. Eye Res.* 144, 46–53. doi: 10.1016/j.exer.2015.08.018

Strauß, O. (2016). Pharmacology of the retinal pigment epithelium, the interface between retina and body system. *Eur. J. Pharmacol.* 787, 84–93. doi: 10.1016/j.ejphar.2016.03.066

Strauss, O. (2005). The retinal pigment epithelium in visual function. *Physiol. Rev.* 85, 845–881. doi: 10.1152/physrev.00021.2004

Sun, Y., and Chen, J. (2008). mTOR signaling: PLD takes center stage. *Cell Cycle* 7, 3118–3123. doi: 10.4161/cc.7.20.6881

Tabatabaian, F., Dougherty, K., Di, F. M., and Gomez-Cambronero, J. (2010). Mammalian target of rapamycin (mTOR) and S6 kinase down-regulate phospholipase D2 basal expression and function. *J. Biol. Chem.* 285, 18991–19001. doi: 10.1074/jbc.M110.111542

Tenconi, P. E., Giusto, N. M., Salvador, G. A., and Mateos, M. V. (2016). Phospholipase D1 modulates protein kinase C-epsilon in retinal pigment epithelium cells during inflammatory response. *Int. J. Biochem. Cell Biol.* 81, 67–75. doi: 10.1016/j.biocel.2016.10.015

Verma, N., and Manna, S. K. (2016). Advanced glycation end products (AGE) potently induce autophagy through activation of raf protein kinase and nuclear factor κB (NF-κB). *J. Biol. Chem.* 291, 1481–1491. doi: 10.1074/jbc.M115.667576

Verma, N., and Manna, S. K. (2017). Advanced glycation end products (AGE) potentiates cell death in p53 negative cells via upregulaion of NF-κ B and impairment of autophagy. *J. Cell. Physiol.* 232, 3598–3610. doi: 10.1002/jcp.25828

Viringipurampeer, I. A., Bashar, A. E., Gregory-Evans, C. Y., Moritz, O. L., and Gregory-Evans, K. (2013). Targeting inflammation in emerging therapies for genetic retinal disease. *Int. J. Inflam.* 2013:581751. doi: 10.1155/2013/581751

Wang, Q. J. (2006). PKD at the crossroads of DAG and PKC signaling. *Trends Pharmacol. Sci.* 27, 317–323. doi: 10.1016/j.tips.2006.04.003

Wang, Y., Hanus, J. W., Abu-Asab, M. S., Shen, D., Ogilvy, A., Ou, J., et al. (2016). NLRP3 upregulation in retinal pigment epithelium in age-related macular degeneration. *Int. J. Mol. Sci.* 17:E73. doi: 10.3390/ijms170 10073

Wang, A. L., Lukas, T. J., Yuan, M., Du, N., Tso, M. O., and Neufeld, A. H. (2009). Autophagy and exosomes in the aged retinal pigment epithelium: possible relevance to drusen formation and age-related macular degeneration. *PLoS One* 4:e4160. doi: 10.1371/journal.pone.0004160

Wang, R., Shen, Z., Yang, L., Yin, M., Zheng, W., Wu, B., et al. (2017). Protective effects of heme oxygenase-1-transduced bone marrow-derived mesenchymal stem cells on reducedsize liver transplantation: role of autophagy regulated by the ERK/mTOR signaling pathway. *Int. J. Mol. Med.* 40, 1537–1548. doi: 10.3892/ijmm.2017.3121

Whitcup, S. M., Nussenblatt, R. B., Lightman, S. L., and Hollander, D. A. (2013). Inflammation in retinal disease. *Int. J. Inflam.* 2013:724648. doi: 10.1155/2013/724648

Willermain, F., Scifo, L., Weber, C., Caspers, L., Perret, J., and Delporte, C. (2018). Potential interplay between hyperosmolarity and inflammation on retinal pigmented epithelium in pathogenesis of diabetic retinopathy. *Int. J. Mol. Sci.* 19:E1056. doi: 10.3390/ijms19041056

Yang, Z., and Klionsky, D. J. (2010). Eaten alive: a history of macroautophagy. *Nat. Cell Biol.* 12, 814–822. doi: 10.1038/ncb0910-814

Zhai, C., Shi, W., Feng, W., Zhu, Y., Wang, J., Li, S., et al. (2018). Activation of AMPK prevents monocrotaline-induced pulmonary arterial hypertension by suppression of NF-κB-mediated autophagy activation. *Life Sci.* 208, 87–95. doi: 10.1016/j.lfs.2018.07.018

Zhong, Z., Umemura, A., Sanchez-Lopez, E., Liang, S., Shalapour, S., Wong, J., et al. (2016). NF-κB restricts inflammasome activation via elimination of damaged mitochondria. *Cell* 164, 896–910. doi: 10.1016/j.cell.2015.12.057

10

# Stress, Dietary Patterns and Cardiovascular Disease

*Luis Pedro Morera[1]*, Georgina Noel Marchiori[2,3], Leonardo Adrián Medrano[1,4] and María Daniela Defagó[2,3]*

*[1] Instituto de Organizaciones Saludables, Universidad Siglo 21, Córdoba, Argentina, [2] Instituto de Investigaciones en Ciencias de la Salud (INICSA), CONICET, Universidad Nacional de Córdoba, Córdoba, Argentina, [3] Escuela de Nutrición, Facultad de Ciencias Médicas, Universidad Nacional de Córdoba, Córdoba, Argentina, [4] Department of Pyschology, Pontificia Universidad Católica Madre y Maestra, Santiago de los Caballeros, Dominican Republic*

***Correspondence:**
*Luis Pedro Morera*
*luis.p.morera@gmail.com*

According to the World Health Organization, an unhealthy diet and insufficient physical activity are the leading global risks to health. Dietary behavior is a modifiable factor in cardiovascular disease (CVD) prevention. Furthermore, the fact that cardiovascular events and stress-related emotional disorders share a common epidemiology may indicate the existence of pathways linking these two diseases (Chauvet-Gelinier and Bonin, 2017). Psychosocial stress can lead to changes in dietary patterns (DP) and under chronic stress conditions, high caloric and hyperpalatable foods are preferred. The interplay between these two factors impacts on several biological pathways: for example, it can prime the hippocampus to produce a potentiated neuroinflammatory response, generating memory deficits; it can also affect gut microbiota composition, ultimately influencing behavior and brain health and creating a predisposition to the development of diseases such as obesity, CVD, diabetes and metabolic syndrome. Though both cognition and emotion can be heavily affected by caloric intake, diet composition and stress, the molecular pathways involved remain elusive (Spencer et al., 2017). In this review, we describe the interplay between stress and DP at a molecular level, and how these factors relate to brain health and mental fitness. Finally, we show how these findings could give rise to novel therapeutic targets for chronic diseases.

**Keywords: stress, cardiovascular disease, dietary patterns, nutrition, microbiome**

## INTRODUCTION

Cardiovascular disease (CVD), is the leading cause of mortality and disability worldwide. According to the Global Burden of Disease study, ischemic heart disease and stroke accounted for 25% of total deaths worldwide in 2013 (Rubinstein et al., 2010; GBD 2013 Mortality and Causes of Death Collaborators, 2015).

The current epidemic of CVD is largely explained by several modifiable risk factors associated with lifestyle, feasible to modify. In this sense, an unbalanced diet, excessive alcohol and tobacco consumption, hypercholesterolemia, diabetes mellitus, high blood pressure, visceral obesity, physical inactivity and psychosocial stress increase the risk of future CVD events and are responsible for an estimated 90% of the population-attributable risk fraction of

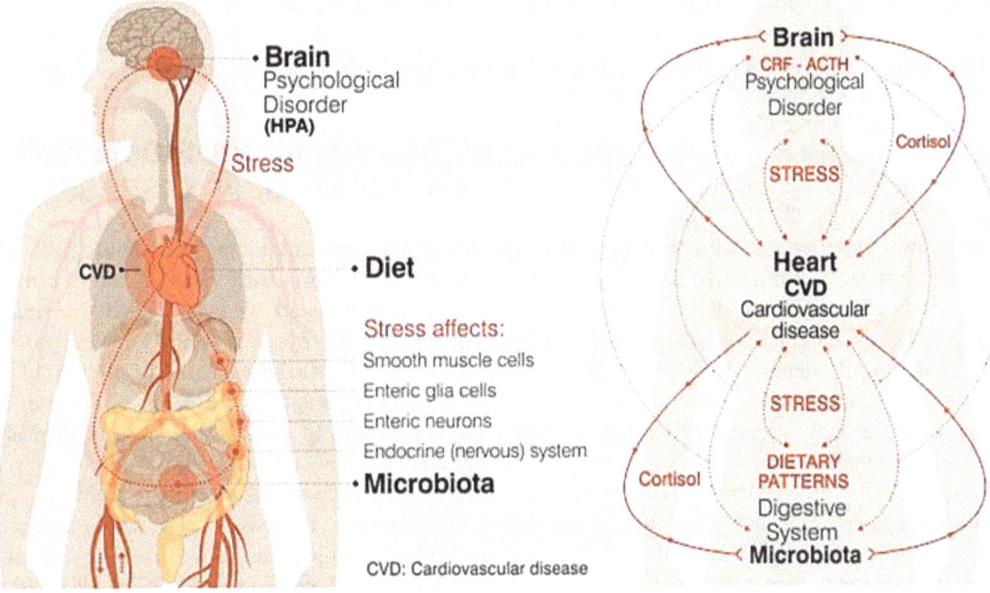


**FIGURE 1** | Relationship between nutritional changes and emotional state and brain health.

ischemic heart disease and stroke worldwide (Schächinger et al., 2000; O'Donnell et al., 2010; Uthman et al., 2014; Karmali et al., 2017). Even more stress-related psychological disorders such as depression show a higher prevalence in patients with coronary artery disease or heart failure compared with the general population (Lane et al., 2002; Ruo et al., 2003; Rutledge et al., 2006).

Chronic or acute exposure to stress (defined as an ongoing or anticipated threat to homeostasis or well-being) favors to the destabilization of the dynamic balance of the organism, and its response promotes the release of chemical mediators that affect the metabolic and behavioral state in humans. Stress-induced activation of the neuroendocrine hypothalamic-pituitary-adrenal axis (HPA), upon exposure to a stressor cortisol is expected to exert widespread metabolic effects, which is mostly necessary to maintain or restore homeostasis. Stress, perhaps, is the trigger in the cascade of neuroendocrine effects that drive the development of the visceral distribution of adipose tissue, resistance to insulin and the consequent hyperinsulinemia, thus leading to the accumulation of cardiovascular risk factors (Serrano Ríos, 2005). Since glucocorticoids favor increased adiposity, mainly, abdominal fat, they can lead to increased appetite, affecting the quantity and quality of the diet (increased sweet and high fat food intake), and body weight gain. Thus, exposure to stress can modify eating behavior. These stress-induced alterations in food intake and energy balance then interacting with emotional state and health cardiovascular, **Figure 1** (Epel et al., 2001; Groesz et al., 2012). Though a relationship between nutritional changes and emotional state and brain health is already known to exist, the exact nature of this relationship has not been established. Research over the last decade has focused on bidirectional communication between gut and brain, termed the gut-brain axis. Dysbiosis and inflammation of the gut have been linked to several mental illnesses including anxiety and depression, although the molecular pathways involved have not yet been elucidated (Clapp et al., 2017).

The aim of this mini-review is to summarize the findings in the literature on how stress influences the molecular pathways affecting behavior, dietary patterns (DP) and their impact on health, and the synergistic effects of this cycle.

**Figure 1** The potential biological mechanisms that connect the observed relationships between DP, stress and mental health could be modulated by the immune and endocrine systems, brain plasticity and the microbiome-gut-brain axis, being key targets for nutritional therapy in future research.

## METHODS

The authors conducted a literature search of available sources describing issues relating to stress, DP and behavior. Research studies were selected based on research topics found in globally acknowledged databases such as Web of Science, PubMed, Springer, and Scopus, from 2010 up to the present time and classified according to their relevancy. The information provided in the selected studies was carefully evaluated and is described and discussed in the following sections.

## NUTRITION AND CARDIOVASCULAR DISEASE

Diet is one of the most studied factors in the pathogenesis of CVD since it affects diverse cardiometabolic risk factors such as obesity, lipid blood profile, blood pressure, glucose-insulin homeostasis, endothelial health, adipocyte metabolism, cardiac function, metabolic expenditure, weight regulation, visceral adiposity, and the microbiome (Mozaffarian, 2016).

Dietary patterns refers to the habitual combinations of foods and meals consumed on a daily basis (Hu, 2002). Several DP have been related to beneficial cardiovascular effects. For example, the Mediterranean DP -characterized by moderate energy intake, high consumption of olive oil, fish, legumes, nuts, fruits, and vegetables; fewer red meats and processed (sodium-preserved) meats; and a regular and moderate consumption of red wine- is associated with low CVD incidence and mortality (Shen et al., 2015; Sanches Machado d'Almeida et al., 2018). This DP and others such as Prudent, DASH or Healthy DP are high in fiber, vitamins, antioxidants, minerals, phenolics, and unsaturated fats, and low in glycemic index, glycemic load, salt, and *trans* fat (Esmaillzadeh et al., 2007; Mozaffarian et al., 2011). The Western DP on the other hand, characterized by a high intake of red meats, fat dairy products, refined grains and sugars, has been positively correlated with higher concentrations of markers of endothelial dysfunction, the first step in CVD: fasting insulin, C peptide, leptin, C reactive protein, homocysteine, tissue plasminogen activator antigen, interleukin 6 (IL-6), E-selectin, intercellular adhesion molecule 1 (sICAM-1) and vascular cells of molecular adhesion 1 (sVCAM-1) (Defagó et al., 2014; Rodríguez-Monforte et al., 2015; Marchiori et al., 2017).

In the long term, not only the quality but also the quantity of nutrients consumed can influence the neural circuits that regulate motivation, emotion and mood. Evidence can be found in literature about the relationship between saturated, *trans* fat intake and the risk of mental disorders (Barnard et al., 2014). Chronic exposure to a high-fat diet may affect the underlying neurobiological pathways of emotion and reward via its action on energy metabolism, endocrine function and immunity. Saturated and *trans* fatty acids favor central fat deposition and have been related with cardiometabolic and neurological diseases (Micha and Mozaffarian, 2008). The omega-3 polyunsaturated fatty acids (PUFAs) participate in modulation inflammation and immunospecific response, cell growth and tissue repair. Omega-3 plays a role in neuronal membrane fluidity and receptor function and lower levels of these PUFAs have been associated with common mental disorders such as depression and generalized anxiety, also with accelerated neurodegeneration (Grant and Guest, 2016).

Acute stress exposure (short term exposure) may shut down appetite by corticotropin-releasing hormone action and epinephrine liberation. However, if the stressor agent persists, the increased cortisol increases appetite and the motivation to eat (Razzoli et al., 2017). Experimental studies have demonstrated how chronic stress exposure increases susceptibility to diet-induced obesity, with induced spontaneous binging and hyperphagia and a preference for highly-palatable food, rich in calories, *trans* fat, salt and sugar (Packard et al., 2014; Ulrich-Lai et al., 2015). Research on human behavior shows a strong link between exposure to stress and binge eating disorder, often associated with development the overweight and obesity. Stress-induced non-nutritive food selection, is often referred to as eating "comfort food" or highly palatable food (Leigh et al., 2018).

## NUTRITION, MICROBIOME AND CARDIOVASCULAR DISEASE

The human gut microbiome contains $10^{14}$ resident micro-organisms, among which bacteria are the most well-studied group, predominated by gram positive *Firmicutes* and gram negative *Bacteroidetes* (Cresci and Bawden, 2015). The collective genome of the microbiome contains millions of genes compared to the approximately 25,000 genes of the human genome and thus contributes to a wide range of biochemical and metabolic functions, such as nutrient acquisition, the harvesting of energy and large numbers of host metabolic pathways.

Inflammatory related diseases has been related to intestinal microbiome composition (bowel and skin diseases, autoimmune arthritis, type 2 diabetes, and atherosclerosis among others) (Buford, 2017). Specifically, an abnormal change in gut flora has been linked to a range of CVD risk factors, including obesity and diabetes. The first analyses on human intestinal microbiota reported a lower amount of *Bacteroidetes* than *Firmicutes* in obese individuals, however, these findings have not been consistently demonstrated in all subsequent metagenomic studies on obesity in humans (Ley, 2010). A lower abundance of butyrate-producing bacteria, in particular *Faecalibacterium prausnitzii,* a major member of the *Firmicutes phylum,* in individuals with obesity-related metabolic disturbances and diabetes has been observed. Furthermore, the presence of this bacterium is inversely correlated with the intake of dietary fat. Other studies have identified increased abundance of *Bifidobacteria* species in healthy individuals compared with individuals with obesity and diabetes (Martín et al., 2017). Dysbiosis has also been linked to CVD and metabolic diseases such as a lower ratio of *Bacteroidetes* to *Firmicutes* in obesity and hypertension, or increased *Collinsella* in atherosclerosis (Brahe et al., 2016).

Several DP have been studied for their ability to modulate the intestinal microbiota. In general terms, a Western DP led to a marked decrease in numbers of total bacteria and beneficial *Bifidobacterium* and *Eubacterium* species, whereas Mediterranean and Prudent DP have been linked to increases in *Lactobacillus, Bifidobacterium,* and *Prevotella,* and decreases in *Clostridium (*Koloverou et al., 2016; Singh et al., 2017*)*. However, dietary manipulation to modify gut microbiome is still at the incipient stage It has been detected that dietary fiber including prebiotics has a beneficial effect on gut microbiota and host health, improving insulin sensitivity, low-grade chronic inflammation, and lipid metabolism (Ahmadmehrabi and Tang, 2017). Prebiotics are non-digestible dietary compounds that stimulate growth or activity of autochthonous microorganisms, resulting in health benefits. They are basically oligo- or polysaccharides of fructose or galactose and also lactulose and lactitol; they promote the development of *bifidobacteria,* which are capable of degrading various complex carbohydrates. Many *Firmicutes* and in particular *Bacteroides* are also able to carry out this function (Suárez, 2013). Prebiotics are naturally present in foods such as wheat, garlic, onion, asparagus, leek, beet, chicory root, and artichoke, among others; they can also be added to products such as milk, yogurt and breakfast cereals. In this regard, adherence to a DP rich in fruits, vegetables and whole grains may modulate the gut microbiome and thus favorably impact on human health.

## GUT BRAIN AXIS AND STRESS

The mechanisms underlying microbiota-gut-brain axis communication involves neuro-immune-endocrine mediators. This interconnected network includes the central nervous system (CNS), the autonomic nervous system, the enteric nervous system and the HPA (Farzi et al., 2018).

In an organism exposed to stress, the hypothalamus stimulates the pituitary by releasing corticotropin-releasing factor (CRF). In the anterior pituitary, CRF causes the release of the adrenocorticotropic hormone (ACTH), which in turn stimulates the adrenals to cause an increased rate of synthesis and release of cortisol (cortisol in humans and corticosterone in rodents) (Foster et al., 2017). Cortisol serves to maintain homeostasis during normal states of activity (regulating cellular function and metabolism) and during periods of stress (Christiansen et al., 2007).

Chronically elevated cortisol levels can disturb brain function, affecting cognition, emotion and motivation, short and long-term memory; sustained HPA axis activation also impairs the immune system response, as has been demonstrated particularly in early life stress (Shirtcliff et al., 2009). Cortisol exerts it's effects trough the interaction with two corticoid receptors, high affinity mineralocorticoid receptors (MR) and low affinity glucocorticoid receptors (GR). A persistently activated HPA axis will eventually lead to a compensatory downregulation of the expression of GR signaling through epigenetic modifications (Weaver et al., 2004). In addition, glucocorticoids increase intestinal permeability, and negatively affects the gut microbiota composition.

Stress-related changes could be also mediated by neuroendocrine hormones, such as norepinephrine (NE) and dopamine (DA); it has long been known that these catecholamines can increase the growth rate of Gram-negative bacteria (Lyte and Ernst, 1992).

In turn, changes in gut microbiome composition has been already related to cognitive disorders and mental illness. There is strong evidence linking major depression and microbiome, and preclinical evidence related to anxiety disorders (Foster and McVey Neufeld, 2013; Malan-Muller et al., 2017).

## LINKING MICROBIOME AND NEURONAL SIGNALING: MECHANISTIC EVIDENCE

Further research is required to elucidate the exact mechanisms and mediators involved in brain-microbiota communication. A central issue that remains unresolved is which mediators the microbiota uses to communicate with the brain and how this network ultimately influences behavior and health.

There are three major systems along with their mediators playing a role in inter-talk between the microbiota and the brain: neuronal communication, endocrine signaling mediators and the immune system mediators. Together, these systems create an integrated molecular network that impact both in gut and brain function.

The gut communicates with the brain through a systemic, central route. The vagus nerve sends information to the brain, where it is processed in the nucleus tractus solitarius; this nucleus then projects to the parabrachial nucleus, which in turns projects to the prefrontal cortex (PFC) and amygdala. These latter are key loci that control anxiety and fear responses. It has been reported that both regions display irregularities in germ free animals (GF), including hypermyelination in the PFC.

Previous papers have shown that the *N*-methyl-D-aspartate (NMDA) receptor subunit (NMDArec2B) has reduced expression in the amygdala of GF animals (Neufeld et al., 2011). Furthermore, it has been demonstrated that feeding prebiotics to these animals elevates their levels of brain-derived neurotrophic factor (BDNF), NMDA receptor subunits, and D-serine in the brain. Moreover, GABA receptor and serotonin 1A receptor are upregulated in the amygdala and hippocampus, respectively, upon supplementing GF animals with a Lactobacillus strain, ultimately regulating behavior in mice (Bravo et al., 2011).

**TABLE 1** | Molecular signaling pathways linking the microbiome with stress-related health outcomes.

| Pathway | Mediator | Microbiome | Health outcome | References |
|---|---|---|---|---|
| Neural pathways | Serotonin | GF vs. specific pathogen-free animals (SPF) | Anxiety-like behavior | Neufeld et al., 2011; Clarke et al., 2012 |
| | GABA | *Bacteroides*, *Parabacteroides* and *Escherichia* species | Depression | Strandwitz et al., 2018 |
| | miRNA | GF vs. GF colonized animals | Anxiety- and fear-related behavior | Hoban et al., 2017 |
| | c-FOS | *Campylobacter jejuni* | Anxiety-like behavior | Lyte et al., 2006; Goehler et al., 2008 |
| | BDNF | GF animals | Brain development | Diaz Heijtz et al., 2011 |
| Endocrine pathways | Cortisol | *Lactobacillus helveticus, Bifidobacteria* | Anxiety-like behavior | Foster et al., 2017 |
| Immune signaling | TNF-α | *Lactobacillus plantarum* PS128 | Improved anxiety-like behavior | Liu et al., 2016 |
| | IL-6 | *Lactobacillus* | Inflammation, overweight, obesity. | Cooper et al., 2016 |
| | IL-1β | *Akkermansia* spp. and *Blautia* spp. | Depression | Marc et al., 2014; Wong et al., 2016 |

The biogenic amine Serotonin [5-hydroxytryptamine (5-HT)] exerts its function in the brain and in the ENS. Most of 5-HT is synthetized by gut mucosal enterochromaffin cells and ENS neurons. Peripherally, 5-HT is involved in gastrointestinal function, smooth muscle contraction and relaxation, and in pain perception. In the brain it is involved in regulating mood and cognition (Yano et al., 2015). Serotonin synthesis depends on the availability of tryptophan, an essential amino acid that must be supplied in the diet, and microbiota plays a central role in the regulation and synthesis of this amine.

Together these findings reinforce the concept that DP can have either a positive or a negative impact on the CNS by regulating critical neurotransmitters implicated in psychiatric disorders, such as depression (Wallace and Milev, 2017; Zalar et al., 2018).

Finally, the immune system plays an important intermediary role between the brain and the gut. Gut-associated lymphoid tissue is the main component of mucosal-associated lymphoid tissue and corresponds to almost 70% of the entire immune system (Vighi et al., 2008). Dysbiosis of the gut microbiota is linked to abnormal immune responses, which are accompanied by irregular cytokine synthesis and release. It has been reported that TNFα and IFNγ production capacity appears to be influenced by the microbiome, whereas cytokines such as IL-1β, IL-6, and Th17-derived IL-17, and IL-22 display fewer, but more specific, associations with the gut microbiota (Schirmer et al., 2016).

**Table 1** Mechanistic pathways, mediators and main microbiome modifications associated with stress related psychological disorders. Molecular signaling pathways linking the microbiome with stress-related health outcomes.

Several studies related to preclinical models of bacterial infections, probiotics treatment and analysis of germ-free (GF) animals suggest that the microbiota can influence the CNS and consequently behavior. Stress-related disorders such as anxiety and depression are among the main psychiatric conditions associated with microbiome changes (Desbonnet et al., 2010, 2015; Bravo et al., 2011).

## CONCLUSION

The treatment of multidimensional diseases such as CVD require multidimensional approaches. Nutritional psychiatry is a growing field of research seeking to provide clinically relevant interventions for multifactorial diseases. This emerging line of inquiry has assembled data on biological pathways such as gastrointestinal microbiota and inflammation, on DP and on how these are modulated by the environment. It has become clear that this intertwined network of environmental factors (such as stress and DP) interacting with the above-mentioned pathways combines to modulate behavior.

Some trending foods and (controversial) diets have brought lasting changes to traditional diets, however, in most cases neither these nor dietary supplements have been subjected to adequate clinical trials to test their safety and efficacy. A better understanding of the interplay between diet, stress, neuronal signaling, phenotypes, and the microbiome will provide important insights into the utility of scientific evidence-based nutrition. Future studies are imperative to proactively avoid cardiovascular events in patient population.

## AUTHOR CONTRIBUTIONS

All authors equally contributed to the drafting, analyses the final version of the manuscript, and read and approved the final version of the manuscript.

## FUNDING

This work was supported by the Ministry of Science and Technology of Córdoba grant GRFT 2017, Universidad Siglo 21 and SECyT Secretary of Science and Technology of the National University of Córdoba (SECyT).

## REFERENCES

Ahmadmehrabi, S., and Tang, W. H. W. (2017). Gut microbiome and its role in cardiovascular diseases. *Curr. Opin. Cardiol.* 32, 761–766. doi: 10.1097/HCO.0000000000000445

Barnard, N. D., Bunner, A. E., and Agarwal, U. (2014). Saturated and trans fats and dementia: a systematic review. *Neurobiol. Aging* 35, S65–S73. doi: 10.1016/j.neurobiolaging.2014.02.030

Brahe, L. K., Astrup, A., and Larsen, L. H. (2016). Can we prevent obesity-related metabolic diseases by dietary modulation of the gut microbiota? *Adv. Nutr.* 7, 90–101. doi: 10.3945/an.115.010587

Bravo, J. A., Forsythe, P., Chew, M. V., Escaravage, E., Savignac, H. M., Dinan, T. G., et al. (2011). Ingestion of *Lactobacillus* strain regulates emotional behavior and central GABA receptor expression in a mouse via the vagus nerve. *Proc. Natl. Acad. Sci. U.S.A.* 108, 16050–16055. doi: 10.1073/pnas.1102999108

Buford, T. W. (2017). Dis trust your gut: the gut microbiome in age-related inflammation, health, and disease. *Microbiome* 5:80. doi: 10.1186/s40168-017-0296-0

Chauvet-Gelinier, J.-C., and Bonin, B. (2017). Stress, anxiety and depression in heart disease patients: a major challenge for cardiac rehabilitation. *Ann. Phys. Rehabil. Med.* 60, 6–12. doi: 10.1016/j.rehab.2016.09.002

Christiansen, J. J., Djurhuus, C. B., Gravholt, C. H., Iversen, P., Christiansen, J. S., Schmitz, O., et al. (2007). Effects of cortisol on carbohydrate, lipid, and protein metabolism: studies of acute cortisol withdrawal in adrenocortical failure. *J. Clin. Endocrinol. Metab.* 92, 3553–3559. doi: 10.1210/jc.2007-0445

Clapp, M., Aurora, N., Herrera, L., Bhatia, M., Wilen, E., and Wakefield, S. (2017). gut microbiota's effect on mental health: the gut-brain axis. *Clin. Pract.* 7:987.

Clarke, G., Grenham, S., Scully, P., Fitzgerald, P., Moloney, R. D., Shanahan, F., et al. (2012). The microbiome-gut-brain axis during early life regulates the hippocampal serotonergic system in a sex-dependent manner. *Mol. Psychiatry* 18, 666–673. doi: 10.1038/mp.2012.77

Cooper, D., Kim, E. B., Marco, M., Rust, B., Welch, L., Horn, W., et al. (2016). Relationship between human gut microbiota and interleukin 6 levels in overweight and obese adults. *FASEB J.* 30:146.

Cresci, G. A., and Bawden, E. (2015). Gut microbiome: what we do and don't know. *Nutr. Clin. Pract.* 30, 734–746.

Defagó, M. D., Elorriaga, N., Irazola, V. E., and Rubinstein, A. L. (2014). Influence of food patterns on endothelial biomarkers: a systematic review. *J. Clin. Hypertens.* 16, 907–913. doi: 10.1111/jch.12431

Desbonnet, L., Clarke, G., Traplin, A., O'sullivan, O., Crispie, F., Moloney, R. D., et al. (2015). Gut microbiota depletion from early adolescence in mice: implications for brain and behaviour. *Brain Behav. Immun.* 48, 165–173. doi: 10.1016/j.bbi.2015.04.004

Desbonnet, L., Garrett, L., Clarke, G., Kiely, B., Cryan, J. F., and Dinan, T. G. (2010). Effects of the probiotic Bifidobacterium infantis in the maternal separation model of depression. *Neuroscience* 170, 1179–1188. doi: 10.1016/j.neuroscience.2010.08.005

Diaz Heijtz, R., Wang, S., Anuar, F., Qian, Y., Björkholm, B., Samuelsson, A., et al. (2011). Normal gut microbiota modulates brain development and behavior. *Proc. Natl. Acad. Sci. U.S.A.* 108, 3047–3052. doi: 10.1073/pnas.1010529108

Epel, E., Lapidus, R., Mcewen, B., and Brownell, K. (2001). Stress may add bite to appetite in women: a laboratory study of stress-induced cortisol and eating behavior. *Psychoneuroendocrinology* 26, 37–49. doi: 10.1016/s0306-4530(00)00035-4

Esmaillzadeh, A., Kimiagar, M., Mehrabi, Y., Azadbakht, L., Hu, F. B., and Willett, W. C. (2007). Dietary patterns and markers of systemic inflammation among iranian women. *J. Nutr.* 137, 992–998. doi: 10.1093/jn/137.4.992

Farzi, A., Fröhlich, E. E., and Holzer, P. (2018). Gut Microbiota and the Neuroendocrine System. *Neurotherapeutics* 15, 5–22. doi: 10.1007/s13311-017-0600-5

Foster, J. A., and McVey Neufeld, K.-A. (2013). Gut-brain axis: how the microbiome influences anxiety and depression. *Trends Neurosci.* 36, 305–312. doi: 10.1016/j.tins.2013.01.005

Foster, J. A., Rinaman, L., and Cryan, J. F. (2017). Stress & the gut-brain axis: regulation by the microbiome. *Neurobiol. Stress* 7, 124–136.

Goehler, L. E., Park, S. M., Opitz, N., Lyte, M., and Gaykema, R. P. A. (2008). Campylobacter jejuni infection increases anxiety-like behavior in the holeboard: possible anatomical substrates for viscerosensory modulation of exploratory behavior. *Brain Behav. Immun.* 22, 354–366. doi: 10.1016/j.bbi.2007.08.009

Grant, R., and Guest, J. (2016). "Role of omega-3 PUFAs in neurobiological health," in *The Benefits of Natural Products for Neurodegenerative Diseases*, eds M.M. Essa, M. Akbar, and G. Guillemin (Cham: Springer International Publishing), 247–274. doi: 10.1007/978-3-319-28383-8_13

Groesz, L. M., Mccoy, S., Carl, J., Saslow, L., Stewart, J., Adler, N., et al. (2012). What is eating you? Stress and the drive to eat. *Appetite* 58, 717–721. doi: 10.1016/j.appet.2011.11.028

Hoban, A. E., Stilling, R. M., Moloney, G., Moloney, R. D., Shanahan, F., Dinan, T. G., et al. (2017). Microbial regulation of microRNA expression in the amygdala and prefrontal cortex. *Microbiome* 5:102. doi: 10.1186/s40168-017-0321-3

Hu, F. B. (2002). Dietary pattern analysis: a new direction in nutritional epidemiology. *Curr. Opin. Lipidol.* 13, 3–9. doi: 10.1097/00041433-200202000-00002

Karmali, K. N., Persell, S. D., Perel, P., Lloyd-Jones, D. M., Berendsen, M. A., and Huffman, M. D. (2017). Risk scoring for the primary prevention of cardiovascular disease. *Cochrane Database Syst. Rev.* 3:CD006887

Koloverou, E., Panagiotakos, D. B., Pitsavos, C., Chrysohoou, C., Georgousopoulou, E. N., Grekas, A., et al. (2016). Adherence to Mediterranean diet and 10-year incidence (2002–2012) of diabetes: correlations with inflammatory and oxidative stress biomarkers in the ATTICA cohort study. *Diabetes Metab. Res. Rev.* 32, 73–81. doi: 10.1002/dmrr.2672

Lane, D., Carroll, D., Ring, C., Beevers, D. G., and Lip, G. Y. H. (2002). The prevalence and persistence of depression and anxiety following myocardial infarction. *Br. J. Health Psychol.* 7, 11–21. doi: 10.1348/135910702169321

Leigh, S. J., Lee, F., and Morris, M. J. (2018). Hyperpalatability and the generation of obesity: roles of environment, stress exposure and individual difference. *Curr. Obes. Rep.* 7, 6–18. doi: 10.1007/s13679-018-0292-0

Ley, R. E. (2010). Obesity and the human microbiome. *Curr. Opin. Gastroenterol.* 26, 5–11. doi: 10.1097/mog.0b013e328333d751

Liu, W.-H., Chuang, H.-L., Huang, Y.-T., Wu, C.-C., Chou, G.-T., Wang, S., et al. (2016). Alteration of behavior and monoamine levels attributable to *Lactobacillus plantarum* PS128 in germ-free mice. *Behav. Brain Res.* 298, 202–209. doi: 10.1016/j.bbr.2015.10.046

Lyte, M., and Ernst, S. (1992). Catecholamine induced growth of gram negative bacteria. *Life Sci.* 50, 203–212. doi: 10.1016/0024-3205(92)90273-r

Lyte, M., Li, W., Opitz, N., Gaykema, R. P. A., and Goehler, L. E. (2006). Induction of anxiety-like behavior in mice during the initial stages of infection with the agent of murine colonic hyperplasia citrobacter rodentium. *Physiol. Behav.* 89, 350–357. doi: 10.1016/j.physbeh.2006.06.019

Malan-Muller, S., Valles-Colomer, M., Raes, J., Lowry, C. A., Seedat, S., and Hemmings, S. M. J. (2017). The gut microbiome and mental health: implications for anxiety- and trauma-related disorders. *J. Int. Biol.* 22, 90–107. doi: 10.1089/omi.2017.0077

Marc, U., Jose, M.-E., Lucile, C., Ricard, N., Magi, F., Eduard, V., et al. (2014). Cytokine-induced depression: current status and novel targets for depression therapy. *CNS Neurol. Disord. Drug Targets* 13, 1066–1074. doi: 10.2174/1871527313666140612121921

Marchiori, G. N., González, A. L., Perovic, N. R., and Defagó, M. D. (2017). Una mirada global sobre la influencia de los patrones alimentarios en las enfermedades cardiovasculares. *Perspect. Nutr. Humana.* 19, 79–92. doi: 10.17533/udea.penh.v19n1a07

Martín, R., Miquel, S., Benevides, L., Bridonneau, C., Robert, V., Hudault, S., et al. (2017). Functional characterization of novel *Faecalibacterium prausnitzii* strains isolated from healthy volunteers: a step forward in the use of f. prausnitzii as a next-generation probiotic. *Front. Microbiol.* 8:1226. doi: 10.3389/fmicb.2017.01226

Micha, R., and Mozaffarian, D. (2008). Trans fatty acids: effects on cardiometabolic health and implications for policy. *Prostaglandins Leukot. Essent. Fatty Acids* 79, 147–152. doi: 10.1016/j.plefa.2008.09.008

GBD 2013 Mortality and Causes of Death Collaborators, (2015). Global, regional, and national age-sex specific all-cause and cause-specific mortality for 240 causes of death, 1990-2013: a systematic analysis for the Global Burden of Disease study 2013. *Lancet* 385, 117–171. doi: 10.1016/s0140-6736(14)61682-2

Mozaffarian, D. (2016). Dietary and policy priorities for cardiovascular disease, diabetes, and obesity: a comprehensive review. *Circulation* 133, 187–225. doi: 10.1161/CIRCULATIONAHA.115.018585

Mozaffarian, D., Appel, L. J., and Horn, L. V. (2011). Components of a cardioprotective diet. *Circulation* 123, 2870–2891. doi: 10.1161/circulationaha.110.968735

Neufeld, K. M., Kang, N., Bienenstock, J., and Foster, J. A. (2011). Reduced anxiety-like behavior and central neurochemical change in germ-free mice. *Neurogastroenterol. Motil.* 23, 255–264. doi: 10.1111/j.1365-2982.2010.01620.x

O'Donnell, M. J., Xavier, D., Liu, L., Zhang, H., Chin, S. L., Rao-Melacini, P., et al. (2010). Risk factors for ischaemic and intracerebral haemorrhagic stroke in 22 countries (the INTERSTROKE study): a case-control study. *Lancet* 376, 112–123. doi: 10.1016/s0140-6736(10)60834-3

Packard, A. E. B., Ghosal, S., Herman, J. P., Woods, S. C., and Ulrich-Lai, Y. M. (2014). Chronic variable stress improves glucose tolerance in rats with sucrose-induced prediabetes. *Psychoneuroendocrinology* 47, 178–188. doi: 10.1016/j.psyneuen.2014.05.016

Razzoli, M., Pearson, C., Crow, S., and Bartolomucci, A. (2017). Stress, overeating, and obesity: insights from human studies and preclinical models. *Neurosci. Biobehav. Rev.* 76, 154–162. doi: 10.1016/j.neubiorev.2017.01.026

Rodríguez-Monforte, M., Flores-Mateo, G., and Sánchez, E. (2015). Dietary patterns and CVD: a systematic review and meta-analysis of observational studies. *Br. J. Nut.* 114, 1341–1359. doi: 10.1017/s0007114515003177

Rubinstein, A., Colantonio, L., Bardach, A., Caporale, J., Garcia Marti, S., Kopitowski, K., et al. (2010). Estimación de la carga de las enfermedades cardiovasculares atribuible a factores de riesgo modificables en Argentina. *Rev. Panam. Salud. Publica* 27, 237–245 doi: 10.1590/s1020-49892010000400001

Ruo, B., Rumsfeld, J. S., Hlatky, M. A., Liu, H., Browner, W. S., and Whooley, M. A. (2003). Depressive symptoms and health-related quality of life: the heart and soul study. JAMA 290, 215–221.

Rutledge, T., Reis, V. A., Linke, S. E., Greenberg, B. H., and Mills, P. J. (2006). Depression in heart failure: a meta-analytic review of prevalence, intervention effects, and associations with clinical outcomes. *J. Am. College Cardiol.* 48, 1527–1537.

Sanches Machado d'Almeida, K., Ronchi Spillere, S., Zuchinali, P., and Corrêa Souza, G. (2018). Mediterranean diet and other dietary patterns in primary prevention of heart failure and changes in cardiac function markers: a systematic review. *Nutrients* 10:58. doi: 10.3390/nu10010058

Schächinger, V., Britten, M. B., and Zeiher, A. M. (2000). Prognostic impact of coronary vasodilator dysfunction on adverse long-term outcome of coronary heart disease. *Circulation* 101, 1899–1906. doi: 10.1161/01.cir.101.16.1899

Schirmer, M., Smeekens, S. P., Vlamakis, H., Jaeger, M., Oosting, M., Franzosa, E. A., et al. (2016). Linking the human gut microbiome to inflammatory cytokine production capacity. *Cell* 167, 1125–1136.e8. doi: 10.1016/j.cell.2016.10.020

Serrano Ríos, M. (2005). El síndrome metabólico: ¿ una versión moderna de la enfermedad ligada al estrés? *Rev. Esp. Cardiol.* 58, 768–771.

Shen, J., Wilmot, K. A., Ghasemzadeh, N., Molloy, D. L., Burkman, G., Mekonnen, G., et al. (2015). Mediterranean dietary patterns and cardiovascular health. *Ann. Rev. Nut.* 35, 425–449.

Shirtcliff, E. A., Coe, C. L., and Pollak, S. D. (2009). Early childhood stress is associated with elevated antibody levels to herpes simplex virus type 1. *Proc. Natl. Acad. Sci. U.S.A.* 106, 2963–2967. doi: 10.1073/pnas.0806660106

Singh, R. K., Chang, H.-W., Yan, D., Lee, K. M., Ucmak, D., Wong, K., et al. (2017). Influence of diet on the gut microbiome and implications for human health. *J. Transl. Med.* 15:73.

Spencer, S. J., Korosi, A., Layé, S., Shukitt-Hale, B., and Barrientos, R. M. (2017). Food for thought: how nutrition impacts cognition and emotion. *npj Science of Food* 1:7.

Strandwitz, P., Kim, K. H., Terekhova, D., Liu, J. K., Sharma, A., Levering, J., et al. (2018). GABA-modulating bacteria of the human gut microbiota. *Nat. Microbiol.* 4, 396–403 doi: 10.1038/s41564-018-0307-3

Suárez, J. E. (2013). Microbiota autóctona, probióticos y prebióticos. *Nutr. Hosp.* 28, 38–41.

Ulrich-Lai, Y. M., Fulton, S., Wilson, M., Petrovich, G., and Rinaman, L. (2015). Stress exposure, food intake and emotional state. *Stress* 18, 381–399.

Uthman, O., Hartley, L., Rees, K., Taylor, F., Volmink, J., Ebrahim, S., et al. (2014). Multiple risk factor interventions for primary prevention of cardiovascular disease in low- and middle-income countries. *Cochrane Database Syst. Rev.* 8:CD011163

Vighi, G., Marcucci, F., Sensi, L., Di Cara, G., and Frati, F. (2008). Allergy and the gastrointestinal system. *Clin. Exp. Immunol.* 153, 3–6. doi: 10.1111/j.1365-2249.2008.03713.x

Wallace, C. J. K., and Milev, R. (2017). The effects of probiotics on depressive symptoms in humans: a systematic review. *Ann. Gen. Psychiatry* 16:14. doi: 10.1186/s12991-017-0138-2

Weaver, I. C. G., Cervoni, N., Champagne, F. A., D'alessio, A. C., Sharma, S., Seckl, J. R., et al. (2004). Epigenetic programming by maternal behavior. *Nat. Neurosci.* 7, 847–854.

Wong, M. L., Inserra, A., Lewis, M. D., Mastronardi, C. A., Leong, L., Choo, J., et al. (2016). Inflammasome signaling affects anxiety- and depressive-like behavior and gut microbiome composition. *Mol. Psychiatry* 21, 797–805. doi: 10.1038/mp.2016.46

Yano, J. M., Yu, K., Donaldson, G. P., Shastri, G. G., Ann, P., Ma, L., et al. (2015). Indigenous bacteria from the gut microbiota regulate host serotonin biosynthesis. *Cell* 161, 264–276. doi: 10.1016/j.cell.2015.02.047

Zalar, B., Haslberger, A., and Peterlin, B. (2018). The role of microbiota in depression - a brief review. *Psychiatr. Danub.* 30, 136–141 doi: 10.24869/psyd.2018.136

11

# TF-ChIP Method for Tissue-Specific Gene Targets

*Amalia Perna[1]* and Lavinia Auber Alberi[1,2]**

*[1] Department of Medicine, University of Fribourg, Fribourg, Switzerland, [2] Swiss Integrative Center for Human Health, Fribourg, Switzerland*

***Correspondence:***
*Amalia Perna*
*amalia.perna@unifr.ch*
*Lavinia Auber Alberi*
*lavinia.alberi@unifr.ch*

Chromatin immunoprecipitation (ChIP) is an assay developed in order to define the dynamic nature of transcription processes. This method has been widely employed to identify methylated and acetylated DNA sequences in a variety of organs both in animals and humans. Nevertheless, this technique is significantly less employed to study transcriptional targets of specific nuclear signaling factors (TFs) and the data published so far have mainly used cell culture material and have been hardly reproduced in *ex-vivo* tissue. As nuclear signaling underlies important adaptive and maladaptive responses in chronic conditions such as cancer and neurodegeneration, there is a need for streamlining the upfront workflow of TF-ChIP for subsequent target sequencing. Based on the typical low concentration of the signaling transcriptional complex and the complexity/length of the ChIP Seq protocol, the field of cellular signaling has been confronted with a major roadblock in identifying clinically relevant targets of pathological and physiological signaling pathways. The present protocol offers a standardized procedure for detecting signaling targets in any whole tissue or specific dissected regions. The advantages of the protocol compared to the existing published methods are: (1) the small amount of starting material; appropriate for tissue subregions; (2) the optimization of DNA fragmentation from whole tissue; (3) suitability for sparsely populated tissues (i.e., brain); (4) the specificity of the TF-targeting readout; and (5) high DNA quality for sequencing or hybridization. The present protocol is highly detailed and can be reproduced using both fresh and fresh-frozen tissue. This is particularly relevant in the clinical setting, where specimen integrity is often the limiting step and where transcriptional target profiling is therapeutically relevant. The method is centered on Notch signaling but can be applied to a variety of nuclear signaling pathways as long as specific antibodies are available for pull down. Taken the superior yield/readout of this procedure, ChIP may finally provide relevant information about dynamic downstream gene changes *in vivo* for use in both basic research and clinical applications.

**Keywords: ChIP, transcription factor, Notch signaling, brain, low amount DNA, region-specific, gene expression**

## INTRODUCTION

Control of gene expression is essential for a cell to assemble the gene products it needs to regulate cellular homeostasis and communication. Virtually, any step of gene expression can be modulated, from the DNA–RNA transcription step (Genuth and Barna, 2018) to transcripts triaging through miRNA, transcript splicing, protein translation through initiation complex, and post-translational modification of a protein (Mansuy and Mohanna, 2011). The various checkpoints of gene expression warrant a finely tuned biological repertoire determining the cellular identity in a context-dependent manner. Direct interaction of a protein with DNA is the simplest and the most direct method by which a protein changes transcription levels conferring the appropriate fitness in response to environmental changes (Olfson and Ross, 2017). In the setting of neurons, transcriptional control is often activity dependent and induces the expression of genes regulating synaptic plasticity and neuronal network function (Flavell and Greenberg, 2008; Engelmann and Haenold, 2016). Under this light, the transcription factor (TF) assumes high relevance. By binding to a specific DNA sequence, a TF controls the rate of transcription of genetic information and it represents the last wheel in the gear chain of a signaling pathway, determining the pathways functional outcome. Nonetheless, most TFs do not work alone. Many large TF families form complex homotypic or heterotypic interactions through dimerization and others may recruit intermediary proteins such as cofactors that modulate the effects of TFs by promoting (activator) or blocking (repressor) the recruitment of RNA polymerase to specific genes and their transcription (Vaquerizas et al., 2009).

Furthermore, despite transcriptional processes are highly conserved, human tissues differ from other mammalian species by gene expression patterns thereby adding another layer of complexity (Qian et al., 2005; Huang et al., 2018).

One of the techniques that has best helped understanding transcriptional factors' biological relevance is chromatin immunoprecipitation (ChIP). ChIP is a powerful technique used to detect, map, and quantify the contacts established between the protein of interest and genomic DNA *in vivo*.

As its name suggests, ChIP relies on the use of antibodies to precipitate or pull-down a DNA-binding protein of interest bound to its genomic locus. These DNA fragments are, then, isolated and characterized in order to draw conclusions about a certain transcriptional process.

Despite a simple working principle, ChIP is notoriously technically challenging, highly sensitive to operational errors and artifacts, and often requires a great deal of upfront optimization before reliable results can be obtained. Moreover, it is expensive and time-consuming.

Here, we present a protocol optimized for TF in brain tissues whose extraordinary complexity is thought to rely on refined transcriptional networks and hierarchies.

In particular, we choose to perform this protocol in the Cornus Ammonis (CA) field of the hippocampus (comparing it with cortex) in order to demonstrate the validity of the technique for a little amount of region-specific starting material and provide a best practice TF-ChIP method for researchers working with whole animal and human tissue.

We decided to focus on Notch1 signaling pathway since it provides a good example for low complexity pathway studies. Notch signaling is a well-known player in the embryonic development but increasing evidence points out a critical role in the mature brain of vertebrates and invertebrates. This pathway appears to be involved in neural progenitor regulation, neuronal connectivity, synaptic plasticity, and learning/memory (Alberi et al., 2013). In addition, Notch was also found aberrantly regulated in neurodegenerative diseases, including Alzheimer's disease and ischemic injury both in rodent models and human tissue (Brai et al., 2016; Marathe et al., 2017) but the mechanistic implication of Notch-dependent targets in this setting remains largely unraveled, limiting its clinical relevance. The signaling is composed by a downstream transcriptional factor, recombining binding protein suppressor of hairless (RBPjK) that normally behaves as a repressor and that needs another protein, Notch intracellular domain (NICD), to be activated and transcribe its target genes. Notch1 signaling has a sophisticated program of gene expression orchestrated by the alternating status of RBPjK. Notch1 is a transmembrane receptor scattered across the cell membrane. Ligand proteins bind to the extracellular domain inducing proteolytic cleavage and release the intracellular domain (NICD), which enters in the nucleus and binds RBPjK. This allows transcription and the subsequent cell response (Siebel and Lendahl, 2017).

The ChIP assay executed in this manuscript is performed specifically in the hippocampal CA fields and involves NICD precipitation in order to assess target genes downstream Notch1 canonical activation.

This work aims to explain in detail the critical steps of the procedure which can be further adapted to any experimental setting using *ex-vivo* tissue (tissues with high extracellular matrix density, secondary factor precipitation, low chromatin yield, signaling pathways with few target genes, etc.) in a very short time.

## MATERIALS AND EQUIPMENT

### Animals

All experiments on mice were performed with permission of the local animal care committee (Canton of Fribourg, Switzerland approved the Protocol no. 2016_32_FR) and according to the present Swiss law and the European Communities Council Directive of 24 November 1986 (86/609/EEC). C57Bl6 male mice were used throughout the experiment. Transgenic Notch Reporter [Tg(C-EGFP) 25 Gaia/Reya; Jax, FL, United States] was used for fluorescent immunohistochemistry (IHC). All animals (3 months of age) were housed on 12 h light–dark cycle with access to food and water *ad libitum*. Mice were euthanized using pentobarbital (120 mg/kg). Once no pinch reflex was assessed, animals were perfused using 0.9% NaCl and either dissected in ice cold saline solution under a stereoscope (Leica, Germany) or immersion fixed using paraformaldehyde (Sigma–Aldrich, United States; P6148).

### ChIP Equipment

Glass dish
Razor blades
Pestle
Eppendorf
Pippettor
Rotating wheel
Prism R$^{TM}$ Refrigerated MicroCentrifuge (Labnet, Switzerland; C2500-R)

Vortex-Genie 2 (Scientific Industries, Inc., United States; SI-0236)
Bioruptor Plus (Diagenode, Belgium; B01020001)
1.5 ml Bioruptor® Plus TPX microtubes (Diagenode, Belgium; C30010010-300)
Qubit Fluorometric Quantitation (Thermo Fisher, United States; Q33226)
ThermoMixer® C (Eppendorf, Germany; #5382000015)
Mupid®-One Electrophoresis System (Eurogentec, Germany)
Omega Lum™ W Imaging System (Aplegen, United States; 81-12120-00)
Biometra TRIO Thermal Cycler Series (Analytik Jena, Germany)
Fragment Analyzer (Advanced Analytical AATI, United States)
Mic qPCR Cycler (Bio Molecular Systems, Australia).

## ChIP Reagents

Formaldehyde solution, 36.5–38% (Sigma-Aldrich, United States; F8775) !caution formaldehyde is toxic by inhalation, ingestion, or contact with skin.
Phosphate-buffered saline (PBS) (10×) pH 7.4 (Thermo Fisher Scientific, United States; AM9625)
Glycine (Sigma-Aldrich, United States; G8898)
Protease inhibitor (PI) cocktail (Sigma-Aldrich, United States; P8340)
Sodium dodecyl sulfate (SDS) (Roth, Germany; CN30.3) !caution SDS is toxic by inhalation, ingestion, or contact with skin.
Ethylenediaminetetraacetic acid (EDTA) (Sigma-Aldrich, United States; E5134)
Tris (Roth, Germany; 5429.3)
4-(2-hydroxyethyl)-1-piperazineethanesulfonic acid (HEPES) (Sigma-Aldrich, United States; H3375)
NaCl (Roth, Germany; 9265.2)
Sodium deoxycholate (Sigma-Aldrich, United States; 30970)
Triton X-100 (Sigma-Aldrich, United States; 93426)
Tris-HCl (Roth, Germany; 9090)
LiCl (Sigma-Aldrich, United States; L9650)
Nonidet P-40 substitute (Sigma-Aldrich, United States; 74385)
Qubit™ dsDNA HS Assay Kit (Thermo Fisher, United States; Q32851)
Pierce™ Protein A/G Agarose (Thermo Fisher, United States; 20421)
Antibodies: Rabbit anti-NICD (Cell Signaling, United States; #4147); Rabbit IgG (Cell Signaling, United States; #2729); and Rabbit anti-Acetyl-Histone H3 (Lys9) (Cell Signaling, United States; #9649)
RNase A solution (Promega, United States; A7974)
Proteinase K (Roche, Switzerland; 03508838103)
Phenol/chloroform/isoamyl alcohol (Roth, Germany; A156) !Caution chloroform is toxic if absorbed through the skin, inhaled or ingested.
Chloroform/isoamyl alcohol (Roth, Germany; X984) !Caution chloroform is toxic if absorbed through the skin, inhaled or ingested.
Sodium acetate (Merck, Germany; 1.06268.0250)
Glycogen (Roche;10901393001)
Isopropanol (Fisher Chemical, United States; P/7500/15)
Ethanol absolute (Fisher Chemical, United States; E/0650DF/15)
Agarose standard (Roth, Germany; 3810)
SYBR™ Safe DNA Gel Stain (Thermo Fisher, United States; S33102)
GoTaq® Hot Start Green Master Mix (Promega, United States; M5122)
GoTaq PCR Master mix (Promega United States; A6001)
GeneRuler 100 bp DNA Ladder, ready-to-use (Thermo Fisher, United States; SM0243)
DNA Gel Loading Dye (6×) (Thermo Fisher, United States; R0611)
DNF-474 High Sensitivity NGS Fragment Analysis Kit (1–6,000 bp) (Advanced Analytical, United States).

## Reagent Setup

Before preparing the final solutions, filter both the water and all the stock solutions. Here volumes are calculated for three precipitations: one for the protein of interest (NICD) plus positive (H3) and negative control (IgG). Scale up if more TFs are planned to be used.

1% FA-PBS (fresh/1 ml for tissue): Mix 972 μl of PBS and 28 μl of FA.

Glycine (2 M stock): Solubilize 1.5 g of glycine in 10 ml of Milli-Q water.

Lysis buffer (fresh/1 ml): Mix 30 μl of SDS [10% (vol/vol) stock solution], 20 μl of EDTA (0.5 M stock solution), 50 μl of Tris pH 8.0 (1 M stock solution), 10 μl of PIs, and fill with filtered Milli-Q water to a final volume of 1 ml. Keep on ice until use. Final concentrations: 0.3% SDS, 10 mM EDTA, 50 mM Tris pH 8.0. ! Critical PI must be added just before use.

IP buffer (10× stock/15 ml): Mix 3 ml of HEPES pH 8.0 (1 M stock solution), 6 ml of NaCl (5 M stock solution), 600 μl of EDTA (0.5 M stock solution), and fill with filtered Milli-Q water to a final volume of 15 ml. Final concentrations: 0.2 M HEPES pH 8.0, 2 M NaCl, 0.02 M EDTA. IP stock solution can be stored in the fridge for several months.

IP buffer (1× fresh/3 ml): Mix 300 μl of high salt IP buffer (10× stock), 30 μl of NaDOC [10% (vol/vol) stock solution], 300 μl of Triton X-100 [10% (vol/vol) stock solution], 30 μl of PIs, and fill with filtered Milli-Q water to a final volume of 3 ml. Keep on ice until use. Final concentrations: 1% high salt IP buffer, 0.1% NaDOC, 1% Triton X-100 ! Critical PI must be added just before use.

Washing buffer – reduced SDS (stock/50 ml): Mix 2.5 ml of HEPES pH 7.6 (1 M stock solution), 1.5 ml of NaCl (5 M stock solution), 5 ml of Triton X-100 [10% (vol/vol) stock solution], 500 μl of NaDOC [10% (vol/vol) stock solution], 250 μl of SDS [20% (vol/vol) stock solution], and fill with filtered Milli-Q water to a final volume of 50 ml. Washing solutions can be stored in the fridge for several months. Final concentrations:

50 mM HEPES pH 7.6, 2 mM NaCl, 1% Triton X-100, 0.1% NaDOC, and 0.1% SDS

Washing buffer – reduced SDS buffer + NaCl (stock/15 ml): Mix 15 ml of reduced SDS buffer and 600 μl of NaCl (5 M stock solution). Washing solutions can be stored in the fridge for several months. Final concentrations: 0.2 M NaCl.

Washing buffer – NP-40 buffer (stock/25 ml): Mix 0.2 ml of Tris–HCl pH 8.0 (1 M stock solution), 0.625 ml of LiCl (8 M stock solution), 40 μl of EDTA (0.5 M stock solution), 1 ml of NP-40 [10% (vol/vol) stock solution], 1 ml of NaDOC [10% (vol/vol) stock solution], and fill with filtered Milli-Q water to a final volume of 25 ml. Washing solutions can be stored in the fridge for several months. Final concentrations: 8 mM Tris–HCl pH 8.0, 2 mM LiCl, 0.8 mM EDTA, 0.4% NP-40, and 0.4% NaDOC.

Washing buffer – TE buffer (stock/50 ml): Mix 0.5 ml of Tris–HCl, pH 8 (1 M stock solution), 100 μl of EDTA (0.5 M stock solution), and fill with filtered Milli-Q water to a final volume of 50 ml. Washing solutions can be stored in the fridge for several months. Final concentrations: 10 mM Tris–HCl, pH 8, 1 mM EDTA.

Elution buffer (fresh/2 ml): Mix 100 μl of Tris, pH 8 (1 M stock solution), 40 μl of EDTA (0.5 M stock solution), 100 μl of SDS [20% (vol/vol) stock solution], and fill with filtered Milli-Q water to a final volume of 2 ml. Elution buffer can be stored in the fridge for several months. Final concentrations: 50 mM Tris pH 8, 10 mM EDTA, and 1% SDS.

Protein A- or protein G-sepharose beads (Pierce™ Protein A/G Agarose; Thermo Fisher, United States; 20421).

## Primers List

Primers were obtained from Microsynth, Switzerland.

| | Forward | Reverse |
|---|---|---|
| Hes5 | 5′-GGG AAA AGG CAG CAT ATT GAG GCG-3′ | 5′-CAC GCT AAA TTG CCT GTG AAT TGG CG-3′ |
| DLL1 | 5′-GTC TCA GGA CCT TCA CAG TAG-3′ | 5′-GAG CAA CCT TCT CCG TAG TAG-3′ |
| GAPDH | 5′-GAT TAC GGG ATG GGT CTG AA-3′ | 5′-GCT GCA CCT CTG GTA ACT CC-3′ |

## Immunohistochemistry

Floating coronal brain sections from the TNR-EGFP mice, exposed to a novel environment (Alberi et al., 2011), were processed for fluorescent IHC according to the previously published protocols (Marathe et al., 2017) using Rabbit anti-NICD (Cell Signaling, United States; #4147) and goat anti-EGFP (Rockland, United States; #600-102-215). Cy3 donkey anti-rabbit (Jackson Immunoresearch, United Kingdom; #711-165-152) and Cy2 donkey anti-goat (Jackson Immunoresearch, United Kingdom; #705-225-147) were used as secondary antibodies. DAPI (Sigma–Aldrich, United States; D9542) was used for nuclear counterstaining.

## Western Blot

Input, unbound, and ChIP-NICD fractions were collected and de-crosslinked by adding 11 μl of 5 M NaCl and 4 μl of RNaseA, and incubating in the thermoshaker for 4 h at 42°C with gentle shaking. Proteins were extracted with Trizol (Trifast; Peqgold, Germany) and resuspended in loading buffer. Twenty-five microliters of protein was loaded onto a 10% polyacrylamide electrophoretic gel. Western blot was conducted as previously described (Marathe et al., 2017) using two primary antibodies: polyclonal goat anti-Notch1 against the c-terminus, 1:1000 (sc-6014; Santa Cruz Biotechnology, United States) and mouse anti-β-actin, 1:2000 (sc-81178; Santa Cruz Biotechnology, United States); and two secondary antibodies diluted 1:2000: Cy3 donkey anti-goat (Jackson Immunoresearch, United Kingdom; # 705-165-147) and Cy2 donkey anti-mouse ( Jackson Immunoresearch, United Kingdom; # 715-225-150). Visualization was performed through a fluorescent imager (Omega Lum G from Aplegen).

# PROCEDURE

## ChIP Protocol Overview

The protocol can be essentially divided into several phases. During the first step, the sample is treated with formaldehyde to cross-link proteins and DNA within ~2 Å of each other. As a result, proteins are covalently bound to their target sequences on the DNA and provide a snapshot of TF occupancy. Later, the chromatin fraction is released from the nucleus by the mean of a lysis buffer, fragmented into small pieces (ranging from 200 to 500 bp) with a sonicator, and then subjected to immunoprecipitation with chosen antibodies. Once immune complexes are obtained, they are separated from the unbound fraction by using protein A- or protein G-sepharose beads (magnetic protein A/G beads can be used instead of sepharose beads, however, washes are performed using an appropriate magnetic tray). After extensive washing to limit the nonspecific binding, the immune-bound complexes are eluted, decrosslinked by proteinase K digestion, and then purified in order to be analyzed (**Figure 1**).

Protein–DNA interactions can, then, be approached fundamentally in two ways: (i) by looking at the presence of specific sequences in the immunoprecipitated DNA by PCR amplification or (ii) by combining genome-wide approaches culminating in a method for deep protein–DNA interactions analysis: ChIP–Seq.

## Considerations Before Starting

- In order to perform a tissue-specific ChIP analysis, it is important to select the specific part of the tissue you are interested in. For peripheral organs, blood could interfere with the purity of your sample, therefore is recommended to transcardially perfuse the animal with saline solution before dissection.

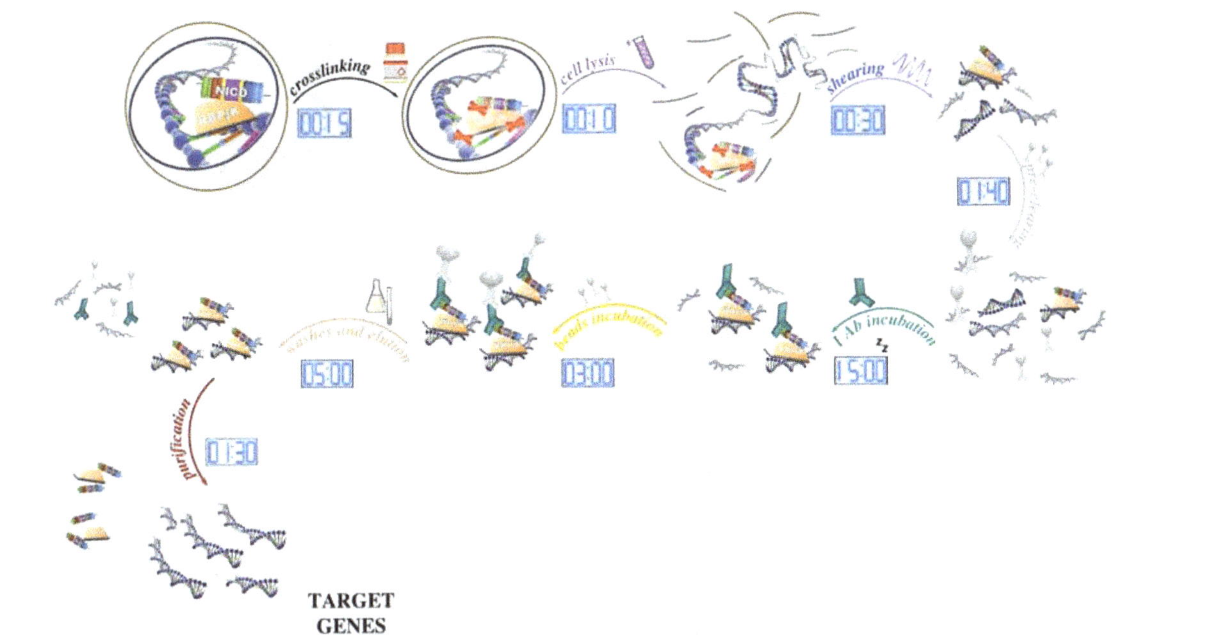


**FIGURE 1 |** Schematic of the ChIP method and its timing. After tissue processing, DNA and proteins are reversibly crosslinked with short formaldehyde incubation (15 min) to maintain the association of proteins with their target DNA sequence. In our ChIP experiment, NICD and RBPjK are first crosslinked with DNA and then cells lysed with ionic lysis buffer (10 min). Chromatin is later fragmented with ultrasounds (30 min) and precleaned with sepharose beads incubation (1 h 40 min). Once all the unspecific DNA fragments are removed, proteins bound to DNA are ready to be targeted by the selected antibody. After ON incubation, antibody–protein–DNA complexes are precipitated using beads (3 h). Washes and elution (5 h) lead to target genes that once purified (5 h) are ready for further applications.

- The tissue could be made of subregions with different cell populations where the signaling behaves differently. It is worth to study *a priori* your tissue anatomy and composition to reduce the background and obtain unequivocal results. In our case, during hippocampus dissection, we carefully removed the dentate gyrus (composed by neuronal progenitor cells and granule cells) and then we selected just the CA field (Sultan, 2013). For the cortex, we removed the white matter to increase the gray matter content for ChIP analysis.
- While planning the experiment, remember to include always a positive control as a very abundant core histone protein (i.e., H3) and a negative control that is a sample treated in the same way as in the immunoprecipitated samples but without Ab or with a non-specific Ab (i.e., IgG).
- For optimal chromatin yield and ChIP results, it is important to use at least 25 mg of tissue for each immunoprecipitation. The chromatin yield does vary between tissue types and some tissues may require more than 25 mg depending on their cell density. Since positive and negative control must be included, at least 75 mg of tissue is required.

## Stepwise Procedure

Crosslinking (timing: ca. 40 min):

Before starting the procedure, prepare all your solutions and keep them refrigerated. Switch on the cold centrifuge and set the Bioruptor sonicator at 4°C. Perform all steps on ice to avoid proteins degradation.

1. After tissue dissection from an anesthetized mouse (**Figure 2A**), snap-freeze the tissue in liquid nitrogen or, if fresh tissue is required, proceed with the protocol.
2. Transfer quickly the tissue in a glass dish already placed in ice.
3. Rapidly put 40 μl of 1% FA-PBS on your tissue piece (this will fix your tissue while it is thawing), start the timer (already set on 15 min), and finely mince the fresh/thawed tissue with two pre-chilled razor blades for 4 min (until it appears slurry and homogeneous).
4. Add 450 μl of 1% FA-PBS in the dish and transfer the tissue to a 1.5 ml tube. Use other 450 μl 1% FA-PBS to harvest tissue residues from the dish and move it into the tube. Incubate for the remaining 10 min at room temperature (RT) on the rotating wheel (make sure to safe-lock the tubes!).
5. Add 63 μl of glycine 2 M to the 940 μl of 1% FA-PBS (final concentration 0.125 M) to terminate cross-linking. Incubate for 10 min at RT on the rotating wheel (make sure to safe-lock the tubes).
6. Wash three times with cold PBS with freshly added PI:

a. Add 500 μl of 1× PBS+PI
b. Invert several times
c. Spin gently at 4°C for 1 min
d. Remove supernatant

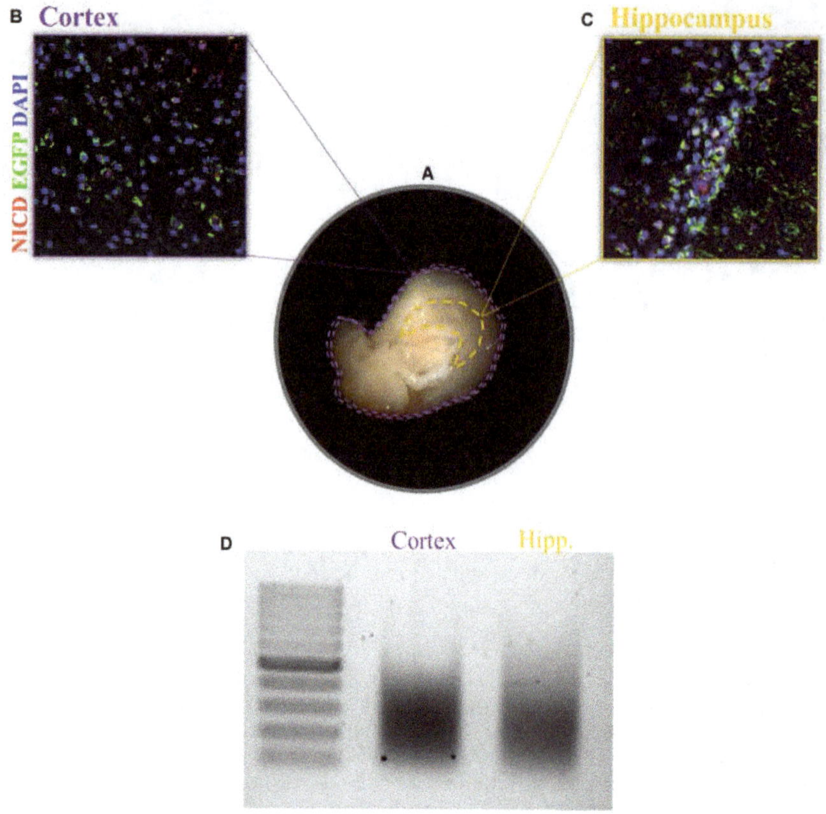


**FIGURE 2 |** Expression of NICD in cortex and hippocampus and chromatin shearing of the two brain tissues. **(A)** Sagittal brain sections, view from the midline, display the hippocampus and cortex. Example of immunofluorescence for NICD (red) in **(B)** cortex and **(C)** hippocampus of the transgenic mouse line (TNR, for transgenic Notch reporter) expressing enhanced green fluorescent protein (EGFP) in cells with Notch canonical signaling activation. Nuclei are stained in blue. **(D)** CA hippocampal fields and cortical tissue 1% formaldehyde fixed are sonicated for 30 cycles (30″ ON/30″ OFF) with the Bioruptor® PLUS at HIGH power setting. All samples were treated with RNase and Proteinase K prior to gel electrophoresis. Scale bar in **B** and **C** is 25 μm.

7. Resuspend the tissue in 600 μl of ice-cold lysis buffer with freshly added PI (first add 200 μl, start to pestle, then add the remaining 400 μl).
8. Smash the tissue with a pestle by going 50 times up and down until the solution is clear and without clumps.
9. Keep the lysate 10 min on ice.

! Safe stop. Samples can be stored at −20°C at this point.

Chromatin sonication (timing ca. 40 min):

Chromatin needs to be fragmented by sonication into not too short and not too long fragments in order to be precipitated.

Extensive sonication could most likely hit TF-binding sequences and impair them, while long fragments obtained with short sonication are difficult to precipitate.

Sonication conditions should be optimized for your experimental settings (see the section "Anticipated Results"). Avoid foaming as this results in a decrease of energy transfer within the solution and will decrease the sonication efficiency.

10. Transfer the lysate in TPX tubes from Diagenode. Prepare three tubes with 200 μl each.
11. Bioruptor Plus (Diagenode, Belgium):
    Power: High
    Runs: 3× 10 cycles
    Interval: 30″ ON/30″ OFF
    Note: Vortex gently and spin down between each run.
    During these 30 min, start washing beads.
12. Centrifuge at 13,500 rpm, 4°C for 10 min.
13. Collect the supernatant and transfer all 600 μl in one 2 ml tube.

! Safe stop. Samples can be stored at −20°C at this point.

Determination of DNA fragment size (timing ca. 5 h):

Sonication is the key step for a successful ChIP experiment and the optimal sonication settings should be determinate for each experimental tissue. Therefore is a good practice to check DNA fragments on agarose gel first times ChIP is performed.

14. Prepare a mix with 60 μl of elution buffer, 4.8 μl of 5 M NaCl, 2 μl RNase A (10 mg/ml), and 40 μl of chromatin. Incubate while shaking at 65°C for 1 h.
15. Add 4 μl proteinase K and incubate 3–4 h at 65°C [this incubation could be extended overnight (ON)].

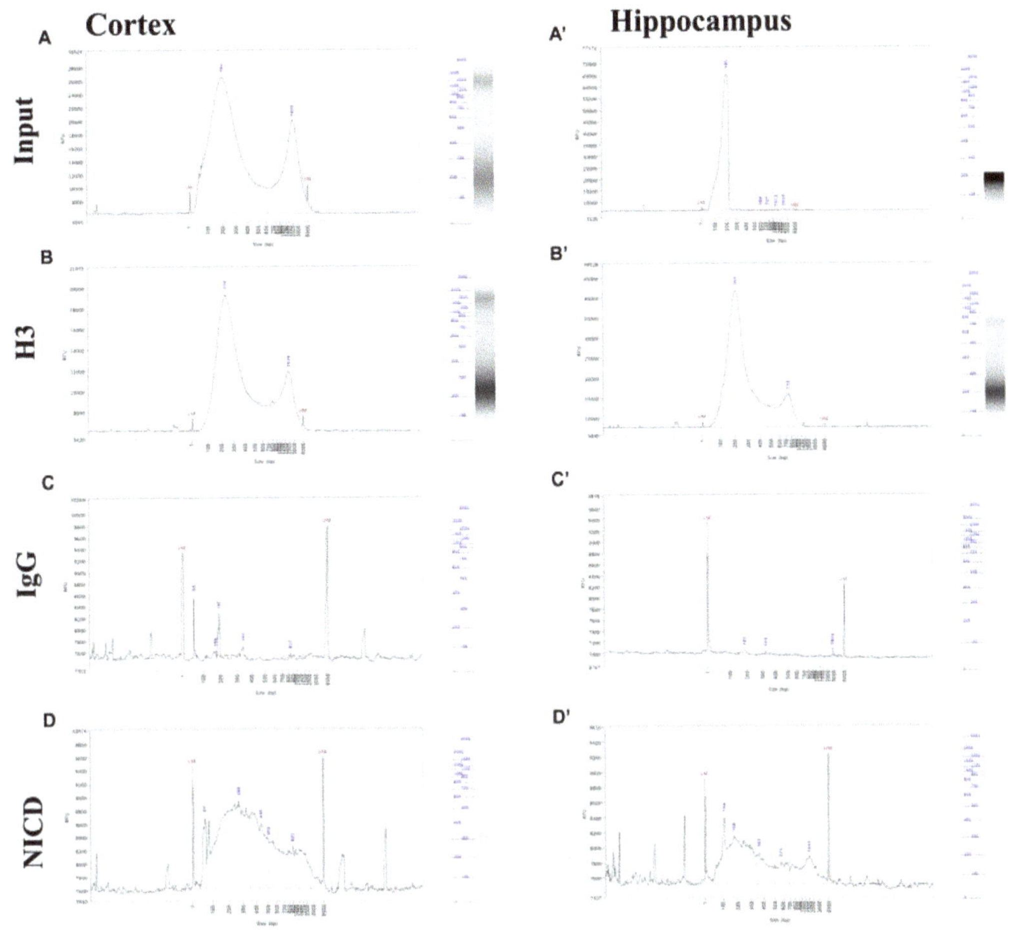


**FIGURE 3 |** Profiling of ChIP fragments. **(A–D)** Electropherograms of automated capillary gel electrophoresis. Size profiles of purified DNA after immunoprecipitations from cortical and hippocampal CA field lysates **(A'–D')** show the fragment length distribution for **(A, A')** input, **(B, B')** H3, and **(C, C')** NICD showing a bimodal distribution and a major peak around 200 bp. **(D, D')** IgG fragment analysis shows a sparse, mostly background peaks. DNA size (bp) is shown.

16. Add 100 μl of phenol/chloroform (1:1), agitate vigorously.
17. Centrifuge for 10 min at 13,500 rpm, 4°C.
18. Collect the aqueous phase.
19. Add 100 μl chloroform/isoamyl alcohol (1:1).
20. Centrifuge for 10 min at 13,500 rpm, 4°C.
21. Collect the aqueous phase.
22. Add 2 μL of glycogen (20 mg/mL) and 30 μl of $NaCH_3COOH$ (3 M).
23. Flick the tube and add 100 μl of isopropanol.
24. Agitate vigorously the tube several times for 1 min.
25. Leave on ice for 10 min or keep in the freezer for 5 min.
26. Centrifuge 20 min at 13,500 rpm, 4°C.
27. Decant supernatant.
28. Wash by adding 500 μl of 75% EtOH. Spin 5 min at 13,500 rpm, 4°C, and decant the supernatant.
29. Air dry and resuspend in 20 μl of $ddH_2O$. Incubate several minutes while shaking at 42°C to dissolve DNA.
30. Run purified DNA in a 1.5% agarose gel with a 100 bp DNA marker to determine fragment size.

Beads washing (timing ca. 15 min):

31. Take the IP buffer 10× from the fridge and make 3 ml of IP buffer 1× and add 20 μl of PI.
32. Transfer 20 μl of beads for preclearing and 40 μl for the IPs. Cut the tip used in order to dispense them. You will have in total two 1.5 ml tubes for preclearing and three for IPs.
33. Wash beads three times with 500 μl PBS: At each step spin down the beads shortly with gentle centrifugation so they don't break, wait until they settle down, and then aspirated gently the PBS with a pump using a 10 μl tip and going progressively down with the tip.
34. Wash one time with 500 μl IP buffer with PI. Keep preclearing beads on ice and store IP beads still in IP buffer in the fridge.

Pre-clearing (timing ca. 1 h 40 min):

Pre-clearing is an optional step but is recommended to reduce non-specific binding to the beads.

SDS presence in the lysis buffer is important since it enhances lysis and sonication but it also interferes with

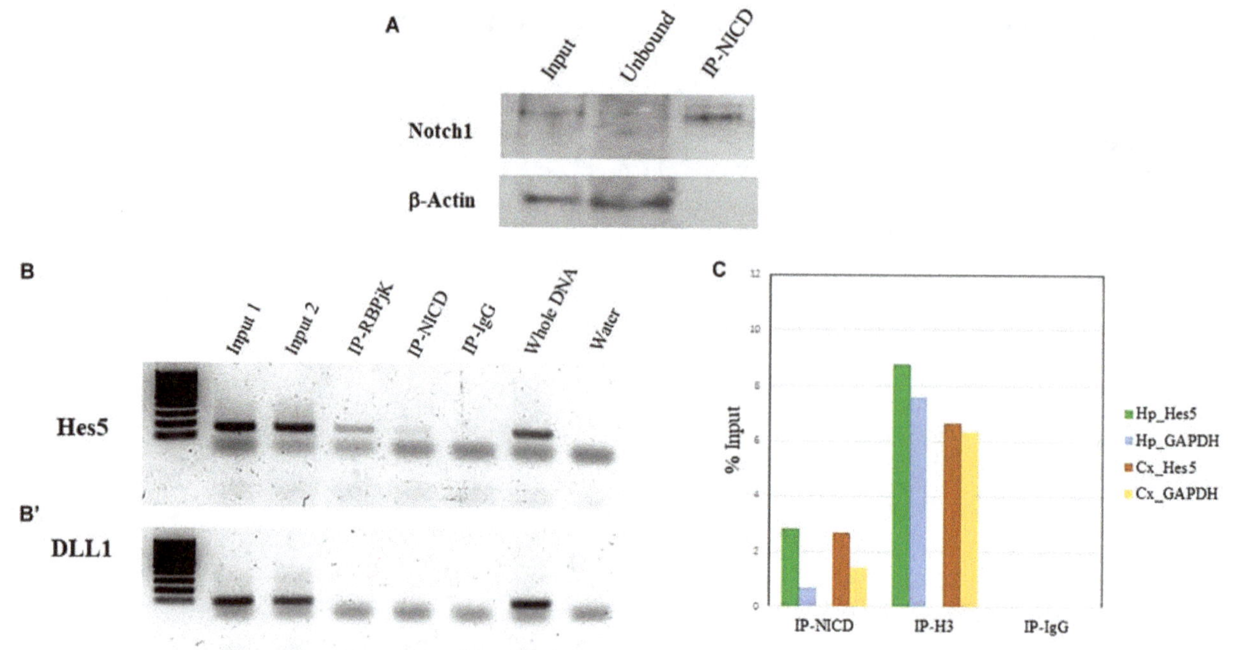


**FIGURE 4 |** ChIP validation. **(A)** Representative western blot of Notch1 protein present in the input, enriched in the ChIP-NICD sample and absent in the unbound solute. β-Actin is used to detect the housekeeping protein in the input and unbound fractions. **(B, B')** PCR analysis of hippocampus ChIPed with antibodies specific for RBPjK and NICD show an amplicon band for the promoter region of the canonical Notch target, Hes5 **(B)**, but no band for the promoter region of DLL1 **(B')**, chosen as a negative control. Inputs and whole DNA are shown as a positive reference and water controls for contaminants. **(C)** Results from real-time qPCR of ChIPed tissue with the NICD antibody shows a fourfold and twofold enrichment of the specific Notch target, Hes5, compared to the GAPDH promoter region in the hippocampus and cortex, respectively. The ChIPed samples with the antibody against acetyl-histone H3 antibodies show the expected amplification of the Hes5 and the GAPDH promoter in both tissues and there is no amplification in the ChIPed samples with IgG.

protein/antibody and antibody/beads binding. Therefore, it has to be diluted up to 0.1%.

35. Add IP buffer to the chromatin in 3:1 proportion (600 μl chromatin + 1200 μl IP buffer)
36. Split the chromatin over the two pre-clearing tubes and add to the 20 μl beads you kept on ice (900 μl each).
37. Incubate for 1–1.5 h @ 4°C on the rotating wheel (make sure to safe-lock the tubes).
38. Spin down the beads from the pre-cleared chromatin, collect the supernatant, and discard the 20 μl beads.
39. Measure the DNA concentration using Qubit.
40. Take 5% of the total volume of pre-cleared chromatin as input material and freeze it.

! Safe stop. Samples can be stored at −20°C at this point.

Immunoprecipitation and washes (timing ca. 16 h):
The optimal antibody concentration should be calibrated for each antibody as this can improve the signal-to-noise ratio of your experiment (see the section "Anticipated Results").

41. Divide the chromatin into three tubes (600 μl per tube) and add the antibodies to each pre-cleared chromatin: (1) specific for the TF, NICD; (2) negative control, IgG; and (3) positive control, histone H3.
42. Put the chromatin with antibodies on a rotating wheel to mix ON at 4°C (make sure to safe-lock the tubes!).
43. Transfer the chromatin + antibodies to the Eppendorf with the 40 μl beads you kept on ice/on the fridge.
44. Rotate for 3 h at 4°C on the rotating wheel (make sure to safe-lock the tubes).
45. Spin down the beads and discard the supernatant.
46. Wash three times with the reduced SDS buffer: At each step, spin down the beads shortly with gentle centrifugation so they don't break, wait until they settle down and then aspirate the buffer with the sucker using a 10 μl tip and going progressively down with the tip.
47. Wash one time with reduced SDS + NaCl buffer.
48. Wash one time with NP-40 buffer.
49. Wash one time with TE buffer.

Eluting the chromatin (timing ca. 15 min):
Prepare fresh elution buffer.

50. Add 500 μl of elution buffer to the beads and 470 μl to the 5% input.
51. Incubate for 12 min at 65°C while shaking. Flick the tube vigorously once during this incubation and once the incubation is finished.
52. Centrifuge 13,500 rpm, 4°C for 1 min.
53. Transfer the supernatant to a new tube, discard the beads.

Reversing the crosslinking (Input and IP-ed Chromatin) (timing ca.4-5 h):

54. Add 11 μl of 5 M NaCl. Flick tubes briefly.

55. Add 4 μl of RNaseA to the eluted chromatin and incubate in the thermoshaker for 1 h at 65°C with gentle shaking.
56. Add 4 μl of proteinase K to the eluted chromatin and incubate in the thermoshaker for 3–4 h at 65°C with gentle shaking (this incubation could be extended ON).
Extraction and purification (timing ca. 1.5 h):
Be careful during the whole extraction and work under a chemical hood.
57. Add 500 μl of phenol/chloroform (1:1), agitate vigorously.
58. Centrifuge for 10 min at 13,500 rpm, 4°C.
59. Collect the aqueous phase.
60. Add 500 μl chloroform/isoamyl alcohol (1:1), agitate vigorously.
61. Centrifuge for 10 min at 13,500 rpm, 4°C.
62. Collect the aqueous phase.
63. Add 50 μl of $NaCH_3COOH$ (3 M).
64. Flick the tube and add 500 μl of isopropanol.
65. Agitate vigorously for 1 min.
66. Keep samples on ice for 10 min or put the samples at −20°C for 5 min.
67. Centrifuge for 20 min at 13,500 rpm, 4°C.
68. Decant the supernatant.
69. Wash by adding 500 μl of 75% EtOH. Spin 5 min at 13,500 rpm, 4°C, and decant the supernatant.
70. Air dry under the hood and resuspend in 10 μl of $ddH_2O$. Incubate several minutes while shaking at 42°C to dissolve DNA.
71. Measure your DNA concentration using Qubit.

### PCR

Primer should be designed bearing in mind that the sequence you precipitated is small and must include the TF-binding sequence. Make sure it is included in your primer design (see the section "Anticipated Results") (**Figure 4B**).

72. Prepare your (Master mix) × *n* samples, using for each sample:

- 7.5 μl hot start GoTaq
- 0.5 μl primers (10 μM)
- $ddH_2O$ up to 15 μl

73. Add at least 1 ng of DNA
74. Use the following ChIP program:

| step | °C | H:mm:ss | Go to |
|---|---|---|---|
| 1 | 94.0 | 0:02:00 | |
| 2 | 94.0 | 0:00:30 | |
| 3 | 56.5 | 0:00:30 | |
| 4 | 72.0 | 0:00:30 | 29× → Step 2 |
| 5 | 72.0 | 0:10:00 | |
| 6 | 4.0 | inf | |

75. Run PCR products in 1.3% agarose gel.

### qPCR

Once a specific amplicon is identified by qualitative PCR, the relative efficiency of chromatin pull down should be evaluated via qPCR (**Figure 4C**).

The primers used for qPCR are the same as for the PCR.

76. Prepare your (Master mix) × *n* samples, using for each sample:

- 7.5 μl Promega GoTaq qPCR master mix
- 0.5 μl Primers (10 μM)
- $ddH_2O$ up to 15 μl

77. Add 1 ng of DNA.
78. Run the standard amplification program according to the manufacturer instructions.

## ANTICIPATED RESULTS

### Starting Material Amount and Crosslinking

Before starting, it is always recommended to check the specificity of the antibody and the activity rate of your TF in the tissue of your interest. One possible way to do this is to perform an IHC of your region of interest. This would help establish the range of starting material to use since this is going to influence the entire experiment. For the experiment we performed in this paper, we found a sparse and nuclear pattern of NICD in cortical tissue as well as in the CA fields of the hippocampus (**Figures 2B,C**). For low concentrations of the TF, as in our case, more chromatin should be used during immunoprecipitation. It is recommended to increase the amount of chromatin rather than the amount of antibody since the latter is going to increase the background. To further confirm the right amount of starting material, it is important to assess the chromatin yield after cell lysis. Each tissue has a different chromatin yield that depends on cell density and tissue composition. Therefore, it is important to measure the DNA concentration with a fluorometric method (Qubit) to evaluate how much tissue and/or lysis buffer is required for the next steps.

Our sample preparation section is well optimized for fresh-frozen samples. In clinical analyses, the vast majority of samples need to be stored at −80°C for later analysis or dispatching to other labs. One of the improvements provided by this protocol is the ongoing fixation while the tissue thaws. This captures chromatin–protein architectural organization in the moment of defrosting and prevents loss of biological content due to cell damage, thus, preserving the integrity of the sample. Furthermore, the mincing step with the razor blades makes fixative penetration uniform and easier and is superior to mechanical treatment that causes cell loss. That said, cross-linking efficiency is empirical and should be tested by modifying either incubation time or formaldehyde concentration prior to performing the whole procedures. Remember that extensive cross-linking may decrease the solubility of any target DNA–protein complex and cause it to be entrapped in the insoluble material removed by sedimentation.

**TABLE 1** | Systematic comparisons of ChIP protocols from tissue.

| Protocol | ChIP on hippocampus | ChIP on brain tissue | Low-cell ChIP | FastChIP | ChIPmentation | TF-ChIP |
|---|---|---|---|---|---|---|
| *Publication title* | Chromatin immunoprecipitation in mouse hippocampal cells and tissues. | Chromatin immunoprecipitation technique for study of transcriptional dysregulation in intact mouse brain. | A rapid micro chromatin immunoprecipitation assay (μChIP). | Protocol for the fast chromatin immunoprecipitation (ChIP) method. | ChIPmentation: fast, robust, low-input ChIP-seq for histones and TFs. | TF-ChIP method for tissue-specific gene targets. |
| *Reference* | Sailaja et al. (2012) | Braveman et al. (2004) | Dahl and Collas (2008) | Nelson et al. (2006) | Schmidl et al. (2015) | This study. |
| *Starting material used* | Mouse whole hippocampus/dissociated hippocampal cells. | One mouse brain hemisphere not perfused. | 1K-100 cells and c.ca 1 $mm^3$ fresh- or frozen-tissue biopsies. | Best results with 2 M cells per IP. | 10 K cells for histone markers 100 K for TF. | 30 mg of tissue (CA1 fields from two hippocampi or bilateral cortex). |
| *Protocol* | General ChIP protocol with Sepharose A/G beads. | Upstate Biotechnology ChIP assay kit for cultured cells adapted to intact mouse brain tissue. | General ChIP protocol using *ab initio* antibody–magnetic bead complexes preparation. | Fast protocol since it shortens two steps:<br>(i) immunoprecipitation time (accelerated by the means of ultrasonic bath)<br>(ii) cross-link reversal and DNA isolation [using a resin-based (Chelex-100)] DNA isolation procedure. | Simple ChIP protocol combined with sequencing library preparation by Tn5 transposase ("tagmentation"). | TF-ChIP protocol with Sepharose A/G beads optimized for pure tissue-specific output. |
| *Histone modification tested* | Not specified | Not tested | H3K9ac, H3K9m2, H3K9m3, H3K27m3, H3K9m3, H3K4m2, H3K4m3. | H3K9Ac, H3K4me2, H3K4m3, H3K27m3. | H3K4me1, H3K4me3, H3K27ac, H3K27me3, H3K36me3. | Not tested. |
| *TF tested* | Not specified | Sp1 | RNAPII | RNA polymerase II, hnRNP K, TBP, CREB and CBP. | CTCF, GATA1, PU.1, and REST. | NICD and RBPjK. |
| *Time estimated* | 3 d | 2–3 d | 1 d | 4–6 h | 2–3 d | 2 d |
| *Advantages* | Optimized for sparsely populated tissues like the brain. | Optimized for sparsely populated tissues like the brain. | (i) Fast procedure;<br>(ii) a small amount of starting material required. | Very fast. | (i) Fast;<br>(ii) low cell numbers for histone marks and relatively low cell numbers for TFs. | (i) Allow detection of dynamic bindings;<br>(ii) tissue-specific;<br>(ii) optimized for low-abundance or not-direct DNA-binding proteins. |
| *Drawbacks* | (i) Needs to be optimized depending on applications;<br>(ii) lack of specific information about TF or histone modification. | (i) ChIP kit needs to be used;<br>(ii) uncertain performance for low-abundance or not-direct DNA-binding proteins. | (i) Not tested for sparsely populated tissues like the brain;<br>(ii) uncertain performance for low-abundance or not-direct DNA-binding proteins;<br>(iii) small yield. Not suitable for analysis of more than one genomic locus. | (i) Not tested for sparsely populated tissues like the brain;<br>(ii) uncertain performance for low-abundance or not-direct DNA-binding proteins. | (i) Additional reagent requirements (transposase);<br>(ii) not tested for tissues;<br>(iii) uncertain performance for low-abundance or not-direct DNA-binding proteins. | Optimization required depending on the tissue density and the TF studied. |
| Advancements with the present protocol. | (i) The antibody for TF has been clearly stated and referenced;<br>(ii) the application has been specified. | (i) Ideally suited for any ChIP-grade antibody, no need for an expensive kit;<br>(ii) designed for co-TF. | (i) Tested and validated for sparsely populated tissue;<br>(ii) designed for co-TF;<br>(iii) high yield from small micro-dissected tissue. | (i) Tested and validated for sparsely populated tissue;<br>(ii) high yield from small micro-dissected tissue. | (i) All reagents are listed;<br>(ii) tested and validated for tissue but also suitable for cell suspension;<br>(iii) high yield from small micro-dissected tissue. | (i) optimized for low expressed-TF-ChIP;<br>(ii) tested and validated to obtain high yields of DNA from sparsely dense tissue;<br>(iii) customizable. |

## Chromatin Shearing

Sonication is very sensitive to changes, and its efficiency depends on several factors such as temperature, cell type, and density, volume, SDS concentration, and the extent of cross-linking. For reproducible results, these parameters should be kept constant.

We use the Bioruptor Plus sonicator from Diagenode equipped with a cooling water bath and a tray holding up to six samples. To shear DNA, ultrasonic waves are transferred through water generating heat. With this system, the temperature is kept at 4°C preserving sample antigenicity. This system is suitable for shearing up to six sample at a time, assuring reproducibility between replicates. Samples' volume, tissue composition, and density impact the sonication outcome. If new tissues are going to be tested with this protocol and there is no previous knowledge of their sonication settings, several optimization steps are required. Samples volumes should be fixed at the beginning and sonication efficiency calibrated by testing several aliquots of the starting material at increasing dilutions in lysis buffer (es. 1×, 2×, 4×, 6×, 8×, 10×). By keeping settings constants, it is possible to retrieve the optimal conditions for your tissue.

We achieved a nice shearing (**Figure 2D**) using 200 μl of both cortical and hippocampal lysates (0.3% of SDS) with a DNA concentration between 6 and 7 ng/μl performing three runs of 10 cycles each with intervals of 30 s ON and 30 s OFF at high power.

It is important to notice that very low SDS concentration and prolonged crosslinking also impact the shearing efficiency. This should be taken into account if any changes are planned to be made.

Shearing was also tested after ChIP by the mean of Fragment Analyzer. We found some inconsistencies between agarose gel and Fragment Analyzer analysis. In both cortex and hippocampus, it is possible to notice a bimodal distribution in the input as well as in immunoprecipitates (**Figure 3**). This may be due to the higher sensitivity of capillary gel electrophoresis to residual contaminants (ions, SDS, proteins, etc.), due to overloading or to conformation/spatial structure of DNA molecules. However, the low peak is predominant in all sample, and the majority of DNA fragments ranging between 200 and 500 bp (**Figures 3A,B,D**). It is also possible to notice that H3 and NICD antibodies show the same behavior in the two tissues (**Figures 3B,B',D,D'**) whereas the mock precipitated IgG sample (the negative control) has barely precipitate fragments (**Figures 3C,C'**).

## PCR Results Analysis

To validate the enrichment of NICD in the ChIP-NICD complex compared to the input and unbound fractions, we performed western blot analysis for Notch1 (c-terminus) and used β-actin as

**TABLE 2 |** Troubleshooting table.

| Problem | Possible reason | Solution |
|---|---|---|
| Fragmented chromatin concentration is too low | 1. Incomplete tissue lysis.<br>2. Not enough tissue used for the chromatin preparation. | 1. Check for single-cell suspension using a microscope.<br>2. If incomplete tissue lysis is excluded, try increasing the starting material amount. |
| Fragments are too large when visualized in Agarose gel. | 1. Samples may have been over-crosslinked.<br>2. Too much input material was processed.<br>3. Insufficient sonication. | 1. Reduce the crosslinking time.<br>2. Reduce the amount of tissues per sonication or dilute it more in Lysis buffer.<br>3. Conduct a sonication time course. |
| Fragments are too short when visualized in Agarose gel. | Samples may have been subjected to excessive shearing by sonication and/or conditions are too harsh. | Conduct a sonication time course. Do not increase the duration of sonication steps, as this could overheat the sample and lead to loss of epitopes. |
| DNA pellets do not solubilize after extraction. | DNA pellet is overdried. | Heat the pellet at 37°C until it is completely solubilized. Try to avoid excessive drying of the DNA pellet. |
| No product or a very little band for the input after PCR reactions. | 1. DNA added to the PCR reaction was not enough. 2. Conditions are not optimal. | 1. Add more DNA to the PCR reaction or increase the number of amplification cycles.<br>2. Optimize the PCR conditions for experimental primer set using purified DNA from cross-linked and fragmented chromatin. |
| No product in the positive control after PCR reactions. | 1. Not enough chromatin or antibody added to the IP reaction.<br>2. DNA could have been lost during washes.<br>3. Incomplete elution of chromatin from beads. | 1. Try to add more chromatin or more antibody.<br>2. Prepare new wash solutions.<br>3. Try increasing elution time and shake tubes more frequently. |
| Visible product in the negative control. | 1. Insufficient washes.<br>2. Too much chromatin added to the IP reaction. | 1. Increase the number and/or stringency of the washes after immunoprecipitation.<br>2. Reduce the amount of negative control antibody or the amount of chromatin. |
| No band for the IP product after PCR reaction. | 1. Not enough antibody added to the IP reaction.<br>2. Not enough DNA added to the PCR reaction.<br>3. Not enough chromatin added to the IP reaction. | 1. Typically a range of 1–5 μg of antibody is added to the IP reaction; however, the exact amount depends greatly on the individual antibody. Try to use ChIP-grade antibodies.<br>2. Increase the number of amplification cycles or add more DNA to the PCR reaction.<br>3. Try to add more chromatin or increase the amount of starting tissue. |

negative control. The ChIP-NICD fraction is enriched in cleaved Notch1 1.6-fold compared to the input. Precipitation is specific to NICD as indicated by the absence of β-actin, which is instead present in the input and unbound fraction (**Figure 4A**).

Downstream assays to investigate protein–DNA interaction at genomic binding sites are polymerase chain reaction (PCR), quantitative polymerase chain reaction (qPCR), DNA microarray (ChIP-on-chip), and massively parallel DNA sequencing (ChIP-seq).

Normal PCR is the easiest but less reliable approach to analyze a ChIP experiment product. It is a fast and cheap method to assess the quality/purity of the immunoprecipitated chromatin, but it is less employed for detection of potential target genes because it is not quantitative. In that case, it is preferable to use qPCR instead since it provides an accurate determination of levels of specific DNA in ChIP-ed samples. In both cases, primers should be designed for a region the TF binds to, the positive control, and for a region, your TF is supposed not to bind, representing the negative control. If there is previous knowledge, it is recommended to first identify the binding site sequence *in silico* in order to accurately amplify the extracted DNA.

If there are no known sites but candidate target genes are available, it is possible to design primers along the length of potential regulatory regions such as promoters and conserved noncoding sequences within intergenic regions. If candidate target genes or potential sites are not available, ChIP-chip (Buck and Lieb, 2004) or ChIP-seq (Fanelli et al., 2011; Furey, 2012) should be considered instead.

In our case, we know that RBPjK-binding motif is CGTGGGAA (Tun et al., 1994). Therefore, we designed a set of primers looking at the presence of these eight nucleotides strings within the sequence of the Hes5 promoter, a canonical Notch signaling target gene. We also chose Delta-like protein 1 (DLL1) promoter as a negative control region since there are no RBPjK-binding motifs. A good example of purity was achieved as demonstrated by the PCR and qPCR results (**Figure 4**). For Hes5 PCR results, we observe amplification in both RBPjK and NICD samples while there is no amplification in IgG lane suggesting that non-specific binding is absent (**Figure 4B**).

On the other hand, the DLL1 PCR shows no amplification (**Figure 4B'**), indicating the specificity of the ChIP for RBPjK and NICD targets.

Quantitative polymerase chain reaction analysis further confirms the specificity obtained using Hes5 as a positive control and GADPH as a negative control (**Figure 4C**). Binding efficiency is expressed by the percent input method that includes normalization for both background levels and input chromatin (Lacazette, 2016).

This protocol is suitable for sequencing (data not shown). From the ChIPed fragments, a library is prepared according to manufacturer's instruction and loaded into the flow-cell for sequencing; trimmed sequence reads are mapped to a reference genome. Next, peaks are found using peak-calling algorithms (Nakato and Shirahige, 2017). To further analyze the data, differential binding or motif analyses are common endpoints of ChIP-seq workflows. The ChIP-Seq procedure allows to map TF-target sequences and provide a functional readout of gene activation in complex tissues, such as the brain, and under different experimental conditions: i.e., environmental enrichment, aging, neurodegeneration, neuroinflammation, etc. Understanding the downstream targets of signaling pathways critical for plasticity and neurodegeneration will facilitate the discrimination of beneficial versus detrimental genes' products that can be employed for developing therapeutic strategies targeting brain diseases.

Concluding, there are already other protocols describing ChIP procedures (**Table 1**; Braveman et al., 2004; Nelson et al., 2006; Dahl and Collas, 2008; Sailaja et al., 2012; Schmidl et al., 2015). However, all these methods are either centered on abundant histone modification or use cells suspensions as starting material. The added value of this protocol is the possibility to perform all the downstream analyses described (i) from a tissue subregion, (ii) precipitating for a rare transcriptional activator (NICD), and (iii) yielding a sufficient amount of DNA with reduced background. The advantage of performing ChIP for NICD, compared to RBPJK, has undisputed advantages as only activated loci under specific conditions will be captured within the tissue revealing active transcriptional targets.

## Troubleshooting

**Table 2** indicates issues which can occur during the procedure with a possible reason and suggestions to solve and avoid them.

## AUTHOR CONTRIBUTIONS

AP conducted the experiments and wrote the manuscript. LA directed the experimentation and co-wrote the manuscript.

## FUNDING

The work is supported by funding of the Swiss National Foundation (31003A_163470, LA).

## ACKNOWLEDGMENTS

We thank Mr. Simon April and Mr. Daniel Brechtold for dedicating time to establish the first steps of this protocols. We thank the animal caretaker at the University of Fribourg, Simone Eichenberger, for helping us sourcing the mice.

## REFERENCES

Alberi, L., Hoey, S. E., Brai, E., Scotti, A. L., and Marathe, S. (2013). Notch signaling in the brain: in good and bad times. *Ageing Res. Rev.* 12, 801–814. doi: 10.1016/j.arr.2013.03.004

Alberi, L., Liu, S., Wang, Y., Badie, R., Smith-Hicks, C., Wu, J., et al. (2011). Activity-induced notch signaling in neurons requires Arc/Arg3.1 and is essential for synaptic plasticity in hippocampal networks. *Neuron* 69, 437–444. doi: 10.1016/j.neuron.2011.01.004

Brai, E., Alina Raio, N., and Alberi, L. (2016). Notch1 hallmarks fibrillary depositions in sporadic alzheimer's disease. *Acta Neuropathol. Commun.* 4:64. doi: 10.1186/s40478-016-0327-2

Braveman, M. W., Chen-Plotkin, A. S., Yohrling, G. J., and Cha, J. H. J. (2004). Chromatin immunoprecipitation technique for study of transcriptional dysregulation in intact mouse brain. *Methods Mol. Biol.* 277, 261–276. doi: 10.1385/1-59259-804-8:261

Buck, M. J., and Lieb, J. D. (2004). ChIP-chip: considerations for the design, analysis, and application of genome-wide chromatin immunoprecipitation experiments. *Genomics* 83, 349–360. doi: 10.1016/j.ygeno.2003.11.004

Dahl, J. A., and Collas, P. (2008). A rapid micro chromatin immunoprecipitation assay (ChIP). *Nat. Protoc.* 3, 1032–1045. doi: 10.1038/nprot.2008.68

Engelmann, C., and Haenold, R. (2016). Transcriptional Control of synaptic plasticity by transcription factor NF-κB. *Neural Plast.* 2016:7027949. doi: 10.1155/2016/7027949

Fanelli, M., Amatori, S., Barozzi, I., and Minucci, S. (2011). Chromatin immunoprecipitation and high-throughput sequencing from paraffin-embedded pathology tissue. *Nat. Protoc.* 6, 1905–1919. doi: 10.1038/nprot.2011.406

Flavell, S. W., and Greenberg, M. E. (2008). Signaling mechanisms linking neuronal activity to gene expression and plasticity of the nervous system. *Annu. Rev. Neurosci.* 31, 563–590. doi: 10.1146/annurev.neuro.31.060407.125631

Furey, T. S. (2012). ChIP-seq and beyond: new and improved methodologies to detect and characterize protein–DNA interactions. *Nat. Rev. Genet.* 13, 840–852. doi: 10.1038/nrg3306

Genuth, N. R., and Barna, M. (2018). Heterogeneity and specialized functions of translation machinery: from genes to organisms. *Nat. Rev. Genet.* 19, 431–452. doi: 10.1038/s41576-018-0008-z

Huang, J., Zheng, J., Yuan, H., and McGinnis, K. (2018). Distinct tissue-specific transcriptional regulation revealed by gene regulatory networks in maize. *BMC Plant Biol.* 18:111. doi: 10.1186/s12870-018-1329-y

Lacazette, E. (2016). A laboratory practical illustrating the use of the ChIP-qPCR method in a robust model: estrogen receptor alpha immunoprecipitation using Mcf-7 culture cells. *Biochem. Mol. Biol. Educ.* 45, 152–160. doi: 10.1002/bmb.20999

Mansuy, I. M., and Mohanna, S. (2011). Epigenetics and the human brain: where nurture meets nature. *Cerebrum* 2011, 1–8.

Marathe, S., Jaquet, M., Annoni, J. -M., and Alberi, L. (2017). Jagged1 is altered in alzheimer's disease and regulates spatial memory processing. *Front. Cell. Neurosci.* 11:220. doi: 10.3389/fncel.2017.00220

Nakato, R., and Shirahige, K. (2017). Recent advances in ChIP-seq analysis: from quality management to whole-genome annotation. *Brief. Bioinform.* 18, 279–290.

Nelson, J. D., Denisenko, O., and Bomsztyk, K. (2006). Protocol for the fast chromatin immunoprecipitation (ChIP) method. *Nat. Protoc.* 1, 179–185. doi: 10.1038/nprot.2006.27

Olfson, E., and Ross, D. A. (2017). Genes orchestrating brain function. *Biol. Psychiatry* 82, e17–e19. doi: 10.1016/j.biopsych.2017.06.003

Qian, J., Esumi, N., Chen, Y., Wang, Q., Chowers, I., and Zack, D. J. (2005). Identification of regulatory targets of tissue-specific transcription factors: application to retina-specific gene regulation. *Nucleic Acids Res.* 33, 3479–3491. doi: 10.1093/nar/gki658

Sailaja, B. S., Takizawa, T., and Meshorer, E. (2012). "Chromatin immunoprecipitation in Mouse hippocampal cells and tissues," in *Transcriptional Regulation: Methods and Protocols*, ed. A. Vancura (New York, NY: Springer New York), 353–364.

Schmidl, C., Rendeiro, A. F., Sheffield, N. C., and Bock, C. (2015). ChIPmentation: fast, robust, low-input ChIP-seq for histones and transcription factors. *Nat. Methods* 12, 963–965. doi: 10.1038/nmeth.3542

Siebel, C., and Lendahl, U. (2017). Notch signaling in development, tissue homeostasis, and disease. *Physiol. Rev.* 97, 1235–1294. doi: 10.1152/physrev.00005.2017

Sultan, F. A. (2013). Dissection of different areas from mouse hippocampus. *Bio Protoc.* 3:e955. doi: 10.21769/BioProtoc.955

Tun, T., Hamaguchi, Y., Matsunami, N., Furukawa, T., Honjo, T., and Kawaichi, M. (1994). Recognition sequence of a highly conserved DNA binding protein RBP-J kappa. *Nucleic Acids Res.* 22, 965–971. doi: 10.1093/nar/22.6.965

Vaquerizas, J. M., Kummerfeld, S. K., Teichmann, S. A., and Luscombe, N. M. (2009). A census of human transcription factors: function, expression and evolution. *Nat. Rev. Genet.* 10, 252–263. doi: 10.1038/nrg2538

# 12

# Lipid Metabolism Crosstalk in the Brain: Glia and Neurons

*Casey N. Barber and Daniel M. Raben**

*Department of Biological Chemistry, The Johns Hopkins University School of Medicine, Baltimore, MD, United States*

***Correspondence:***
*Daniel M. Raben*
*draben@jhmi.edu*

Until recently, glial cells have been considered mainly support cells for neurons in the mammalian brain. However, many studies have unveiled a variety of glial functions including electrolyte homeostasis, inflammation, synapse formation, metabolism, and the regulation of neurotransmission. The importance of these functions illuminates significant crosstalk between glial and neuronal cells. Importantly, it is known that astrocytes secrete signals that can modulate both presynaptic and postsynaptic function. It is also known that the lipid compositions of the pre- and post-synaptic membranes of neurons greatly impact functions such as vesicle fusion and receptor mobility. These data suggest an essential lipid-mediated communication between glial cells and neurons. Little is known, however, about how the lipid metabolism of both cell types may interact. In this review, we discuss neuronal and glial lipid metabolism and suggest how they might interact to impact neurotransmission.

**Keywords: neurons, lipids, glial, CNS, communication**

Research on glial cells began in 1846, when Rudolf Virchow described a "substance" in which the various parts of the nervous system were embedded. In subsequent years, different kinds of glial cells were discovered and classified. Even though Santiago Ramon y Cajal was the first to propose a wide and diverse list of the functions of glia, these cells were viewed as simple neuronal support cells (García-Marín et al., 2007). In the last 20 years, however, studies have illuminated many functions of glia, highlighting their significance within the nervous system. In addition to providing many homeostatic functions to neurons, glial cells play a large role in regulating neurotransmission. Currently, much is known about lipid metabolism within neurons and glia separately, but little is known about potential lipid metabolic crosstalk between the two cell types. Here, we propose that lipid metabolism specifically from glial cells affects neurotransmission by regulating the rates of synaptic vesicle exo- and endocytosis. We will describe the known functions of glia and their lipid metabolism and then describe how glial lipid metabolism can possibly interact with neuronal lipid metabolism to regulate neurotransmission within the mammalian central nervous system.

Glial cells are the predominant cell type in the mammalian brain. They can contribute to 33–66% of the brain's total mass. Glial cells are segregated into three main classifications: astrocytes, microglia, and oligodendrocytes. Importantly, each cell type performs critical functions that sustain the health and function of the surrounding neurons. Astrocytes have many functions, among them are regulating water transport and ion levels in neurons, maintaining the blood brain barrier, and clearing glutamate from synapses to prevent neurotoxicity (Jäkel and Dimou, 2017). Microglia act as neuroprotectors by engulfing debris and cells in the process of apoptosis. Microglia actively surveil and respond to the state of functional synapses, such that they can sense dysfunctional synapses and influence information circuitry by either contributing to the repair or removal of a cell (Graeber and Streit, 2010). In the developing brain, microglia actively phagocytose some synaptic material and have a critical role in synaptic pruning during maturation (Paolicelli et al., 2011). Oligodendrocytes are well-known as the myelin-producing glial cells that insulate axons to ensure rapid electrical conduction and also provide trophic support to neurons (Simons and Trajkovic, 2006). Together glial cells provide an abundance of support to neurons, and defects in glial cells are implicated in many neurological diseases such as Alzheimer's disease, amyotrophic lateral sclerosis, and herpes encephalitis (Tracey et al., 2018).

As mentioned above, much is known about the variety of functions performed by these non-neuronal cells within the mammalian brain. Specifically, there is a wealth of information regarding the brain's energy utilization and how glial cells and neurons work together to support the brain's energy demands (Pellerin et al., 2007; Bélanger et al., 2011; Bruce et al., 2017; Tracey et al., 2018). This is crucial, as 20% of the body's total ATP consumption occurs in the brain, primarily for restoring ion gradients and motor-driven transport, as well as other functions (Bélanger et al., 2011). However, not nearly as much is known about lipid metabolism within glial cells and its potential neuronal implications. Here, we would like to propose that there is significant lipid metabolic crosstalk between glia and neurons that could influence neuronal function and neurotransmission. This could be yet another example of how glial cells regulate synaptic transmission and brain function overall.

Lipid molecules are key components of the brain's complex structure and function, with lipids comprising around 50% of the brain's dry weight. The lipid composition of neuronal and glial cell membranes has been shown to affect cell function and neurotransmission (O'Brien and Sampson, 1965; Puchkov and Haucke, 2013). The brain is mainly comprised of long-chain polyunsaturated fatty acids (LC-PUFAs) such as eicosapentaenoic acid, docosahexaenoic acid, and arachidonic acid. Importantly, several recent studies provide evidence that fatty acids, including essential fatty acids which must be obtained from the diet, can cross the blood-brain barrier (BBB) and be taken up by neurons via fatty acid transporters. Both neurons and astrocytes express several fatty acid transporters such as FATP1, FATP4, and CD36. It was recently shown that fatty acid binding protein 7 (FABP7) knockout mice exhibit schizophrenic phenotypes, such as deficits in prepulse inhibition, related to mutated spine morphology. Neurons from these mice had a reduction in dendritic complexity, spine density, and maturity of spines of pyramidal neurons (Watanabe et al., 2007; Ebrahimi et al., 2016; Bruce et al., 2017).

It is also widely thought that neurons receive metabolic support from astrocytes in a number of ways, one of which being that fatty acid oxidation primarily occurs in astrocytes. After which, the metabolites (ketones, NADH, acetyl CoA, $FADH_2$) are taken up and utilized by neurons. Neurons are not energy-storing cells and do not normally contain a significant pool of lipid droplets or glycogen. Therefore, the available energy is depleted rapidly. This is one factor that makes them especially sensitive to stressful conditions such as continued stimulation. This is because the consumption of glycogen or fatty acids from lipid droplets is used in many other cell types as energy reserves. Periods of such high stimulation lead to increased reactive oxygen species (ROS) levels, which causes a buildup of peroxidated fatty acids. This is extremely harmful to neurons and must be prevented by removing or destroying the peroxidated fatty acids. In contrast to neurons, astrocytes store energy in the form of lipid droplets and act as a buffer to periods of toxic stimulation to neurons. Studies have shown that periods of high stress in neurons induce the formation of lipid droplets in nearby astrocytes, implying that overstimulated neurons may shuttle their peroxidated fatty acids to neighboring astrocytes (Bailey et al., 2015; Liu et al., 2015). This effect was found to be dependent on lipoproteins, the proteins responsible for trafficking fatty acids. In support of these studies, Ioannou et al. (2018) found that stressed neurons release peroxidated fatty acids bound to lipoproteins that are secreted by astrocytes or neurons. Neighboring astrocytes endocytose these lipoprotein-fatty acid particles and store the fatty acids in their lipid droplets. Astrocytes also react to overstimulated neurons by breaking down their lipid droplets and shuttling them to their own mitochondria for oxidative phosphorylation. Taken together, these data support the notion that astrocytes provide defense for overstimulated neurons by preventing fatty acid toxicity (Ioannou et al., 2018).

In addition to the metabolism of peroxidated lipids by astrocytes, most of the research regarding astrocytic lipid metabolism has been conducted specifically on cholesterol, and further research is required to study the metabolism of other lipids within astrocytes. Astrocytes and neurons both make cholesterol *de novo* but differ greatly in the pathways of cholesterol homeostasis and trafficking. Currently cholesterol metabolism within astrocytes serves as a model to illustrate the differences within neurons and astrocytes in pathways of synthesis, utilization, and efflux. Chen et al. (2013) found that astrocytes expel cholesterol with both lipid-free apolipoproteins and lipoproteins, while cholesterol efflux from neurons is induced only by lipoproteins. Lipoproteins are synthesized specifically by astrocytes and not neurons. While these proteins take cholesterol from neurons, they are also able to bind lipoprotein receptors within neuronal membranes that induce synaptogenesis (Chen et al., 2013).

Cholesterol is particularly enriched in synaptic membranes and affects a number of properties including endo- and exocytosis, lipid raft formation, and membrane fluidity, all of which greatly regulate neurotransmission. Therefore, the synthesis and transport of cholesterol is a modulating factor of synaptic signaling. Camargo et al. (2012) found that the synthesis of cholesterol, as well as fatty acids, within astrocytes is dependent on sterol regulatory element binding proteins (SREBPs). It was later found that components of the SREBP pathway are most highly expressed in hippocampal astrocytes. Importantly, a decrease in SREBP activity in astrocytes leads to a defect in synaptic function and plasticity. Mutated proteins within the astrocyte SREBP pathway caused a defect in synaptic structure, vesicle populations, and presynaptic function. Specifically, synapses in mice in which the SREBP cleavage-activating protein (SCAP) was deleted from GFAP-expressing

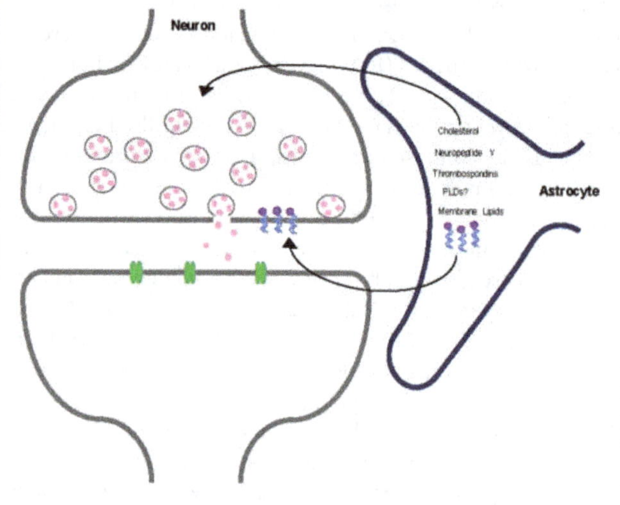


**FIGURE 1 |** Astrocytes secrete many factors that are critical to neuron function such as cholesterol, neuropeptide Y, thrombospondins, and other metabolic intermediates. We hypothesize that membrane lipids are also secreted by astrocytes and taken up by neurons to regulate neurotransmission. Additionally, PLDs selectively expressed within astrocytes may contribute to this astrocytic lipid metabolism.

cells were found to have lower levels of SNAP-25, a crucial SNARE protein involved in vesicle fusion with the presynaptic membrane (van Deijk et al., 2017). This is a critical example of how elements produced within glial cells can be transferred to neurons to affect synaptic transmission.

The phospholipid composition of presynaptic membranes contributes to the regulation of the rates of synaptic vesicle exo- and endocytosis. The shapes of particular lipids affect the membrane curvature and make the architecture more or less susceptible to vesicle fusion. Cholesterol, diacylglycerol, and phosphatidic acid are cone-shaped lipids and induce negative membrane curvature, promoting membrane fusion (Ammar et al., 2013). In addition to affecting membrane curvature, these lipids also bind important protein regulators of vesicle fusion, such as syntaxin-1A, NSF, and small GTPases (Jang et al., 2012). Therefore, portions of the membrane that are more highly enriched in these cone-shaped lipids are potentially more likely to undergo vesicle fusion, highlighting the phospholipid composition of synaptic membranes as a regulating factor of synaptic vesicle cycling.

So how is the lipid composition of membranes determined? What factors play a role in regulating the relative amounts of lipids within membranes? One of the most important factors are lipid-metabolizing enzymes, such as diacylglycerol kinases (DGKs) and phospholipases, that catalyze the conversion of these lipids. For example, DGKs and phospholipases D (PLDs) both produce phosphatidic acid from different substrates (Puchkov and Haucke, 2013). As phosphatidic acid is highly implicated in vesicle fusion, these enzymes are thought to be regulators of the synaptic vesicle cycle. In 2016, Goldschmidt et al. found that knockout of a particular DGK, DGKθ, in neurons resulted in significantly decreased rates of endocytosis after stimulation, in comparison to wildtype neurons. This is just one study, in addition to many others, that has discovered proteins with a regulatory role in the synaptic vesicle cycle (Rosahl et al., 1995; Südhof and Rizo, 1996; Wang et al., 1997; Turner et al., 1999; Reim et al., 2001; Pechstein et al., 2010; Lai et al., 2017). Many of these characterized proteins can be categorized by their mechanism of action on the SV cycle: regulation of calcium influx, regulation of SNARE dynamics, changes in membrane curvature, or synaptic vesicle priming. However, in some cases, the exact molecular actions of regulatory proteins have not been discovered. Being that the lipid membrane is the physical barrier between an intact synaptic vesicle and the synaptic cleft, it is not hard to imagine that the last regulatory step of vesicle fusion could be the lipid composition of the presynaptic membrane. This being so, the hypothesis that many SV regulatory proteins are lipid-metabolizing proteins is not inconceivable.

In addition to proteins, other factors influence the phospholipid composition of membranes. As discussed above, astrocytes synthesize lipids, and traffic them to neurons, offering another point of regulation by astrocytes. Also, they secrete signals that can influence synaptic transmission. These are often signaling factors that have downstream effects that influence synaptic vesicle fusion (Jäkel and Dimou, 2017). What about astrocytic factors that have a more direct impact on the synaptic vesicle cycle? We hypothesize that astrocytes have a direct role in regulating synaptic transmission via astrocyte lipid metabolism followed by transport to neurons. We suggest that astrocytes might be responsible for making some of the lipids that are directly inserted into the presynaptic plasma membrane. Other proteins, such as flippases, are likely involved that flip lipids into the inner membrane leaflet and sort these lipids into microdomains that make certain areas of the membrane susceptible for fusing with synaptic vesicles (Andersen et al., 2016). Astrocytes are involved in the transportation of several molecules and proteins to neurons, so membrane lipids such as phosphatidic acid could feasibly be transferred directly or indirectly from astrocytes to neurons. In fact, Tabernero et al. (2001) found that astrocytes secrete oleic acid and suggested that this is taken up by neurons for the process of phospholipid synthesis during neuronal differentiation. In addition to lipids, studies have also found that astrocytes secrete or release: large vesicles containing functional mitochondria, ATP, and lipid droplets (Falchi et al., 2013); dense-core vesicles containing neuropeptide Y (Ramamoorthy and Whim, 2008); glucose, lactate, glutamine, and glutamate through gap junctions connecting astrocytes (Giaume et al., 1997; Gandhi et al., 2009); thrombospondins and hevin, which act on neurons to promote synaptogenesis (Christopherson et al., 2005; Kucukdereli et al., 2011); and many other molecules and proteins such as glypicans, Wnts, and tumor necrosis factor α (TNFα) (Allen, 2014). Therefore, there is much evidence that astrocytes release many factors that affect neurons, and we propose that lipids are also an important astrocyte-secreted factor.

Astrocytic processes are intimately involved with synapses, comprising the tripartite synapse. Astrocytes have a wide, radial branching morphology, allowing them to physically protrude into the synaptic cleft between pre- and postsynaptic boutons and exchange information with these elements, contributing to synaptic physiology (Perea et al., 2009). Therefore, it is conceivable that lipids may be transferred within the synaptic region of the neuron because of how closely related neurons and astrocytes are in physical space. In support of this hypothesis, Zhu et al. (2016) found that phosphatidic acid produced specifically from astrocytes regulates neurite outgrowth and dendritic branching in neurons. This study found that knockdown of PLD1 only in astrocytes led to a reduction in secretion of phosphatidic acid and a decrease in dendritic branching of neurons. Furthermore, neurons grown in the presence of conditioned media from astrocytes with PLD1 knockdown had significantly decreased dendritic branching. This study is an example of how secreted lipids from astrocytes can affect functional aspects of neurons.

Astrocytes could also synthesize other proteins that have regulatory roles in the synaptic vesicle cycle, thereby having a more indirect effect on neurotransmission. For instance, it is possible that specific lipid-metabolizing enzymes could be expressed only within glial cells and that mechanisms transfer the products of the reactions they catalyze from glial cells to neurons to affect membrane architecture. We hypothesize that PLD may be implicated in synaptic vesicle exocytosis. The localization and expression of PLD is currently unclear (Saito et al., 2000; Ammar et al., 2015; Vermeren et al., 2016), although some studies suggest that PLDs are localized within glial cells (Jin et al., 2002; Zhang et al., 2004; Zhu et al., 2016). The localization and expression pattern of PLDs in the brain needs to be clarified, but it is possible that PLDs are selectively expressed in astrocytes. If this is the case, astrocytes could produce phosphatidic acid by PLD that is trafficked to or taken up by neurons to influence the dynamics of synaptic vesicle fusion (**Figure 1**).

In conclusion, we believe that glial cells have a specific role in regulating synaptic transmission in neurons via lipid metabolism. The relative amount of certain lipids within neuronal membranes impacts the efficiency of endo- and exocytosis, and this could be developed by lipid synthesis or metabolism within glial cells. Further research is required to determine the expression of lipid-metabolizing enzymes within glial cells and pathways of lipid metabolism and trafficking. Regardless, astrocytes, microglia, and oligodendrocytes are vital components of the nervous system that contribute to regulating many neuronal functions, including synaptic transmission.

## AUTHOR CONTRIBUTIONS

All authors listed have made a substantial, direct and intellectual contribution to the work, and approved it for publication.

## FUNDING

This work was supported by grant from the National Institutes of Health (R01NS077923, DR).

## REFERENCES

Allen, N. J. (2014). Astrocyte regulation of synaptic behavior. *Cell Dev. Biol.* 30, 439–463. doi: 10.1146/annurev-cellbio-100913-013053

Ammar, M., Kassas, N., Chasserot-Golaz, S., Bader, M. F., and Vitale, N. (2013). Lipids in regulated exocytosis: what are they doing? *Front. Endocrinol.* 4:125. doi: 10.3389/fendo.2013.00125

Ammar, M. R., Thahouly, T., Hanauer, A., Stegner, D., Nieswandt, B., and Vitale, N. (2015). PLD1 participates in BDNF-induced signalling in cortical neurons. *Sci. Rep.* 5:14778. doi: 10.1038/srep14778

Andersen, J. P., Vestergaard, A. L., Mikkelsen, S. A., Mogensen, L. S., Chalat, M., and Molday, R. S. (2016). P4-ATPases as phospholipid flippases—structure, function, and enigmas. *Front. Physiol.* 7:275. doi: 10.3389/fphys.2016.00275

Bailey, A. P., Koster, G., Guillermier, C., Hirst, E. M., MacRae, J. I., Lechene, C. P., et al. (2015). Antioxidant role for lipid droplets in a stem cell niche of drosophila. *Cell* 163, 340–353. doi: 10.1016/j.cell.2015.09.020

Bélanger, M., Allaman, I., and Magistretti, P. J. (2011). Brain Energy metabolism: focus on astrocyte-neuron metabolic cooperation. *Cell Metab.* 14, 724–738. doi: 10.1016/j.cmet.2011.08.016

Bruce, K. D., Zsombok, A., and Eckel, R. H. (2017). Lipid processing in the brain: a key regulator of systemic metabolism. *Front. Endocrinol.* 8:60. doi: 10.3389/fendo.2017.00060

Camargo, N., Brouwers, J. F., Loos, M., Gutmann, D. H., Smit, A. B., and Verheijen, M. H. (2012). High-fat diet ameliorates neurological deficits caused by defective astrocyte lipid metabolism. *FASEB J.* 26, 4302–4315. doi: 10.1096/fj.12-205807

Chen, J., Zhang, X., Kusumo, H., Costa, L. G., and Guizzetti, M. (2013). Cholesterol efflux is differentially regulated in neurons and astrocytes: implications for brain cholesterol homeostasis. *Biochim. Biophys. Acta Mol. Cell. Biol. Lipids* 1831, 263–275. doi: 10.1016/j.bbalip.2012.09.007

Christopherson, K. S., Ullian, E. M., Stokes, C. C., Mullowney, C. E., Hell, J. W., Agah, A., et al. (2005). Thrombospondins are astrocyte secreted proteins that promote CNS synaptogenesis. *Cell* 120, 421–433. doi: 10.1016/j.cell.2004.12.020

Ebrahimi, M., Yamamoto, Y., Sharifi, K., Kida, H., Kagawa, Y., Yasumoto, Y., et al. (2016). Astrocyte-expressed FABP7 regulates dendritic morphology and excitatory synaptic function of cortical neurons. *Glia* 64, 48–62. doi: 10.1002/glia.22902

Falchi, A. M., Sogos, V., Saba, F., Piras, M., Congiu, T., and Piludu, M. (2013). Astrocytes shed large membrane vesicles that contain mitochondria, lipid droplets and ATP. *Histochem. Cell Biol.* 139, 221–231. doi: 10.1007/s00418-012-1045-x

Gandhi, G. K., Cruz, N. F., Ball, K. K., Theus, S. A., and Dienel, G. A. (2009). Selective astrocytic gap junctional trafficking of molecules involved in the glycolytic pathway: impact on cellular brain imaging. *J. Neurochem.* 110, 857–869. doi: 10.1111/j.1471-4159.2009.06173.x

García-Marín, V., García-López, P., and Freire, M. (2007). Cajal's contributions to glia research. *Trends Neurosci.* 30, 479–487. doi: 10.1016/j.tins.2007.06.008

Giaume, C., Tabernero, A., and Medina, J. M. (1997). Metabolic trafficking through astrocytic gap junctions. *Glia* 21, 114–123. doi: 10.1002/(SICI)1098-1136(199709)21:1<114::AID-GLIA13>3.0.CO;2-V

Graeber, M. B., and Streit, W. J. (2010). Microglia: biology and pathology. *Acta Neuropathol.* 119, 89–105. doi: 10.1007/s00401-009-0622-0

Ioannou, M., Jackson, J., Sheu, S.-H., Chang, C.-L., Weigel, A. V., Liu, H., et al. (2018). Neuron-astrocyte metabolic coupling during neuronal stimulation protects against fatty acid toxicity. *Biorxiv* 465237. doi: 10.1101/465237

Jäkel, S., and Dimou, L. (2017). Glial cells and their function in the adult brain: a journey through the history of their ablation. *Front. Cell Neurosci.* 11:24. doi: 10.3389/fncel.2017.00024

Jang, J. H., Lee, C. S., Hwang, D., and Ryu, S. H. (2012). Understanding of the roles of phospholipase D and phosphatidic acid through their binding partners. *Prog. Lipid Res.* 51, 71–81. doi: 10.1016/j.plipres.2011.12.003

Jin, S., Schatter, B., Weichel, O., Walev, I., Ryu, S., and Klein, J. (2002). Stability of phospholipase D in primary astrocytes. *Biochem. Biophys. Res. Co* 297, 545–551. doi: 10.1016/S0006-291X(02)02231-3

Kucukdereli, H., Allen, N. J., Lee, A. T., Feng, A., Ozlu, M. I., Conatser, L. M., et al. (2011). Control of excitatory CNS synaptogenesis by astrocyte-secreted proteins Hevin and SPARC. *Proc. Natl. Acad. Sci. USA.* 108, E440–E49. doi: 10.1073/pnas.1104977108

Lai, Y., Choi, U. B., Leitz, J., Rhee, H. J., Lee, C., Altas, B., et al. (2017). Molecular mechanisms of synaptic vesicle priming by Munc13 and Munc18. *Neuron* 95, 591–607.e10. doi: 10.1016/j.neuron.2017.07.004

Liu, L., Zhang, K., Sandoval, H., Yamamoto, S., Jaiswal, M., Sanz, E., et al. (2015). Glial lipid droplets and ROS induced by mitochondrial defects promote neurodegeneration. *Cell* 160, 177–190. doi: 10.1016/j.cell.2014.12.019

O'Brien, J. S., and Sampson, E. L. (1965). Lipid composition of the normal human brain: gray matter, white matter, and myelin. *J. Lipid Res.* 6, 537–544.

Paolicelli, R. C., Bolasco, G., Pagani, F., Maggi, L., Scianni, M., Panzanelli, P., et al. (2011). Synaptic pruning by microglia is necessary for normal brain development. *Science* 333, 1456–1458. doi: 10.1126/science.1202529

Pechstein, A., Shupliakov, O., and Haucke, V. (2010). Intersectin 1: a versatile actor in the synaptic vesicle cycle. *Biochem. Soc. T* 38, 181–186. doi: 10.1042/BST0380181

Pellerin, L., Bouzier-Sore, A. K., Aubert, A., Serres, S., Merle, M., Costalat, R., et al. (2007). Activity-dependent regulation of energy metabolism by astrocytes: an update. *Glia* 55, 1251–1262. doi: 10.1002/glia.20528

Perea, G., Navarrete, M., and Araque, A. (2009). Tripartite synapses: astrocytes process and control synaptic information. *Trends Neurosci.* 32, 421–431. doi: 10.1016/j.tins.2009.05.001

Puchkov, D., and Haucke, V. (2013). Greasing the synaptic vesicle cycle by membrane lipids.*Trends Cell Biol.* 23, 493–503. doi: 10.1016/j.tcb.2013.05.002

Ramamoorthy, P., and Whim, M. D. (2008). Trafficking and fusion of neuropeptide Y-containing dense-core granules in astrocytes. *J. Neurosci.* 28, 13815–13827. doi: 10.1523/JNEUROSCI.5361-07.2008

Reim, K., Mansour, M., Varoqueaux, F., McMahon, H. T., Südhof, T. C., Brose, N., et al. (2001). Complexins regulate a late step in Ca2+-dependent neurotransmitter release. *Cell* 104, 71–81. doi: 10.1016/S0092-8674(01)0 0192-1

Rosahl, T. W., Spillane, D., Missler, M., Herz, J., Selig, D. K., Wolff, J. R., et al. (1995). Essential functions of synapsins I and II in synaptic vesicle regulation. *Nature* 375, 488–493. doi: 10.1038/375488a0

Saito, S., Sakagami, H., and Kondo, H. (2000). Localization of mRNAs for phospholipase D (PLD) type 1 and 2 in the brain of developing and mature rat. *Dev. Brain Res.* 120, 41–47. doi: 10.1016/S0165-3806(99)0 0189-3

Simons, M., and Trajkovic, K. (2006). Neuron-glia communication in the control of oligodendrocyte function and myelin biogenesis. *J. Cell Sci.* 119, 4381–4389. doi: 10.1242/jcs.03242

Südhof, T. C., and Rizo, J. (1996). Synaptotagmins: C2-domain proteins that regulate membrane traffic. *Neuron* 17, 379–388. doi: 10.1016/S0896-6273(00)80171-3

Tabernero, A., Lavado, E. M., Granda, B., Velasco, A., and Medina, J. M. (2001). Neuronal differentiation is triggered by oleic acid synthesized and released by astrocytes. *J. Neurochem.* 79, 606–616. doi: 10.1046/j.1471-4159.2001.00598.x

Tracey, T. J., Steyn, F. J., Wolvetang, E. J., and Ngo, S. T. (2018). Neuronal lipid metabolism: multiple pathways driving functional outcomes in health and disease. *Front. Mol. Neurosci.* 11:10. doi: 10.3389/fnmol.2018.00010

Turner, K. M., Burgoyne, R. D., and Morgan, A. (1999). Protein phosphorylation and the regulation of synaptic membrane traffic.*Trends Neurosci.* 22, 459–464. doi: 10.1016/S0166-2236(99)01436-8

van Deijk, A. F., Camargo, N., Timmerman, J., Heistek, T., Brouwers, J. F., Mogavero, F., et al. (2017). Astrocyte lipid metabolism is critical for synapse development and function *in vivo*. *Glia* 65, 670–682. doi: 10.1002/glia.23120

Vermeren, M. M., Zhang, Q., Smethurst, E., Segonds-Pichon, A., Schrewe, H., and Wakelam, M. J. (2016). The phospholipase D2 knock out mouse has ectopic purkinje cells and suffers from early adult-onset anosmia. *PLoS ONE* 11:e0162814. doi: 10.1371/journal.pone.0162814

Wang, Y., Okamoto, M., Schmitz, F., Hofmann, K., and Südhof, T. C. (1997). Rim is a putative Rab3 effector in regulating synaptic-vesicle fusion. *Nature* 388, 593–598. doi: 10.1038/41580

Watanabe, A., Toyota, T., Owada, Y., Hayashi, T., Iwayama, Y., Matsumata, M., et al. (2007). Fabp7 maps to a quantitative trait locus for a schizophrenia endophenotype. *PLoS Biol.* 5:e297. doi: 10.1371/journal.pbio.0050297

Zhang, Y., Huang, P., Du, G., Kanaho, Y., Frohman, M. A., and Tsirka, S. E. (2004). Increased expression of two phospholipase D isoforms during experimentally induced hippocampal mossy fiber outgrowth. *Glia* 46, 74–83. doi: 10.1002/glia.10322

Zhu, Y. B., Gao, W., Zhang, Y., Jia, F., Zhang, H. L., Liu, Y. Z., et al. (2016). Astrocyte-derived phosphatidic acid promotes dendritic branching. *Sci. Rep.* 6:21096. doi: 10.1038/srep21096

# 13

# Ambroxol Hydrochloride Improves Motor Functions and Extends Survival in a Mouse Model of Familial Amyotrophic Lateral Sclerosis

*Alexandra Bouscary[1,2], Cyril Quessada[1,2], Althéa Mosbach[1,2], Noëlle Callizot[3], Michael Spedding[4]*, Jean-Philippe Loeffler[1,2]* and Alexandre Henriques[1,2,4]*†*

*[1] Université de Strasbourg, UMR_S 1118, Fédération de Médecine Translationnelle, Strasbourg, France, [2] INSERM, U1118, Mécanismes Centraux et Périphériques de la Neurodégénérescence, Strasbourg, France, [3] Neuro-sys SAS, Gardanne, France, [4] Spedding Research Solutions SAS, Le Vesinet, France*

***Correspondence:**
Michael Spedding
michael@speddingresearchsolutions.fr
Jean-Philippe Loeffler
loeffler@unistra.fr
Alexandre Henriques
alexandre.henriques@neuro-sys.com

**†Present address:**
Alexandre Henriques
Neuro-sys SAS, Gardanne, France

Amyotrophic lateral sclerosis (ALS) is a multifactorial and fatal neurodegenerative disease. Growing evidence connects sphingolipid metabolism to the pathophysiology of ALS. In particular, levels of ceramides, glucosylceramides, and gangliosides are dysregulated in the central nervous system and at the neuromuscular junctions of both animal models and patients. Glucosylceramide is the main precursor of complex glycosphingolipids that is degraded by lysosomal (GBA1) or non-lysosomal (GBA2) glucocerebrosidase. Here, we report that GBA2, but not GBA1, activity is markedly increased in the spinal cord, of SOD1$^{G86R}$ mice, an animal model of familial ALS, even before disease onset. We therefore investigated the effects of ambroxol hydrochloride, a known GBA2 inhibitor, in SOD1$^{G86R}$ mice. A presymptomatic administration of ambroxol hydrochloride, in the drinking water, delayed disease onset, protecting neuromuscular junctions, and the number of functional spinal motor neurons. When administered at disease onset, ambroxol hydrochloride delayed motor function decline, protected neuromuscular junctions, and extended overall survival of the SOD1$^{G86R}$ mice. In addition, ambroxol hydrochloride improved motor recovery and muscle re-innervation after transient sciatic nerve injury in non-transgenic mice and promoted axonal elongation in an *in vitro* model of motor unit. Our study suggests that ambroxol hydrochloride promotes and protects motor units and improves axonal plasticity, and that this generic compound is a promising drug candidate for ALS.

**Keywords: ambroxol, GBA2, glucocerebrosidase, ALS, neuromuscular junction, glucosylceramide**

## INTRODUCTION

Amyotrophic lateral sclerosis (ALS) is a fatal neurodegenerative disease characterized by a loss of cortical motor neurons in the motor cortex and spinal motor neurons located in the brainstem and in the spinal cord with denervation. Considered to be the most common motor neuron disease in adults, ALS leads to progressive paralysis, muscle atrophy, fasciculation, and spasticity and affects the central nervous system and peripheral organs (Schmitt et al., 2014). ALS is associated with sporadic forms (90%) and familial form (10%). Mutations on genes encoding superoxide dismutase 1 (SOD1), TAR DNA-binding protein of 43 kDa (TDP-43) and fused in sarcoma (FUS), and repeat expansions in chromosome 9 open reading frame 72 (C9ORF72) (Lattante et al., 2015) are now documented. It is reported that lipid metabolism in ALS patient has a major impact on the disease severity. A high incidence of dyslipidemia and hypermetabolism is present in ALS patients (Desport et al., 2001; Funalot et al., 2009) and hypermetabolism and high low-density lipoprotein (LDL)/high-density lipoprotein (HDL) ratios or high body mass index are associated with better prognosis and slower disease progression (Dupuis et al., 2008; Paganoni et al., 2011; Jésus et al., 2018). The causes of the metabolic dysfunctions in ALS remain unknown and could result from central pathologies combined with peripheral alterations.

Metabolomic studies have now shown that recent human evolution has marked changes in lipid metabolism in muscle and brain to support increased metabolic activity (Noakes and Spedding, 2012; Bozek et al., 2014). Beyond their role in energy metabolism, lipids and particularly sphingolipids are modulators of cellular signaling pathways and participate in the maintenance and repair of the various components of the motor axis such as neurons and muscles. Our transcriptomic studies on muscle biopsies in ALS patients showed a significant increase in the expression of the UGCG gene (UDP-glucose ceramide glucosyltransferase), encoding the sphingolipid metabolism enzyme that synthesizes glucosylceramide (GlcCer) (Henriques et al., 2015; Dodge, 2017; Henriques et al., 2017). It has been shown in ALS that GlcCer and ceramide levels are deregulated (Cutler et al., 2002; Dodge et al., 2015; Henriques et al., 2015; Henriques et al., 2018). These data suggest that GlcCer plays a key role in the pathophysiology of ALS. We performed a lipidomic analysis of different tissues of SOD1$^{G86R}$ mice, an animal model of ALS, and we observed a complete rearrangement of the main lipid classes, including sphingolipids like GlcCer and ceramides in the muscles and spinal cords of SOD1$^{G86R}$ mice, before the onset of the disease. Inhibition of GlcCer synthesis by administration of a UGCG inhibitor (AMP-DMN) significantly delays functional recovery after sciatic nerve injury (Henriques et al., 2015; Henriques et al., 2018). GlcCer is the precursor of gangliosides, and this hydrolysis is performed by GBA1 and GBA2, two beta-glucocerebrosidases (GCases).

Our previous results have shown a beneficial effect for SOD1$^{G86R}$ mice after inhibition of GlcCer degradation (Henriques et al., 2017). Partial inhibition of GlcCer degradation with a low dose of conduritol B epoxide (CBE) (10 mg/kg/d) delays disease onset and improves motor functions in presymptomatic and in symptomatic SOD1$^{G86R}$ mice. Pharmacological inhibition of GCase by CBE preserves motor neuron number and the neuromuscular junctions (NMJs) in SOD1$^{G86R}$ mice. Furthermore, CBE promotes recovery after sciatic nerve injury *in vivo* (Henriques et al., 2017). Conversely, a high dose CBE (100 mg/kg/d) induced neuronal toxicity and can be used to inhibit the lysosomal GCase to induce a chemical model of Gaucher's diseases (Kanfer et al., 1975; Vardi et al., 2016). Indeed, CBE is an inhibitor of lysosomal GCase (GBA1) and, less potently, of the non-lysosomal GCase (GBA2) (Ridley et al., 2013). Moreover, loss-of-function mutations of GBA1 are a major cause of hereditary Parkinson's Disease (PD), while the activation of beta-GCase increases alpha-synuclein clearance and lysosomal function in dopaminergic neurons (Schapira, 2015; Mazzulli et al., 2016; Stojkovska et al., 2018); thus, there may be a risk of PD with GBA1 inhibitors.

GBA2 is localized at the plasma membrane and as a membrane-associated protein at the Golgi apparatus and at the endoplasmic reticulum (Woeste and Wachten, 2017). Loss of function of GBA2 is associated with hereditary spastic paraplegia suggesting that the regulation of GlcCer at the plasma membrane and/or at intracellular organelles is important for the maintenance of motor functions, even if the role of GBA2 in the central nervous system remains poorly understood.

Our approach was therefore to inhibit the non-lysosomal GBA2 without inhibiting GBA1. Among the safe molecules able to cross the blood–brain barrier (BBB), ambroxol hydrochloride (AMB) has been extensively studied (Albin and Dauer, 2014; McNeill et al., 2014; Ambrosi et al., 2015; Migdalska-Richards et al., 2016b; Migdalska-Richards et al., 2017; O'Regan et al., 2017). In our study, we confirmed that AMB inhibited GBA2 activity. We have then investigated the effects of AMB *in vivo*, in a transgenic model of ALS and on non-transgenic mice to determine whether it could improve the lifespan of SOD1$^{G86R}$ mice and stimulate the plasticity of the neuromuscular junctions (NMJs).

## RESULTS

### GBA2 Activity Is Increased in Pre-Symptomatic SOD1$^{G86R}$ Mice

GlcCer is a precursor of complex glycosphingolipids. It is synthetized from ceramide by the GlcCer synthase and degraded by GBA1 or GBA2, two GCases. We previously reported that inhibition of GCase activity by a low dose of CBE is neuroprotective in the SOD1$^{G86R}$ mice (Henriques et al., 2017). CBE has inhibitory activities on lysosomal and GBA2 activity (Ridley et al., 2013).

Here, we sought to measure GCase activities at specific pH, and in presence or absence of detergent, to determine whether GBA1 (pH = 4.6, with detergent) and GBA2 (pH = 5.8, no detergent) activities are dysregulated in tissues of SOD1$^{G86R}$ mice (Witte et al., 2010). At a symptomatic disease stage, characterized by moderate motor dysfunctions, GBA1 activity was not significantly altered in SOD1$^{G86R}$ when compared to control non-transgenic mice (**Figure 1A**). However, GBA2 activity was strongly increased in the spinal cord of SOD1$^{G86R}$ mice at 105d (symptomatic) but not in muscle or in liver. This increase in GBA2 activity was also observed in presymptomatic SOD1$^{G86R}$ mice (**Supplementary Figure 1A**). The GBA1 activity was not changed at either time point. GBA1 and GBA2 share common enzymatic activity but differ in structure, thus allowing the use of specific inhibitors. The effects of AMB on GCase activities *in vitro* have been compared to those of CBE. As previously reported (Ridley et al., 2013), CBE had a strong inhibitory effect on the GBA1 activity being 10-fold less potent on GBA2 activity (**Figure 1B**). AMB has been reported to inhibit the GBA2 activity (Maegawa et al., 2009), which was confirmed in a dose-dependent manner (**Figure 1C**). Taken together, these results show that GBA2 activity is increased in SOD1$^{G86R}$ mice, already

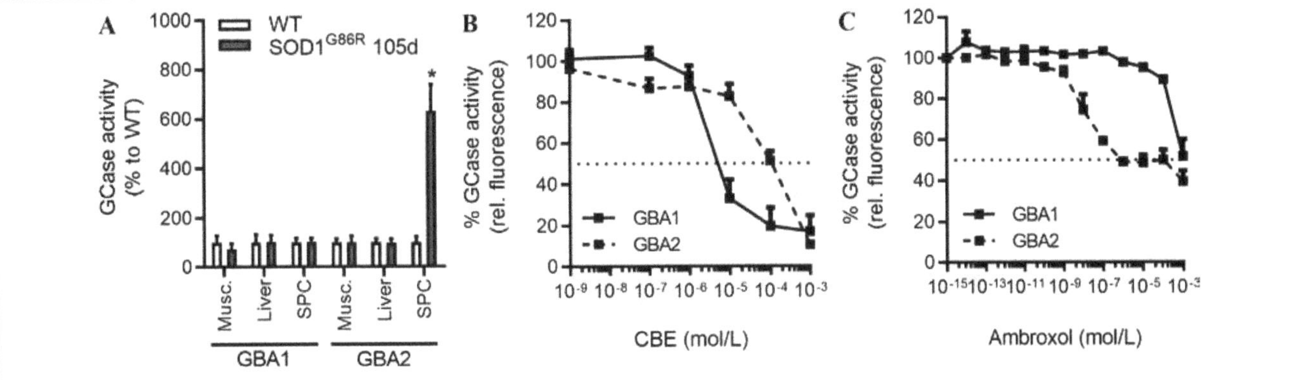


**FIGURE 1 |** GCase activities in symptomatic SOD1$^{G86R}$ mice. **(A)** GCase activity in different tissues of SOD1$^{G86R}$ and wild type (WT) mice at 105d ($n$ = 5–9/tissues, $^{*}p < 0.05$). **(B)** GCase [glucocerebrosidase (GBA)] activity after conduritol B epoxide (CBE) dose-response ($n$ = 6/group). **(C)** GCase (GBA) activity after ambroxol hydrochloride (AMB) dose-response in liver tissue ($n$ = 4/group).

at pre-symptomatic disease stage, and that AMB can inhibit its activity.

## Ambroxol Hydrochloride Delays Disease Onset, Preserve the Integrity of Motor Units, and Increases Survival of SOD1$^{G86R}$ Mice

AMB was administrated to presymptomatic SOD1$^{G86R}$ mice, to determine whether it could influence disease onset and loss of motor functions in a preventive manner. Grip strength was used as an indicator of muscle strength. SOD1$^{G86R}$ mice were treated from 75 days to 95 days of age, and body mass and muscle strength were evaluated every other day (**Figure 2**). In the first cohort of presymptomatic SOD1$^{G86R}$ mice, AMB had no significant effects on the body mass of treated mice (**Figure 2A**); however, it strongly improved the muscle strength of SOD1$^{G86R}$ mice and significantly delayed of disease onset, defined as a drop of more than 20% of the mouse maximal strength (**Figure 2B**). These results were replicated in a separate cohort of SOD1$^{G86R}$ mice, using the same experimental conditions (**Supplementary Figure 2**). Indeed, an improved muscle strength and a delayed disease onset were observed after AMB administration in the second cohort.

At 95 days of age, neurodegeneration of motor neurons is detected in the lumbar region of the spinal cord of SOD1$^{G86R}$ mice (Henriques et al., 2017). As compared to the WT mice, 40% of motor neurons (MNs) are lost at this time point. The number of MNs in the lumbar region of the spinal cord was significantly higher in SOD1$^{G86R}$ mice treated with AMB (**Figures 2C, D**), suggesting that presymptomatic administration of AMB delays neurodegeneration. In order to determine whether the spared MNs have axonal projection to hind limb muscles, fluorogold, a retrograde tracer, has been injected in gastrocnemius and tibialis anterior muscles. SOD1$^{G86R}$ mice treated with AMB had more MNs-positive for fluorogold (**Figures 2E, F**).

Muscle strength is dependent on the innervation status of muscles. The integrity of NMJs was assessed by immunohistochemistry with the overlapping of post-synaptic cluster of nicotinic acetylcholine receptors (nAChR) and the axonal markers neurofilament and synaptophysin. AMB has significantly protected muscle innervation in SOD1$^{G86R}$ mice, as they had almost two times more NMJs than the vehicle group, at 95 days of age (**Figure 2G, H**). These results suggest that presymptomatic administration of AMB delays disease onset by improving the integrity of the motor units.

Next, we sought to determine whether a later administration of AMB, at disease onset, could slow down disease progression and improve survival of SOD1$^{G86R}$ mice. AMB was administrated to SOD1$^{G86R}$ mice and wild-type littermates, starting at 95 days of age. From 95 days of age, motor symptoms progress rapidly in SOD1$^{G86R}$ mice, and they reach disease end stage around 110 days of age. Body mass, muscle strength, and overall survival were monitored to follow the progression of ALS symptoms (**Figure 3**). After administration of AMB, the decline in body mass was limited, and SOD1$^{G86R}$ mice were heavier, although this effect was transient (**Figure 3A**). A clear improvement of muscle strength was observed, starting from day 101, in SOD1$^{G86R}$ mice treated with AMB when compared to the SOD1$^{G86R}$ vehicle group (**Figure 3B**). Most importantly, survival of SOD1$^{G86R}$ mice was significantly increased by 6 days after administration of AMB (**Figure 3C**).

Altogether, these results show that AMB delays disease progression when the treatment is initiated at disease onset.

## Ambroxol Hydrochloride Improves Motor Recovery After Sciatic Nerve Injury in Non-Transgenic Mice

We have previously demonstrated that partial inhibition of GCase activity with CBE improves axonal elongation *in vitro* and *in vivo* recoveries after sciatic nerve injury (Henriques et al., 2017).

We hypothesized that AMB could exert similar pro-regenerative effects. First, we investigated whether AMB could enhance axonal elongation and the formation of NMJs, in an *in vitro* model of motor units, based on a co-culture of myoblasts and spinal cord explants (Combes et al., 2015). This *in vitro* model allows the maturation of axons and the formation of NMJs, as

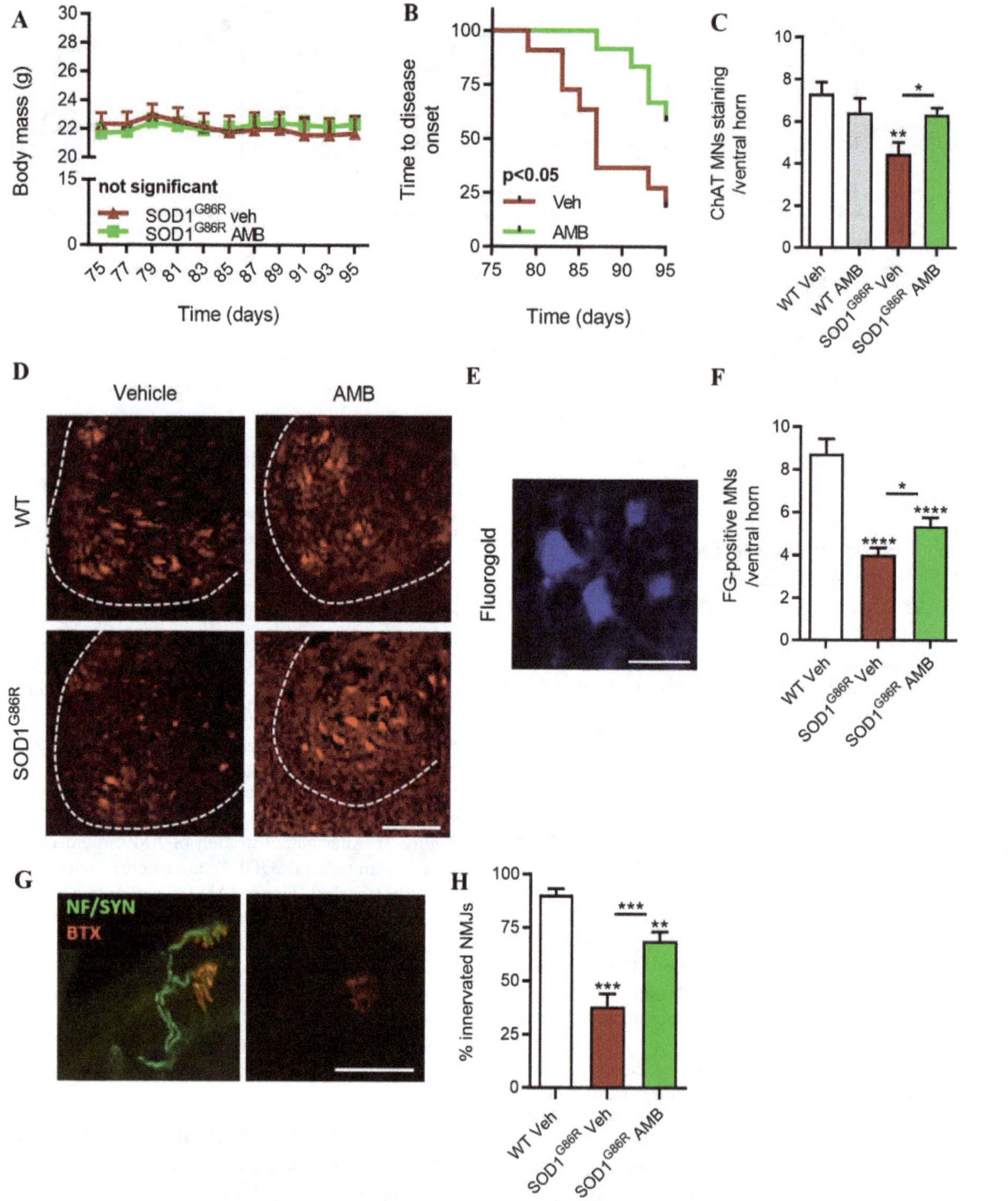


**FIGURE 2 |** AMB improves motor functions and preserves neuromuscular junction and the functional motor neurons (MNs) in pre-symptomatic SOD1$^{G86R}$ mice. **(A)** Body mass evolution in SOD1$^{G86R}$ mice after AMB treatment (not significant, $n$ = 11–12/group). **(B)** Kaplan–Meier showing time to onset of muscle strength loss in SOD1$^{G86R}$ mice ($p$ < 0.05, $n$ = 11–12/group). **(C)** Quantification of choline acetyl transferase (ChAT)-positive cells located in the ventral horn of the spinal cord and having a size bigger than 400 µm$^2$ ($n$ = 5/group). **(D)** Representative pictures of the ventral horn of the L1–L3 lumbar area, after immunostaining with ChAT (red), a marker specific for spinal motor neurons. Ventral horns are delimited by dashed lines. Scale bar = 100 µm. **(E)** Representative picture of retrogradely labeled spinal MNs after fluorogold (FG) injection in hindlimb muscles. Scale bar = 50 µm. **(F)** Quantification of FG-positive MNs in ventral horn of the spinal cord ($n$ = 10/group, $^*p$ < 0.05; $^{****}p$ < 0.00001, one-way ANOVA test). **(G)** Representative pictures of innervated (left panel) and denervated (right panel) of neuromuscular junctions in SOD1$^{G86R}$ mice (bungarotoxin, BTX, red; neurofilament and synaptophysin, green). Scale bar = 50 µm. **(H)** Neuromuscular junctions (NMJ) integrity in tibialis anterior muscle ($^{**}p$ < 0.01; $^{***}p$ < 0.001).

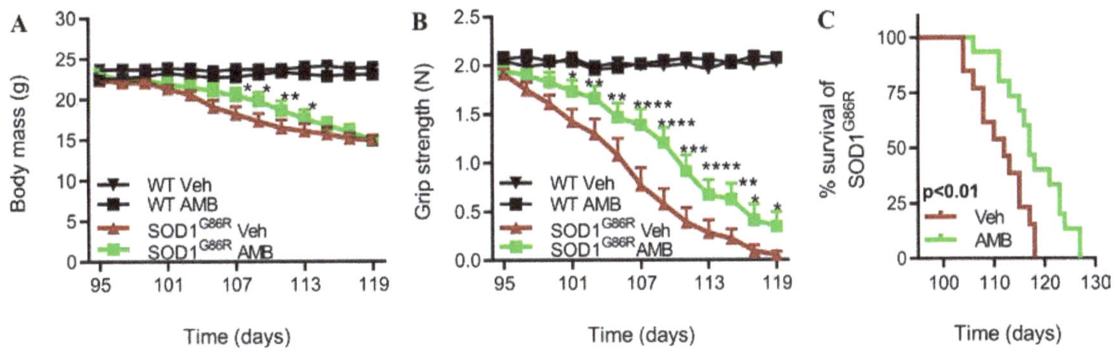


**FIGURE 3 |** AMB delays disease onset and improves motor functions in symptomatic SOD1$^{G86R}$ mice. **(A)** Body mass evolution in SOD1$^{G86R}$ and WT mice ($n$ = 12–15/group). **(B)** Muscle strength evolution in SOD1$^{G86R}$ and WT ($n$ = 12–15/group). **(C)** Kaplan–Meier analysis of SOD1$^{G86R}$ mice survival ($n$ = 13–15/group, $^{*}p < 0.05$; $^{**}p < 0.01$; $^{***}p < 0.001$; $^{****}p < 0.0001$).

observed by muscle contraction triggered by the application of acetylcholine. The presence of NMJs was confirmed by the colocalization of the axonal neurofilament and the presence of post-synaptic nicotinic acetylcholine receptors (**Figure 4A, Supplementary Figure 3**).

The neurite network was significantly longer in presence of the highest dose of AMB (100 µM) (**Figure 4B**). This effect corresponds to a +45% increase when compared to the vehicle group. Lower doses of AMB did not promote neurite elongation.

AMB was able to significantly increase the number of *in vitro* NMJs, determined by the number clusterized nAChRs, in a linear dose-dependent manner, at doses ranging from 10 to 100 µM. The effect of AMB was therefore stronger on the formation of NMJs than on the elongation of axons, in this model (**Figure 4C**).

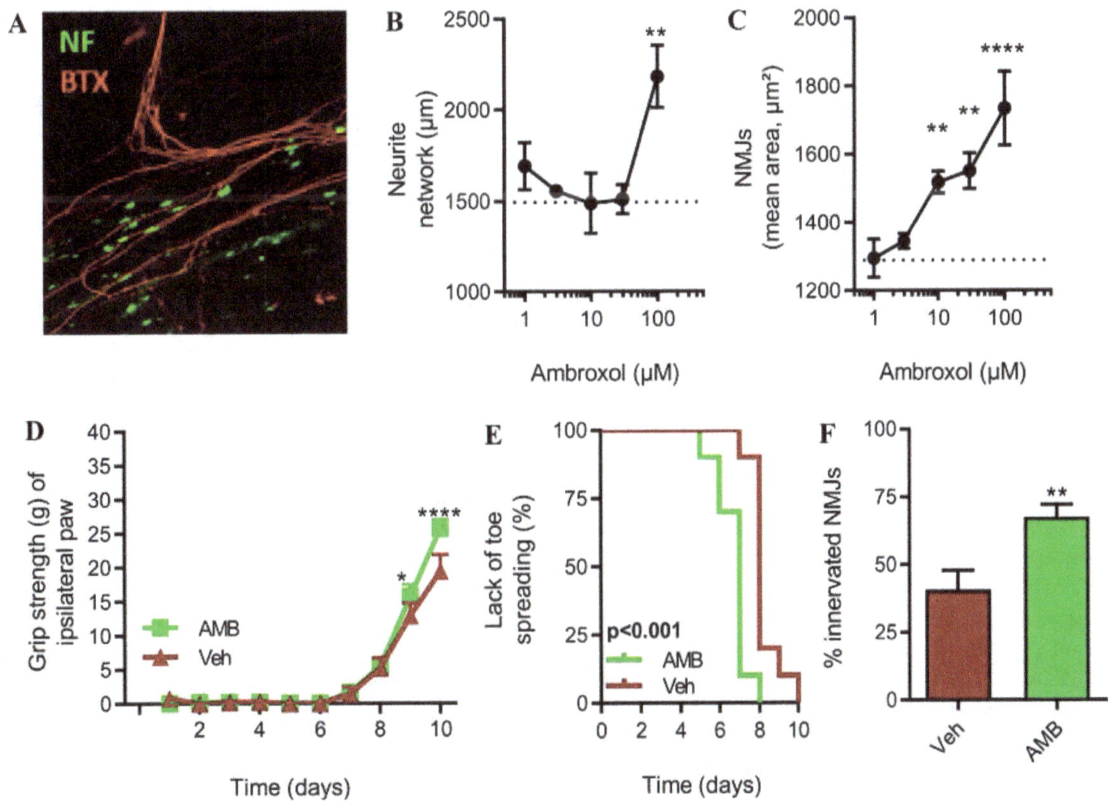


**FIGURE 4 |** Inhibition of GlcCer degradation by AMB improves *in vivo* axonal plasticity and nerve regeneration after sciatic nerve crush study in non-transgenic mice. **(A)** Representative picture of *in vitro* neuromuscular junctions (NMJs). **(B)** Total length of neurofilament-positive neurites and **(C)** total area NMJs ($n$ = 5/group). **(D)** Muscle strength of ipsilateral hind paws ($n$ = 10/group, $^{*}p < 0.05$; $^{****}p < 0.0001$). **(E)** Kaplan–Meier showing time to observable toe spreading after sciatic nerve injury ($n$ = 10/group, $p < 0.001$). **(F)** NMJ integrity in tibialis anterior muscle ($n$ = 10/group, $^{**}p < 0.01$).

To further evaluate the pro-regenerative effect of AMB on the motor units, we have subjected non-transgenic mice to peripheral nerve injury, to follow-up functional recovery, such as muscle strength and toe spreading, and the number of functional NMJs after treatment with AMB. Upon treatment, mice recovered significantly faster when compared to the control group. Indeed, on days 9 and 10, muscle strength of the injured hindlimb was statistically higher after application of AMB (**Figure 4D**). In a second and independent cohort, we have confirmed the beneficial effect of AMB (3 mM) on functional recovery after sciatic injury. The regenerative effect of AMB was also observed at a dose of 1 mM in this model (**Supplementary Figure 4**). Spontaneous toe spreading is lost after hindlimb muscle denervation. The recovery of toe spreading is a proxy for early sign of reinnervation and was monitored every day. AMB caused a modest but significant effect, as the mice recovered between 1 to 2 days earlier as compared to the control group (**Figure 4E**). Most importantly, 10 days after injury, the number of innervated neuromuscular junctions was 70% greater after application of AMB, suggesting that AMB promotes the formation of new NMJs, which may strongly participate in the pro-regenerative effect of this compound (**Figure 4F**).

## DISCUSSION

### Glycosphingolipids and Motor Axis

Dysregulation of GlcCer and other glycosphingolipids (e.g., GM1a) was previously reported by us and others in ALS patients and in animal models (Dodge et al., 2015; Henriques et al., 2015; Dodge, 2017; Henriques et al., 2017; Henriques et al., 2018).

GlcCer is degraded by GBA1 or GBA2 beta-GCases. Growing evidence suggests a tight connection between GBA2 activity and motor functions, as full loss of function of GBA2 is a cause of hereditary spastic paraplegia type 46 (SPG46) (Woeste and Wachten, 2017; Woeste et al., 2019). Conversely, pharmacological inhibition of GBA2 activity has been shown to improve the motor phenotype (e.g., motor coordination) of an animal model of Niemann's Pick disease (Marques et al., 2015). Moreover, GM1a, a downstream metabolite of GlcCer, is detected on the cell surface of motor axons and at nerve endings in NMJs. The presence of anti-GM1 autoantibodies has been associated with multifocal motor neuropathy and the acute motor axonal form of Guillain-Barré, suggesting a key role for glycosphingolipids in the maintenance of motor axons and possibly NMJs.

We have shown that inhibition of GCase by CBE causes a concentration-dependent increase in GlcCer, and in the downstream glycosphingolipid GM1a, which was associated with pro-survival and pro-regenerative effects. Treatment with CBE fully prevented loss of GM1a/CTB staining at NMJs in tibialis anterior muscle of SOD1$^{G86R}$ mice, associated with delayed loss in grip strength (Henriques et al., 2017). Interestingly, the inhibition of GlcCer synthase (GCS) accelerates functional decline. Inhibition of GCS also delays the recovery to spinal crush in non-transgenic mice. Thus, a coherent picture emerges in ALS where inhibiting GCase activity and increasing the pool of glycosphingolipids, presumably at the NMJs, are beneficial.

### Ambroxol Improved Motor Function in SOD1$^{G86R}$ Mice

Our results showed that GBA2 activity is increased in the spinal cord of SOD1$^{G86R}$ mice, even at the presymptomatic disease stage, which could impair the metabolism of glycosphingolipids and later contribute to the development of motor dysfunctions. Here, we propose ambroxol as a drug candidate for ALS. Ambroxol is known to inhibit of GBA2 activity, mainly catalyzed by GBA2. By inhibiting GBA2, we aimed to prevent the hydrolysis of GlcCer located outside the lysosome, mainly at the plasma membrane, the endoplasmic reticulum, and/or at the Golgi apparatus (Maegawa et al., 2009; Shanmuganathan and Britz-McKibbin, 2011). Our study showed that ambroxol delayed the decline of motor functions and protected motor neurons from degeneration in a transgenic animal model of ALS. Most importantly, ambroxol was able to maintain the functionality of spinal motor neurons in the SOD1$^{G86R}$ mice. For these promising pre-clinical effects, ambroxol has recently been given orphan drug status for ALS by the European Medical Agency.

### Clinical Relevance of Ambroxol for ALS

Ambroxol is marketed as an expectorant and mucolytic for lung diseases and for sore throat, with local anesthetic effects. In the CNS, ambroxol is potentially an inhibitor of sodium (Nav1.8) and calcium channels, with claimed anti-glutamatergic properties. Evidence suggests that ambroxol has direct anti-oxidative properties which could translate into beneficial effects in ALS (reviewed by Weiser, 2008).

In addition to its effects on GBA2, ambroxol is also known to bind the enzyme GBA1 in the cytosol and to correct enzyme folding and to improve its addressing to the acidic environment of the lysosome where the drug dissociates, thereby increasing GBA1 activity. The chaperone effect on ambroxol on GBA1 is combined with a positive modulation of GBA1 expression level (Magalhaes et al., 2018). It cannot be excluded that ambroxol could stimulate lysosomal-dependent pathway of protein clearance in ALS (Boland et al., 2018), as ambroxol reduces the alpha-synucleinopathy in an *in vivo* model of PD (Migdalska-Richards et al., 2016b).

Gaucher's disease is caused by genetic mutations of GBA1, resulting in the loss of GBA1 activity (Kanfer et al., 1975; Vardi et al., 2016). In addition, mutations on GBA1 and/or reduced expression of the protein are an important risk factor of PD (Barrett et al., 2013).

Recently, high dose of ambroxol was able to decrease the severity of neurological symptoms of patients with the neuropathic form of Gaucher's disease, suggesting that oral administration of ambroxol successfully target the metabolism of glycosphingolipids in the central nervous system (Narita et al., 2016). Two other clinical trials are currently investigating the effects of ambroxol in PD (NCT02941822; NCT02914366).

## Ambroxol Improved the Plasticity of Motor Units

We have also shown that ambroxol hastened functional recovery in a non-transgenic animal model of sciatic nerve injury. Given the modest effect on the kinetic of recovery, the effects of ambroxol are most likely due to an increased ability to rebuilt NMJs. Indeed, in presence of ambroxol, the percentage of re-innervated NMJs was twice higher than that in the vehicle group. Moreover, the *in vitro* co-culture model of motor units provided similar results as ambroxol strongly increased the formation of NMJs but modestly promoted axonal elongation. It indicates that ambroxol was able to stimulate the formation of NMJs. This effect could explain the beneficial outcomes in the SOD1$^{G86R}$ mice through motor axonal sprouting and muscle re-innervation.

Altogether, our results further connected the glycosphingolipid metabolism to the pathophysiology of ALS and indicated that inhibition of GBA2 may be a novel target for ALS.

# METHODS

## Animal Care and Maintenance

FVB/N non-transgenic female mice derived from Charles River were used to perform nerve sciatic injury experiment.

For others' experiments, FVB/N female mice, overexpressing the SOD1$^{G86R}$ (Ripps et al., 1995), were generated and maintained in our animal facility at 23°C with 12-h light/dark cycle. They had water and regular A04 rodent chow *ad libitum*. AMB (3 mM, Sigma-Aldrich) was given by drinking water for mice treated, and vehicle mice was treated with animal facility water. For the presymptomatic stage study, the treatment started at 75 days of age and stopped at 95 days of age. For the symptomatic stage study (survival experiment), the treatment started to 95 days of age and stopped when mice were euthanized. Mice showing strong motor dysfunction at 93 days of age were not included in the symptomatic cohort. Mice were euthanized when animals were paralyzed and unable to roll over within 5 s after being pushed on their back. For euthanasia, mice were intracardially perfused with PBS 1X at 4°C after intraperitoneal injection with Dolethal (120 mg/kg).

## Motor Assessment

Body mass was analyzed on a daily basis. Muscle strength (mean of three tests, grip test, Bioseb, Chaville, France) and the inverted grid test to assess the motor performance and coordination of mice were analyzed every 2 days. Onset of muscle strength loss was defined as a drop of more than 10% of the mouse maximal strength.

## Sciatic Nerve Injury

Peripheral nerve injury was performed in order to induce muscle denervation and axonal regeneration. Wild-type mice were anesthetized with ketamine chlorohydrate (100 mg/kg) and xylazine (5 mg/kg). The sciatic nerve was exposed at mid-thigh level and lesioned with fine forceps for 30 s. The skin incision was sutured, and mice were allowed to recover. The hind limb, contralateral to the lesion, served as control. Mice were treated with AMB (3 mM) for 13 days, starting the day before surgery. Mice were followed on a daily basis. Mice were sacrificed by intraperitoneal injection with Doléthal (120 mg/kg) and intracardially perfused with PBS at 4°C.

## Retrograde Labeling

Mice were treated with AMB (3 mM in drinking water) or with the vehicle solution (regular drinking water) from 75d of age at 95d of age. Mice were anesthetized at 94 days of age with ketamine chlorohydrate (100 mg/kg) and xylazine (5 mg/kg), and their hind limb muscles were injected with fluorogold (hydroxystilbamidine bis[methanesulfonate], Sigma-Aldrich; 10 mg/ml in PBS, 10% DMSO) FG with Hamilton seringue (26 gauge, 10 μl), and tissues were collected 24 h after injection.

## Motor Neurons Counting

Tissues were fixed paraformaldehyde 4% and stored in PBS at 4°C until further use. Lumbar segments L1–L3 fixed in paraformaldehyde 4% were used for studying the number of motor neurons innervating hind limb muscle. After cryoprotection in 30% sucrose, coronal sections 16 μm thick from L1–L3 spinal segment were realized with a cryostat and were either stained with an anti-choline acetylcholine transferase (1/100, Millipore, France) and an alexa594-conjugated goat (1/200, Jackson ImmunoResearch, Suffolk, UK) antibodies, either mount on slides for Fluorogold counting. All neurons located in the ventral horn, which were >400 μm$^2$ in size and ChAT-positive, were considered as alpha motor neurons. 10 sections of spinal cord were counted, and cell area of motor neurons was measured with ApoTome 2 (Zeiss) microscope.

## Neuromuscular Junction Labeling

Tissues were fixed paraformaldehyde 4% and stored in PBS at 4°C until further use. Under a binocular microscope, tibialis anterior muscle fibers were prepared into thin bundles. Neuromuscular junction morphology was studied by labeling of the acetylcholine receptors with rhodamine-conjugated α-bungarotoxin (1/400, Sigma-Aldrich), and labeling of nerve terminals was performed with a rabbit polyclonal anti-synaptophysin antibody diluted 1/50 (Abcam, Cambridge, UK), and anti-neurofilament diluted 1/50. For immunofluorescence of terminal nerve, Alexa-conjugated goat anti-rabbit IgG diluted 1/500 (Jackson ImmunoResearch, Suffolk, UK) was used. Muscle bundles were mounted into slides, prior to fluorescence microscopy (ApoTome 2, Zeiss). NMJs were considered as denervated when the presynaptic nerve terminal was absent from the postsynaptic region.

## Beta-Glucosidase Activity

Tissues were snap frozen in liquid nitrogen and stored at −80°C until further use. Frozen tissues were lysed with a TissuLyser (Qiagen, CA) and suspended in phosphate potassium (pH7) buffer extraction. After centrifugation (12,000 rpm for 15 min at 4°C), the supernatants were transferred to new tubes and stored at −80°C. The bicinchoninic acid assay (BCA) method, a colorimetric assay method, was used to measured protein level with a BCA range (Interchim). A GBA buffer was used and adapted according to the enzymatic activity desired (McIlvaine buffer, 150 mM). For GBA1, enzymatic reaction was carried out with the GBA buffer pH4.6 and adding 0.1% triton and 0.1% BSA. For GBA2, enzymatic reaction was carried out with the GBA buffer pH5.8 and adding 0.1% BSA. After inhibitor addition and fluorescent agent 4-methylumbelliferone addition (4-MU, Sigma-Aldrich), samples were incubated 2 h at 37°C. For reading results, excitation was carried out at 360-nm excitation, and absorbance was measured at 445 nm emission (TriStar LB 941, Berthold Technologies).

### Co-Culture of Spinal Cord Explants and Myoblasts

The rat spinal cord–human muscle co-culture was performed as described previously (Combes et al., 2015). Human myoblast was grown on 96-well plate in a mix of MEM and M199 medium, supplemented with glutamine 2 mM, insulin, epidermal growth factor, basic fibroblast growth factor, fetal bovine serum 10%, and penicillin/streptomycin. Spinal cord explants with dorsal roots of 13-day-old Wistar rat embryos (Janvier, Le Genest-St-IsIe, France) were dissected and grown on the muscle monolayer. The co-cultures were maintained in a mix medium (MEM/M199), with 5% fetal calf serum, insulin, glutamine, and penicillin streptomycin. Ambroxol treatment was initiated when the spinal cord explants were added to the muscle monolayer and lasted 27 days. The treatment was renewed every other day during medium change. A total of 10 wells per conditions have been initiated. *In vitro* NMJs and neurite network were identified by immunostaining with alpha-bungarotoxin coupled with Alexa 488 and with a primary antibody against neurofilament 200 kD from mouse revealed with an anti-mouse Alexa 568. Sixty pictures have been automatically taken using same acquisition parameter with ImageXpress (Molecular Device) at 10× magnification and were analyzed with MetaXpress (Molecular Device). After segmentation of the pictures (**Supplementary Figure 3**), the total length of the neurite network and the total area of clustered nAChR were measured.

## AUTHOR CONTRIBUTIONS

Conceived and designed the experiments: AB, J-PL, AH; Performed the experiments: AB, CQ, AM, AH; Analysis and interpretation of the data: AB, NC, MS, J-PL, AH; Contributed reagents/materials/analysis tools: MS, J-PL; Wrote, discussed and approved the final version of the manuscript: AB, CQ, AM, NC, MS, J-PL, AH.

## FUNDING

The work was funded by "Association pour la Recherche et le Développement de Moyens de Lutte contre les Maladies Neurodégénératives" (AREMANE, J.P.L.), the "Association française contre les myopathies" (AFM, JPL). SRS contributed with salary and reagents. J-PL and MS are currently receiving funds from Fight MND foundation.

## ACKNOWLEDGEMENTS

We thank Annie Picchinenna for her help in the project.

### Statistical Analysis

Data are expressed as the mean ± SEM and were analyzed with GraphPad Prism version 6.0 software. Student's *t* test was used to compare two groups, and ANOVA followed by Fisher's LSD test was applied to compare more than two groups. Grip strength curves were analyzed with two-way ANOVA, and survival curves were analyzed with log-rank test. Differences with *p*-values of <0.05 were considered significant.

## REFERENCES

Albin, R. L., and Dauer, W. T. (2014). Magic shotgun for Parkinson's disease? *Brain* 137, 1274–1275. doi: 10.1093/brain/awu076

Ambrosi, G., Ghezzi, C., Zangaglia, R., Levandis, G., Pacchetti, C., and Blandini, F. (2015). Ambroxol-induced rescue of defective glucocerebrosidase is associated with increased LIMP-2 and saposin C levels in GBA1 mutant Parkinson's disease cells. *Neurobiol. Dis.* 82, 235–242. doi: 10.1016/j.nbd.2015.06.008

Barrett, M. J., Giraldo, P., Capablo, J. L., Alfonso, P., Irun, P., Garcia-Rodriguez, B., et al. (2013). Greater risk of parkinsonism associated with non-N370S GBA1 mutations. *J. Inherit. Metab. Dis.* 36, 575–580. doi: 10.1007/s10545-012-9527-5

Boland, B., Yu, W. H., Corti, O., Mollereau, B., Henriques, A., Bezard, E., et al. (2018). Promoting the clearance of neurotoxic proteins in neurodegenerative disorders of ageing. *Nat. Rev. Drug Discov.* 17, 660–688. doi: 10.1038/nrd.2018.109

Bozek, K., Wei, Y., Yan, Z., Liu, X., Xiong, J., Sugimoto, M., et al. (2014). Exceptional evolutionary divergence of human muscle and brain metabolomes parallels human cognitive and physical uniqueness. *PLoS Biol.* 12, e1001871. doi: 10.1371/journal.pbio.1001871

Combes, M., Poindron, P., and Callizot, N. (2015). Glutamate protects neuromuscular junctions from deleterious effects of β-amyloid peptide and conversely: an in vitro study in a nerve-muscle coculture. *J. Neurosci. Res.* 93, 633–643. doi: 10.1002/jnr.23524

Cutler, R. G., Pedersen, W. A., Camandola, S., Rothstein, J. D., and Mattson, M. P. (2002). Evidence that accumulation of ceramides and cholesterol esters mediates oxidative stress–induced death of motor neurons in amyotrophic lateral sclerosis. *Ann. Neurol.* 52, 448–457. doi: 10.1002/ana.10312

Desport, J. C., Preux, P. M., Magy, L., Boirie, Y., Vallat, J. M., Beaufrère, B., et al. (2001). Factors correlated with hypermetabolism in patients with amyotrophic lateral sclerosis. *Am. J. Clin. Nutr.* 74, 328–334. doi: 10.1093/ajcn/74.3.328

Dodge, J. C. (2017). Lipid involvement in neurodegenerative diseases of the motor system: insights from lysosomal storage diseases. *Front. Mol. Neurosci.* 10 (356), 1–14. doi: 10.3389/fnmol.2017.00356

Dodge, J. C., Treleaven, C. M., Pacheco, J., Cooper, S., Bao, C., Abraham, M., et al. (2015). Glycosphingolipids are modulators of disease pathogenesis in amyotrophic lateral sclerosis. *Proc. Natl. Acad. Sci.* 112, 8100–8105. doi: 10.1073/pnas.1508767112

Dupuis, L., Corcia, P., Fergani, A., Gonzalez De Aguilar, J. L., Bonnefont-Rousselot, D., Bittar, R., et al. (2008). Dyslipidemia is a protective factor in amyotrophic lateral sclerosis. *Neurology* 70 (13), 1004–1009. doi: 10.1212/01.wnl.0000285080.70324.27

Funalot, B., Desport, J.-C., Sturtz, F., Camu, W., and Couratier, P. (2009). High metabolic level in patients with familial amyotrophic lateral sclerosis. *Amyotroph. Lateral Scler.* 10, 113–117. doi: 10.1080/17482960802295192

Henriques, A., Croixmarie, V., Bouscary, A., Mosbach, A., Keime, C., Boursier-Neyret, C., et al. (2018). Sphingolipid metabolism is dysregulated at transcriptomic and metabolic levels in the spinal cord of an animal model of amyotrophic lateral sclerosis. *Front. Mol. Neurosci.* 10 (433), 1–14. doi: 10.3389/fnmol.2017.00433

Henriques, A., Croixmarie, V., Priestman, D. A., Rosenbohm, A., Dirrig-Grosch, S., D'Ambra, E., et al. (2015). Amyotrophic lateral sclerosis and denervation alter sphingolipids and up-regulate glucosylceramide synthase. *Hum. Mol. Genet.* 24, 7390–7405. doi: 10.1093/hmg/ddv439

Henriques, A., Huebecker, M., Blasco, H., Keime, C., Andres, C. R., Corcia, P., et al. (2017). Inhibition of β-glucocerebrosidase activity preserves motor unit integrity in a mouse model of amyotrophic lateral sclerosis. *Sci. Rep.* 7 (5235), 1–15. doi: 10.1038/s41598-017-05313-0

Jésus, P., Fayemendy, P., Nicol, M., Lautrette, G., Sourisseau, H., Preux, P.-M., et al. (2018). Hypermetabolism is a deleterious prognostic factor in patients with amyotrophic lateral sclerosis. *Eur. J. Neurol.* 25, 97–104. doi: 10.1111/ene.13468

Kanfer, J. N., Legler, G., Sullivan, J., Raghavan, S. S., and Mumford, R. A. (1975). The Gaucher mouse. *Biochem. Biophys. Res. Commun.* 67, 85–90. doi: 10.1016/0006-291X(75)90286-7

Lattante, S., Ciura, S., Rouleau, G. A., and Kabashi, E. (2015). Defining the genetic connection linking amyotrophic lateral sclerosis (ALS) with frontotemporal dementia (FTD). *Trends Genet.* 31, 263–273. doi: 10.1016/j.tig.2015.03.005

Maegawa, G. H. B., Tropak, M. B., Buttner, J. D., Rigat, B. A., Fuller, M., Pandit, D., et al. (2009). Identification and characterization of ambroxol as an enzyme enhancement agent for gaucher disease. *J. Biol. Chem.* 284, 23502–23516. doi: 10.1074/jbc.M109.012393

Magalhaes, J., Gegg, M. E., Migdalska-Richards, A., and Schapira, A. H. (2018). Effects of ambroxol on the autophagy-lysosome pathway and mitochondria in primary cortical neurons. *Sci. Rep.* 8, 1385. doi: 10.1038/s41598-018-19479-8

Marques, A. R. A., Aten, J., Ottenhoff, R., van Roomen, C. P. A. A., Herrera Moro, D., Claessen, N., et al. (2015). Reducing GBA2 activity ameliorates neuropathology in niemann-pick Type C mice. *PLoS One* 10, e0135889. doi: 10.1371/journal.pone.0135889

Mazzulli, J. R., Zunke, F., Tsunemi, T., Toker, N. J., Jeon, S., Burbulla, L. F., et al. (2016). Activation of -glucocerebrosidase reduces pathological -synuclein and restores lysosomal function in parkinson's patient midbrain neurons. *J. Neurosci.* 36, 7693–7706. doi: 10.1523/JNEUROSCI.0628-16.2016

McNeill, A., Magalhaes, J., Shen, C., Chau, K.-Y., Hughes, D., Mehta, A., et al. (2014). Ambroxol improves lysosomal biochemistry in glucocerebrosidase mutation-linked Parkinson disease cells. *Brain* 137, 1481–1495. doi: 10.1093/brain/awu020

Migdalska-Richards, A., Daly, L., Bezard, E., and Schapira, A. H. V. (2016b). Ambroxol effects in glucocerebrosidase and α-synuclein transgenic mice: ambroxol in transgenic mice. *Ann. Neurol.* 80, 766–775. doi: 10.1002/ana.24790

Migdalska-Richards, A., Ko, W. K. D., Li, Q., Bezard, E., and Schapira, A. H. V. (2017). Oral ambroxol increases brain glucocerebrosidase activity in a nonhuman primate. *Synapse* 71, e21967. doi: 10.1002/syn.21967

Narita, A., Shirai, K., Itamura, S., Matsuda, A., Ishihara, A., Matsushita, K., et al. (2016). Ambroxol chaperone therapy for neuronopathic Gaucher disease: a pilot study. *Ann. Clin. Transl. Neurol.* 3, 200–215. doi: 10.1002/acn3.292

Noakes, T., and Spedding, M. (2012). Olympics: run for your life. *Nature* 487, 295–296. doi: 10.1038/487295a

O'Regan, G., deSouza, R.-M., Balestrino, R., and Schapira, A. H. (2017). Glucocerebrosidase Mutations in Parkinson Disease. *J. Park. Dis.* 7, 411–422. doi: 10.3233/JPD-171092

Paganoni, S., Deng, J., Jaffa, M., Cudkowicz, M. E., and Wills, A.-M. (2011). Body mass index, not dyslipidemia, is an independent predictor of survival in amyotrophic lateral sclerosis. *Muscle Nerve* 44, 20–24. doi: 10.1002/mus.22114

Ridley, C. M., Thur, K. E., Shanahan, J., Thillaiappan, N. B., Shen, A., Uhl, K., et al. (2013). β-Glucosidase 2 (GBA2) Activity and Imino Sugar Pharmacology. *J. Biol. Chem.* 288, 26052–26066. doi: 10.1074/jbc.M113.463562

Ripps, M. E., Huntley, G. W., Hof, P. R., Morrison, J. H., and Gordon, J. W. (1995). Transgenic mice expressing an altered murine superoxide dismutase gene provide an animal model of amyotrophic lateral sclerosis. *Proc. Natl. Acad. Sci.* 92, 689–693. doi: 10.1073/pnas.92.3.689

Schapira, A. H. V. (2015). Glucocerebrosidase and Parkinson disease: recent advances. *Mol. Cell. Neurosci.* 66, 37–42. doi: 10.1016/j.mcn.2015.03.013

Schmitt, F., Hussain, G., Dupuis, L., Loeffler, J.-P., and Henriques, A. (2014). A plural role for lipids in motor neuron diseases: energy, signaling and structure. *Front. Cell. Neurosci.* 8 (52), 1–10. doi: 10.3389/fncel.2014.00025

Shanmuganathan, M., and Britz-McKibbin, P. (2011). Inhibitor screening of pharmacological chaperones for lysosomal β-glucocerebrosidase by capillary electrophoresis. *Anal. Bioanal. Chem.* 399, 2843–2853. doi: 10.1007/s00216-011-4671-6

Stojkovska, I., Krainc, D., and Mazzulli, J. R. (2018). Molecular mechanisms of α-synuclein and GBA1 in Parkinson's disease. *Cell Tissue Res.* 373, 51–60. doi: 10.1007/s00441-017-2704-y

Vardi, A., Zigdon, H., Meshcheriakova, A., Klein, A. D., Yaacobi, C., Eilam,R., et al. (2016). Delineating pathological pathways in a chemically induced mouse model of Gaucher disease. *J. Pathol.* 239, 496–509. doi: 10.1002/path.4751

Weiser, T. (2008). Ambroxol: a CNS drug? *CNS Neurosci. Ther.* 14, 17–24. doi: 10.1111/j.1527-3458.2007.00032.x

Witte, M. D., Kallemeijn, W. W., Aten, J., Li, K.-Y., Strijland, A., Donker-Koopman, W. E., et al. (2010). Ultrasensitive in situ visualization of active glucocerebrosidase molecules. *Nat. Chem. Biol.* 6, 907–913. doi: 10.1038/nchembio.466

Woeste, M. A., and Wachten, D. (2017). The Enigmatic Role of GBA2 in controlling locomotor function. *Front. Mol. Neurosci.* 10 (386), 1–9. doi: 10.3389/fnmol.2017.00386

Woeste, M. A., Stern, S., Raju, D. N., Grahn, E., Dittmann, D., Gutbrod, K., et al. (2019). Species-specific differences in non-lysosomal glucosylceramidase GBA2 function underlie locomotor dysfunction arising from loss-of-function mutations. *J. Biol. Chem.* 294 (11), 3853–3871. doi: 10.1074/jbc.RA118.006311

14

# Novel Cellular Functions of Very Long Chain-Fatty Acids: Insight From ELOVL4 Mutations

*Ferenc Deák[1,2,3], Robert E. Anderson[1,2,4,5,6], Jennifer L. Fessler[6] and David M. Sherry[2,6,7]**

*[1] Department of Geriatric Medicine, Reynolds Oklahoma Center on Aging, University of Oklahoma Health Sciences Center, Oklahoma City, OK, United States, [2] Oklahoma Center for Neurosciences, University of Oklahoma Health Sciences Center, Oklahoma City, OK, United States, [3] Harold Hamm Diabetes Center, University of Oklahoma Health Sciences Center, Oklahoma City, OK, United States, [4] Dean McGee Eye Institute, University of Oklahoma Health Sciences Center, Oklahoma City, OK, United States, [5] Department of Ophthalmology, University of Oklahoma Health Sciences Center, Oklahoma City, OK, United States, [6] Department of Cell Biology, University of Oklahoma Health Sciences Center, Oklahoma City, OK, United States, [7] Department of Pharmaceutical Sciences, University of Oklahoma Health Sciences Center, Oklahoma City, OK, United States*

***Correspondence:***
*David M. Sherry*
*david-sherry@ouhsc.edu*

Elongation of Very Long chain fatty acids-4 (ELOVL4) protein is a member of the ELOVL family of fatty acid elongases that is collectively responsible for catalyzing formation of long chain fatty acids. ELOVL4 is the only family member that catalyzes production of Very Long Chain Saturated Fatty Acids (VLC-SFA) and Very Long Chain Polyunsaturated Fatty Acids (VLC-PUFA) with chain lengths ≥28 carbons. ELOVL4 and its VLC-SFA and VLC-PUFA products are emerging as important regulators of synaptic signaling and neuronal survival in the central nervous system (CNS). Distinct sets of mutations in *ELOVL4* cause three different neurological diseases in humans. Heterozygous inheritance of one set of autosomal dominant *ELOVL4* mutations that leads to truncation of the ELOVL4 protein causes Stargardt-like macular dystrophy (STGD3), an aggressive juvenile-onset retinal degeneration. Heterozygous inheritance of a different set of autosomal dominant *ELOVL4* mutations that leads to a full-length protein with single amino acid substitutions causes spinocerebellar ataxia 34 (SCA34), a late-onset neurodegenerative disease characterized by gait ataxia and cerebellar atrophy. Homozygous inheritance of a different set of *ELOVL4* mutations causes a more severe disease with infantile onset characterized by seizures, spasticity, intellectual disability, ichthyosis, and premature death. ELOVL4 is expressed widely in the CNS and is found primarily in neurons. ELOVL4 is expressed in cell-specific patterns within different regions of the CNS that are likely to be related to disease symptoms. In the retina, ELOVL4 is expressed exclusively in photoreceptors and produces VLC-PUFA that are incorporated into phosphatidylcholine and enriched in the light sensitive membrane disks of the photoreceptor outer segments. VLC-PUFA are enzymatically converted into "elovanoid" compounds that appear to provide paracrine signals that promote photoreceptor and neuronal survival. In the brain, the main ELOVL4 products are VLC-SFA that are incorporated into sphingolipids and enriched in synaptic vesicles, where they regulate kinetics of presynaptic neurotransmitter release. Understanding the function of ELOVL4 and its VLC-SFA and VLC-PUFA products will advance our understanding of basic mechanisms in neural signaling and has potential for developing novel therapies for seizure and neurodegenerative diseases.

**Keywords: very long chain-fatty acids, seizure, neurodegeneration, spinocerebellar ataxia, Stargardt's-like macular dystrophy**

## INTRODUCTION

Lipids are critical biochemical components of the central nervous system (CNS) that are essential for proper CNS function. The lipid composition of the brain is unique and exceedingly diverse (Sastry, 1985; Bozek et al., 2015; Hopiavuori et al., 2017; Hopiavuori et al., 2018). Aberrant lipid composition, metabolism, and signaling in the CNS is associated with neuropsychiatric and neurodegenerative diseases. Aging also is known to alter lipid composition in the brain (see Sebastiao et al., 2013; Muller et al., 2015; Lauwers et al., 2016; Spassieva et al., 2016). In general, lipids are known as key participants in membrane structures and for their role in cell signaling (Bazinet and Laye, 2014; Sanchez-Alegria et al., 2018). Recently, lipids also have been suggested to serve as regulators of synaptic transmission (Marza et al., 2008; Brodde et al., 2012; Sebastiao et al., 2013; Carta et al., 2014; Lauwers et al., 2016), and a number of lipid metabolism enzymes have been localized to synaptic terminals where they would be positioned to provide local regulation of synaptic transmission (Cremona et al., 1999; Di Paolo et al., 2004; Rohrbough et al., 2004). However, these studies focused primarily on lipids with fatty acid chains of 16–22 carbons in length. Our understanding of the functions of fatty acids with longer chain lengths in the nervous system is more limited.

Recent studies have revealed novel functions for Very Long Chain-Fatty Acids (VLC-FA), defined by a chain length of 28 or more carbons, in neural signaling (Bennett et al., 2014a,b; Bhattacharjee et al., 2017; Jun et al., 2017; Hopiavuori et al., 2018). This review will discuss the seven known members of the Elongation of Very Long Chain-Fatty Acids (ELOVL) family of enzymes responsible for elongation of saturated and polyunsaturated fatty acids (**Figure 1**). In particular, we will focus on ELOVL4 and the role of its Very Long Chain-Saturated Fatty Acids (VLC-SFA) and Very Long Chain-PolyUnsaturated Fatty Acids (VLC-PUFA) products in neurological disease, synaptic transmission, and neuronal survival in the CNS. By convention, *ELOVL4* refers to the human gene, *Elovl4* to the non-human mammalian gene, and *elovl4* to non-mammalian gene. ELOVL4 refers to the protein in all species.

### The ELOVL Family of Fatty Acid Elongases

The ELOVL family of enzymes in mammals is comprised of seven members that all reside in the endoplasmic reticulum (ER) and are thought to form a multimeric complex (Okuda et al., 2010). Together, the ELOVL family is responsible for the elongation of saturated and unsaturated fatty acids (Guillou et al., 2010; Kihara, 2012; Yu et al., 2012). ELOVL4, specifically, is essential for the biosynthesis of VLC-SFA and VLC-PUFA (Agbaga et al., 2008). Each member of the ELOVL family is a multi-pass transmembrane protein containing a large ELO domain with a high degree of homology to a family of fatty acid elongases in yeast (Zhang et al., 2003), an N-linked glycosylation near the N-terminus, a catalytic histidine motif (HXXHH) that is essential for the elongase function (Logan et al., 2014), and a di-lysine ER-retention motif (KXKXX) located in the C-terminus domain that is required for proper localization to the ER (Logan et al., 2013). The initial topological model of ELOVL protein structure, based on ELOVL4, predicted five transmembrane domains (SOUSI model; **Figure 2A**; Zhang et al., 2001; Molday and Zhang, 2010). More recent modeling, using a variety of bioinformatics tools (MEMSAT-SVM, MEM-SAT3; ENSEMBLE, Phobius, and TMHMM2 models; **Figure 2B**), predicts seven transmembrane domains (Ozaki et al., 2015). In both models, the N-terminus and N-linked glycosylation site are located in the ER lumen, and the C-terminus ER-retention motif is located on the cytoplasmic side of the ER membrane. A key difference between the 5- and 7-membrane spanning topologies is the placement of the catalytic histidine motif. The five transmembrane spanning topology places this motif in or near the ER lumen close to the start of the third transmembrane domain. The seven transmembrane spanning topology places this motif near the beginning of the fourth transmembrane domain on the cytoplasmic side of the ER membrane. The precise structure of the ELOVL proteins remains unresolved as no crystal structures of any full-length ELOVL proteins are available to date.

Fatty acid elongation occurs by cycling through a four step process (condensation, reduction, dehydration, and reduction), with two carbon atoms added through each cycle. Members of the ELOVL family catalyze the first step, a condensation reaction between a fatty acyl-CoA and malonyl-CoA (Pereira et al., 2004; Jakobsson et al., 2006). The second and fourth reduction steps are catalyzed by 3-ketoacyl-CoA and trans-2,3-enoyl-CoA reductases (KAR and TER), respectively, the third dehydration step is catalyzed by 3-hydroxyacyl-CoA dehydratases (HACD1-4) (**Figure 3**; Moon and Horton, 2003; Konishi et al., 2010). The ELOVL family proteins are thought to form hetero-oligomeric complexes in the ER (Okuda et al., 2010).

Complexing of ELOVL proteins is important to their function (Okuda et al., 2010; Logan et al., 2014). ELOVL4 is known to homodimerize, with dimerization of WT and STDG3 mutant ELOVL4 causing mislocalization of the complex away from the ER (Grayson and Molday, 2005; Molday and Zhang, 2010) and exerting a dominant negative effect on enzyme function

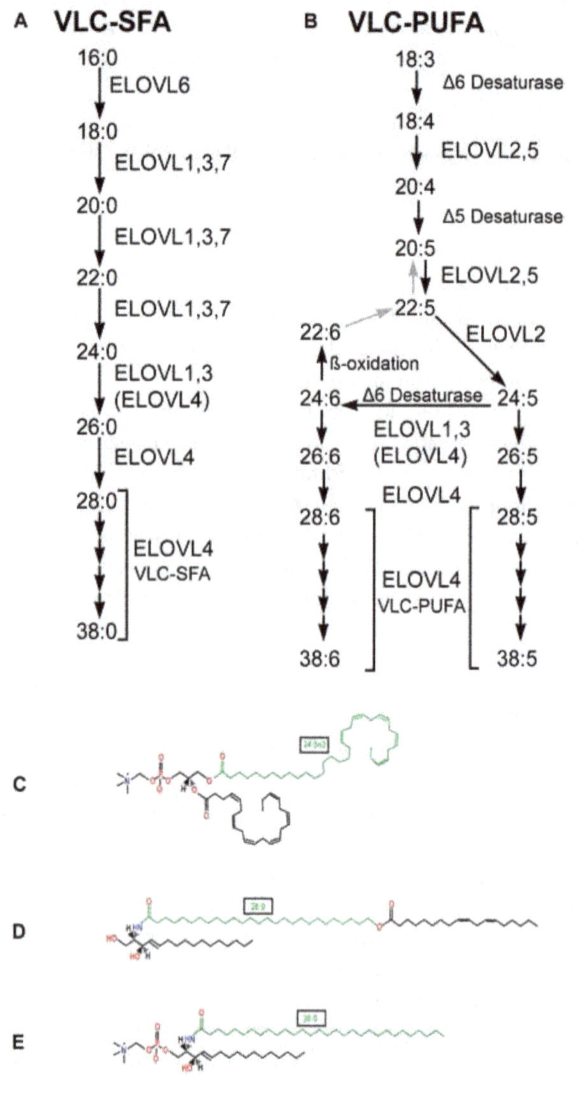


**FIGURE 1** | VLC-SFA and VLC-PUFA elongation pathways. **(A)** VLC-SFA biosynthesis pathway. Elongation steps are performed by ELOVL1-7. Although some ELOVL family members catalyze specific steps in VLC-SFA synthesis, others are multifunctional and may catalyze multiple steps. Elongation of C24 substrates also may be performed by ELOVL4 (ELOVL4). **(B)** VLC-PUFA biosynthesis pathway. Desaturation and elongation steps are performed by ELOVL1-5, Δ5 Desaturase (fatty acid desaturase-1, FADS1), and Δ6 desaturase (fatty acid desaturase-2, FADS2) as indicated. Although some ELOVL family members catalyze specific steps in VLC-PUFA synthesis, others are multifunctional and may catalyze multiple steps. Elongation of C24 substrates also may be performed by ELOVL4 (ELOVL4). **(C)** VLC-PUFA are incorporated into phosphatidylcholine in the retina. Example shown contains the VLC-PUFA, 34:5n3 (green), and the long chain-PUFA, 22:6n3 (DHA). **(D)** VLC-SFA are incorporated into ω-O-acylceramides in the skin. Example shown contains the VLC-SFA, 28:0 (green) ω-O-linked with 18:2n3. **(E)** VLC-SFA are incorporated into sphingolipids in the brain. Example shown shows sphingomyelin containing the VLC-SFA, 30:0 (green) (panels C–E from Hopiavuori et al., 2019, used with permission).

(Logan et al., 2014). In addition, ELOVL4 can hetero-oligomerize with other ELOVL family members and also can complex with other enzymes associated with VLC-FA elongation (Okuda et al., 2010). Furthermore, STDG3 mutants of ELOVL4 interact with other ELOVL family elongases and other VLC-FA-associated enzymes more strongly that WT ELOVL4, suggesting that mutant forms of ELOVL4 also might affect synthesis of other fatty acid species in addition to VLC-FA (Okuda et al., 2010).

The ELOVL family of elongases is involved in elongation of many different lipid species. Importantly, some ELOVL family elongases show distinct substrate selectivity and mediate very specific elongation reactions, while other members of the family show broader substrate selectivity and can show functional redundancy (Guillou et al., 2010; Kihara, 2012; Yu et al., 2012). Thus, the ELOVL family mediates a wide range of fatty acid elongation reactions leading to a diverse array of PUFA and SFA products.

ELOVL4 mediates elongation of long chain PUFA and SFA to form VLC-PUFA and VLC-SFA of 28 carbon chain length, respectively (**Figure 1**). ELOVL4 can then further elongate VLC-PUFA and VLC-SFA of 28 carbon chain length to produce VLC-PUFA and VLC-SFA species with chain lengths up to 38 carbons (Agbaga et al., 2008, 2010b). With respect to formation of VLC-PUFA, both 20:5n3 (eicosapentaenoic acid, EPA) and 22:5n3 (docosapentaenoic acid, DPA) precursors support downstream synthesis of VLC-PUFA (Agbaga et al., 2008). EPA is preferred as a substrate for elongation to VLC-PUFA over 20:4n6 (arachidonic acid, AA) and 22:6n3 (docosahexaenoic acid, DHA) (Yu et al., 2012). Importantly, ELOVL4 does not elongate shorter chain polyunsaturated fatty acids to DHA (Agbaga et al., 2010a). Formation of VLC-SFA is accomplished by ELOVL4-mediated elongation of 26:0–28:0, which can then be elongated further by ELOVL4 to produce VLC-SFA with longer carbon chains (Guillou et al., 2010; Kihara, 2012). The major VLC-SFA products of ELOVL4 in the brain are 28:0 and 30:0 (Hopiavuori et al., 2018).

The extreme length of the VLC-SFA and VLC-PUFA confers unique properties to the complex lipids and membranes into which they are incorporated. The very long, linear carbon chain of VLC-SFA confers a high melting temperature and would increase membrane stiffness through Van der Waals interactions between adjacent alkyl chains. Furthermore, the linear structure of VLC-SFA would be of sufficient length to span across the leaflets of the lipid bilayer, further affecting membrane properties (Hopiavuori et al., 2018, discussed further below). In contrast, VLC-PUFA, due to their length and multiple methylene interrupted *cis* double bonds, lead to locally disordered phospholipid packing in the membrane, increased fluidity, and potentially affect membrane curvature (Antonny et al., 2015; Lauwers et al., 2016).

The VLC-PUFA and VLC-SFA products of ELOVL4 are generated in a tissue-specific manner and are incorporated into more complex lipids in a tissue-specific manner. In the skin, the major products of ELOVL4 are VLC-SFA, as shown by the fact that epidermal fatty acids longer than C26 are virtually absent in newborn mice lacking a functional Elovl4 protein (Cameron et al., 2007). The molecular species of skin ceramides and glucosylceramides (GlcCer) contain VLC-SFA in non-hydroxy, α-hydroxy, and ω-hydroxy forms, the latter occurring in non-esterified and esterified forms (mostly with

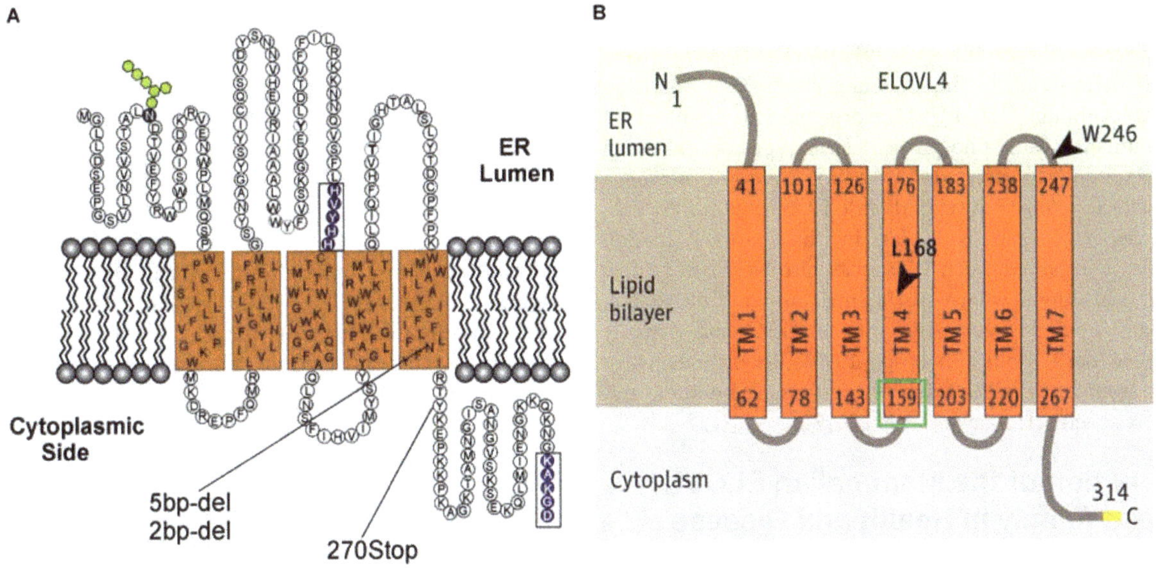


**FIGURE 2 |** Predicted transmembrane topology for ELOVL4. **(A)** Predicted five transmembrane-spanning topology for ELOVL4 (Zhang et al., 2001; Molday and Zhang, 2010). **(B)** Predicted seven transmembrane-spanning topology for ELOVL4 (Ozaki et al., 2015; figures used with permission).

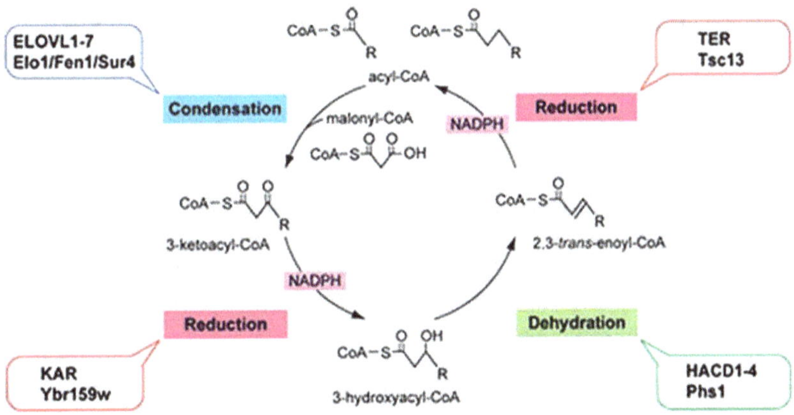


**FIGURE 3 |** Fatty acid elongation by the ELOVL family of enzymes. Diagram of the four-step fatty acid elongation cycle indicating the mammalian (ALL CAPITALS) and the yeast enzymes involved in each step. The ELOVL family elongasaes catalyze the initial condensation reaction (Kihara, 2012; figure used with permission).

18:2) (**Figure 1**). Strikingly, the skin of Elovl4$^{-/-}$ mice is devoid of the epidermal unique ω-O-acylceramides (> C30) (McMahon et al., 2007; Vasireddy et al., 2007). Part of the ω-hydroxy-Ceramide and GlcCer species are esterified to specific skin proteins (Amen et al., 2013), and are critical to establishing the extremely hydrophobic extracellular lipid lamellae of the stratum corneum that serves as the water barrier for the skin. Similarly, ELOVL4 in the Meibomian gland also generates VLC-SFA that are incorporated into ω-O-acylceramides, which are essential components of the lipid layer that covers the aqueous tear film and prevents evaporation (McMahon et al., 2014). In the testes, ELOVL4 produces VLC-PUFA (Santiago Valtierra et al., 2018), which are incorporated into sphingolipid products via ceramide synthase 3 (CerS3) (Rabionet et al., 2008). Conditional deletion of CerS3 leads to the absence of virtually all of sphingolipid products that contain VLC-PUFA, and infertility due to enhanced apoptosis during meiosis and spermatogenic arrest (Rabionet et al., 2015). VLC-PUFA are likely to be important to human fertility, as decreased VLC-PUFA levels in sperm are associated with decreased sperm quantity and quality (Craig et al., 2019).

In the CNS, ELOVL4 produces both VLC-SFA and VLC-PUFA in a region-specific manner. In the brain, the main ELOVL4 products are VLC-SFA, which are incorporated in sphingolipids that are enriched in synaptic vesicles and regulate presynaptic release (Hopiavuori et al., 2018). In retina, the main ELOVL4 products are VLC-PUFA (Agbaga et al., 2008, 2010b), which are incorporated into phosphatidylcholine and enriched in the light sensitive photoreceptor outer segments

(Aveldano, 1987). VLC-PUFA are critical to photoreceptor health and survival (Agbaga et al., 2008, 2010b; Bennett et al., 2014a,b; Bhattacharjee et al., 2017; Jun et al., 2017). VLC-PUFA have been reported previously in the brain (Poulos et al., 1988; Robinson et al., 1990). Although VLC-PUFA are present in the brain only in trace amounts in health, phosphatidylcholine species containing VLC-PUFA were reported previously in the brain of newborn children affected with Zellweger disease (Poulos et al., 1988), a rare peroxisomal biogenesis disorder in which in the oxidation of VLC-FA is impaired. Such PC species also were detected in the brain of healthy newborn rats in small amounts, decreasing substantially from postnatal days 1 to 16 and being virtually absent at 60 days (Robinson et al., 1990). Recent exhaustive lipidomic studies of healthy wildtype adult mouse brain did not detect these species (Hopiavuori et al., 2017).

## The Function of the Mammalian ELOVL Elongase Family in Health and Disease

The mammalian ELOVL family of elongases has a number of important functions in the body and, as a group, are particularly important to CNS function, the epidermal water barrier, systemic metabolic functions, and also are likely to be important to fertility. Mutations affecting *ELOVL1*, *-4*, *-5*, and *-7* are associated with neurological disease. Importantly, the diseases caused by these mutations have some shared characteristics that suggest fatty acid elongation in general is particularly critical to the health of the CNS. No disease causing mutations in *ELOVL2*, *-3*, or *-6* have been reported to date. The synthetic activities and functions of each ELOVL family member are summarized below.

### ELOVL1

ELOVL1 elongates SFA with chain lengths of 18–24 carbons and shows functional redundancy with ELOVL3 and ELOVL7 (**Figure 1**; Guillou et al., 2010; Ohno et al., 2010; Kihara, 2012). Deletion of *Elovl1* in mice causes disruption of the lamellae in the stratum corneum of the skin and disrupts the water barrier of the skin leading to perinatal lethality (Sassa et al., 2013). *Elovl1* mutant mice also show deficiency of VLC-SFA and VLC-mono-unsaturated fatty acids in the tear film (Sassa et al., 2018). *ELOVL1* is expressed at moderate levels in the brain (Tvrdik et al., 2000). An autosomal dominant mutation in human *ELOVL1* has recently been reported that produces ichthyosis, hypomyelination, spastic paraplegia, partial deafness, and optic atrophy (Mueller et al., 2019). This syndrome shares some symptoms with the neuro-ichtyotic syndrome caused by autosomal recessive mutations in *ELOVL4* (Aldahmesh et al., 2011; Mir et al., 2014; discussed below).

### ELOVL2

ELOVL2 elongates PUFA with 20–22 carbon and SFA with 18–20 carbon chains (**Figure 1**; Guillou et al., 2010; Zadravec et al., 2011; Kihara, 2012)and has low expression in the brain (Tvrdik et al., 2000). Knockout studies in mice indicate that *Elovl2* is essential for normal lipid homeostasis (Pauter et al., 2014). No human diseases arising from *ELOVL2* mutations have been reported to date, although polymorphisms with genetic linkage to autism have been reported recently (Sun et al., 2018). Interestingly, human epigenetic screening indicates that the *ELOVL2* gene shows a progressive increase in methylation that begins at an early stage of life and is a promising biomarker for aging in all tissues (Garagnani et al., 2012; Gopalan et al., 2017; Slieker et al., 2018; Jung et al., 2019) that can be used for forensic age determination (Spolnicka et al., 2018).

### ELOVL3

ELOVL3 elongates SFA with chain lengths of 18–24 carbons and can be functionally redundant with ELOVL1 and ELOVL7 (**Figure 1**; Westerberg et al., 2004; Guillou et al., 2010; Kihara, 2012). Knockout of *Elovl3* in mice disrupts the water barrier of the skin and causes hyperplasia of the sebaceous glands and hair loss (Westerberg et al., 2004; Kihara, 2012). No linkage to CNS disease in humans has been reported for ELOVL3.

### ELOVL4

ELOVL4 elongates long-chain PUFA and long-chain SFA of 24 carbon length to VLC-PUFA and VLC-SFA (≥26 carbons; **Figure 1**; Agbaga et al., 2008, 2010b; Guillou et al., 2010; Kihara, 2012). ELOVL4 also can further elongate VLC-PUFA and VLC-SFA up to 38 carbons in length. No other ELOVL family member performs this function. Thus, there is no compensation for mutations that compromise the ability of ELOVL4 to synthesize VLC-PUFA or VLC-SFA. Mutations in *ELOVL4* cause three different human diseases with tissue-specific characteristics: Stargardt-like macular dystrophy (STGD3), spinocerebellar ataxia 34 (SCA34), and a neuro-ichthyotic syndrome. All of these diseases have profound effects on the CNS and are discussed in more detail in several sections below.

### ELOVL5

ELOVL5 mediates elongation of long chain-PUFA and long chain-SFA between 18 and 22 carbons in length (**Figure 1**; Leonard et al., 2002; Guillou et al., 2010; Kihara, 2012). Two different mutations in *ELOVL5* cause spinocerebellar ataxia 38 (SCA38) in humans, which is characterized by gait ataxia, nystagmus, anosmia, and cerebellar atrophy (Di Gregorio et al., 2014). In the cerebellum, ELOVL5 is highly expressed in Purkinje cells, which provide the sole output from the cerebellar cortex, and in some cells of unidentified type located in the granule cell layer (Di Gregorio et al., 2014; Hoxha et al., 2017).

### ELOVL6

ELOVL6 has been suggested to mediate the first, rate-limiting step in fatty acid elongation of saturated and unsaturated/polyunsaturated fatty acids with chain length of 16 carbons, and is expressed at high levels in the liver, adipose tissue, and brain (**Figure 1**; Moon et al., 2001; Guillou et al., 2010; Kihara, 2012; Moon et al., 2014). *Elovl6* knockout mice are insulin resistant and develop obesity and hepatosteatosis when fed a high fat diet (Matsuzaka et al., 2007), indicating that ELOVL6 is important to normal metabolic regulation. The activity of ELOVL6 can also regulate thermogenic activity in brown fat adipocytes (Tan et al., 2015) and chondrocyte growth (Kikuchi et al., 2016). No direct causal linkage of *ELOVL6* mutations to human disease has been established.

### ELOVL7

ELOVL7 elongates SFA with chain lengths of 18–22 carbons and shows some functional redundancy with ELOVL1 and ELOVL3 (Guillou et al., 2010; Naganuma et al., 2011; Kihara, 2012). No direct causal relationship between ELOVL7 and human disease has been established. However, association of single nucleotide polymorphisms in *ELOVL7* with early onset Parkinson's disease has been reported (Li et al., 2018). A case of apparent mitochondrial encephalomyopathy arising from homozygous deletion of the contiguous *NDUFAF2*, *ERCC8*, and *ELOVL7* genes on chromosome 5 has been reported (Janssen et al., 2009). No changes in fatty acid synthesis were found, suggesting that deletion of *ELOVL7* is unlikely to be the root cause of the disease.

## Non-mammalian ELOVL Family Fatty Acid Elongases

ELOVL family fatty acid elongases in fish also have been of particular interest because of their function as source of polyunsaturated fatty acids. As indicated above, ELOVL family elongases are highly conserved across eukaryotes, and homologs of mammalian ELOVL2, ELOVL4, and ELOVL5 have been identified and characterized functionally in several species of teleost fish, including zebrafish, Salmon, cobia, and Chu's croaker (Hastings et al., 2004; Morais et al., 2009; Monroig et al., 2010, 2011; Carmona-Antonanzas et al., 2011; Lin et al., 2018). For more detailed discussion of ELOVL gene evolution (see Castro et al., 2016). A single isoform of ELOVL2 has been identified in fish (Morais et al., 2009). ELOVL5 is expressed in a single isoform in some fish species (i.e., Chu's croaker, Lin et al., 2018), while other species express two functionally similar isoforms (ELOVL5a and b) (i.e., Atlantic salmon, Hastings et al., 2004; Morais et al., 2009). ELOVL2 and ELOVL5 are functionally redundant with one another and serve functions similar to their mammalian homologs: ELOVL2 elongates C20 and C22 PUFA to C24 PUFA; ELOVL5a and 5b elongate C18 and C20 PUFA to C22 PUFA (Carmona-Antonanzas et al., 2011).

Similar to mammals, ELOVL4 in fish is highly expressed in brain, retina, and gonads and is essential for formation of VLC-SFA and VLC-PUFA (Monroig et al., 2010, 2011; Carmona-Antonanzas et al., 2011). However, ELOVL4 in fish can be expressed in a single isoform (i.e., Atlantic salmon, cobia Carmona-Antonanzas et al., 2011; Monroig et al., 2011) or two isoforms (ELOVL4a and b) that are encoded by separate genes (i.e., zebrafish, Monroig et al., 2010). ELOVL4a and ELOVL4b show very distinct substrate specificities: ELOVL4b readily elongates both VLC-SFA and VLC-PUFA, but ELOVL4a elongates only VLC-SFA (Monroig et al., 2010). In fish that express only a single ELOVL4 isoform, ELOVL4 shows activity similar to zebrafish ELOVL4b and elongates both VLC-SFA and VC-PUFA (Monroig et al., 2010; Carmona-Antonanzas et al., 2011). Fish ELOVL4 also can elongate C20 and C22 substrates, making it functionally redundant with ELOVL2 and to a lesser extent ELOVL5 (Carmona-Antonanzas et al., 2011), in contrast to mammalian ELOVL4. Importantly, this broad substrate selectivity could allow fish ELOVL2 and ELOVL4 to participate in the synthesis of DHA, as these enzymes can catalyze synthesis of 24:5n-3 from 22:5n-3, allowing for subsequent desaturation and β-oxidation to form DHA (Hastings et al., 2004; Monroig et al., 2010, 2011; Carmona-Antonanzas et al., 2011).

## Distribution of the ELOVL Family in the CNS

Several members of the ELOVL family are expressed in the CNS (ELOVL1, -3, -4, -5, and -6), but their expression levels differ across brain regions (Tvrdik et al., 2000; Lein et al., 2007; Hoxha et al., 2017; Sherry et al., 2017). ELOVL2 and ELOVL7 are expressed at very low levels in mammalian brain, if at all (Tvrdik et al., 2000; Lein et al., 2007), although ELOVL2 is expressed highly in the brain of non-mammals (Oboh et al., 2016). The best characterized ELOVL family members in the mammalian brain are ELOVL4 and ELOVL5 (Hoxha et al., 2017; Sherry et al., 2017; Hopiavuori et al., 2018). Mutations in either *ELOVL4* or *ELOVL5* cause neurological disease in humans (see below and **Table 1**). Interestingly, zebrafish ELOVL4a, which catalyzes formation of VLC-SFA only, is highly expressed in brain, and ELOVL4b, which catalyzes production of VLC-PUFA as well as VLC-SFA, is highly expressed in retina (Monroig et al., 2010; Carmona-Antonanzas et al., 2011). This distribution of ELOVL4 isoforms would result in similar patterns of VLC-SFA and VLC-PUFA production in the brains and retinae of teleost fish and mammals. ELOVL5 also is expressed at high levels in the fish brain (Kohlhardt, 1989), similar to mammalian brain.

### ELOVL4 Distribution in the Brain

ELOVL4 is the most highly expressed and widely distributed member of the ELOVL family in the brain as shown by immunolabeling and *in situ* hybridization (see **Figure 4**). ELOVL4 expression varies in a region- and cell type-specific manner (Lein et al., 2007; Sherry et al., 2017; Hopiavuori et al., 2018) which is likely to be related to the dysfunctions observed in diseases arising from *Elovl4* mutations. Expression of ELOVL4 is especially prominent in the olfactory bulb, hippocampus, cerebral cortex, thalamus, and cerebellum, although most other brain regions also show substantial levels of ELOVL4. An exception to this pattern is the basal ganglia, which show very little ELOVL4 expression (Sherry et al., 2017). At the cellular level, ELOVL4 expression is primarily neuronal, although small ELOVL4-positive cells have been observed in brain white matter suggesting potential expression in oligodendrocytes (Sherry et al., 2017). Among neurons, ELOVL4 expression is present in glutamatergic as well as GABAergic neurons (Sherry et al., 2017), and also may occur in neurons that utilize other neurotransmitters.

Within a region, ELOVL4 expression is cell-specific (**Figure 5**). In the retina, ELOVL4 is expressed exclusively by photoreceptor cells (Agbaga et al., 2008), consistent with the photoreceptor degeneration associated with ELOVL4 mutations that cause Stargardt's-like macular dystrophy (STGD3) (Bernstein et al., 2001; Edwards et al., 2001; Zhang et al., 2001; Maugeri et al., 2004; Bardak et al., 2016; Donato et al., 2018). In the cerebellum, ELOVL4 levels are extremely high in granule cells, moderate in basket and stellate cells, and low in Purkinje cells (Sherry et al., 2017). These cell-specific differences

**TABLE 1 |** Summary of human disease-causing *ELOVL4* mutations.

| Human disease | Inheritance | Genomic mutation | Protein mutation/structure /function | Retinal symptoms | Other CNS symptoms | Skin symptoms | Onset/Progression | References |
|---|---|---|---|---|---|---|---|---|
| Wildtype ELOVL4. | Homozygous | Wildtype (no mutation) | Wildtype. Intrinsic endoplasmic reticulum membrane protein. 314 AA length | – | – | – | – | Edwards et al., 2001; Zhang et al., 2001 |
| Stargardt's-like macular dystrophy (STGD3) | Autosomal dominant | 790–794 del AACTT "5 bp deletion" | Exon 6, N264Lfs10X | Macular degeneration | None reported | None | Juvenile onset. Rapid progression. | Edwards et al., 2001; Zhang et al., 2001 |
| Stargardt's-like macular dystrophy (STGD3) | Autosomal dominant | 789 del T *plus* 794 del T "2 bp deletion" | Exon 6, N264Tfs9X | Macular degeneration | None reported | None | Juvenile onset. Rapid progression. | Bernstein et al., 2001 |
| Stargardt's-like macular dystrophy (STGD3) | Autosomal dominant | c.810C > G | Exon 6, Y270X | Macular degeneration | None reported | None | Juvenile onset. Rapid progression. | Maugeri et al., 2004 |
| Stargardt's-like macular dystrophy (STGD3) | Autosomal dominant | c.814G > C | Exon 6, E272Q | Macular degeneration | None reported | None reported | Juvenile onset. Rapid progression. | Bardak et al., 2016 |
| Stargardt's-like macular dystrophy (STGD3) | Autosomal dominant | c.895A > G | Exon 6, M299V | Macular degeneration | None reported | None reported | Juvenile onset. Rapid progression. | Bardak et al., 2016 |
| Stargardt's-like macular dystrophy (STGD3) | Autosomal dominant | c.-90 G > C | Promoter, rs62407622 | Macular degeneration | None reported | None reported | Juvenile onset. Rapid progression. | Donato et al., 2018 |
| Stargardt's-like macular dystrophy (STGD3) | Autosomal dominant | c.-236 C > T | Promoter, rs240307 | Macular degeneration | None reported | None reported | Juvenile onset. Rapid progression. | Donato et al., 2018 |
| Spinocerebellar ataxia (SCA34) | Autosomal dominant | c.504G > C | Exon 4, L168F Full-length protein | Not reported | Gait and limb ataxia. Dysarthria. Nystagmus and eye movement deficits. Abnormal tendon reflexes. No autonomic disturbance. Cerebellar and pontine atrophy. | Erythrokerato-dermia Variabilis | Avg. onset: 51 years of age. Onset in 4th to 5th decade. Slow progression. | Cadieux-Dion et al., 2014 |

*(Continued)*

**TABLE 1** | Continued

| Human disease | Inheritance | Genomic mutation | Protein mutation/structure /function | Retinal symptoms | Other CNS symptoms | Skin symptoms | Onset/Progression | References |
|---|---|---|---|---|---|---|---|---|
| Spinocerebellar ataxia (SCA34) | Autosomal dominant | c.736T > G | Exon 4, W246G Full-length protein | Normal | Gait and limb ataxia. Dysarthria. Nystagmus and eye movement deficits. Abnormal tendon reflexes. Babinski reflex may be present. Autonomic disturbance sometimes present. Cerebellar and pontine atrophy. | None | Avg. onset: 34 years of age (range: 2nd–6th decade). Slow progression. | Ozaki et al., 2015 |
| Spinocerebellar ataxia (SCA34) | Autosomal dominant | c.539A > C | Exon 4, Q180P Full length protein | None reported | Gait ataxia more pronounced than limb ataxia. Dysarthria. Nystagmus and eye movement deficits. Moderate cerebellar and pontine atrophy. | Erythrokerato-dermia Variabilis | Onset in middle 20 s (1 case known). Progression unclear at present | Bourassa et al., 2015 |
| Spinocerebellar ataxia (SCA34) | Autosomal dominant | c698C > T | Exon 4, T233M Full length protein | None reported | Gait ataxia (no limb ataxia). No dysarthria. No nystagmus, but abnormal eye movements present. Hyporeflexia. Mild cerebellar and pontine atrophy. | Erythrokerato-dermia Variabilis | 15 years of age (1 case known). Slow progression | Bourque et al., 2018 |
| ELOVL4 Neuro-ichthyotic syndrome | Homozygous recessive | c.689delT | Exon 6, I230MfsX22 | Normal fundus and flicker ERG | Seizures, intellectual disability, spastic quadriplegia | Ichthyosis | Infancy (Gestation?) Developmental delay | Aldahmesh et al., 2011 |
| ELOVL4 Neuro-ichthyotic syndrome | Homozygous recessive | c.646C > T | Exon 5, R216X | Not reported | Seizures, intellectual disability, spastic quadriplegia | Ichthyosis | Infancy (Gestation?) Developmental delay | Aldahmesh et al., 2011 |
| ELOVL4 Neuro-ichthyotic syndrome | Homozygous recessive | c.78C > G | Exon 1, Y26X | Not reported | Seizures, intellectual disability, spastic quadriplegia | Ichthyosis | Infancy (Gestation?) Developmental delay | Mir et al., 2014 |

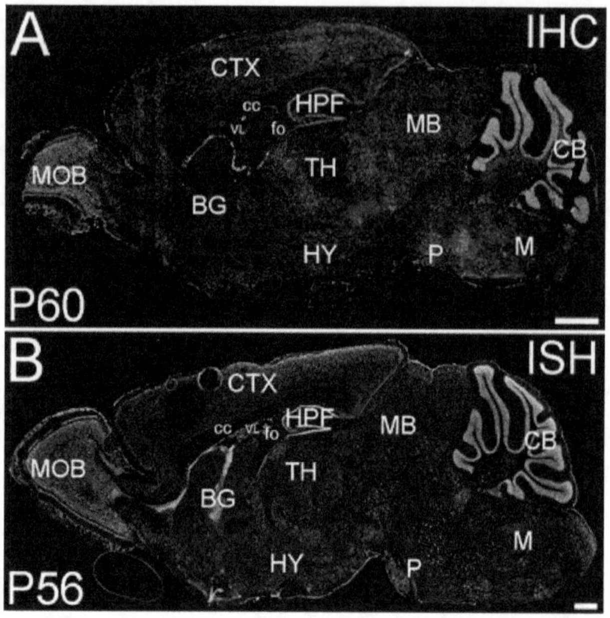


**FIGURE 4 |** ELOVL4 protein and mRNA distribution in the adult mouse brain. **(A)** Immunofluorescent labeling for ELOVL4 in the postnatal day 60 mouse brain is widely distributed, but shows cell-specific distribution in different regions of the brain. **(B)** *In situ* hybridization (ISH) for *Elovl4* mRNA in the mouse brain at P56 shows distribution similar to that of ELOVL4 protein. (Image from: Allen Institute for Brain Science Allen Mouse Brain Atlas for the P56 mouse brain, image number 69059903_134; http://mouse.brain-map.org). CB, cerebellum; BG, basal ganglia; CTX, cerebral cortex; HPF, hippocampal formation; HY, hypothalamus; M, medulla; MB, midbrain; MOB, main olfactory bulb; P, pons; cc, corpus callosum; fo, fornix; VL, lateral ventricle. Scale bars = 1 mm (figure from Sherry et al., 2017).

in ELOVL4 expression may be related to the symptoms and progression of spinocerebellar ataxia-34 (SCA34), which is caused by human *ELOVL4* mutations (Cadieux-Dion et al., 2014; Bourassa et al., 2015; Ozaki et al., 2015; Bourque et al., 2018). In the hippocampus, the highest levels of ELOVL4 in neurons in the CA3 and CA4 regions, with low expression in CA1 and dentate gyrus (Sherry et al., 2017; Hopiavuori et al., 2018), consistent with the severe, spontaneous epileptiform bursting and seizure activity observed in mice homozygous for the 5bp deletion STGD3 mutant *ELOVL4* alleles (Hopiavuori et al., 2018). This phenotype is also consistent with the seizure activity reported in the recessive human *ELOVL4* neuro-ichthyotic syndrome (Aldahmesh et al., 2011; Mir et al., 2014).

Expression of ELOVL4 in the brain is developmentally regulated, with *Elovl4* mRNA expression levels peaking around the time of birth and then steadily falling as the brain matures, reaching a steady state level by about postnatal day 30 in mice (Mandal et al., 2004). Immunolabeling studies of the developing mouse brain between embryonic day 18 (E18) and postnatal day 60 (P60) show that ELOVL4 is very highly expressed in regions such as the subventricular zone, the dentate gyrus of the hippocampus, and the internal and external granular layers of the cerebellum during periods of neurogenesis (Sherry et al., 2017). ELOVL4 expression in these regions declines as neurogenesis declines, suggesting some role for ELOVL4 and its VLC-FA products in neurogenesis.

### ELOVL5 Distribution in the Brain

ELOVL5 distribution has been characterized in the cerebellum, using immunolabeling of wildtype mouse cerebellum (Di Gregorio et al., 2014) and β-galactosidase reporter labeling in transgenic *Elovl5* knockout mice (Hoxha et al., 2017). ELOVL5 is expressed in cerebellar Purkinje cells, stellate and basket cells in the molecular layer, and at lower levels in a sparse, unidentified cell population in the granule cell layer of the cerebellar cortex and in cells in the deep cerebellar nuclei (Di Gregorio et al., 2014; Hoxha et al., 2017). Two different missense mutations in *ELOVL5* (c.214C > G, p.Leu72Val and c.689G > T, p.Gly230Val) cause SCA38, which is characterized by gait ataxia, dysarthria, abnormal eye movements, and cerebellar atrophy with onset in the third or fourth decade (Di Gregorio et al., 2014). ELOVL5 expression also was noted in small cells located in the white matter, most likely representing myelin-producing oligodendrocytes (Hoxha et al., 2017). Elsewhere in the brain, ELOVL5 is expressed by the mitral cells of the olfactory bulb, consistent with the anosmia (loss of the sense of smell) reported in *Elovl5* knockout mice, and in various sites in the brainstem (Hoxha et al., 2017). ELOVL5 also is expressed in other regions of the brain, but this has not been characterized in detail.

Thus, ELOVL4 and ELOVL5, and possibly other ELOVL enzyme family members, are expressed in a region- and cell-specific manner in the CNS, which would lead to cell-specific profiles of fatty acid synthesis and incorporation into complex lipids (Agbaga et al., 2018). This suggests that the effects of mutations on the enzymatic activity of ELOVL4, ELOVL5, and other lipid metabolizing enzymes are likely to be key determinants of the neurological symptoms associated with specific mutations in these enzymes. Developing a better understanding of the lipid profiles of specific cell types in the CNS will be important to advancing our mechanistic understanding of the role of VLC-FA in the healthy CNS and in neurological disease.

## Diseases Associated With ELOVL4

Several disease-causing mutations in the human *ELOVL4* gene have been identified to date (Bernstein et al., 2001; Edwards et al., 2001; Zhang et al., 2001; Maugeri et al., 2004; Aldahmesh et al., 2011; Cadieux-Dion et al., 2014; Mir et al., 2014; Bourassa et al., 2015; Ozaki et al., 2015; Bardak et al., 2016; Bourque et al., 2018; Donato et al., 2018; **Table 1** and **Figure 6**). Mutations in *ELOVL4* cause three distinct neurodegenerative diseases that depend on the specific mutation and its pattern of inheritance: Stargardt-like macular dystrophy (STGD3), spinocerebellar ataxia-34 (SCA34) with or without erythrokeratodermia variabilis (EKV), and a severe neuro-ichthyotic syndrome. Each disease is discussed below.

### STGD3

Six different heterozygous mutations in *ELOVL4* cause autosomal dominant STGD3, an aggressive degeneration striking the macular region of the retina with juvenile onset and rapid

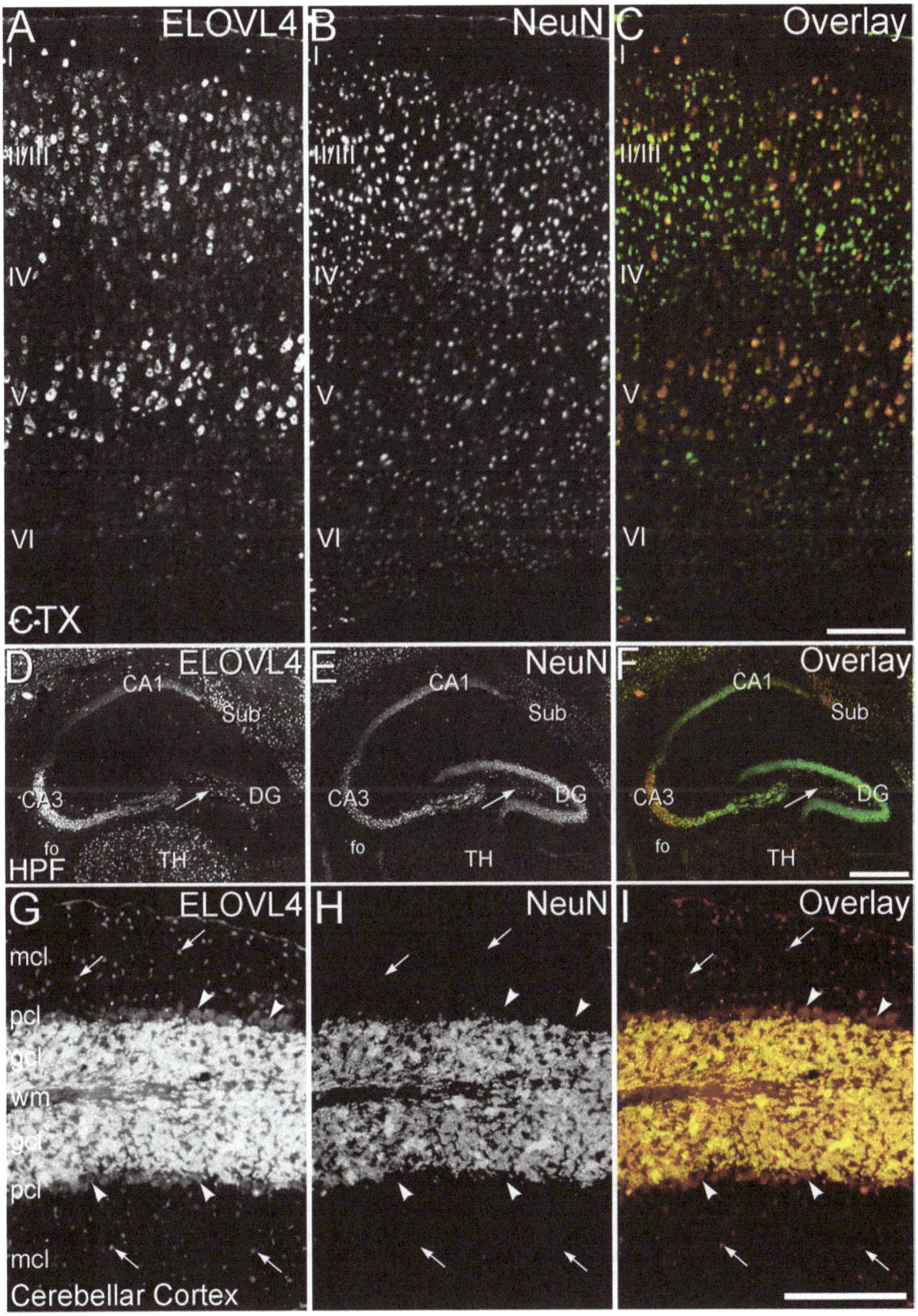


**FIGURE 5** | Continued

**FIGURE 5 |** Cell-specific expression of ELOVL4 in isocortex, hippocampus and cerebellum. **(A–C)** Cerebral Cortex (CTX). **(A)** Labeling for ELOVL4 is present in all layers of the cerebral cortex (CTX). Cells in the pyramidal layers (II/III and V) are most prominently labeled, but ELOVL4-positive cells also are present in the molecular layer (I), layer 4 (IV) and layer 6 (VI). **(B)** Labeling for the neuronal marker, NeuN. **(C)** Overlay of panels A and B shows close correspondence of ELOVL4 (red) and NeuN labeling (green). **(D–F)** Hippocampal formation (HPF). **(D)** Labeling for ELOVL4 is present in the cellular layers of the HPF, including the Cornu Ammonis, with field 1 (CA1) showing less prominent labeling than field 3 (CA3). Prominent ELOVL4 labeling also is present in the subiculum (sub) and interneurons in the polymorph layer (arrow). Cells along the inner margin of the dentate gyrus (DG) show moderate ELOVL4 labeling, but most dentate granule cells show little ELOVL4 labeling. **(E)** Labeling for the neuronal marker, NeuN. **(F).** Overlay of **(D,E)** shows close correspondence of ELOVL4 (red) and NeuN (green) labeling. TH, Thalamus. **(G–I)** Cerebellar cortex. **(G)** Cross section through a cerebellar folium showing ELOVL4 expression in the cerebellar cortex. Neurons (arrows) in the molecular cell layer (mcl) show strong ELOVL4 labeling, but the Purkinje cells (arrowheads) in the Purkinje cell layer (pcl) show only moderate levels of ELOVL4 labeling. The densely packed cells of the granule cell layer (gcl) show very intense labeling. **(H)** Labeling for the neuronal marker, NeuN, strongly labels neurons in the gcl, but not Purkinje cells, as appropriate. **(I)** Overlay of **(G,H)** shows close correspondence of intense ELOVL4 (red) and NeuN (green) labeling resulting in an orange color in the gcl. wm, white matter of the arbor vitae. Scale bars = 200 μm for **(A–C,G–I)**; 500 μm for **(D–F)**.

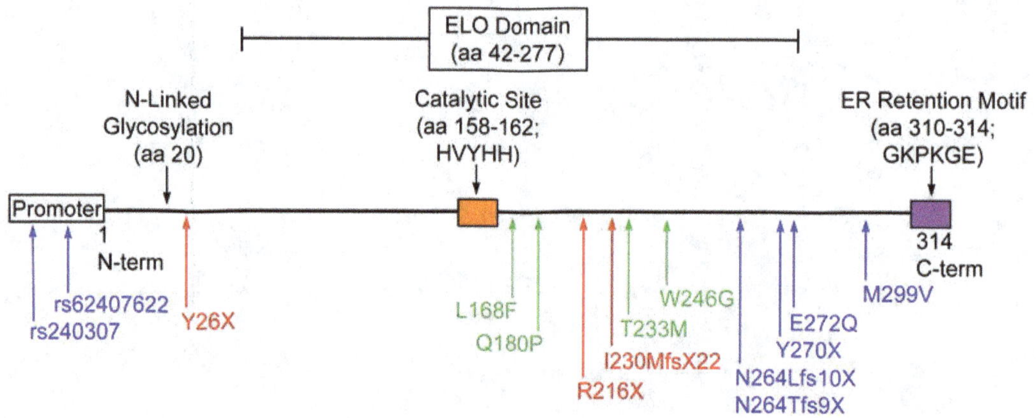


**FIGURE 6 |** Disease-causing mutations in ELOVL4. STGD3-causing mutations (blue) result in early truncation of ELOVL4 and the loss of the C-terminal ER retention motif or, in the case of the promoter mutations, severely suppress *ELOVL4* expression. SCA34-causing mutations (green) result in amino acid substitutions but still produce a full-length protein. ELOVL4 Neuro-ichthyosis-causing mutations (red) cause very early termination of the protein that would truncate substantial portions of transmembrane domains in either the 5-transmembrane or 7-transmembrane models of ELOVL4 topology in addition to deleting the ER retention motif.

progression (Bernstein et al., 2001; Edwards et al., 2001; Zhang et al., 2001; Maugeri et al., 2004; Bardak et al., 2016; Donato et al., 2018). Symptoms associated with STGD3 are limited to the retina, as STGD3 patients show no additional CNS disease or skin abnormalities (Bernstein et al., 2001; Edwards et al., 2001; Zhang et al., 2001). Importantly, STGD3-causing *ELOVL4* mutations result in a loss of function. STGD3 arises from several different mutations in exon 6 that result in premature termination of the protein and cause the loss of the C-terminal ER retention motif (Bernstein et al., 2001; Edwards et al., 2001; Zhang et al., 2001; Maugeri et al., 2004; Bardak et al., 2016). The 5 bp deletion STDG3 mutant form of ELOVL4 exerts a dominant-negative effect on the enzyme and leads to mislocalization of ELOVL4 away from the ER (Logan et al., 2013; Logan et al., 2014). Two additional STGD3-causing mutations in the *ELOVL4* promoter that suppress *ELOVL4* expression have been identified recently (Donato et al., 2018).

## SCA34

Four different heterozygous mutations in the *ELOVL4* gene cause autosomal dominant spinocerebellar ataxia-34 (SCA34), a late-onset degenerative disease of the cerebellum that may present with or without erythrokeratodermia variabilis (EKV; red thickened skin) (Cadieux-Dion et al., 2014; Bourassa et al., 2015; Ozaki et al., 2015; Bourque et al., 2018). The gait ataxia and cerebellar degeneration that are characteristic of the disease appear in the second to sixth decade of life, with symptom onset varying according to the specific mutation. Other CNS symptoms also may be present, including dysarthria (difficulty speaking), abnormal eye movements, and abnormal tendon reflexes. Patients with SCA34 do not show any clinical retinal deficits. All of the known mutations that cause SCA34 are mutations in exon 4 that result in a single amino acid substitution and produce a full-length protein. The presence of neural deficits and degeneration in the brain appear in the absence of retinal symptoms in SCA34 patients, suggesting that SCA34-causing mutations in *ELOVL4* may preferentially affect synthesis of VLC-SFA, rather than VLC-PUFA. A recent study suggests that SCA34 patients with the p.T233M SCA34 mutation also may experience multi-system neurodegeneration beyond the cerebellum, neuropsychiatric disturbances, and dementia, in addition to the known motor deficits of SCA34 (Ozaki et al., 2019).

## ELOVL4 Neuro-Ichthyotic Syndrome

Three different homozygous mutations in the *ELOVL4* gene cause a severe neuro-ichthyotic syndrome (Aldahmesh et al., 2011; Mir et al., 2014). The neural components of this syndrome include severe seizures, intellectual disability, spasticity, and neurodegeneration in the brain. These neurological impairments are accompanied by ichthyosis (a scaly thickening of the skin), developmental delay, and premature death. Mutations that cause this severe syndrome may be associated with truncation of the protein, whether affecting just the first few amino acids at the N-terminal (Mir et al., 2014), or the last C-terminal third of the protein (Aldahmesh et al., 2011), which includes the critical ER retention motif of ELOVL4. Interestingly, homozygous inheritance of STDG3 alleles in transgenic mice in which ELOVL4 has been rescued in the skin to prevent perinatal death due to dehydration, causes a syndrome characterized by severe seizures and early death about postnatal days 20–21 (Hopiavuori et al., 2018). No cases of homozygous inheritance of STGD3 or SCA34 *ELOVL4* alleles in humans have been reported to date.

## Neurophysiological Role of ELOVL4, Its Products, and Their Functions in the CNS and at the Synapse

Despite the obvious importance of ELOVL4 to the health and function of the CNS, the precise role and mechanisms of action of its main fatty acid products, VLC-PUFA and VLC-SFA, are incompletely understood. Recent evidence suggests that specific lipid species that contain each of these types of very-long acyl chains may have important roles, with VLC-PUFA serving as precursors of metabolites involved in homeostatic signals and VLC-SFA serving as modulators of synaptic transmission.

### VLC-PUFA as Homeostatic Survival Signals

Recently, elegant studies of VLC-PUFA by the Bazan laboratory identified a new class of bioactive fatty acids they named "elovanoids" (Bhattacharjee et al., 2017; Jun et al., 2017; Bazan, 2018). These compounds, hydroxylated derivatives of 32:6n-3 and 34:6n-3 produced by a form of lipoxygenase, were described as neuroprotective in the retina., The primary products of ELOVL4 in the retina are VLC-PUFA that are incorporated into phosphatidylcholine and enriched in the disc membranes of the light-sensitive photoreceptor outer segments (Aveldano, 1987). Each morning, photoreceptors shed a portion of the discs at the distal tip of the outer segment, which are phagocytosed by the overlying retinal pigmented epithelium (RPE) and degraded. The VLC-PUFA in the shed outer segment membranes serve as the precursors for production of oxygenated elovanoid derivatives in RPE cells. Elovanoids then provide a neuroprotective feedback signal to enhance expression of pro-survival proteins by the photoreceptors to compensate for high levels of oxidative stress (Jun et al., 2017). In good agreement with these findings, elovanoids also have been shown to have protective effects in neurons subjected to oxygen and glucose deprivation or to induced excitotoxicity in culture, and in an animal model of ischemic stroke (Bhattacharjee et al., 2017). Together, these data revealed a novel pro-homeostatic and neuroprotective lipid-signaling mechanism that helps to sustain the integrity of neuronal cells. For more information on omega-3 and omega-6 unsaturated fatty acids, DHA, docosanoids, elovanoids and their biological functions, we refer to an excellent recent review from Bazan (2018).

### VLC-SFA as Modulators of Synaptic Function

An emerging understanding suggests that VLC-SFA are important for normal synaptic function and that VLC-SFA deficiency arising from ELOVL4 mutations impairs synaptic transmission and causes synaptopathy. Recent studies performed using mice homozygous for the 5 bp deletion STDG3 mutation, which effectively renders ELOVL4 inactive, showed that VLC-SFA are important, novel modulators of presynaptic release kinetics (Hopiavuori et al., 2018). Of the potential roles that VLC-SFA may play in the CNS, we will consider two major areas below: as structural elements and as signaling molecule and signal modifiers. We also provide thoughts on future research directions to better understand the function of VLC-FA and their potential clinical relevance.

## Structural Role of VLC-SFA

Although much remains unknown about the role of ELOLV4 and its VLC-SFA products in neurophysiology, we suggest that VLC-SFA incorporated into sphingolipids in the synaptic vesicle membrane may potentially serve as membrane stabilizers, anchor points for proteins, and lipid raft-like components.

### Potential Role for VLC-SFA in Membrane Fusion

One of the most precisely regulated membrane fusion events known occurs during neurotransmission in the synaptic terminal (Südhof, 2004; Südhof and Rothman, 2009). Membrane fusion is a fundamental step in neurotransmitter release when synaptic vesicles (SV) fuse with the plasma membrane at the active zone to release their neurotransmitter content into the synaptic cleft. Receptors on the postsynaptic side bind the transmitter and relay the signal to the next neuron. This process, which is the basis for information processing in the brain, has received considerable attention in human cognitive research and in neurodegenerative diseases such as Alzheimer's and Parkinson's diseases (Dickson, 1997; Selkoe, 2001, 2002; Petersen, 2004; Nguyen et al., 2006). The core machinery required for action potential evoked synchronized transmitter release and the molecular components needed for neurotransmission are now identified. This core complex contains three SNARE (soluble NSF attachment protein -SNAP- receptor) proteins (Sollner et al., 1993): the synaptic vesicle protein, synaptobrevin (also known as VAMP, Vesicle Associated Membrane Protein), and the target membrane bound syntaxin and SNAP-25 proteins. The coiled motifs of these three proteins form a four helical complex structure, thus bringing the membranes in close proximity (McNew et al., 2000; Melia et al., 2002). During action potentials, the fusion of the vesicular and active zone membranes is triggered by binding of calcium ions to synaptotagmin1, another vesicular protein, which binds preferentially to phospholipids (Perin et al., 1990; Fernandez-Chacon et al., 2001). Recently, an array of synaptic proteins (Munc13, Munc18, Rabphilin, and Complexin) that interact with the core complex and assist in the precise regulation of synaptic release have been discovered (Hata et al., 1993; Rizo and Sudhof, 2002; Deák et al., 2006b;

Deák et al., 2009; Südhof and Rothman, 2009). Recently, the exact stoichiometry of these and other SV proteins and SV lipids was reported, and biophysical characterization of SV membranes was performed (Takamori et al., 2006; Hopiavuori et al., 2017; Hopiavuori et al., 2018). Regarding lipids, these authors showed that an average 40 nm diameter SV contains some 7000 phospholipid and 5-6000 cholesterol molecules. Together, the glycerophospholipids phosphatidylcholine, phosphatidylethanolamine, and phosphatidylserine comprise more than 90% of the phospholipid content, part of the rest being phosphatidylinositol, sphingomyelin, and hexosylceramide (Takamori et al., 2006). The most abundant VLC-SFA components of the SV membrane lipid were 28:0 and 30:0 incorporated into sphingolipids (Hopiavuori et al., 2018).

During exocytosis, the membrane lipid bilayers merge in a stepwise process. First, the membrane leaflets exposed to the cytoplasm make contact each other and then, if forced with sufficient energy, will merge. Only after this process is initiated, and at least partially completed, can the other membrane leaflets – in the case of synaptic neurotransmission, the luminal leaflet of the synaptic vesicle and the extracellular leaflet of the plasma membrane – contact each other. Thus, an intermediate state – called hemifusion – exists when the outer leaflets of the vesicle and plasma membrane form a temporary new bilayer. After these outer leaflets merge, the vesicular lumen and the synaptic cleft remain separate. Next, after a fusion pore is formed, the release of neurotransmitter is initiated (**Figure 7**).

VLC-SFA potentially could change the structure of the lipid bilayer and its biophysical properties, thereby affecting the process of membrane fusion. The SV membrane contains 28:0 and 30:0 as components of sphingolipids (Hopiavuori et al., 2018). These very long saturated acyl chains are of sufficient length to traverse both leaflets of the SV lipid bilayer. We hypothesize that the hydrophobic van der Walls interactions between these very long chains stabilize the SV lipid bilayer, hindering the separation of the two leaflets during hemifusion and fusion pore formation. The enrichment of VLC-SFA in SV membranes, therefore, would increase the energy required to initiate vesicular fusion, stabilizing the membranes and reducing random spontaneous fusion events unrelated to action-potential mediated synaptic release. According to this model, acyl-acyl hydrophobic interactions across the lipid bilayer would increase the van der Waals forces within the bilayer, thereby stabilizing the membrane and inhibiting fusion with other membranes. Assuming that the energy source driving membrane fusion is constant, the vesicular release process would be slowed in SVs with high VLC-SFA content. The VLC-SFA in the vesicle membrane could thereby provide a biophysical resistance to the activation of SNARE complexes, which is essential for $Ca^{2+}$-regulated exocytosis of synaptic vesicles (Deák et al., 2006a, 2009; Südhof and Rothman, 2009; Südhof and Rizo, 2011; Imig et al., 2014; Shen et al., 2015), slowing SV fusion. We suggest that this increased barrier may help to regulate the timing of vesicular release. *Elovl4* mutations that cause seizures (STDG3 and ELOVL4 neuro-ichthyotic syndrome) effectively eliminate the enzymatic function of ELOVL4 and, thus, lead to SVs that lack VLC-SFA. The absence of the van der Waals forces generated by the VLC-SFA within the SV lipid bilayer would therefore be expected to increase the probability of spontaneous release events by removing a barrier to fusion. In this case, the precise timing of synaptic release would be compromised, leading to bursting activity and seizures, as seen in the hippocampus of knock-in mice homozygous for the 5bp deletion STGD3 *ELOVL4* mutation (**Figure 8**; Hopiavuori et al., 2018). Consistent with this hypothesis, hippocampal neurons cultured from mice homozygous for the 5bp deletion STGD3 *ELOVL4* mutation show accelerated synaptic release kinetics (Hopiavuori et al., 2018). Critically, supplementation of a mixture of 28:0 and 30:0 VLC-SFA to these neurons via the culture medium restored normal synaptic release kinetics (**Figure 9**; Hopiavuori et al., 2018).

The length and saturation of VLC-SFA also may enable them to sterically inhibit protein-protein interactions in the vesicular release machinery. However, interactions between VLC-SFA and the vesicle fusion machinery remain unknown at present. VLC-SFA interactions are also likely to keep the membrane bilayers highly ordered and stable, thus hindering the effects of synaptobrevin juxta- and trans-membrane regions in disturbing outer leaflet lipid ordering and changing curvature of membrane (Tarafdar et al., 2015). It is also plausible for charged phospholipids (e.g., sphingolipids) containing VLC-SFA to interact with the release proteins via a strongly charged segment in synaptobrevin/VAMP located next to its transmembrane domain outside of the SV (Quetglas et al., 2000).

What other functional consequences might result from the presence of VLC-SFA in the SV membrane? It is well established that the SNARE protein syntaxin1A forms clusters in the active zone (Takamori et al., 2006; Khuong et al., 2013). Interestingly, the syntaxin1A clusters are dispersed in the absence of $PI(3,4,5)P_3$ at *Drosophila* larval neuromuscular junction (Khuong et al., 2013). Could VLC-SFA containing sphingolipids, similarly, cluster synaptobrevin/VAMPs, the vesicular SNARE binding partners of syntaxins in the SV membrane? Although an intriguing possibility, it is unlikely that islands of VLC-SFA in the membrane would serve as anchoring points for vesicular SNAREs, as the expected effect of VLC-SFA deficiency would be to disorganize the VAMPs, which would lead to slower release. Exactly the opposite of the observed effect of VLC-SFA deficiency in the mouse model (Hopiavuori et al., 2018). The presence of VLC-SFA could impose some ordering of proteins at the fusion site beyond the SNARE proteins, though, as many accessory or modulatory vesicular proteins have transmembrane domains (e.g., Synaptotagmins) or membrane anchoring lipid modifications. Interestingly, the role of VLC-SFA in synaptic release is markedly different from that described for cholesterol, which facilitates synchronized evoked transmitter release (Wasser et al., 2007; Linetti et al., 2010; Teixeira et al., 2012). Miniature synaptic potentials arise from single SV release in the absence of action potentials (Katz and Miledi, 1979; Sara et al., 2005). Therefore, these events are useful direct indicators of membrane fusion dynamics; future studies could address the effect of VLC-SFA on miniature release.

Alternatively, the effect of VLC-SFA anchoring points should be considered for vesicular events that do not complete

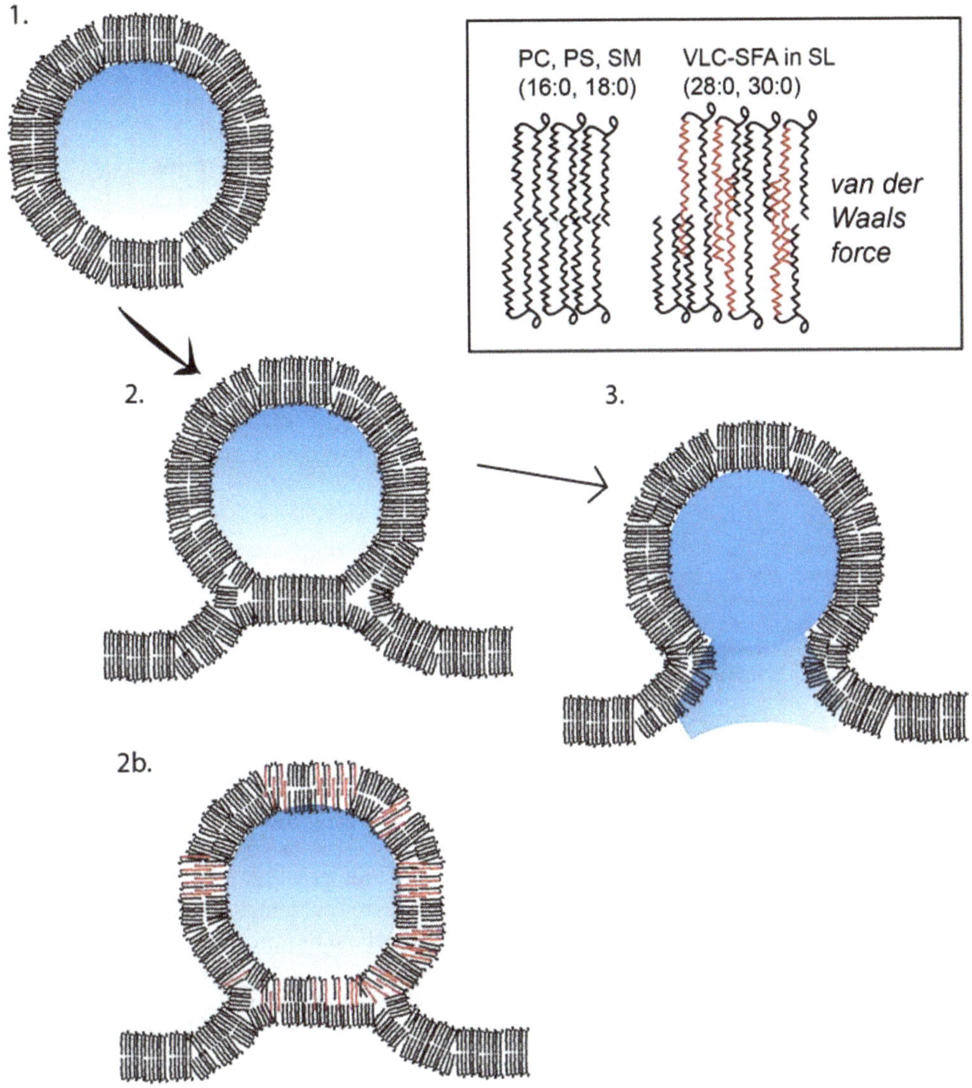


**FIGURE 7 |** Model of membrane fusion between a VLC-SFA-rich synaptic vesicle and presynaptic active zone membrane. In this cartoon, a synaptic vesicle (SV) containing lipids with common fatty acids (phosphatidylcholine or phosphatidylserine molecules with palmitic, 16:0, and stearic acids, 18:0) is used as a model to illustrate the three stages of synaptic vesicular exocytosis, namely, (1) undocked vesicle; (2) docked and hemifused vesicle stage, with deformation tilt of the membranes and stalk formation; and (3) membrane fusion and contents release stage. In (2b), an SV is depicted with lipids containing, in addition, VLC-SFA (typically 28:0 or 30:0 fatty acid chains, see inset). We have shown that the normal presence of these fatty acids in the SV membrane renders it more stable than do the shorter LC fatty acids, thereby fusing and releasing at comparatively lower rates (Hopiavuori et al., 2018) (PS, phosphatidylserine; PC, phosphatidylcholine; SM, sphingomyelin; SL, sphingolipids; see text for more details).

fusion and intermixing of vesicular membrane with the plasma membrane. Neurophysiologists call such partial fusion events as "Kiss and run" (Fesce et al., 1994; Stevens and Williams, 2000) when the fusion pore is reversibly closed and the vesicle escapes intact without merging fully into the active zone membrane (Gandhi and Stevens, 2003; Südhof and Rizo, 2011). It remains to be tested whether VLC-SFA alter the preference for the fusion mode from total exocytosis to kiss-and-run events.

Another intriguing question is whether VLC-SFA are components of lipid rafts. Lipid rafts are specific microdomains of the plasma membrane, which differ in their composition from the rest of the plasma membrane (Jacobson et al., 2007). Formation of rafts requires cholesterol, and these cholesterol- and sphingolipid-rich plasma membrane microdomains play important roles in compartmentalization of cellular functions. Lipid rafts, which range in size from 10 to 200 nm in diameter, comprise various fractions of the plasma membrane depending on the cell type, and provide a mechanism for ordering clusters of proteins within them (Hao et al., 2001). The detergent-insoluble lipid rafts contain proteins that are modified posttranslationally by acylation or glycosylphosphatidylinositol (GPI) modification. Some as yet unidentified interactions between VLC-SFA and other components of the lipid rafts could increase the stability of the raft domains. Alternatively, the long acyl chain length of

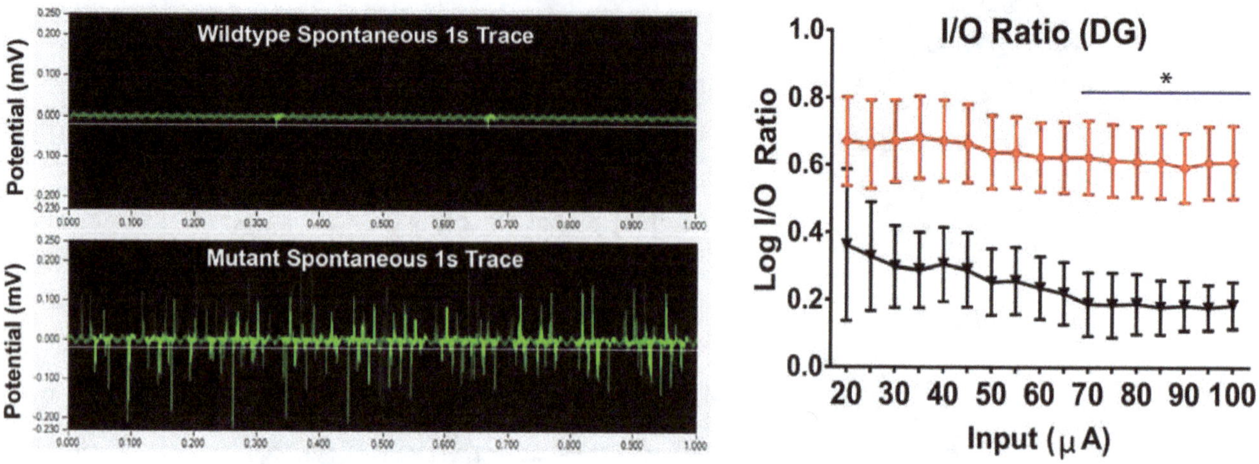


**FIGURE 8** | Seizure activity resulting from STGD3 deletion. **Left:** Spontaneous bursting activity in hippocampal slices from $S^{+}$*Elovl4*$^{mut/mut}$ mice with knock-in of the 5 bp STGD3 mutation and skin-specific rescue of wildtype (WT) *ELOVL4* function to prevent perinatal lethality, and $S^{+}$*Elovl4*$^{wt/wt}$ control mice expressing the WT *ELOVL4* gene under baseline conditions. Representative traces of field potentials from postnatal day 19 $S^{+}$*Elovl4*$^{wt/wt}$ **(upper trace)** and $S^{+}$*Elovl4*$^{mut/mut}$ mice **(lower trace)**. Each trace represents the first 1 s of a single channel chosen from a 10 min recording taken using a 64 channel multi-electrode array. The $S^{+}$*Elovl4*$^{mut/mut}$ slice shows a dramatic increase in spontaneous neuronal activity compared to WT littermates. **Right:** Stepwise increased stimulations to perforant path synapses in dentate gyrus (DG) revealed a markedly enhanced input/output (I/O) ratio indicating a boost in synaptic strength in the main input pathway from the entorhinal cortex of $S^{+}$*Elovl4*$^{mut/mut}$ mice (red) compared to $S^{+}$*Elovl4*$^{wt/wt}$ control mice (statistics: two-way RM ANOVA, *$p < 0.05$ from 70 to 100 μA).

VLC-SFA are suited perfectly to the increased width of the lipid bilayer in the rafts.

VLC-PUFA also are potential modulators of synaptic function. Due to their polyunsaturated structure and large size, VLC-PUFA could regulate membrane fluidity and curvature by disrupting phospholipid packing of the lipid bilayer of synaptic membranes, similarly, to DHA and other PUFA (Antonny et al., 2015; Lauwers et al., 2016). The retina provides one example for such a role of VLC-PUFA: depletion of VLC-PUFA from mouse photoreceptors by conditional knockout of *Elovl4* reduced photoreceptor synaptic vesicle diameter compared to synaptic vesicle diameter in wildtype photoreceptors (Bennett et al., 2014b). This change in diameter potentially could affect vesicle fusion or transmitter content. Consistent with this notion, the amplitude of signals in the electroretinogram that reflect transmission of rod photoreceptor signals to the inner retina, also was reduced in the conditional *Elovl4* knockout mice (Bennett et al., 2014a). For more detailed insight on VLC-FA function in the retina and vision, we refer to our colleague's most recent review (Hopiavuori et al., 2019).

## Potential Signaling Functions of VLC-SFA and VLC-PUFA

VLC-SFA and VLC-PUFA potentially also might tune synaptic transmission through inter-neuronal interactions. As discussed above, elegant studies by the Bazan laboratory identified a new class of bioactive oxygenated VLC-PUFA derivatives they named elovanoids, including mono-hydroxy 32:6n3, the stable derivative of the hydroperoxy precursor of elovanoid-N32, which has neuroprotective activity in the retina (**Figure 10**; Jun et al., 2017). Alternatively, VLC-SFA or VLC-PUFA could potentially serve as an initial substrate for novel messenger pathways to provide either intracellular or trans-synaptic signals that would modulate synaptic function. For example, endocannabinoids provide retrograde signals to modulate presynaptic function via receptor-mediated signaling (Wilson and Nicoll, 2002; Fan and Yazulla, 2004). Another example to be considered is intracellular signaling via the PLC-PIP2-IP3/DAG pathway.

Proper intracellular membrane trafficking depends on the phosphatidylinositol-phosphate (PIP) system. Although PIPs are a minor fraction of the membrane lipids, they are essential for proper targeting of vesicular traffic and for synaptic endocytosis (Di Paolo et al., 2004; Zoncu et al., 2007). The cytoplasmic side of cellular membranes acquires an asymmetrical PIP profile through an elaborate regulatory system of selective PI kinases, including PIPKgamma (Wenk et al., 2001), PIPK4 (Guo et al., 2003), and phosphatases. Importantly, PIPs also interact with various ion channels. For instance, modulation of transient receptor potential (TRP) channels by phosphoinositides, especially $PIP_2$, is well established (Rohacs and Nilius, 2007; Rohacs, 2015). Whether VLC-FA can exert similar effects on integral membrane proteins such as ion channels is a fascinating untested question.

## Open Questions, Future Directions

### Trafficking of VLC-SFA-Containing Membranes From Endoplasmic Reticulum (ER) to SV

Although there is abundant information on ER trafficking from yeast and other single cell organisms (Novick and Schekman, 1979; Balch et al., 1984; Kaiser and Schekman, 1990), the details of

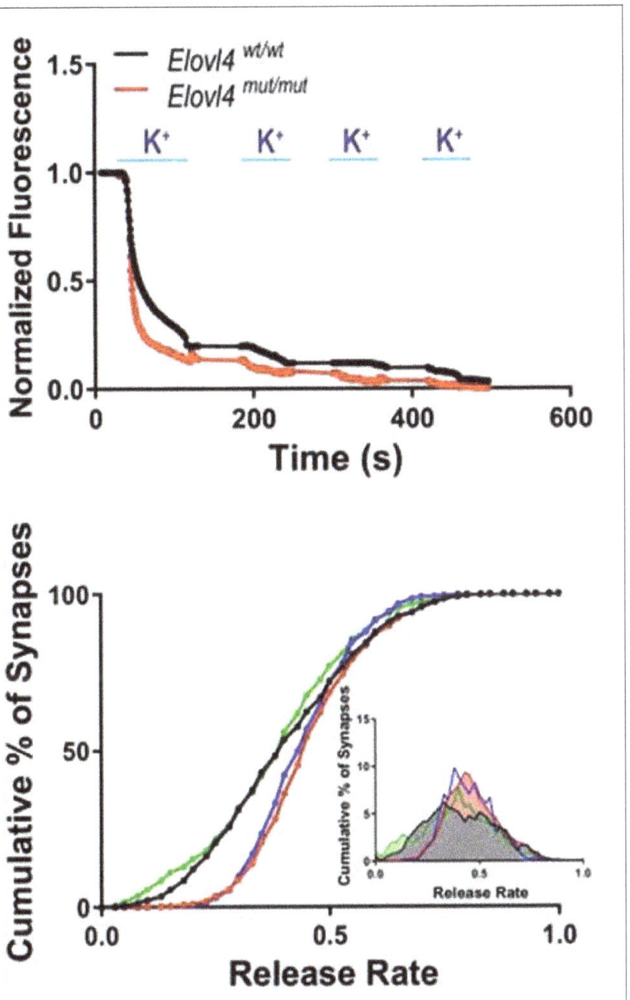


**FIGURE 9 |** Accelerated synaptic vesicle release in *Elovl4* mutant neurons and its rescue by VLC-SFA. **Top panel:** Faster synaptic release in $Elovl4^{mut/mut}$ hippocampal synapses (red) compared to WT control synapses (black), as detected with FM1-43 dye. Representative traces of average synaptic release activated by four rounds of high $K^+$ depolarization. **Bottom panel:** Cumulative graph depicts the fraction of total releasable synaptic vesicle pool exocytosed after 15 s depolarization (WT = black line). Vesicle release kinetics was recorded by FM1-43 fluorescence from 900 to 1200 synapses. Note the robust right shift of the cumulative distribution for $Elovl4^{mut/mut}$ synapses (red), which is rescued by supplementation with 28:0 and 30:0 SFAs (green) but not by 24:0 (blue). Inset: Frequency distribution of responses with slowest responding synapses on the left, and the fastest on the right on the curve.

SV formation are incompletely understood. Because the enzymes that elongate fatty acids, including ELOVL4, localize to the ER, questions arise about how lipids containing the VLC-SFA get selectively incorporated into synaptic vesicles, during the step of vesicle budding and fusion that precedes the release of vesicles from the ER. Before vesicle budding, v-SNARE and transmembrane cargo proteins from the ER membrane collect into the ER budding zone and recruit the proximal and distal coat assembly, leading to a vesicle bound by a neck to the ER membrane (Bonifacino and Glick, 2004). The cargo then becomes concentrated, membrane curvature increases, and vesicle scission occurs. It is tempting to speculate that there may be interaction between lipids containing VLC-SFA and specific transmembrane cargo proteins of the ER. It may also be envisaged that specific proteins of the proximal coat assembly, which regulate the coordinated sorting of vesicles, play a role in selectively trapping the lipids with VLC-SFA into vesicle populations destined to become SVs.

Targeting of vesicles to different organelles requires highly coordinated modification of the PIPs in their membranes. For instance, PIPK4 phosphorylates $PIP_2$ in SV (Guo et al., 2003). Interestingly, contact sites between virtually every organelle and the ER have been identified, and the functional importance of these small, specialized membrane domains is increasingly recognized. Recent developments have highlighted the role of PI-4-P gradients as critical determinants of the non-vesicular transport of various lipids from the ER to other organelles such as the Golgi or plasma membrane (Balla, 2018).

In addition to the ER at the soma, a well-developed smooth ER (SER) in neuronal axons has been known for nearly half a century (Droz et al., 1975). The axonal ER has important biosynthetic functions including synthesis of axonal proteins and nerve ending components (Luarte et al., 2018). An interesting possibility is that the lipid composition of SVs originating from the somatic ER might be modified at the axonal SER during their axonal transport. One can also hypothesize that VLC-SFA may be synthesized there and added to sphingosine (by one of the Cer synthases) or exchanged with an ordinary (16:0) FA-containing sphingolipid at the SER by lipid remodeling. It is clear that most ELOVL4 is localized to the somatic SER, but the possibility that a small fraction of ELOVL4 might be present in axonal SER outposts cannot be ruled out.

## Further Clinical Implications of VLC-FA

### Epilepsy and Ketogenic Diet

Epilepsy patients are prescribed a ketogenic diet – a fat-rich diet that is low in sugars – when all anti-convulsive drugs fail to reduce seizures (Cervenka et al., 2013; Sharma and Tripathi, 2013). The clinical effectiveness of the ketogenic diet (including medium-chain triglyceride diet) has been confirmed in a number of clinical trials carried out mainly on children (Liu, 2008; Kayyali et al., 2014; Kossoff et al., 2018), but its application may be limited by the number of early (gastrointestinal distress, acidosis, hypoglycaemia, dehydration and lethargy), and late adverse effects (hyperuricemia, hyperlipidaemia, kidney stones, easy bruising, and decreases in height and weight) (Ballaban-Gil et al., 1998; Kang et al., 2004; Ulamek-Koziol et al., 2016). With strict monitoring and adapting the diet to the needs of the individual patient according to recently updated guidelines (Kossoff et al., 2018), it is possible to avoid most of these complications. The mechanism by which the ketogenic diet helps to control seizures remains unknown (Kayyali et al., 2014). Assessing changes of VLC-FA levels in the CNS associated with ketogenic diet and seizure disorders could provide valuable insight into the pathophysiology of epilepsy and help to develop more effective therapies.

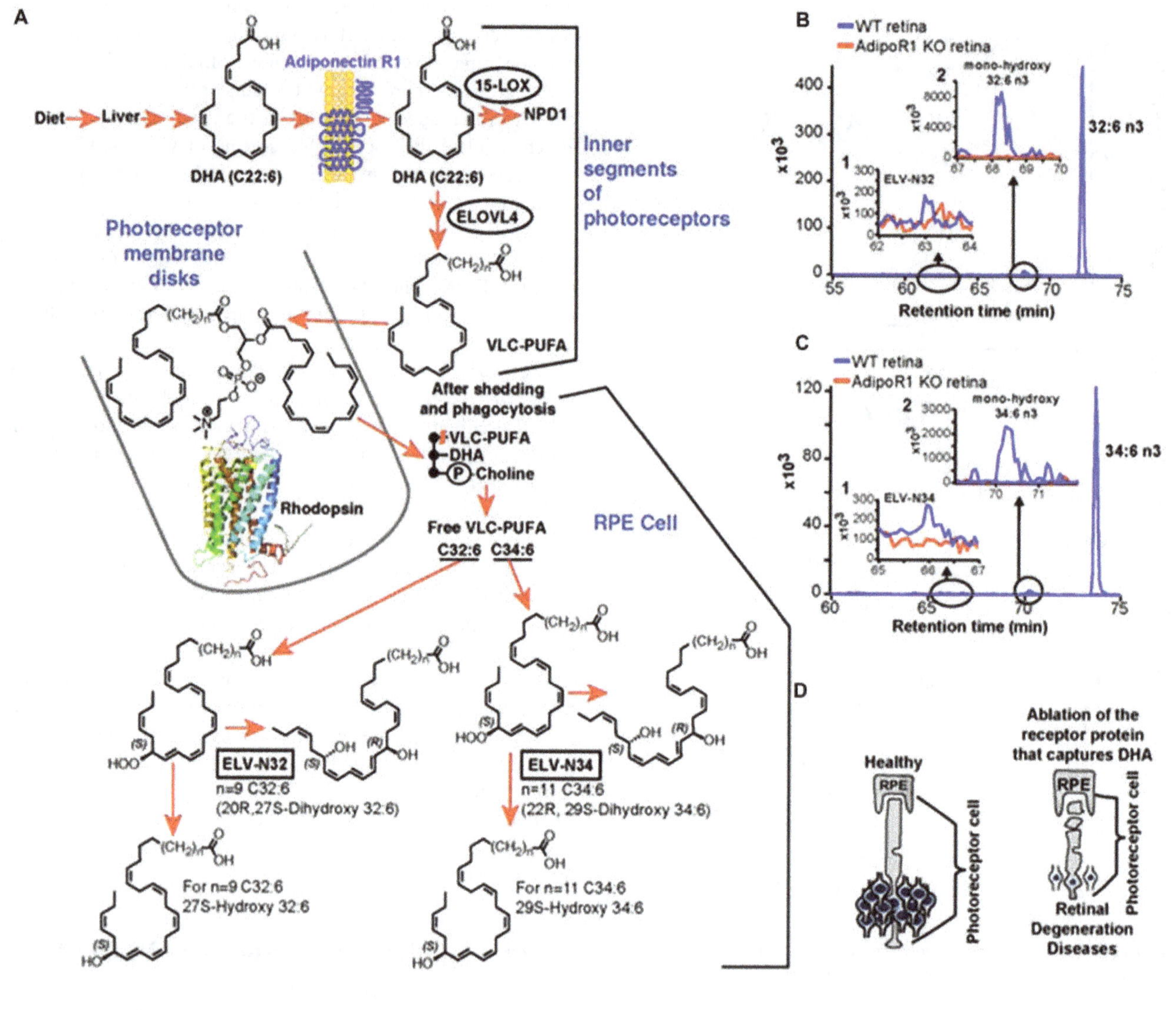


**FIGURE 10 |** Elovanoid signaling derivatives of VLC-PUFA. Genetic ablation of adiponectin receptor 1 leads to depletion of VLC-PUFAs and its derivatives in retina. **(A)** Dietary DHA, or that derived from dietary 18:3n3, is supplied by the liver and captured by adiponectin receptor 1 (AdipoR1), followed by elongation in the inner segment of PRC by ELOVL4 to VLC-PUFA and incorporation into phosphatidylcholine molecular species, which also contains DHA. During daily PRC outer segment renewal, these phosphatidylcholine molecular species interact with rhodopsin and, after shedding and phagocytosis, become part of RPE cells. UOS or other disruptors of homeostasis trigger the release of VLC-PUFAs. 32:6n3 and 34:6n3 are depicted generating hydroperoxy forms, and then ELV-N32 or ELV-N34, respectively. **(B)** The pool size of free 32:6n3 in retinas of AdipoR1 knockout (KO) mice (red) is decreased as compared with that in wild type (WT) (blue). Insert (1) shows ELV-N32 in KO (red) and WT (blue); insert (2) shows mono-hydroxy 32:6n3, the stable derivative of the hydroperoxy precursor of ELV-N32, in WT (blue) and lack of detectable signal in the KO (red). **(C)** Similarly, the pool size of free 34:6n3 in retinas of AdipoR1 KO mice (red) is decreased as compared with that in WT (blue). Insert (1) shows ELV-N32 in KO (red) and WT (blue); insert (2) shows mono-hydroxy 34:6n3, the stable derivative of the hydroperoxy precursor of ELV-N34, in WT (blue) and lack of detectable signal in the KO (red). **(D)** RPE cells sustain PRC functional integrity (left); right, the ablation of AdipoR1 switches off DHA availability, and PRC degeneration ensues.

## Dementia and Alzheimer's Disease

There is tremendous interest in nutritional interventions to prevent cognitive impairment in the elderly, including the potential of fatty acids to prevent or slow cognitive impairment (Bazan et al., 2002; Sinn et al., 2010; Calon, 2011; Jiao et al., 2014; Burckhardt et al., 2016; Rangel-Huerta and Gil, 2018). Change in cell membrane lipid composition has been suggested to be associated with cognitive impairment in Alzheimer's disease (Drolle et al., 2017; Diaz et al., 2018; Penke et al., 2018). Moreover, association between beta-amyloid (Aβ), a main pathological hallmark of Alzheimer's, and arachidonic acid in erythrocyte membrane was found to be specific to Apolipoprotein E ε4 non-carrier patients (Hooper et al., 2017). Treatments with DHA or other PUFAs have not provided significant protection from cognitive decline in the elderly thus far (Carrie et al., 2009; Dacks et al., 2013; Jiao et al., 2014; Phillips et al., 2015;

Nishihira et al., 2016; Zhang et al., 2016), however, assessment of treatments including lipids with longer fatty acids than DHA have started only recently. Ongoing massive clinical trials, like the Cognitive Ageing, Nutrition, and Neurogenesis (CANN) trial, are presently testing potential benefits of combined dietary intervention with long-chain n-3 PUFA and flavonoids on cognition in older adults with mild cognitive impairment or subjective memory impairment (Irvine et al., 2018). The studies summarized in this review pose a number of stimulating questions and open future research directions to explore the potential applicability of VLC-FA to the treatment of specific human brain and retina diseases, like cognitive impairment, epileptic seizures and macular degeneration.

## IN SUMMARY

Recent studies reveal novel functional roles for ELOVL4 and its VLC-FA products in the CNS, including retina and brain, in health and disease. VLC-PUFA play vital functions in the CNS as precursors of compounds that serve newly recognized roles in homeostatic signaling and regulation of neuronal survival. Most recently it was shown that VLC-SFA have essential functions in synaptic transmission, with disruption of VLC-SFA synthesis leading to seizures and neurodegeneration both in patients lacking ELOVL4 and in mouse models of ELOVL4 mutations. A better understanding of VLC-SFA and VLC-PUFA metabolism and their functions in the CNS holds great promise for development of new therapeutic avenues for treatment of seizures and neurodegenerative diseases.

## AUTHOR CONTRIBUTIONS

FD, RA, JF, and DS contributed to the writing and editing of the manuscript.

## FUNDING

This work was supported by a Presbyterian Health Foundation Team Science grant to FD, RA, and DS and NIH grant P30AG050911-04S1. FD was supported by a bridge grant from the Presbyterian Health Foundation and NIH grant P30AG050911-04S1. JF was supported by the OUHSC Department of Cell Biology and a Presbyterian Health Foundation Seed Grant to DS. RA was supported by the NIH grants R01EY04149, P30EY021725, and R21NS090117.

## ACKNOWLEDGMENTS

The authors are thankful to Dr. Martin-Paul Agbaga, Dr. Blake Hopiavuori, Dr. Raghavendra Y. Nagaraja, Gyening Yeboah, Richard Brush, Megan Stiles, and Dr. Feng Li for their insights and discussion.

## REFERENCES


Agbaga, M. P., Brush, R. S., Mandal, M. N., Elliott, M. H., Al-Ubaidi, M. R., and Anderson, R. E. (2010a). Role of ELOVL4 protein in the biosynthesis of docosahexaenoic acid. *Adv. Exp. Med. Biol.* 664, 233–242. doi: 10.1007/978-1-4419-1399-9-27

Agbaga, M. P., Mandal, M. N., and Anderson, R. E. (2010b). Retinal very long-chain PUFAs: new insights from studies on ELOVL4 protein. *J. Lipid Res.* 51, 1624–1642. doi: 10.1194/jlr.R005025

Agbaga, M. P., Brush, R. S., Mandal, M. N., Henry, K., Elliott, M. H., and Anderson, R. E. (2008). Role of Stargardt-3 macular dystrophy protein (ELOVL4) in the biosynthesis of very long chain fatty acids. *Proc. Natl. Acad. Sci. U.S.A.* 105, 12843–12848. doi: 10.1073/pnas.0802607105

Agbaga, M. P., Merriman, D. K., Brush, R. S., Lydic, T. A., Conley, S. M., Naash, M. I., et al. (2018). Differential composition of DHA and very-long-chain PUFAs in rod and cone photoreceptors. *J. Lipid Res.* 59, 1586–1596. doi: 10.1194/jlr.M082495

Aldahmesh, M. A., Mohamed, J. Y., Alkuraya, H. S., Verma, I. C., Puri, R. D., Alaiya, A. A., et al. (2011). Recessive mutations in ELOVL4 cause ichthyosis, intellectual disability, and spastic quadriplegia. *Am. J. Hum. Genet.* 89, 745–750. doi: 10.1016/j.ajhg.2011.10.011

Amen, N., Mathow, D., Rabionet, M., Sandhoff, R., Langbein, L., Gretz, N., et al. (2013). Differentiation of epidermal keratinocytes is dependent on glucosylceramide:ceramide processing. *Hum. Mol. Genet.* 22, 4164–4179. doi: 10.1093/hmg/ddt264

Antonny, B., Vanni, S., Shindou, H., and Ferreira, T. (2015). From zero to six double bonds: phospholipid unsaturation and organelle function. *Trends Cell Biol.* 25, 427–436. doi: 10.1016/j.tcb.2015.03.004

Aveldano, M. I. (1987). A novel group of very long chain polyenoic fatty acids in dipolyunsaturated phosphatidylcholines from vertebrate retina. *J. Biol. Chem.* 262, 1172–1179.

Balch, W. E., Dunphy, W. G., Braell, W. A., and Rothman, J. E. (1984). Reconstitution of the transport of protein between successive compartments of the Golgi measured by the coupled incorporation of N-acetylglucosamine. *Cell* 39(2 Pt 1), 405–416. doi: 10.1016/0092-8674(84)90019-9

Balla, T. (2018). Ca(2+) and lipid signals hold hands at endoplasmic reticulum-plasma membrane contact sites. *J. Physiol.* 596, 2709–2716. doi: 10.1113/JP274957

Ballaban-Gil, K., Callahan, C., O'Dell, C., Pappo, M., Moshe, S., and Shinnar, S. (1998). Complications of the ketogenic diet. *Epilepsia* 39, 744–748.

Bardak, H., Gunay, M., Ercalik, Y., Bardak, Y., Ozbas, H., Bagci, O., et al. (2016). Analysis of ELOVL4 and PRPH2 genes in turkish stargardt disease patients. *Genet. Mol. Res.* 15, 1-6. doi: 10.4238/gmr15048774

Bazan, N. G. (2018). Docosanoids and elovanoids from omega-3 fatty acids are pro-homeostatic modulators of inflammatory responses, cell damage and neuroprotection. *Mol. Aspects Med.* 64, 18–33. doi: 10.1016/j.mam.2018.09.003

Bazan, N. G., Colangelo, V., and Lukiw, W. J. (2002). Prostaglandins and other lipid mediators in Alzheimer's disease. *Prostaglandins Other Lipid Mediat.* 6, 197–210. doi: 10.1016/s0090-6980(02)00031-x

Bazinet, R. P., and Laye, S. (2014). Polyunsaturated fatty acids and their metabolites in brain function and disease. *Nat. Rev. Neurosci.* 15, 771–785. doi: 10.1038/nrn3820

Bennett, L. D., Brush, R. S., Chan, M., Lydic, T. A., Reese, K., Reid, G. E., et al. (2014a). Effect of reduced retinal VLC-PUFA on rod and cone photoreceptors. *Invest. Ophthalmol. Vis. Sci.* 55, 3150–3157. doi: 10.1167/iovs.14-13995

Bennett, L. D., Hopiavuori, B. R., Brush, R. S., Chan, M., Van Hook, M. J., Thoreson, W. B., et al. (2014b). Examination of VLC-PUFA-deficient photoreceptor terminals. *Invest Ophthalmol. Vis. Sci.* 55, 4063–4072. doi: 10.1167/iovs.14-13997

Bernstein, P. S., Tammur, J., Singh, N., Hutchinson, A., Dixon, M., Pappas, C. M., et al. (2001). Diverse macular dystrophy phenotype caused by a novel complex mutation in the ELOVL4 gene. *Invest. Ophthalmol. Vis. Sci.* 42, 3331–3336.

Bhattacharjee, S., Jun, B., Belayev, L., Heap, J., Kautzmann, M. A., Obenaus, A., et al. (2017). Elovanoids are a novel class of homeostatic lipid mediators that protect neural cell integrity upon injury. *Sci. Adv.* 3:e1700735. doi: 10.1126/sciadv.1700735

Bonifacino, J. S., and Glick, B. S. (2004). The mechanisms of vesicle budding and fusion. *Cell* 116, 153–166. doi: 10.1016/s0092-8674(03)01079-1

Bourassa, C. V., Raskin, S., Serafini, S., Teive, H. A., Dion, P. A., and Rouleau, G. A. (2015). A new ELOVL4 mutation in a case of spinocerebellar ataxia with erythrokeratodermia. *JAMA Neurol.* 72, 942–943. doi: 10.1001/jamaneurol.2015.0888

Bourque, P. R., Warman-Chardon, J., Lelli, D. A., LaBerge, L., Kirshen, C., Bradshaw, S. H., et al. (2018). Novel ELOVL4 mutation associated with erythrokeratodermia and spinocerebellar ataxia (SCA 34). *Neurol. Genet.* 4:e263. doi: 10.1212/NXG.0000000000000263

Bozek, K., Wei, Y., Yan, Z., Liu, X., Xiong, J., Sugimoto, M., et al. (2015). Organization and evolution of brain lipidome revealed by large-scale analysis of human, chimpanzee, macaque, and mouse tissues. *Neuron* 85, 695–702. doi: 10.1016/j.neuron.2015.01.003

Brodde, A., Teigler, A., Brugger, B., Lehmann, W. D., Wieland, F., Berger, J., et al. (2012). Impaired neurotransmission in ether lipid-deficient nerve terminals. *Hum. Mol. Genet.* 21, 2713–2724. doi: 10.1093/hmg/dds097

Burckhardt, M., Herke, M., Wustmann, T., Watzke, S., Langer, G., and Fink, A. (2016). Omega-3 fatty acids for the treatment of dementia. *Cochrane Database Syst. Rev.* 4:CD009002. doi: 10.1002/14651858.CD009002.pub3

Cadieux-Dion, M., Turcotte-Gauthier, M., Noreau, A., Martin, C., Meloche, C., Gravel, M., et al. (2014). Expanding the clinical phenotype associated with ELOVL4 mutation: study of a large french-canadian family with autosomal dominant spinocerebellar ataxia and erythrokeratodermia. *JAMA Neurol.* 71, 470–475. doi: 10.1001/jamaneurol.2013.6337

Calon, F. (2011). Omega-3 polyunsaturated fatty acids in Alzheimer's disease: key questions and partial answers. *Curr. Alzheimer Res.* 8, 470–478. doi: 10.2174/156720511796391881

Cameron, D. J., Tong, Z., Yang, Z., Kaminoh, J., Kamiyah, S., Chen, H., et al. (2007). Essential role of Elovl4 in very long chain fatty acid synthesis, skin permeability barrier function, and neonatal survival. *Int. J. Biol. Sci.* 3, 111–119. doi: 10.7150/ijbs.3.111

Carmona-Antonanzas, G., Monroig, O., Dick, J. R., Davie, A., and Tocher, D. R. (2011). Biosynthesis of very long-chain fatty acids (C>24) in atlantic salmon: cloning, functional characterisation, and tissue distribution of an Elovl4 elongase. *Comp. Biochem. Physiol. B Biochem. Mol. Biol.* 159, 122–129. doi: 10.1016/j.cbpb.2011.02.007

Carrie, I., Abellan Van Kan, G., Rolland, Y., Gillette-Guyonnet, S., and Vellas, B. (2009). PUFA for prevention and treatment of dementia? *Curr. Pharm. Des.* 15, 4173–4185. doi: 10.2174/138161209789909764

Carta, M., Lanore, F., Rebola, N., Szabo, Z., Da Silva, S. V., Lourenco, J., et al. (2014). Membrane lipids tune synaptic transmission by direct modulation of presynaptic potassium channels. *Neuron* 81, 787–799. doi: 10.1016/j.neuron.2013.12.028

Castro, L. F., Tocher, D. R., and Monroig, O. (2016). Long-chain polyunsaturated fatty acid biosynthesis in chordates: insights into the evolution of Fads and Elovl gene repertoire. *Prog. Lipid Res.* 62, 25–40. doi: 10.1016/j.plipres.2016.01.001

Cervenka, M. C., Henry, B., Nathan, J., Wood, S., and Volek, J. S. (2013). Worldwide dietary therapies for adults with epilepsy and other disorders. *J. Child Neurol.* 28, 1034–1040. doi: 10.1177/0883073813488671

Craig, L. B., Brush, R. S., Sullivan, M. T., Zavy, M. T., Agbaga, M. P., and Anderson, R. E. (2019). Decreased very long chain polyunsaturated fatty acids in sperm correlates with sperm quantity and quality. *J. Assist. Reprod. Genet.* 36, 1379–1385. doi: 10.1007/s10815-019-01464-3

Cremona, O., Di Paolo, G., Wenk, M. R., Luthi, A., Kim, W. T., Takei, K., et al. (1999). Essential role of phosphoinositide metabolism in synaptic vesicle recycling. *Cell* 99, 179–188. doi: 10.1016/s0092-8674(00)81649-9

Dacks, P. A., Shineman, D. W., and Fillit, H. M. (2013). Current evidence for the clinical use of long-chain polyunsaturated n-3 fatty acids to prevent age-related cognitive decline and Alzheimer's disease. *J. Nutr. Health Aging* 17, 240–251. doi: 10.1007/s12603-012-0431-3

Deák, F., Shin, O. H., Kavalali, E. T., and Sudhof, T. C. (2006a). Structural determinants of synaptobrevin 2 function in synaptic vesicle fusion. *J. Neurosci.* 26, 6668–6676. doi: 10.1523/JNEUROSCI.5272-05.2006

Deák, F., Shin, O. H., Tang, J., Hanson, P., Ubach, J., Jahn, R., et al. (2006b). Rabphilin regulates SNARE-dependent re-priming of synaptic vesicles for fusion. *EMBO J.* 25, 2856–2866. doi: 10.1038/sj.emboj.7601165

Deák, F., Xu, Y., Chang, W. P., Dulubova, I., Khvotchev, M., Liu, X., et al. (2009). Munc18-1 binding to the neuronal SNARE complex controls synaptic vesicle priming. *J. Cell Biol.* 184, 751–764. doi: 10.1083/jcb.200812026

Di Gregorio, E., Borroni, B., Giorgio, E., Lacerenza, D., Ferrero, M., Lo Buono, N., et al. (2014). ELOVL5 mutations cause spinocerebellar ataxia 38. *Am. J. Hum. Genet.* 95, 209–217. doi: 10.1016/j.ajhg.2014.07.001

Di Paolo, G., Moskowitz, H. S., Gipson, K., Wenk, M. R., Voronov, S., Obayashi, M., et al. (2004). Impaired PtdIns(4,5)P2 synthesis in nerve terminals produces defects in synaptic vesicle trafficking. *Nature* 431, 415–422. doi: 10.1038/nature02896

Diaz, M., Fabelo, N., Ferrer, I., and Marin, R. (2018). "Lipid raft aging" in the human frontal cortex during nonpathological aging: gender influences and potential implications in Alzheimer's disease. *Neurobiol. Aging* 67, 42–52. doi: 10.1016/j.neurobiolaging.2018.02.022

Dickson, D. W. (1997). The pathogenesis of senile plaques. *J. Neuropathol. Exp. Neurol.* 56, 321–339. doi: 10.1097/00005072-199704000-00001

Donato, L., Scimone, C., Rinaldi, C., Aragona, P., Briuglia, S., D'Ascola, A., et al. (2018). Stargardt phenotype associated with two ELOVL4 promoter variants and ELOVL4 downregulation: new possible perspective to etiopathogenesis? *Invest. Ophthalmol. Vis. Sci.* 59, 843–857. doi: 10.1167/iovs.17-22962

Drolle, E., Negoda, A., Hammond, K., Pavlov, E., and Leonenko, Z. (2017). Changes in lipid membranes may trigger amyloid toxicity in Alzheimer's disease. *PLoS One* 12:e0182194. doi: 10.1371/journal.pone.0182194

Droz, B., Rambourg, A., and Koenig, H. L. (1975). The smooth endoplasmic reticulum: structure and role in the renewal of axonal membrane and synaptic vesicles by fast axonal transport. *Brain Res.* 93, 1–13. doi: 10.1016/0006-8993(75)90282-6

Edwards, A. O., Donoso, L. A., and Ritter, R. (2001). A novel gene for autosomal dominant Stargardt-like macular dystrophy with homology to the SUR4 protein family. *Invest. Ophthalmol. Vis. Sci.* 42, 2652–2663.

Fan, S. F., and Yazulla, S. (2004). Inhibitory interaction of cannabinoid CB1 receptor and dopamine D2 receptor agonists on voltage-gated currents of goldfish cones. *Vis. Neurosci.* 21, 69–77. doi: 10.1017/s0952523804041070

Fernandez-Chacon, R., Konigstorfer, A., Gerber, S. H., Garcia, J., Matos, M. F., Stevens, C. F., et al. (2001). Synaptotagmin I functions as a calcium regulator of release probability. *Nature* 410, 41–49. doi: 10.1038/35065004

Fesce, R., Grohovaz, F., Valtorta, F., and Meldolesi, J. (1994). Neurotransmitter release: fusion or 'kiss-and-run'? *Trends Cell Biol.* 4, 1–4. doi: 10.1016/0962-8924(94)90025-6

Gandhi, S. P., and Stevens, C. F. (2003). Three modes of synaptic vesicular recycling revealed by single-vesicle imaging. *Nature* 423, 607–613. doi: 10.1038/nature01677

Garagnani, P., Bacalini, M. G., Pirazzini, C., Gori, D., Giuliani, C., Mari, D., et al. (2012). Methylation of ELOVL2 gene as a new epigenetic marker of age. *Aging Cell* 11, 1132–1134. doi: 10.1111/acel.12005

Gopalan, S., Carja, O., Fagny, M., Patin, E., Myrick, J. W., McEwen, L. M., et al. (2017). Trends in DNA methylation with age replicate across diverse human populations. *Genetics* 206, 1659–1674. doi: 10.1534/genetics.116.195594

Grayson, C., and Molday, R. S. (2005). Dominant negative mechanism underlies autosomal dominant stargardt-like macular dystrophy linked to mutations in ELOVL4. *J. Biol. Chem.* 280, 32521–32530. doi: 10.1074/jbc.M503411200

Guillou, H., Zadravec, D., Martin, P. G., and Jacobsson, A. (2010). The key roles of elongases and desaturases in mammalian fatty acid metabolism: insights from transgenic mice. *Prog. Lipid Res.* 49, 186–199. doi: 10.1016/j.plipres.2009.12.002

Guo, J., Wenk, M. R., Pellegrini, L., Onofri, F., Benfenati, F., and De Camilli, P. (2003). Phosphatidylinositol 4-kinase type IIalpha is responsible for the phosphatidylinositol 4-kinase activity associated with synaptic vesicles. *Proc. Natl. Acad. Sci. U.S.A.* 100, 3995–4000. doi: 10.1073/pnas.0230488100

Hao, M., Mukherjee, S., and Maxfield, F. R. (2001). Cholesterol depletion induces large scale domain segregation in living cell membranes. *Proc. Natl. Acad. Sci. U.S.A.* 98, 13072–13077. doi: 10.1073/pnas.231377398

Hastings, N., Agaba, M. K., Tocher, D. R., Zheng, X., Dickson, C. A., Dick, J. R., et al. (2004). Molecular cloning and functional characterization of fatty acyl desaturase and elongase cDNAs involved in the production of eicosapentaenoic and docosahexaenoic acids from alpha-linolenic acid in Atlantic salmon (salmo salar). *Mar. Biotechnol.* 6, 463–474. doi: 10.1007/s10126-004-3002-8

Hata, Y., Slaughter, C. A., and Sudhof, T. C. (1993). Synaptic vesicle fusion complex contains unc-18 homologue bound to syntaxin. *Nature* 366, 347–351. doi: 10.1038/366347a0

Hooper, C., De Souto Barreto, P., Payoux, P., Salabert, A. S., Guyonnet, S., Andrieu, S., et al. (2017). Cross-sectional associations of cortical beta-amyloid with erythrocyte membrane long-chain polyunsaturated fatty acids in older adults with subjective memory complaints. *J. Neurochem.* 142, 589–596. doi: 10.1111/jnc.14062

Hopiavuori, B. R., Agbaga, M. P., Brush, R. S., Sullivan, M. T., Sonntag, W. E., and Anderson, R. E. (2017). Regional changes in CNS and retinal glycerophospholipid profiles with age: a molecular blueprint. *J. Lipid Res.* 58, 668–680. doi: 10.1194/jlr.M070714

Hopiavuori, B. R., Anderson, R. E., and Agbaga, M. P. (2019). ELOVL4: very long-chain fatty acids serve an eclectic role in mammalian health and function. *Prog. Retin. Eye Res.* 69, 137–158. doi: 10.1016/j.preteyeres.2018.10.004

Hopiavuori, B. R., Deak, F., Wilkerson, J. L., Brush, R. S., Rocha-Hopiavuori, N. A., Hopiavuori, A. R., et al. (2018). Homozygous expression of mutant ELOVL4 leads to seizures and death in a novel animal model of very long-chain fatty acid deficiency. *Mol. Neurobiol.* 55, 1795–1813. doi: 10.1007/s12035-017-0824-8

Hoxha, E., Gabriele, R. M. C., Balbo, I., Ravera, F., Masante, L., Zambelli, V., et al. (2017). Motor deficits and cerebellar atrophy in Elovl5 knock out mice. *Front. Cell Neurosci.* 11:343. doi: 10.3389/fncel.2017.00343

Imig, C., Min, S. W., Krinner, S., Arancillo, M., Rosenmund, C., Sudhof, T. C., et al. (2014). The morphological and molecular nature of synaptic vesicle priming at presynaptic active zones. *Neuron* 84, 416–431. doi: 10.1016/j.neuron.2014.10.009

Irvine, M. A., Scholey, A., King, R., Gillings, R., Vauzour, D., Demichele, S. J., et al. (2018). The cognitive ageing, nutrition and neurogenesis (CANN) trial: design and progress. *Alzheimers Dement.* 4, 591–601. doi: 10.1016/j.trci.2018.08.001

Jacobson, K., Mouritsen, O. G., and Anderson, R. G. (2007). Lipid rafts: at a crossroad between cell biology and physics. *Nat. Cell Biol.* 9, 7–14. doi: 10.1038/ncb0107-7

Jakobsson, A., Westerberg, R., and Jacobsson, A. (2006). Fatty acid elongases in mammals: their regulation and roles in metabolism. *Prog. Lipid Res.* 45, 237–249. doi: 10.1016/j.plipres.2006.01.004

Janssen, R. J., Distelmaier, F., Smeets, R., Wijnhoven, T., Ostergaard, E., Jaspers, N. G., et al. (2009). Contiguous gene deletion of ELOVL7, ERCC8 and NDUFAF2 in a patient with a fatal multisystem disorder. *Hum. Mol. Genet.* 18, 3365–3374. doi: 10.1093/hmg/ddp276

Jiao, J., Li, Q., Chu, J., Zeng, W., Yang, M., and Zhu, S. (2014). Effect of n-3 PUFA supplementation on cognitive function throughout the life span from infancy to old age: a systematic review and meta-analysis of randomized controlled trials. *Am. J. Clin. Nutr.* 100, 1422–1436. doi: 10.3945/ajcn.114.095315

Jun, B., Mukherjee, P. K., Asatryan, A., Kautzmann, M. A., Heap, J., Gordon, W. C., et al. (2017). Elovanoids are novel cell-specific lipid mediators necessary for neuroprotective signaling for photoreceptor cell integrity. *Sci. Rep.* 7:5279. doi: 10.1038/s41598-017-05433-7

Jung, S. E., Lim, S. M., Hong, S. R., Lee, E. H., Shin, K. J., and Lee, H. Y. (2019). DNA methylation of the ELOVL2, FHL2, KLF14, C1orf132/MIR29B2C, and TRIM59 genes for age prediction from blood, saliva, and buccal swab samples. *Forensic. Sci. Int. Genet.* 38, 1–8. doi: 10.1016/j.fsigen.2018.09.010

Kaiser, C. A., and Schekman, R. (1990). Distinct sets of SEC genes govern transport vesicle formation and fusion early in the secretory pathway. *Cell* 61, 723–733. doi: 10.1016/0092-8674(90)90483-u

Kang, H. C., Chung, D. E., Kim, D. W., and Kim, H. D. (2004). Early- and late-onset complications of the ketogenic diet for intractable epilepsy. *Epilepsia* 45, 1116–1123. doi: 10.1111/j.0013-9580.2004.10004.x

Katz, B., and Miledi, R. (1979). Estimates of quantal content during 'chemical potentiation' of transmitter release. *Proc. R. Soc. Lond. B Biol. Sci.* 205, 369–378. doi: 10.1098/rspb.1979.0070

Kayyali, H. R., Gustafson, M., Myers, T., Thompson, L., Williams, M., and Abdelmoity, A. (2014). Ketogenic diet efficacy in the treatment of intractable epileptic spasms. *Pediatr. Neurol.* 50, 224–227. doi: 10.1016/j.pediatrneurol.2013.11.021

Khuong, T. M., Habets, R. L., Kuenen, S., Witkowska, A., Kasprowicz, J., Swerts, J., et al. (2013). Synaptic PI(3,4,5)P3 is required for syntaxin1a clustering and neurotransmitter release. *Neuron* 77, 1097–1108. doi: 10.1016/j.neuron.2013.01.025

Kihara, A. (2012). Very long-chain fatty acids: elongation, physiology and related disorders. *J. Biochem.* 152, 387–395. doi: 10.1093/jb/mvs105

Kikuchi, M., Shimada, M., Matsuzaka, T., Ishii, K., Nakagawa, Y., Takayanagi, M., et al. (2016). Crucial role of Elovl6 in chondrocyte growth and differentiation during growth plate development in mice. *PLoS One* 11:e0159375. doi: 10.1371/journal.pone.0159375

Kohlhardt, M. (1989). Insensitivity of the open state of (-)-DPI-modified cardiac Na+ channels to the blocking effects of the (+) enantiomer. *Eur. J. Pharmacol.* 168, 115–118. doi: 10.1016/0014-2999(89)90642-0

Konishi, H., Okuda, A., Ohno, Y., and Kihara, A. (2010). Characterization of HACD1 K64Q mutant found in arrhythmogenic right ventricular dysplasia patients. *J. Biochem.* 148, 617–622. doi: 10.1093/jb/mvq092

Kossoff, E. H., Zupec-Kania, B. A., Auvin, S., Ballaban-Gil, K. R., Christina Bergqvist, A. G., Blackford, R., et al. (2018). Optimal clinical management of children receiving dietary therapies for epilepsy: updated recommendations of the International ketogenic diet study group. *Epilepsia Open* 3, 175–192. doi: 10.1002/epi4.12225

Lauwers, E., Goodchild, R., and Verstreken, P. (2016). Membrane lipids in presynaptic function and disease. *Neuron* 90, 11–25. doi: 10.1016/j.neuron.2016.02.033

Lein, E. S., Hawrylycz, M. J., Ao, N., Ayres, M., Bensinger, A., Bernard, A., et al. (2007). Genome-wide atlas of gene expression in the adult mouse brain. *Nature* 445, 168–176. doi: 10.1038/nature05453

Leonard, A. E., Kelder, B., Bobik, E. G., Chuang, L. T., Lewis, C. J., Kopchick, J. J., et al. (2002). Identification and expression of mammalian long-chain PUFA elongation enzymes. *Lipids* 37, 733–740. doi: 10.1007/s11745-002-0955-6

Li, G., Cui, S., Du, J., Liu, J., Zhang, P., Fu, Y., et al. (2018). Association of GALC, ZNF184, IL1R2 and ELOVL7 with parkinson's disease in southern chinese. *Front. Aging Neurosci.* 10:402. doi: 10.3389/fnagi.2018.00402

Lin, Z., Huang, Y., Zou, W., Rong, H., Hao, M., and Wen, X. (2018). Cloning, tissue distribution, functional characterization and nutritional regulation of a fatty acyl Elovl5 elongase in chu's croaker Nibea coibor. *Gene* 659, 11–21. doi: 10.1016/j.gene.2018.03.046

Linetti, A., Fratangeli, A., Taverna, E., Valnegri, P., Francolini, M., Cappello, V., et al. (2010). Cholesterol reduction impairs exocytosis of synaptic vesicles. *J. Cell Sci.* 123(Pt 4), 595–605. doi: 10.1242/jcs.060681

Liu, Y. M. (2008). Medium-chain triglyceride (MCT) ketogenic therapy. *Epilepsia* 49(Suppl. 8), 33–36. doi: 10.1111/j.1528-1167.2008.01830.x

Logan, S., Agbaga, M. P., Chan, M. D., Brush, R. S., and Anderson, R. E. (2014). Endoplasmic reticulum microenvironment and conserved histidines govern ELOVL4 fatty acid elongase activity. *J. Lipid Res.* 55, 698–708. doi: 10.1194/jlr.M045443

Logan, S., Agbaga, M. P., Chan, M. D., Kabir, N., Mandal, N. A., Brush, R. S., et al. (2013). Deciphering mutant ELOVL4 activity in autosomal-dominant stargardt macular dystrophy. *Proc. Natl. Acad. Sci. U.S.A.* 110, 5446–5451. doi: 10.1073/pnas.1217251110

Luarte, A., Cornejo, V. H., Bertin, F., Gallardo, J., and Couve, A. (2018). The axonal endoplasmic reticulum: one organelle-many functions in development, maintenance, and plasticity. *Dev. Neurobiol.* 78, 181–208. doi: 10.1002/dneu.22560

Mandal, M. N., Ambasudhan, R., Wong, P. W., Gage, P. J., Sieving, P. A., and Ayyagari, R. (2004). Characterization of mouse orthologue of ELOVL4: genomic organization and spatial and temporal expression. *Genomics* 83, 626–635. doi: 10.1016/j.ygeno.2003.09.020

Marza, E., Long, T., Saiardi, A., Sumakovic, M., Eimer, S., Hall, D. H., et al. (2008). Polyunsaturated fatty acids influence synaptojanin localization to regulate synaptic vesicle recycling. *Mol. Biol Cell.* 19, 833–842. doi: 10.1091/mbc.e07-07-0719

Matsuzaka, T., Shimano, H., Yahagi, N., Kato, T., Atsumi, A., Yamamoto, T., et al. (2007). Crucial role of a long-chain fatty acid elongase, Elovl6, in obesity-induced insulin resistance. *Nat. Med.* 13, 1193–1202. doi: 10.1038/nm1662

Maugeri, A., Meire, F., Hoyng, C. B., Vink, C., Van Regemorter, N., Karan, G., et al. (2004). A novel mutation in the ELOVL4 gene causes autosomal dominant Stargardt-like macular dystrophy. *Invest. Ophthalmol. Vis. Sci.* 45, 4263–4267. doi: 10.1167/iovs.04-0078

McMahon, A., Butovich, I. A., Mata, N. L., Klein, M., Ritter, R. III, Richardson, J., et al. (2007). Retinal pathology and skin barrier defect in mice carrying a stargardt disease-3 mutation in elongase of very long chain fatty acids-4. *Mol. Vis.* 13, 258–272.

McMahon, A., Lu, H., and Butovich, I. A. (2014). A role for ELOVL4 in the mouse meibomian gland and sebocyte cell biology. *Invest. Ophthalmol. Vis. Sci.* 55, 2832–2840. doi: 10.1167/iovs.13-13335

McNew, J. A., Weber, T., Parlati, F., Johnston, R. J., Melia, T. J., Sollner, T. H., et al. (2000). Close is not enough: SNARE-dependent membrane fusion requires an active mechanism that transduces force to membrane anchors. *J. Cell Biol.* 150, 105–117.

Melia, T. J., Weber, T., McNew, J. A., Fisher, L. E., Johnston, R. J., Parlati, F., et al. (2002). Regulation of membrane fusion by the membrane-proximal coil of the t-SNARE during zippering of SNAREpins. *J. Cell Biol.* 158, 929–940. doi: 10.1083/jcb.200112081

Mir, H., Raza, S. I., Touseef, M., Memon, M. M., Khan, M. N., Jaffar, S., et al. (2014). A novel recessive mutation in the gene ELOVL4 causes a neuro-ichthyotic disorder with variable expressivity. *BMC Med. Genet.* 15:25. doi: 10.1186/1471-2350-15-25

Molday, R. S., and Zhang, K. (2010). Defective lipid transport and biosynthesis in recessive and dominant stargardt macular degeneration. *Prog. Lipid Res.* 49, 476–492. doi: 10.1016/j.plipres.2010.07.002

Monroig, O., Rotllant, J., Cerda-Reverter, J. M., Dick, J. R., Figueras, A., and Tocher, D. R. (2010). Expression and role of Elovl4 elongases in biosynthesis of very long-chain fatty acids during zebrafish danio rerio early embryonic development. *Biochim. Biophys. Acta* 1801, 1145–1154. doi: 10.1016/j.bbalip.2010.06.005

Monroig, Ó, Webb, K., Ibarra-Castro, L., Holt, G. J., and Tocher, D. R. (2011). Biosynthesis of long-chain polyunsaturated fatty acids in marine fish: characterization of an Elovl4-like elongase from cobia rachycentron canadum and activation of the pathway during early life stages. *Aquaculture* 312, 145–153. doi: 10.1016/j.aquaculture.2010.12.024

Moon, Y. A., and Horton, J. D. (2003). Identification of two mammalian reductases involved in the two-carbon fatty acyl elongation cascade. *J. Biol. Chem.* 278, 7335–7343. doi: 10.1074/jbc.M211684200

Moon, Y. A., Ochoa, C. R., Mitsche, M. A., Hammer, R. E., and Horton, J. D. (2014). Deletion of ELOVL6 blocks the synthesis of oleic acid but does not prevent the development of fatty liver or insulin resistance. *J. Lipid Res.* 55, 2597–2605. doi: 10.1194/jlr.M054353

Moon, Y. A., Shah, N. A., Mohapatra, S., Warrington, J. A., and Horton, J. D. (2001). Identification of a mammalian long chain fatty acyl elongase regulated by sterol regulatory element-binding proteins. *J. Biol. Chem.* 276, 45358–45366. doi: 10.1074/jbc.M108413200

Morais, S., Monroig, O., Zheng, X., Leaver, M. J., and Tocher, D. R. (2009). Highly unsaturated fatty acid synthesis in Atlantic salmon: characterization of ELOVL5- and ELOVL2-like elongases. *Mar. Biotechnol.* 11, 627–639. doi: 10.1007/s10126-009-9179-0

Mueller, N., Sassa, T., Morales-Gonzalez, S., Schneider, J., Salchow, D. J., Seelow, D., et al. (2019). De novo mutation in ELOVL1 causes ichthyosis, acanthosis nigricans, hypomyelination, spastic paraplegia, high frequency deafness and optic atrophy. *J. Med. Genet.* 56, 164–175. doi: 10.1136/jmedgenet-2018-105711

Muller, C. P., Reichel, M., Muhle, C., Rhein, C., Gulbins, E., and Kornhuber, J. (2015). Brain membrane lipids in major depression and anxiety disorders. *Biochim. Biophys. Acta* 1851, 1052–1065. doi: 10.1016/j.bbalip.2014.12.014

Naganuma, T., Sato, Y., Sassa, T., Ohno, Y., and Kihara, A. (2011). Biochemical characterization of the very long-chain fatty acid elongase ELOVL7. *FEBS Lett.* 585, 3337–3341. doi: 10.1016/j.febslet.2011.09.024

Nguyen, J. H., Yamamoto, S., Steers, J., Sevlever, D., Lin, W., Shimojima, N., et al. (2006). Matrix metalloproteinase-9 contributes to brain extravasation and edema in fulminant hepatic failure mice. *J. Hepatol.* 44, 1105–1114. doi: 10.1016/j.jhep.2005.09.019

Nishihira, J., Tokashiki, T., Higashiuesato, Y., Willcox, D. C., Mattek, N., Shinto, L., et al. (2016). Associations between serum omega-3 fatty acid levels and cognitive functions among community-dwelling octogenarians in okinawa, Japan: the KOCOA study. *J. Alzheimers Dis.* 51, 857–866. doi: 10.3233/JAD-150910

Novick, P., and Schekman, R. (1979). Secretion and cell-surface growth are blocked in a temperature-sensitive mutant of *Saccharomyces cerevisiae*. *Proc. Natl. Acad. Sci. U.S.A.* 76, 1858–1862. doi: 10.1073/pnas.76.4.1858

Oboh, A., Betancor, M. B., Tocher, D. R., and Monroig, O. (2016). Biosynthesis of long-chain polyunsaturated fatty acids in the African catfish *Clarias gariepinus*: molecular cloning and functional characterisation of fatty acyl desaturase (fads2) and elongase (elovl2) cDNAs7. *Aquaculture* 462, 70–79. doi: 10.1016/j.aquaculture.2016.05.018

Ohno, Y., Suto, S., Yamanaka, M., Mizutani, Y., Mitsutake, S., Igarashi, Y., et al. (2010). ELOVL1 production of C24 acyl-CoAs is linked to C24 sphingolipid synthesis. *Proc. Natl. Acad. Sci. U.S.A.* 107, 18439–18444. doi: 10.1073/pnas.1005572107

Okuda, A., Naganuma, T., Ohno, Y., Abe, K., Yamagata, M., Igarashi, Y., et al. (2010). Hetero-oligomeric interactions of an ELOVL4 mutant protein: implications in the molecular mechanism of stargardt-3 macular dystrophy. *Mol. Vis.* 16, 2438–2445.

Ozaki, K., Ansai, A., Nobuhara, K., Araki, T., Kubodera, T., Ishii, T., et al. (2019). Prevalence and clinicoradiological features of spinocerebellar ataxia type 34 in a Japanese ataxia cohort. *Parkinsonism Relat. Disord.* doi: 10.1016/j.parkreldis.2019.05.019 [Epub ahead of print].

Ozaki, K., Doi, H., Mitsui, J., Sato, N., Iikuni, Y., Majima, T., et al. (2015). A Novel Mutation in ELOVL4 leading to spinocerebellar ataxia (SCA) with the hot cross bun sign but lacking erythrokeratodermia: a broadened spectrum of SCA34. *JAMA Neurol.* 72, 797–805. doi: 10.1001/jamaneurol.2015.0610

Pauter, A. M., Olsson, P., Asadi, A., Herslof, B., Csikasz, R. I., Zadravec, D., et al. (2014). Elovl2 ablation demonstrates that systemic DHA is endogenously produced and is essential for lipid homeostasis in mice. *J. Lipid Res.* 55, 718–728. doi: 10.1194/jlr.M046151

Penke, B., Paragi, G., Gera, J., Berkecz, R., Kovacs, Z., Crul, T., et al. (2018). The role of lipids and membranes in the pathogenesis of Alzheimer's disease: a comprehensive view. *Curr. Alzheimer Res.* 15, 1191–1212. doi: 10.2174/1567205015666180911151716

Pereira, S. L., Leonard, A. E., Huang, Y. S., Chuang, L. T., and Mukerji, P. (2004). Identification of two novel microalgal enzymes involved in the conversion of the omega3-fatty acid, eicosapentaenoic acid, into docosahexaenoic acid. *Biochem. J.* 384(Pt 2), 357–366. doi: 10.1042/BJ20040970

Perin, M. S., Fried, V. A., Mignery, G. A., Jahn, R., and Sudhof, T. C. (1990). Phospholipid binding by a synaptic vesicle protein homologous to the regulatory region of protein kinase C. *Nature* 345, 260–263. doi: 10.1038/345260a0

Petersen, R. C. (2004). Mild cognitive impairment as a diagnostic entity. *J. Intern. Med.* 256, 183–194. doi: 10.1111/j.1365-2796.2004.01388.x

Phillips, M. A., Childs, C. E., Calder, P. C., and Rogers, P. J. (2015). No effect of omega-3 fatty acid supplementation on cognition and mood in individuals with cognitive impairment and probable alzheimer's disease: a randomised controlled trial. *Int. J. Mol. Sci.* 16, 24600–24613. doi: 10.3390/ijms161024600

Poulos, A., Sharp, P., Johnson, D., and Easton, C. (1988). The occurrence of polyenoic very long chain fatty acids with greater than 32 carbon atoms in molecular species of phosphatidylcholine in normal and peroxisome-deficient (Zellweger's syndrome) brain. *Biochem. J.* 253, 645–650. doi: 10.1042/bj2530645

Quetglas, S., Leveque, C., Miquelis, R., Sato, K., and Seagar, M. (2000). Ca2+-dependent regulation of synaptic SNARE complex assembly via a calmodulin- and phospholipid-binding domain of synaptobrevin. *Proc. Natl. Acad. Sci. U.S.A.* 97, 9695–9700. doi: 10.1073/pnas.97.17.9695

Rabionet, M., Bayerle, A., Jennemann, R., Heid, H., Fuchser, J., Marsching, C., et al. (2015). Male meiotic cytokinesis requires ceramide synthase 3-dependent sphingolipids with unique membrane anchors. *Hum. Mol. Genet.* 24, 4792–4808. doi: 10.1093/hmg/ddv204

Rabionet, M., van der Spoel, A. C., Chuang, C. C., von Tumpling-Radosta, B., Litjens, M., Bouwmeester, D., et al. (2008). Male germ cells require polyenoic sphingolipids with complex glycosylation for completion of meiosis: a link to ceramide synthase-3. *J. Biol. Chem.* 283, 13357–13369. doi: 10.1074/jbc.M800870200

Rangel-Huerta, O. D., and Gil, A. (2018). Effect of omega-3 fatty acids on cognition: an updated systematic review of randomized clinical trials. *Nutr. Rev.* 76, 1–20. doi: 10.1093/nutrit/nux064

Rizo, J., and Sudhof, T. C. (2002). Snares and munc18 in synaptic vesicle fusion. *Nat. Rev. Neurosci.* 3, 641–653. doi: 10.1038/nrn898

Robinson, B. S., Johnson, D. W., and Poulos, A. (1990). Unique molecular species of phosphatidylcholine containing very-long-chain (C24-C38) polyenoic fatty acids in rat brain. *Biochem. J.* 265, 763–767. doi: 10.1042/bj2650763

Rohacs, T. (2015). Phosphoinositide regulation of TRPV1 revisited. *Pflugers Arch.* 467, 1851–1869. doi: 10.1007/s00424-015-1695-3

Rohacs, T., and Nilius, B. (2007). Regulation of transient receptor potential (TRP) channels by phosphoinositides. *Pflugers Arch.* 455, 157–168. doi: 10.1007/s00424-007-0275-6

Rohrbough, J., Rushton, E., Palanker, L., Woodruff, E., Matthies, H. J., Acharya, U., et al. (2004). Ceramidase regulates synaptic vesicle exocytosis and trafficking. *J. Neurosci.* 24, 7789–7803. doi: 10.1523/JNEUROSCI.1146-04.2004

Sanchez-Alegria, K., Flores-Leon, M., Avila-Munoz, E., Rodriguez-Corona, N., and Arias, C. (2018). PI3K signaling in neurons: a central node for the control of multiple functions. *Int. J. Mol. Sci.* 19, E3725. doi: 10.3390/ijms19123725

Santiago Valtierra, F. X., Penalva, D. A., Luquez, J. M., Furland, N. E., Vasquez, C., Reyes, J. G., et al. (2018). Elovl4 and Fa2h expression during rat spermatogenesis: a link to the very-long-chain PUFAs typical of germ cell sphingolipids. *J. Lipid Res.* 59, 1175–1189. doi: 10.1194/jlr.M081885

Sara, Y., Virmani, T., Deak, F., Liu, X., and Kavalali, E. T. (2005). An isolated pool of vesicles recycles at rest and drives spontaneous neurotransmission. *Neuron* 45, 563–573. doi: 10.1016/j.neuron.2004.12.056

Sassa, T., Ohno, Y., Suzuki, S., Nomura, T., Nishioka, C., Kashiwagi, T., et al. (2013). Impaired epidermal permeability barrier in mice lacking elovl1, the gene responsible for very-long-chain fatty acid production. *Mol. Cell Biol.* 33, 2787–2796. doi: 10.1128/MCB.00192-13

Sassa, T., Tadaki, M., Kiyonari, H., and Kihara, A. (2018). Very long-chain tear film lipids produced by fatty acid elongase ELOVL1 prevent dry eye disease in mice. *FASEB J.* 32, 2966–2978. doi: 10.1096/fj.201700947R

Sastry, P. S. (1985). Lipids of nervous tissue: composition and metabolism. *Prog. Lipid Res.* 24, 69–176. doi: 10.1016/0163-7827(85)90011-6

Sebastiao, A. M., Colino-Oliveira, M., Assaife-Lopes, N., Dias, R. B., and Ribeiro, J. A. (2013). Lipid rafts, synaptic transmission and plasticity: impact in age-related neurodegenerative diseases. *Neuropharmacology* 64, 97–107. doi: 10.1016/j.neuropharm.2012.06.053

Selkoe, D. J. (2001). Alzheimer's disease: genes, proteins, and therapy. *Physiol. Rev.* 81, 741–766.

Selkoe, D. J. (2002). Alzheimer's disease is a synaptic failure. *Science* 298, 789–791.

Sharma, S., and Tripathi, M. (2013). Ketogenic diet in epileptic encephalopathies. *Epilepsy Res. Treat.* 2013:652052. doi: 10.1155/2013/652052

Shen, D. N., Zhang, L. H., Wei, E. Q., and Yang, Y. (2015). Autophagy in synaptic development, function, and pathology. *Neurosci. Bull.* 31, 416–426. doi: 10.1007/s12264-015-1536-6

Sherry, D. M., Hopiavuori, B. R., Stiles, M. A., Rahman, N. S., Ozan, K. G., Deak, F., et al. (2017). Distribution of ELOVL4 in the developing and adult mouse brain. *Front. Neuroanat.* 11:38. doi: 10.3389/fnana.2017.00038

Sinn, N., Milte, C., and Howe, P. R. (2010). Oiling the brain: a review of randomized controlled trials of omega-3 fatty acids in psychopathology across the lifespan. *Nutrients* 2, 128–170. doi: 10.3390/nu2020128

Slieker, R. C., Relton, C. L., Gaunt, T. R., Slagboom, P. E., and Heijmans, B. T. (2018). Age-related DNA methylation changes are tissue-specific with ELOVL2 promoter methylation as exception. *Epigenetics Chromatin* 11:25. doi: 10.1186/s13072-018-0191-3

Sollner, T., Whiteheart, S. W., Brunner, M., Erdjument-Bromage, H., Geromanos, S., Tempst, P., et al. (1993). SNAP receptors implicated in vesicle targeting and fusion. *Nature* 362, 318–324. doi: 10.1038/362318a0

Spassieva, S. D., Ji, X., Liu, Y., Gable, K., Bielawski, J., Dunn, T. M., et al. (2016). Ectopic expression of ceramide synthase 2 in neurons suppresses neurodegeneration induced by ceramide synthase 1 deficiency. *Proc. Natl. Acad. Sci. U.S.A.* 113, 5928–5933. doi: 10.1073/pnas.1522071113

Spolnicka, M., Pospiech, E., Peplonska, B., Zbiec-Piekarska, R., Makowska, Z., Pieta, A., et al. (2018). DNA methylation in ELOVL2 and C1orf132 correctly predicted chronological age of individuals from three disease groups. *Int. J. Legal. Med.* 132, 1–11. doi: 10.1007/s00414-017-1636-0

Stevens, C. F., and Williams, J. H. (2000). "Kiss and run" exocytosis at hippocampal synapses. *Proc. Natl. Acad. Sci. U.S.A.* 97, 12828–12833. doi: 10.1073/pnas.230438697

Südhof, T. C. (2004). The synaptic vesicle cycle. *Annu. Rev. Neurosci.* 27, 509–547. doi: 10.1146/annurev.neuro.26.041002.131412

Südhof, T. C., and Rizo, J. (2011). Synaptic vesicle exocytosis. *Cold Spring Harb. Perspect. Biol.* 3:a005637. doi: 10.1101/cshperspect.a005637

Südhof, T. C., and Rothman, J. E. (2009). Membrane fusion: grappling with SNARE and SM proteins. *Science* 323, 474–477. doi: 10.1126/science.1161748

Sun, C., Zou, M., Wang, X., Xia, W., Ma, Y., Liang, S., et al. (2018). FADS1-FADS2 and ELOVL2 gene polymorphisms in susceptibility to autism spectrum disorders in Chinese children. *BMC Psychiatr.* 18:283. doi: 10.1186/s12888-018-1868-7

Takamori, S., Holt, M., Stenius, K., Lemke, E. A., Gronborg, M., Riedel, D., et al. (2006). Molecular anatomy of a trafficking organelle. *Cell* 127, 831–846. doi: 10.1016/j.cell.2006.10.030

Tan, C. Y., Virtue, S., Bidault, G., Dale, M., Hagen, R., Griffin, J. L., et al. (2015). Brown adipose tissue thermogenic capacity is regulated by Elovl6. *Cell Rep.* 13, 2039–2047. doi: 10.1016/j.celrep.2015.11.004

Tarafdar, P. K., Chakraborty, H., Bruno, M. J., and Lentz, B. R. (2015). Phosphatidylserine-dependent catalysis of stalk and pore formation by synaptobrevin JMR-TMD peptide. *Biophys. J.* 109, 1863–1872. doi: 10.1016/j.bpj.2015.08.051

Teixeira, G., Vieira, L. B., Gomez, M. V., and Guatimosim, C. (2012). Cholesterol as a key player in the balance of evoked and spontaneous glutamate release in rat brain cortical synaptosomes. *Neurochem. Int.* 61, 1151–1159. doi: 10.1016/j.neuint.2012.08.008

Tvrdik, P., Westerberg, R., Silve, S., Asadi, A., Jakobsson, A., Cannon, B., et al. (2000). Role of a new mammalian gene family in the biosynthesis of very long chain fatty acids and sphingolipids. *J. Cell Biol.* 149, 707–718. doi: 10.1083/jcb.149.3.707

Ulamek-Koziol, M., Pluta, R., Bogucka-Kocka, A., and Czuczwar, S. J. (2016). To treat or not to treat drug-refractory epilepsy by the ketogenic diet? that is the question. *Ann. Agric. Environ. Med.* 23, 533–536. doi: 10.5604/12321966.1226841

Vasireddy, V., Uchida, Y., Salem, N. Jr., Kim, S. Y., Mandal, M. N., Reddy, G. B., et al. (2007). Loss of functional ELOVL4 depletes very long-chain fatty acids (> or =C28) and the unique omega-O-acylceramides in skin leading to neonatal death. *Hum. Mol. Genet.* 16, 471–482. doi: 10.1093/hmg/ddl480

Wasser, C. R., Ertunc, M., Liu, X., and Kavalali, E. T. (2007). Cholesterol-dependent balance between evoked and spontaneous synaptic vesicle recycling. *J. Physiol.* 579(Pt 2), 413–429. doi: 10.1113/jphysiol.2006.123133

Wenk, M. R., Pellegrini, L., Klenchin, V. A., Di Paolo, G., Chang, S., Daniell, L., et al. (2001). PIP kinase Igamma is the major PI(4,5)P(2) synthesizing enzyme at the synapse. *Neuron* 32, 79–88. doi: 10.1016/s0896-6273(01)00456-1

Westerberg, R., Tvrdik, P., Unden, A. B., Mansson, J. E., Norlen, L., Jakobsson, A., et al. (2004). Role for ELOVL3 and fatty acid chain length in development of hair and skin function. *J. Biol. Chem.* 279, 5621–5629. doi: 10.1074/jbc.M310529200

Wilson, R. I., and Nicoll, R. A. (2002). Endocannabinoid signaling in the brain. *Science* 296, 678–682. doi: 10.1126/science.1063545

Yu, M., Benham, A., Logan, S., Brush, R. S., Mandal, M. N., Anderson, R. E., et al. (2012). ELOVL4 protein preferentially elongates 20:5n3 to very long chain PUFAs over 20:4n6 and 22:6n3. *J. Lipid Res.* 53, 494–504. doi: 10.1194/jlr.M021386

Zadravec, D., Tvrdik, P., Guillou, H., Haslam, R., Kobayashi, T., Napier, J. A., et al. (2011). ELOVL2 controls the level of n-6 28:5 and 30:5 fatty acids in testis, a prerequisite for male fertility and sperm maturation in mice. *J. Lipid Res.* 52, 245–255. doi: 10.1194/jlr.M011346

Zhang, K., Kniazeva, M., Han, M., Li, W., Yu, Z., Yang, Z., et al. (2001). A 5-bp deletion in ELOVL4 is associated with two related forms of autosomal dominant macular dystrophy. *Nat. Genet.* 27, 89–93. doi: 10.1038/83817

Zhang, X. M., Yang, Z., Karan, G., Hashimoto, T., Baehr, W., Yang, X. J., et al. (2003). Elovl4 mRNA distribution in the developing mouse retina and phylogenetic conservation of Elovl4 genes. *Mol. Vis.* 9, 301–307.

Zhang, Y., Chen, J., Qiu, J., Li, Y., Wang, J., and Jiao, J. (2016). Intakes of fish and polyunsaturated fatty acids and mild-to-severe cognitive impairment risks: a dose-response meta-analysis of 21 cohort studies. *Am. J. Clin. Nutr.* 103, 330–340. doi: 10.3945/ajcn.115.124081

Zoncu, R., Perera, R. M., Sebastian, R., Nakatsu, F., Chen, H., Balla, T., et al. (2007). Loss of endocytic clathrin-coated pits upon acute depletion of phosphatidylinositol 4,5-bisphosphate. *Proc. Natl. Acad. Sci. U.S.A.* 104, 3793–3798. doi: 10.1073/pnas.0611733104

15

# Oxidative Stress in Retinal Degeneration Promoted by Constant LED Light

*Maria M. Benedetto* [1,2] *and Maria A. Contin* [1,2*]

[1]*Departamento de Química Biológica Ranwel Caputto, Facultad de Ciencias Químicas, Universidad Nacional de Córdoba, Córdoba, Argentina,* [2]*Centro de Investigaciones en Química Biológica de Córdoba (CIQUIBIC), CONICET, Universidad Nacional de Córdoba, Córdoba, Argentina*

***Correspondence:**
*Maria A. Contin*
*mcontin@fcq.unc.edu.ar;*
*maria.ana.contin@unc.edu.ar*

Light pollution by artificial light, might accelerate retinal diseases and circadian asynchrony. The excess of light exposure is a growing problem in societies, so studies on the consequences of long-term exposure to low levels of light are needed to determine the effects on vision. The possibility to understand the molecular mechanisms of light damage will contribute to the knowledge about visual disorders related to defects in the phototransduction. Several animal models have been used to study retinal degeneration (RD) by light; however, some important aspects remain to be established. Previously, we demonstrated that cool white treatment of 200 lux light-emitting diode (LED) induces retinal transformation with rods and cones cell death and significant changes in opsin expression in the inner nuclear layer (INL) and ganglion cell layer (GCL). Therefore, to further develop describing the molecular pathways of RD, we have examined here the oxidative stress and the fatty acid composition in rat retinas maintained at constant light. We demonstrated the existence of oxidative reactions after 5 days in outer nuclear layer (ONL), corresponding to classical photoreceptors; catalase (CAT) enzyme activity did not show significant differences in all times studied and the fatty acid study showed that docosahexaenoic acid decreased after 4 days. Remarkably, the docosahexaenoic acid diminution showed a correlation with the rise in stearic acid indicating a possible association between them. We assumed that the reduction in docosahexaenoic acid may be affected by the oxidative stress in photoreceptors outer segment which in turn affects the stearic acid composition with consequences in the membrane properties. All these miss-regulation affects the photoreceptor survival through unknown mechanisms involved. We consider that oxidative stress might be one of the pathways implicated in RD promoted by light.

**Keywords: retinal light damage, LED light, oxidative stress, fatty acid, electroretinogram**

## INTRODUCTION

The disturbance between the amount of reactive oxygen species (ROS) and antioxidants production is defined as oxidative stress. This imbalance produces tissue injury (Halliwell, 1994). The retina carries out the capture of light photons, and for this, it is exposed to suffer oxidative stress. However, it has many mechanisms to counteract these processes through the action of antioxidant enzymes as superoxide dismutase (SOD), catalase (CAT) and glutathione peroxidase (GSHPx) and vitamins as ascorbic acid, vitamin E, melanin (Iusifov et al., 1980; Scibior and Czeczot, 2006; Pavarino et al., 2013). The overexposure to light may be one of the many factors that can induce the interruption of this homeostasis, promoting the injury of eye tissues, cell death or stimulating simultaneously antioxidant protection by up-regulation of antioxidant enzymes (Yusifov et al., 2000); however, when the equilibrium is broken the consequence is the induction of retinal degeneration (RD). In mammals, in normal light conditions, the retina fulfills two main roles: the vision over rods and cones activity and the non-image forming tasks including circadian entrainment, pupillary response to light, secretion of melatonin and sleep regulation (Berson et al., 2002; Rollag et al., 2003; Guido et al., 2010; Sikka et al., 2014). Light stimulates photoreceptor cells activating the phototransduction cascade which promotes hyperpolarization (Sung and Chuang, 2010). Light overexposure-induced RD might induce retinal task deficits with consequences in the secretion of melatonin, desynchronization of rhythms such as sleep/wake, among others. The use of different sources of artificial light is increasing in actual society but this promotes changes in human behavior. Furthermore, the use of technologies such as light-emitting diode (LED), smart TVs and cell-phones, promote an excess of blue light exposure especially at night. Albeit the effects of artificial illumination are unknown, it may have a strong impact on retinal functions with negative consequences on people's health. Considering that the excess of light exposure constitutes an upcoming polluter, it is clearly an emerging public health issue. Different animal models have been used by researchers in order to study the processes of RD promoted by light exposure. Even though Noell et al. (1966) suggested that exposure to light produces retinal changes, this phenomenon has not been fully clarified yet (Shear et al., 1973; Rapp and Williams, 1979; Sperling et al., 1980; Semple-Rowland and Dawson, 1987; Remé et al., 2000; Organisciak and Vaughan, 2010; Roehlecke et al., 2013; Shang et al., 2014). In retina and retinal pigment epithelium (RPE) cells, the exposure to blue light inhibits the mitochondrial enzymes and cytochrome oxidase expression inducing retinal damage (Chen, 1993; Cai et al., 2000; Roehlecke et al., 2011) suggesting the existence of oxidative stress mechanisms as part of the retinal cell death mechanism induced by light exposure. Recently, Nakamura et al. (2017) established that LED light exposure during 2 h (800 lx) induced retinal damage where oxidative stress was partially involved. However, the consequences of constant low light exposure in which the phototransduction mechanism is constantly activated for long time remain unknown. In this regard, we have established and characterized a model of RD induced by a constant exposure to LED. We have showed that classical photoreceptor cell death without caspase-3 activation and a gradual increase in levels of rhodopsin-phospho-Ser334 as a result of light exposure, suggesting that constant light produces changes in the regulation of phototransduction in rods (Contín et al., 2013).

However, retinal ganglion cells (RGCs) do not die after constant light treatment (LL), suggesting a neuroprotection mechanism also involved in our model (Benedetto et al., 2017). So, the key questions in the present work are: does the overexposure at constant low levels of LED light yield oxidative stress? What is the kinetic of oxidative stress production if the exposure is constant? Therefore, the goals of this work were to investigate the existence of oxidative stress, fatty acid composition and retinal function during the different days of LL stimulation in retinas of Wistar rats.

## MATERIALS AND METHODS

### Animals

All animal procedures were performed in accordance with the protocol approved by the local animal committee (School of Chemistry, UNC, Exp. 2018-740), in accordance with the ARVO statement for the use of animals in ophthalmic and vision research. Wistar rats from 12 to 15 weeks of age were maintained with food and water *ad libitum* and illumination cycle from 12:12 h (light/dark) with white fluorescent light on (~50 lux) from Zeitgeber time (ZT) 0–12 from the time they were born, up to the experiment.

### Light Damage

#### Constant Light

RD was induced as described by Contín et al. (2013). Briefly, rats were exposed to constant light in boxes with LED lamps (EVERLIGHT Electronic Co., Ltd. T-13/4 3294-15/T2C9-1HMB, color temperature of 5,500 K) in the inner upper surface and temperature-controlled at 24 ± 1°C. At the level of the rats' eyes, 200 lx were measured with a light meter (model 401036; Extech Instruments Corp., Waltham, MA, USA). After 1 to 8 days of constant light stimulation (LL1–LL8) the animals were killed in a $CO_2$ chamber at ZT6. Controls in light dark cycle (LD), with LED or fluorescent light (RT) and constant darkness (DD) were exposed for 7 days.

#### Dark Period Protocol

Animals were subjected to a constant light during 8 days with periods of dark during 2, 4, 6, 10 and 12 h every day at the beginning of the subjective night (ZT6) under identical conditions as animals exposed to LL, in the temperature-controlled stress box at 24 ± 1°C.

### Electroretinograms (ERGs)

The methods employed for Scotopic electroretinogram (ERG) were as previously described by Dorfman et al. (2014) using an ERG machine (Akonic BIOPC, Buenos Aires, Argentina). Briefly, first animals were adapted to dark for 20 min. Then, they were anesthetized with an intraperitoneal injection containing a solution of xylazine hydrochloride (2 mg/kg) and ketamine hydrochloride (150 mg/kg). Pupils were dilated with tropicamide (1% Alcon Laboratories) and, in order to prevent eye dehydration and permit electrical contact activity when the electrode is recording, the cornea was irrigated with proparacaine hydrochloride (0.5% Alcon Laboratories). Both eyes were recorded simultaneously applying flashes of white light (5 ms, 0.1 Hz) from a photostimulator set at maximum brightness (3 cd s/m$^2$ without filter). Then, the recordings were amplified and filtered (1.5 Hz low-pass filter, 300 Hz high-pass filter, notch filter activated). An average of 10 responses for each eye was measured. Mean "a" and "b" waves peak latencies and amplitudes of the responses from each group of rats were compared.

## Outer Nuclear Layer Analysis

The retinal fixation method, sectioning and nuclear quantification were as previously described (Contín et al., 2013). Briefly, rats' eyes were fixed overnight at 4°C in 4% (W/V) paraformaldehyde in 100 mM sodium phosphate buffer (PBS, pH 7.3). Then, they were cryoprotected in sucrose and mounted in an optimal cutting temperature compound (OCT; Tissue-Tek® Sakura). Retinal sections were cut along the horizontal meridian (nasal-temporal). The sections were stained with 1% Hoechst (33258 Sigma Aldrich) for 5 min and photographed using a confocal microscope (Olympus FV1200, Japan) at 40× magnification. The nuclei were counted in "left, middle left, middle right and right" designated areas from five different animals per treatment using the software ImageJ (v. 1.45) and the plugin "Automatic Nuclei Counter".

## Superoxide Production

Dihydroethidium [(DHE; sigma 37291-25 mg dihydroethidium at 10-mg/mL stock solution in dimethylsulfoxide)], a redox-sensitive probe, was used to detect superoxide generation as previously described (Peng et al., 2011). Briefly, eyes were removed, washed in PBS solution and then incubated with 1 mM DHE for 12 h at room temperature in PBS. Then the eyes were incubated in paraformaldehyde 4% for 12 h at room temperature, harvested and quikly frozen in liquid nitrogen for cryosection (Leica CM 1950, Leica Microsystems Ltd, Wetzlar, Germany). The cryosections (10 μm) were analyzed by confocal microscopy (Olympus FV300, Japan). The DHE molecules enter the cells and are oxidized by superoxide contained inside cells, to ethidium (Et) which is fluorescent. This product is retained in the cell allowing the estimation of cellular superoxide production.

## Oxidative Stress Quantification

ROS molecules were determined by flow cytometry with 2′,7′-dichlorofluorescein diacetate (DCFH-DA) probe (D6883 Sigma). DCFH-DA is sensitive to oxidation and is nonfluorescent, it may be oxidized by ROS and peroxides and become a fluorescent molecule, DCFH (Gomes et al., 2005). Briefly, retinas dissected and dissociated in 0.25% (W/V) trypsin (Life Technology, Inc., Carlsbad, CA, USA) for 7 min at 37°C were centrifuged at 3,000 rpm for 3 min, incubated with 200 μl of trypsin inhibitor (STI) for 3 min and washed twice with PBS 1×. Then, they were suspended in 200 μl of PBS 1×, incubated with DCFH-DA (5 μM) for 60 min at 37°C in dark, washed twice with PBS 1× and analyzed on a Becton-Dickinson FACS flow cytometer; the excitation and emission wavelengths were set at 488 and 525 nm, respectively. Data were analyzed with FlowJo software (LC, Ashland, Ore). Three independent experiments were performed and the results were expressed as mean ± standard error (SE) in arbitrary units of DCFH fluorescence intensity.

## Catalase Activity Detection

Catalase (CAT) activity was assessed according to Aebi (1984). Briefly, individual retinas were homogenized in PBS 1×. Then, 1.3 ml of Buffer Phosphate (50 mM, pH 7.4) and 1.25 ml of distilled $H_2O$ were added to 300 μl of previously homogenized sample. Subsequently, 150 μl of $H_2O_2$ (300 mM) was added and the spectrophotometric changes were detected by measuring the absorbance at 240 nm for 1 min. The protein concentration was determined by Bradford (1976).

## Lipid Extraction From Rat Retinas

Lipids were extracted from the samples as Folch' method slightly modified (Folch et al., 1957). Briefly, collected retinas were homogenized in 200 μl of MiliQ $H_2O$ and 3 ml of a combination of Chloroform: methanol [(2:1; v/v)] and 600 μl of MiliQ $H_2O$ were added and vortexed vigorously for 5 min and centrifuged at 2,000 rpm at 15°C for 10 min. The layer containing chloroform was collected and 1.5 ml of a mixture of chloroform: methanol: $H_2O$ [(3:48:47; v/v/v)] was added, mixed gently and centrifuged 10 min at 2,000 rpm. Finally, chloroform was dried under a stream of $N_2$ and the extracts stored for further experiments.

### Fatty Acid Methyl Esters Analysis by Gas Chromatography/Mass Spectrometry With Ion-Trap Detector

Extracted lipids were transmethylated to fatty acid methyl esters (FAMEs) with sodium methoxide and toluene [(2:1; v/v)] overnight at 4°C. FAMEs were then extracted with hexane and analyzed by using a GC/MS (Saturn® 2000 GC/MS, Agilent, Santa Clara, USA) equipped with an ion-trap detector and a fused capillary column (HP-5MS, 30 mm × 0.25 mm i.d × 0.25 μm film thickness, Agilent, Santa Clara, USA). The carrier gas used was Helium (flow rate 1.0 ml/min); the detector and injector temperature were maintained at 150°C and 300°C, respectively. The injection (split-splitless injector) volume of the sample was 1 μl with a split ratio of 1:50. The oven was programmed as follows: 170°C for 3 min—200°C at the rate of 1.2°C/min—10°C/min to 240°C—80°C/min to 280°C and 80°C/min to 300°C with a final hold for 46.7 min.

The column temperature was programmed as follows: 170°C; 1.2°/min to 200°C—10°/min to 240°C—80°/min to 2,800°C—80°/min to 300°C and hold at 300°C for 4 min. Then, FAMEs were identified comparing mass spectra with dates in the library (National Institute of Standards and Technology, Gaithersburg, MD, USA). Furthermore, we compared FAMEs retention times with the commercial standard Supelco 37-Component FAME Mix (Sigma Aldrich, St. Louis, MO, USA).

## Statistical Analysis

Statistical analysis was carried out using the Infostat software (Version 2017, InfoStat Group, FCA, National University of Córdoba, Argentina). One-way analysis of variance (ANOVA) was used for statistical comparisons. In the text and figure, data are expressed as mean ± SD or SE. It was considered

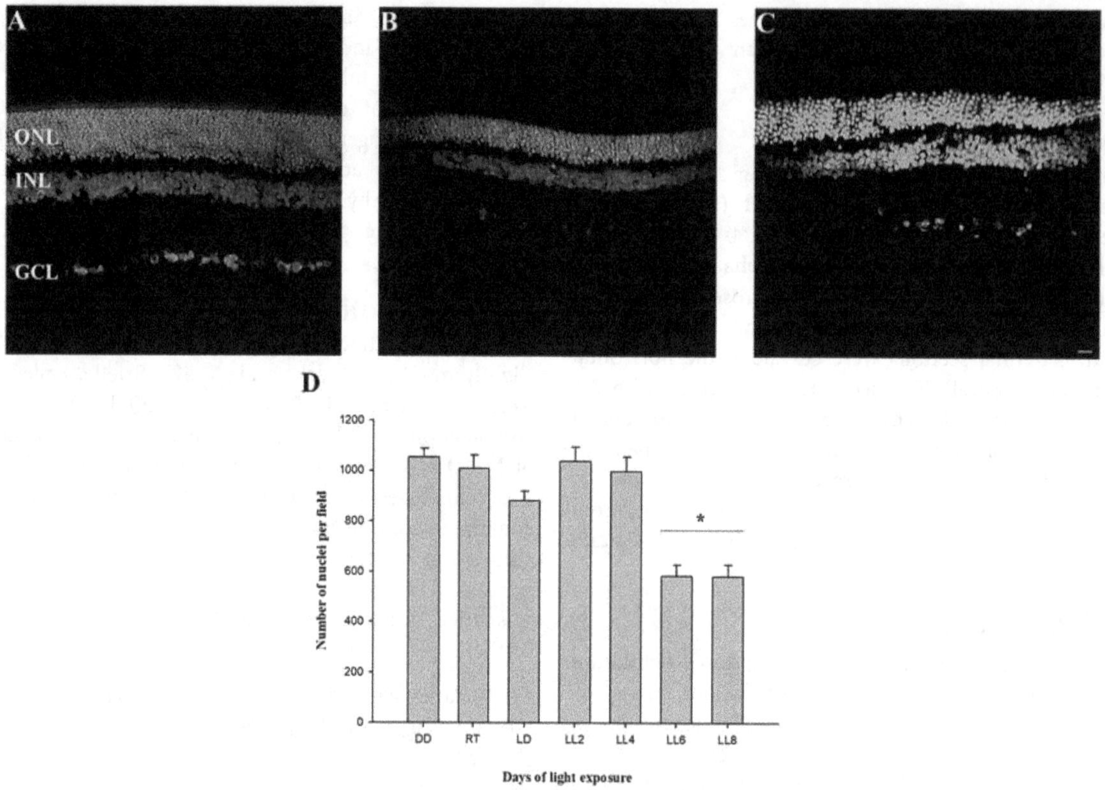


**FIGURE 1** | Outer nuclear layer analysis. **(A)** Rat retinas maintained in dark for 7 days (DD). **(B–C)** Retinas from rats exposed 6 (LL6) or 8 (LL8) days to constant light (200 lx). **(D)** Quantification of ONL nuclei; rat retina images corresponding to controls [(LD cycle, RT cycle and non-exposure to light (DD)] or exposure to 200 lx LED light (LL) for 2, 4, 6, and 8 days were analyzed to quantify photoreceptor survival. Data are mean ± standard error (SE), $n = 2$ animals/group from five independent experiments, $*p < 0.05$ vs. DD and RT by one-way analysis of variance (ANOVA) and Duncan's *post hoc* test. ONL, outer nuclear layer; INL, inner nuclear layer; GCL, ganglion cell layer. Scale bar indicates 30 μm.

statistically significant a *p*-value < 0.05. The normality and homogeneity of the variance assumptions were proved with Shapiro–Wilks and Levene tests, respectively. Duncan *post hoc* test with a *p* value < 0.05 were considered statistically significant. A non-parametric Kruskal-Wallis test was performed when the data did not comply with the assumptions of the ANOVA. Spearman correlation coefficients were calculated to determine associations between the content of fatty acids.

# RESULTS

## Structural Retinal Analysis

In order to know the kinetic of cell death events we analyzed the retinal layers, oxidative stress, CAT activity, fatty acid composition and ERG activity in animals exposed to constant light. The analysis of retinal structure revealed a reduction in outer nuclear layer (ONL) thickness at LL6 and LL8 compared with animals reared in DD (**Figures 1A–C**). The quantification of nuclei in this area showed a significant reduction after 6 and 8 days of constant light (583.04 ± 45.31 and 580.10 ± 45.31 nuclei, respectively) compared with DD and RT [(1052.19 ± 38.41 and 1007.63 ± 54.32 nuclei, respectively, $p < 0.005$, **Figure 1D**)]; indicating that between LL0 to LL6 are being carried out the photoreceptor cell death pathways.

## Oxidative Stress Study

### DHE Determination

In order to know if retinas from animals exposed to constant light have oxidative stress, DHE was measured in retinal sections as indicated in "Materials and Methods" section. DHE and superoxide anion reaction produces ethidium (E), which binds to DNA rising the fluorescence in the cells (Gomes et al., 2005; Fernandes et al., 2006). Here, we show that retinas from animals exposed for 2 days of LL (LL2) have fluorescent label in few cells in ONL; however, at 8 days of LL (LL8) a significant increment of DHE label was observed (**Figures 2A–C**), correlating with ONL cell reduction (**Figure 1**). Besides the clear staining in ONL, no positive labeled in other retinal layer were observed in any time of LL studied, indicating the existence of oxidized products specifically in this layer.

### Reactive Oxygen Species Quantification

To determine the kinetic of oxidative stress events occurred in ONL of retinas exposed to LL, ROS production was determined

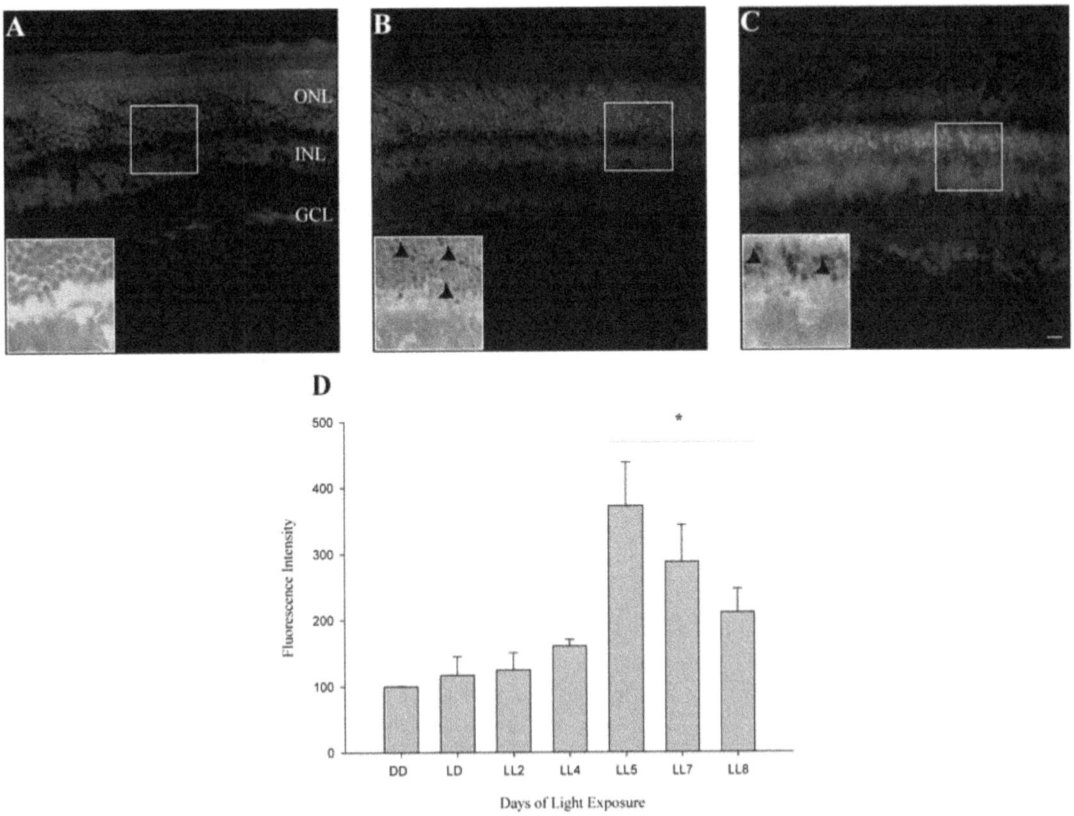


**FIGURE 2** | Oxidative stress study. **(A–C)** DHE staining at DD, LL2 and 8 days of light-emitting diode (LED) light exposure. Arrowheads show DHE positive cells in the ONL. **(D)** Reactive oxygen species (ROS) production detection by Flow cytometry using the DCFH-DA probe in controls (DD and LD) and in animals exposed to 2, 4, 5, 7 and 8 days to constant light (LL2–8). Data are mean ± SE, $n = 1$ animal/group from three independent experiments, $*p < 0.05$ vs. DD by Kruskal Wallis. ONL, outer nuclear layer; INL, inner nuclear layer; GCL, ganglion cell layer. Scale bar indicates 30 μm.

by flow cytometry using the DCFH-DA probe as indicated in "Materials and Methods" section. At 2 and 4 days of LL no significant increases in fluorescence were observed (124.70 ± 44.94 and 160.69 ± 16.9%, respectively). However, constant light treatment increases the levels of fluorescence, showing significant changes after 5 days of LL (LL5) where the production of ROS was maximal (372.16 ± 113.44%) respect to control in DD (100%). Although at 7 and 8 days of LL the fluorescence production decreased in correlation with cell death in the ONL (287.97 ± 221.55 and 211.00 ± 80.80%, respectively), ROS production was greater than in DD (**Figure 2D**).

## Catalase Activity Determination

CAT enzyme is known to contribute to $H_2O_2$ detoxification in the retina and the inhibition of its activity increases $H_2O_2$ concentration 2.5-fold, which cannot make up for the GPX activity (Ohta et al., 1996) the enzyme being an antioxidant factor in retina. In order to investigate the CAT activity and its association in the prevention of oxidative stress in constant light exposed rats, it was assessed as indicated in "Materials and Methods" section. Although constant light stimuli increased lightly CAT activity at 6 and 8 days of LL (7.22 ± 3.95 and 5.96 ± 3.27, respectively) with respect to LL 2 and 4 (3.38 ± 1.44 and 4.35 ± 2.24, respectively), reaching the levels of DD and RT (5.82 ± 2.55 and 6.96 ± 4.30, respectively) there were no significant differences in any times of LL measured (**Figure 3**), suggesting that CAT is affected by the desynchronization of animals by constant light exposure.

## Retinal Fatty Acid

The outer segment membrane of retinal rods and cones contain high polyunsaturated fatty acids (PUFAs) where docosahexaenoic (22–6 n-3, DHA) and arachidonic acid (20:4 n-6, AA) are the major species present. Because PUFAs are a target for oxidation, the analysis by GC-MS in rat retinas from animal exposure to different LL allow us to determine if there are changes in the membrane components during RD as a result of light exposure. Individual fatty acids were identified comparing the mass spectra with those present in the NIST library and their retention time with a commercial standard (see "Materials and Methods"). Representative GC/MS analyses of fatty acids from retinas of control animals and exposed to light (LL) are shown in **Figure 4A**. Palmitic (16:0, PA) and arachidonic acid (20:4 n-6, AA), did not show statistical differences in any times of LL studied (**Figures 4B,D**). However, stearic acid (18:0, EA) shows increased levels with respect to control at LL4, maintaining this higher level at LL6 and LL8 (**Figure 4C**) in association with the DHA decrease which was significant at LL 4 and 8

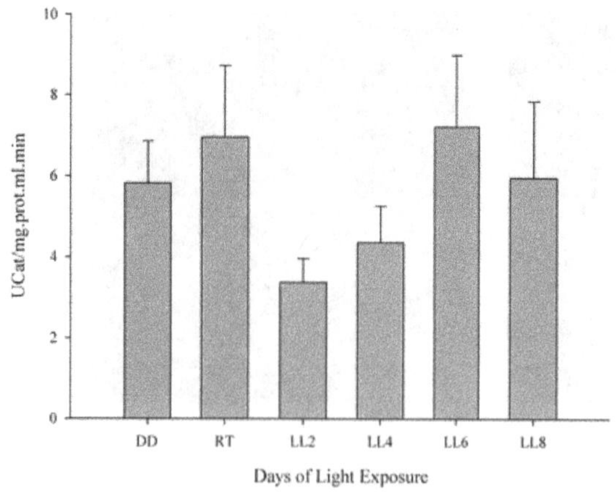


**FIGURE 3 |** Catalase activity study in retinal light damage. CAT activity expressed as U/mg prot.ml.min in controls (DD and RT) and rats exposed at different days of LL. Data are mean ± SE, $n = 1$ animal/group from three independent experiments, $p = 0.216$ by one-way ANOVA and Duncan's *post hoc* test.

(**Figure 4E**). In order to determine if the variations were related, we perform a correlation analysis between EA and DHA in control animals (DD) and animals exposed to 4, 6 and 8 days to LL. **Figures 5A–D** show no correlation in control animals maintained in dark (DD) and in LL6, however, there is a positive correlation in LL4 ($\rho = 1$) and negative correlation in LL8 ($\rho = -0.8$).

## Electroretinograms Responses

Previously we demonstrated retinal functional alterations in the scotopic ERG responses, showing that throughout the days of LL, the two principal waves "a" and "b" tend to decrease their amplitudes and increase their latency time, reaching abolished records after LL4, indicating that photoreceptor cells fail between the first 4 days of LL (Quintana et al., 2016). Here, to study the effects of light interruption by darkness, the animals were exposed to constant light with 2, 4, 6, 10 or 12 h of dark during the subjective night as indicated in "Materials and Methods" section. As shown in **Figure 5**, with 2, 4 and 6 h of rest in darkness per day during subjective night, the ERG show abolished records as we described before, however, at 8 and 10 h of dark the ERG began to restore, reaching normal values at 12 h. This result indicates that including hours of rest in darkness during the subjective night the effects of light exposure may be less harmful than constant stimuli.

# DISCUSSION

The excess of artificial light exposure constitutes a problem that is emergent worldwide. The behavior of excessive exposure to light might have effects on the vision, promoting RD and circadian asynchrony in healthy population. We have previously characterized a RD model that may provide the possibility to study specific events associated with RD under conditions of low light with LED sources, at constant or long-term periods of exposure (LP context). We demonstrated that photoreceptor cells died along the days of continuous light stimuli through a caspase-3 independent mechanism. Rhodopsin analysis did not show a reduction in protein levels, however, rhodopsin-phospho-Ser334 increased gradually with the days of LL exposure indicating increasing levels in the phosphorylation. The study of rhodopsin allows us to investigate the role of phototransduction mechanism in the RD model suggesting that rhodopsin dysregulation could be involved in one of the ways of RD (Contín et al., 2013). Furthermore, in the inner retina, we demonstrated a relocation of non-visual photopigments (OPN4 and OPN5); however, inner retinal cells survival were not affected, indicating a compensatory mechanism of protection with possible changes in synchronization of circadian rhythms (Benedetto et al., 2017). To further describe the molecular pathways of cell death, in this work, we have examined the oxidative stress involvement in the effects of constant exposure to LED sources. Results from both DHE and DCFH-DA probe analysis demonstrate the existence of oxidative reactions in LL exposed rats (**Figure 2**). The ONL label of DHE indicates the occurrence of oxidative stress only in this layer, discarding stress mechanisms in other cells of the retina, coinciding with cell death study. DCFH-DA analysis shows that the production of ROS increases significantly after LL5 with higher levels at this day of LL (**Figure 2D**) indicating oxidative stress from 5 days of constant light. Powerful defenses against oxidative stress are the effect of Vitamin E, Ascorbic Acid, and melanin as well as the activity of antioxidant enzyme superoxide dismutase (SOD), CAT and GSHPx (Yusifov et al., 2000). Here, we demonstrated that CAT activity does not present significant differences in all times studied (**Figure 3**) showing a light diminution at LL2 to LL4 with respect to controls in DD and LD treatments; however, at LL6 and LL8 the CAT activity increases showing levels similar to the controls. Previous studies have demonstrated that CAT enzyme is finely regulated by the circadian rhythms; CAT bioinformatic and mRNA studies have been shown putative E-box sites in CAT and GPx regulatory regions; furthermore, CAT mRNA expression and enzyme activity shows circadian rhythmicity with higher levels at the end of the day (Navigatore Fonzo et al., 2009; Kharwar and Haldar, 2012; Lacoste et al., 2017). Sani et al. (2006) have demonstrated that CAT activity shows changes across a 24-h period in mouse. Thus, we hypothesize that constant light might produce a complex and multifactorial biological process inducing progressive desynchronization of circadian rhythm with concomitant antioxidant function altered; and therefore, the break of the equilibrium between ROS over-production and antioxidant processes. However, further studies are necessary in order to conclude an association between them.

The vertebrate retina contains high concentration of PUFA; particularly, in the outer segment membrane of retinal rod and cones, the PUFAs DHA and AA are the major species examined (Fliesler and Anderson, 1983; Giusto et al., 2000; SanGiovanni and Chew, 2005). PUFAs are essential for maintaining the appropriate fluidity of the membrane, necessary for efficient phototransduction cascade (Brown, 1994; Gawrisch and Soubias, 2008). The composition of membrane lipids and their direct interaction with proteins

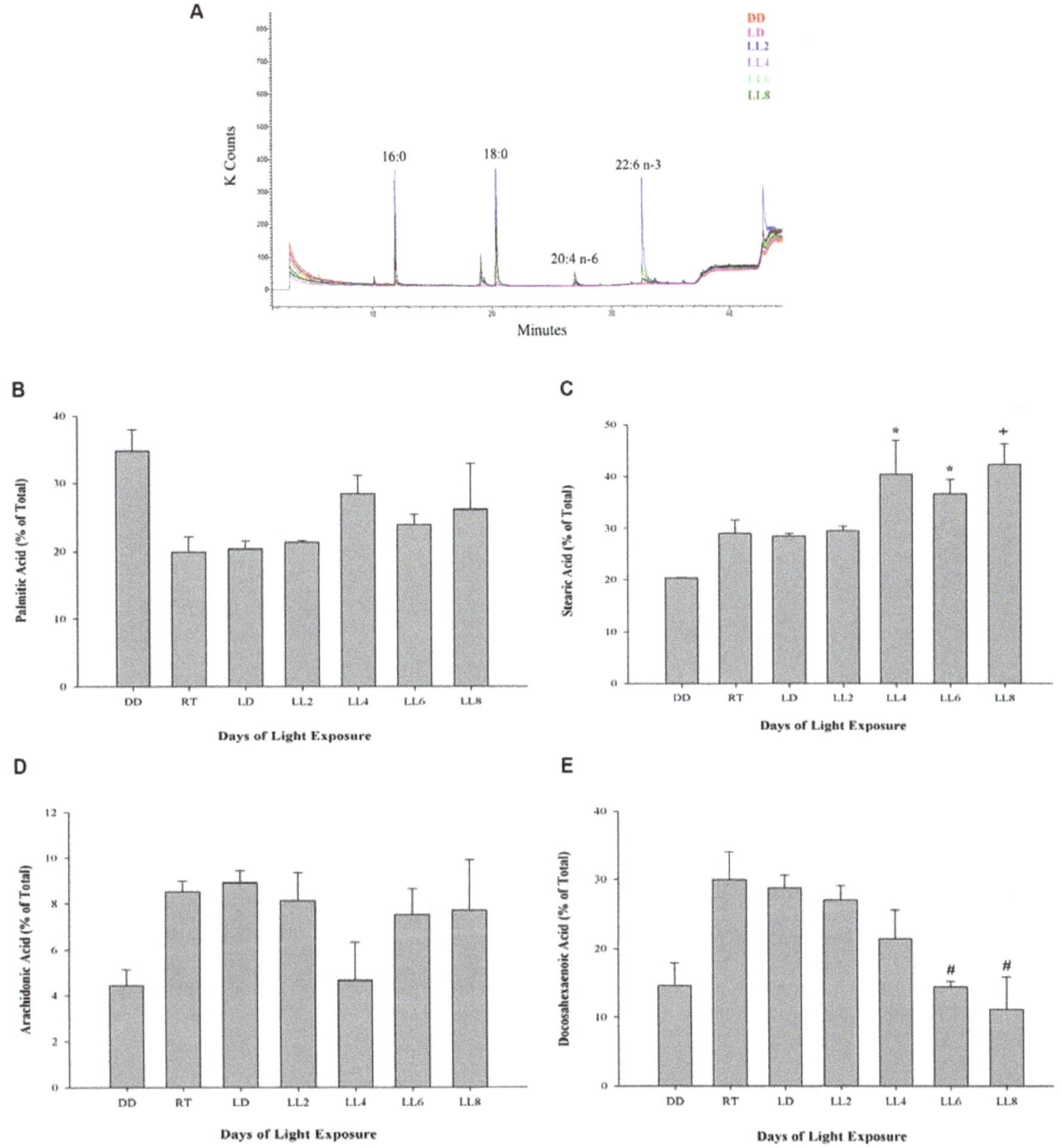


**FIGURE 4** | Fatty acid composition in light-treated rat retinas. **(A)** Full scan GC-MS total ion chromatograms of rat retina from controls (DD and LD) and rats exposed to 2, 4, 6 and 8 days of LL. 16:0, palmitic acid; 18:0, stearic acid; 20:4 n-6, arachidonic acid; 22:6 n-3, docosahexaenoic acid. **(B–E)** Quantification of palmitic **(B)**, stearic **(C)**, arachidonic **(D)** and docosahexaenoic acid **(E)** from controls (DD, RT and LD) and animals exposed for 2, 4, 6 and 8 days of constant light (LL), expressed as a percentage of total fatty acids, respectively. Data are mean ± SE, $n = 1$ animal/group from three independent experiments, $^{*}p < 0.05$ vs. DD and LD; $^{+}p < 0.05$ vs. DD; $^{\#}p < 0.05$ vs. RT and LD, by Kruskal-Wallis.

play an important role in the modulation of the rhodopsin function (Salas-Estrada et al., 2018). A good retinal function is subject to adequate membrane structure which contains high levels of DHA. Anderson and Penn (2004) proposed, as neuroprotective adaptive responses, changes in DHA levels at different environmental conditions with the aim to control the number of photons captured by rhodopsin molecule. In the fatty acid n-3-deficient rod outer segment, it has been shown that reduced rhodopsin transducin (Gt) coupling, reduced cGMP phosphodiesterase activity, and slower formation of metarhodopsin II-Gt complex, relative to the animals fed with n-3-adequate diet, explained the reduced activity of rod phototransduction in these animals (Anderson and Penn, 2004). These findings support the so called "photostasis" which infers the morphological and biochemistry adaptation to capture a constant number of photons. The constant light exposure may

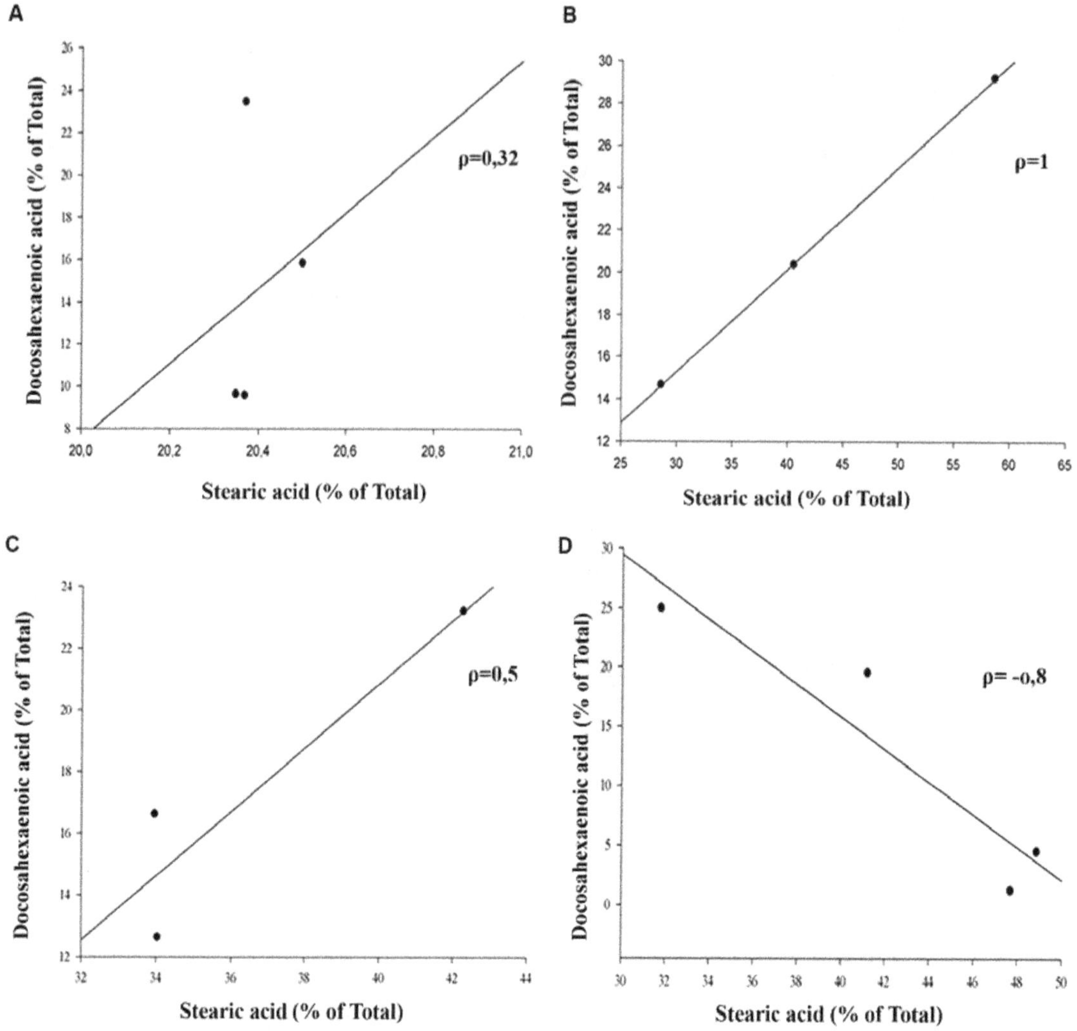


**FIGURE 5 |** Linear correlation analysis between stearic and docosahexaenoic acid in light-treated retinas. **(A)** Control animals maintained in DD. **(B–D)** Animals maintained for 4, 6 and 8 days at constant light, respectively. ρ: pearson correlation coefficient, $n = 1$ animal/group from three independent experiments.

break the adaptive mechanism and promote several pathways of cell death.

DHA and AA are obtained from two ways: (a) the diet or (b) synthesized from alpha-linolenic (18:3n3) and linoleic acids (18:2n6). DHA is transported from the liver to the RPE cells (Scott and Bazan, 1989). In rat rods, DHA is essential for normal development of function (Benolken et al., 1973; Wheeler et al., 1975) where rat deficient in PUFA showed reduced ERG responses (Jeffrey et al., 2002). DHA located mainly in photoreceptors represents 50% of the total fatty acid and recently it has been demonstrated that the membrane of rod outer segment has higher levels of PUFA and Very Long Chain-PUFA (VLC-PUFA) in rod-dominant rats than cone-dominant, suggesting that rods and cones do not have equal lipid requirements (Agbaga et al., 2018). The cell membranes are susceptible to oxidation due to high level of unsaturation of PUFAs, furthermore, retina membranes exposed to light, elevate the concentration of oxygen with the presence of rhodopsin photo-bleached products that increment the risk (Kagan et al., 1981; Wiegand et al., 1983; Rózanowska and Sarna, 2005; Hunter et al., 2012). Earlier study revealed that lipid peroxidation reactions in light-induced RD induce the specific loss of DHA from rod outer segment membranes during constant illumination with an increase in the production of lipid hydroperoxides. None of the other fatty acids, including the AA, changed significantly over the 3-day time periods; concluding that light mediates the peroxidation of PUFAS in outer segment membrane acids and supporting the hypothesis that peroxidation is involved in retinal light degeneration (Wiegand et al., 1983). So, as we exposed the rat retinas to constant light at 200 lux, and we demonstrated increase in ROS significantly at LL5, we decided to study if fatty acid composition is altered belonging to the days in LL, specially by oxidative stress processes. Results from GC-MS analysis shows that PA (saturated) and AA (unsaturated) do not show statistical changes with the days of LL. However, DHA (unsaturated) decreased with the LL exposure with statistical significance at LL4, 6 and 8 compared with controls in LD and RT (**Figure 4E**). Remarkably, the decrease of DHA draws a parallel with an SA increase at the same day of LL (**Figure 4C**). The study of the correlation between both fatty acids shows an association between them in LL-treated retinas; instead, we did not find any association in control animals (DD). We assumed that the reduction in DHA may be affected by the oxidative stress in photoreceptor outer segment which in turn affects the photoreceptor survival through unknown different miss-regulation mechanism involved. The hepatic metabolism, through desaturation and elongation steps, influences the fatty acid composition (Engler et al., 2000). Diabetes, atherosclerosis, neurological disorders, cancer and others are enhanced by the disturbances in fatty acid content (see Zolfaghari and Ross, 2003). One fatty acid biosynthesis pathway begins with the desaturation of PA and SA; in this way, delta-9-desaturase (Δ9-desaturase) is the key enzyme necessary for the conversion from palmitic to palmitoleic acid (16:1n-7) and stearic to oleic acid (18:1n-9). Δ6 and Δ5-desaturase enzymes are required for the metabolism of essential fatty acids, linoleic (18:2n-6) and alpha-linolenic (18:3n-3), to long-chain PUFAs (LCP-DHA). Hormonal, dietary factors, peroxisomal proliferators and developmental processes can affect the activity of Δ9-desaturase, which alters monounsaturated and PUFA composition (Ntambi, 1995, 1999). In hypertensive rats, DHA-fed Δ9-desaturase activity decreases at 53% suggesting that dietary DHA influences properties and function of cellular membranes due to changes in fatty acid composition (Engler et al., 2000). Animals with Δ9-desaturase activity dysregulation show changes in the relation of stearic:oleic acid with effects over membrane fluidity and function (Ntambi, 1995, 1999). Lai et al. (2010) saw that patients with BCD (Bietti crystalline dystrophy; a retinal degenerative disease) have higher concentration of stearic acid and lower octadecadienoic acid (18:1n-9) than healthy animals. Furthermore, the activity of Δ9-desaturase and the concentration of monounsaturated fatty acids were lower in BCD animals suggesting abnormalities in lipid metabolism demonstrating a direct relation between rising levels of stearic acid, lowering fatty acid concentration and retinal dysfunction (Lai et al., 2010). We think that reduction of DHA levels by oxidation in LL rats may affect the desaturase activity in retina causing the rising of stearic acid accumulation which might affect the membrane proprieties giving more rigidity to the outer segment. It may explain part of the cell death mechanism induced by oxidative stress. Furthermore, the excess of light may alter the levels of Neuroprotectin D1 (NPD1) due to the DHA oxidation. NPD1 is a biologically active DHA derivative which induces downstream pro-survival pathways such as gene expression, pro-apoptotic gene suppression and pro-inflammatory responses, among others. The diminution of DHA may alter these ways across inducing photoreceptor cell death (see Asatryan and Bazan, 2017). Other studies are required to better understand the effects of DHA reduction; nevertheless, analyzing the time course of oxidative stress, we consider that it is not the only pathway involved, because the production of DHE and ROS have a maximum expression after LL5-6 (**Figure 2**), and the reduction of ONL occurs between LL6 and LL8; however, the two principal waves of ERG, a and b, tend to decrease the amplitudes and increase the latency time during light stimuli, reaching abolished records at LL4 (Quintana et al., 2016). All these results suggest that a dysfunction of retinal electrical activity occurs previously to redox imbalance. It has been demonstrated that low intensities of light stimuli need the activation of photopigments and phototransduction to induce RD (Hao et al., 2002; Grimm and Remé, 2013), suggesting that impairment of the phototransduction mechanism could be responsible for cell death. Besides, previously we demonstrated the existence of more phosphorylated rhodopsin (rhodopsin-phospho-Ser$^{334}$) after LL2 with a higher level at LL7, supporting the idea that changes in phototransduction cascade are also involved (Contín et al., 2013). Here, we show scotopic ERG responses abolished until 6 h of rest darkness during subjective night; however, after 8 h of dark the activity begin to restore, reaching normal values at 12 h (**Figure 6**). These results suggest that the existence of regulatory mechanisms tend to revert or prevent the process of cell death when the retina is maintained in rest (notice the difference between 10 and 12 h of darkness); nevertheless, when light exposure is prolonged a threshold is exceeded promoting a chain of different cell death pathways. Further studies are necessary to determine the role of opsin-mediated RD processes in this model; however, we think that retinal dysfunction during the 1st days of LL (LL1-LL4) is promoted by phototransduction processes which may induce other pathways of cell death as the oxidative stress occurr. Therefore, prevention therapies with antioxidants would not completely solve RD by LED light.

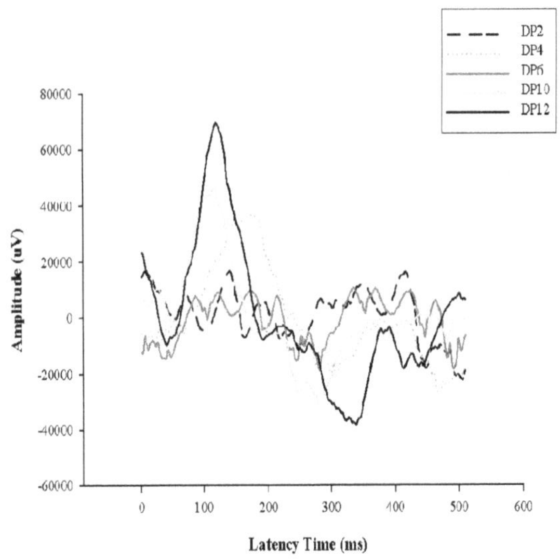


**FIGURE 6** | Electroretinogram (ERG) analysis in animals exposed to dark period. Animals exposed for 8 days of constant light with dark periods of 2, 4, 6, 10 and 12 h per day during subjective night (DP 2–8); DD, constant dark. DP, dark period.

## AUTHOR CONTRIBUTIONS

MB has contributed with the hypothesis, has performed the experiments, the analysis of the results and discussion. MC is the corresponding author, and had written the manuscript.

## FUNDING

This work has been supported by Consejo Nacional de Investigaciones Científicas y Tecnológicas de la República Argentina (CONICET), Secretaria de Ciencia y Tecnología—Universidad Nacional de Córdoba (SeCyT-UNC) and by Agencia Nacional de Promoción Científica y Técnica (FONCyT, PICT 2012 No. 021).

## ACKNOWLEDGMENTS

We are grateful to Dr Pablo Yunes, Dr Carlos R. Mas and Dr Cecilia Sampedro for technical support and Rosa Andrada for animal facility management and to Lucia Carlota Pedraza for doing the language quality check of this manuscript.

## REFERENCES

Aebi, H. (1984). Catalase *in vitro*. *Methods Enzymol.* 105, 121–126. doi: 10.1016/S0076-6879(84)05016-3

Agbaga, M. P., Merriman, D. K., Brush, R. S., Lydic, T. A., Conley, S. M., Naash, M. I., et al. (2018). Differential composition of DHA and very-long-chain PUFAs in rod and cone photoreceptors. *J. Lipid Res.* 59, 1586–1596. doi: 10.1194/jlr.M082495

Anderson, R. E., and Penn, J. S. (2004). Environmental light and heredity are associated with adaptive changes in retinal DHA levels that affect retinal functionz. *Lipids* 39, 1121–1124. doi: 10.1007/s11745-004-1338-8

Asatryan, A., and Bazan, N. G. (2017). Molecular mechanisms of signaling via the docosanoid neuroprotectin D1 for cellular homeostasis and neuroprotection. *J. Biol. Chem.* 292, 12390–12397. doi: 10.1074/jbc.r117.783076

Benedetto, M. M., Guido, M. E., and Contin, M. A. (2017). Non-visual photopigments effects of constant light-emitting diode light exposure on the inner retina of Wistar rats. *Front. Neurol.* 8:417. doi: 10.3389/fneur.2017.00417

Benolken, R. M., Anderson, R. E., and Wheeler, T. G. (1973). Membrane fatty acids associated with the electrical response in visual excitation. *Science* 182, 1253–1254. doi: 10.1126/science.182.4118.1253

Berson, D. M., Dunn, F. A., and Takao, M. (2002). Phototransduction by retinal ganglion cells that set the circadian clock. *Science* 295, 1070–1073. doi: 10.1126/science.1067262

Bradford, M. M. (1976). A rapid and sensitive method for the quantitation of microgram quantities of protein utilizing the principle of protein-dye binding. *Anal. Biochem.* 72, 248–254. doi: 10.1006/abio.1976.9999

Brown, M. F. (1994). Modulation of rhodopsin function by properties of the membrane bilayer. *Chem. Phys. Lipids* 73, 159–180. doi: 10.1016/0009-3084(94)90180-5

Cai, J., Nelson, K. C., Wu, M., Sternberg, P. Jr., and Jones, D. P. (2000). Oxidative damage and protection of the RPE. *Prog. Retin. Eye Res.* 19, 205–221. doi: 10.1016/s1350-9462(99)00009-9

Chen, E. (1993). Inhibition of cytochrome oxidase and blue-light damage in rat retina. *Graefes Arch. Clin. Exp. Ophthalmol.* 231, 416–423. doi: 10.1007/bf00919652

Contín, M. A., Arietti, M. M., Benedetto, M. M., Bussi, C., and Guido, M. E. (2013). Photoreceptor damage induced by low-intensity light: model of retinal degeneration in mammals. *Mol. Vis.* 19, 1614–1625.

Dorfman, D., Aranda, M. L., González Fleitas, M. F., Chianelli, M. S., Fernandez, D. C., Sande, P. H., et al. (2014). Environmental enrichment protects the retina from early diabetic damage in adult rats. *PLoS One* 9:e101829. doi: 10.1371/journal.pone.0101829

Engler, M. M., Bellenger-Germain, S. H., Engler, M. B., Narce, M. M., and Poisson, J. P. G. (2000). Dietary docosahexaenoic acid affects stearic acid desaturation in spontaneously hypertensive rats. *Lipids* 35, 1011–1015. doi: 10.1007/s11745-000-0612-0

Fernandes, D. C., Wosniak, J., Pescatore, L. A., Bertoline, M. A., Liberman, M., Laurindo, F. R. M., et al. (2006). Analysis of DHE-derived oxidation products by HPLC in the assessment of superoxide production and NADPH oxidase activity in vascular systems. *Am. J. Physiol. Cell Physiol.* 292, C413–C422. doi: 10.1152/ajpcell.00188.2006

Fliesler, S. J., and Anderson, R. E. (1983). Chemistry and metabolism of lipids in the vertebrate retina. *Prog. Lipid Res.* 22, 79–131. doi: 10.1016/0163-7827(83)90004-8

Folch, J., Lees, M., and Sloane Stanley, G. H. (1957). A simple method for the isolation and purification of total lipides from animal tissues. *J. Biol. Chem.* 226, 497–509.

Gawrisch, K., and Soubias, O. (2008). Structure and dynamics of polyunsaturated hydrocarbon chains in lipid bilayers-significance for GPCR function. *Chem. Phys. Lipids* 153, 64–75. doi: 10.1016/j.chemphyslip.2008.02.016

Giusto, N. M., Pasquaré, S. J., Salvador, G. A., Castagnet, P. I., Roque, M. E., and Ilincheta de Boschero, M. G. (2000). Lipid metabolism in vertebrate retinal rod outer segments. *Prog. Lipid Res.* 39, 315–391. doi: 10.1016/s0163-7827(00)00009-6

Gomes, A., Fernandes, E., and Lima, J. L. (2005). Fluorescence probes used for detection of reactive oxygen species. *J. Biochem. Biophys. Methods* 65, 45–80. doi: 10.1016/j.jbbm.2005.10.003

Grimm, C., and Remé, C. E. (2013). Light damage as a model of retinal degeneration. *Methods Mol. Biol.* 935, 87–97. doi: 10.1007/978-1-62703-080-9_6

Guido, M. E., Garbarino-Pico, E., Contin, M. A., Valdez, D. J., Nieto, P. S., Verra, D. M., et al. (2010). Inner retinal circadian clocks and non-visual photoreceptors: novel players in the circadian system. *Prog. Neurobiol.* 92, 484–504. doi: 10.1016/j.pneurobio.2010.08.005

Halliwell, B. (1994). Free radicals, antioxidants, and human disease: curiosity, cause, or consequence? *Lancet* 344, 721–724. doi: 10.1016/s0140-6736(94)92211-x

Hao, W., Wenzel, A., Obin, M. S., Chen, C. K., Brill, E., Krasnoperova, N. V., et al. (2002). Evidence for two apoptotic pathways in light-induced retinal degeneration. *Nat. Genet.* 32, 254–260. doi: 10.1038/ng984

Hunter, J. J., Morgan, J. I., Merigan, W. H., Sliney, D. H., Sparrow, J. R., and Williams, D. R. (2012). The susceptibility of the retina to photochemical damage from visible light. *Prog. Retin. Eye Res.* 31, 28–42. doi: 10.1016/j.preteyeres.2011.11.001

Iusifov, E. I., Sakina, N. L., and Dontsov, A. E. (1980). Glutathione peroxidase activity of frog eye pigment epithelium. *Biokhimiia* 45, 1470–1475.

Jeffrey, B. G., Mitchell, D. C., Hibbeln, J. R., Gibson, R. A., Chedester, A. L., and Salem, N. (2002). Visual acuity and retinal function in infant monkeys fed long-chain PUFA. *Lipids* 37, 839–848. doi: 10.1007/s11745-002-0969-0

Kagan, V. E., Kuliev, I. Y., Spirichev, V. B., Shvedova, A. A., and Kozlov, Y. P. (1981). Accumulation of lipid peroxidation products and depression of retinal electrical activity in vitamin E-deficient rats exposed to high-intensity light. *Bull. Exp. Biol. Med.* 91, 144–147. doi: 10.1007/bf00835390

Kharwar, R. K., and Haldar, C. (2012). Daily variation in antioxidant enzymes and lipid peroxidation in lungs of a tropical bird Perdicula asiatica: role of melatonin and nuclear receptor RORα. *Comp. Biochem. Physiol. Part A Mol. Integr. Physiol.* 162, 296–302. doi: 10.1016/j.cbpa.2012.01.021

Lacoste, M. G., Ponce, I. T., Golini, R. L., Delgado, S. M., and Anzulovich, A. C. (2017). Aging modifies daily variation of antioxidant enzymes and oxidative status in the hippocampus. *Exp. Gerontol.* 88, 42–50. doi: 10.1016/j.exger.2016.12.002

Lai, T. Y. Y., Chu, K. O., Chan, K. P., Ng, T. K., Yam, G. H. F., Lam, D. S. C., et al. (2010). Alterations in serum fatty acid concentrations and desaturase activities in Bietti crystalline dystrophy unaffected by CYP4V2 genotypes. *Invest. Ophthalmol. Vis. Sci.* 51, 1092–1097. doi: 10.1167/iovs.09-3665

Nakamura, M., Kuse, Y., Tsuruma, K., Shimazawa, M., and Hara, H. (2017). The involvement of the oxidative stress in murine blue LED light-induced retinal damage model. *Biol. Pharm. Bull.* 40, 1219–1225. doi: 10.1248/bpb.b16-01008

Navigatore Fonzo, L. S., Golini, R. S., Delgado, S. M., Ponce, I. T., Bonomi, M. R., Rezza, I. G., et al. (2009). Temporal patterns of lipoperoxidation and antioxidant enzymes are modified in the hippocampus of vitamin A-deficient rats. *Hippocampus* 19, 869–880. doi: 10.1002/hipo.20571

Noell, W. K., Walker, V. S., Kang, B. S., and Berman, S. (1966). Retinal damage by light in rats. *Invest. Ophthalmol.* 5, 450–473.

Ntambi, J. M. (1995). The regulation of stearoyl-CoA desaturase (SCD). *Prog. Lipid Res.* 34, 139–150. doi: 10.1016/0163-7827(94)00010-j

Ntambi, J. M. (1999). Regulation of stearoyl-CoA desaturase by polyunsaturated fatty acids and cholesterol. *J. Lipid Res.* 40, 1549–1558.

Ohta, Y., Yamasaki, T., Niwa, T., Niimi, K., Majima, Y., and Ishiguro, I. (1996). Role of catalase in retinal antioxidant defence system: its comparative study among rabbits, guinea pigs and rats. *Ophthalmic Res.* 28, 336–342. doi: 10.1159/000267925

Organisciak, D. T., and Vaughan, D. K. (2010). Retinal light damage: mechanisms and protection. *Prog. Retin. Eye Res.* 29, 113–134. doi: 10.1016/j.preteyeres.2009.11.004

Pavarino, É. C., Russo, A., Galbiatti, A. L. S., Almeida, W. P., and Goloni-Bertollo, E. M. (2013). "Glutathione: biosynthesis and mechanism of action," in *Glutathione: Biochemistry, Mechanisms of Action and Biotechnological Implications*, 1st Edn. eds N. Labrou and E. Flemetakis (New York, NY: Nova Science Publishers, Inc.), 1–34.

Peng, Y. W., Zallocchi, M., Wang, W. M., Delimont, D., and Cosgrove, D. (2011). Moderate light-induced degeneration of rod photoreceptors with delayed transducin translocation in shaker1 mice. *Invest. Ophthalmol. Vis. Sci.* 52, 6421–6427. doi: 10.1167/iovs.10-6557

Quintana, Q., Benedetto, M. L., Maldonado, M. M., Vera de Payer, E. A. C., and Contin, M. A. (2016). Electroretinography: a biopotential to assess the function/dysfunction of the retina. *J. Phys. Conf. Ser.* 705:012053. doi: 10.1088/1742-6596/705/1/012053

Rapp, L. M., and Williams, T. P. (1979). Damage to the albino rat retina produced by low intensity light. *Photochem. Photobiol.* 29, 731–733. doi: 10.1111/j.1751-1097.1979.tb07758.x

Remé, C. E., Grimm, C., Hafezi, F., Wenzel, A., and Williams, T. P. (2000). Apoptosis in the retina: the silent death of vision. *News Physiol. Sci.* 15, 120–124. doi: 10.1152/physiologyonline.2000.15.3.120

Roehlecke, C., Schumann, U., Ader, M., Brunssen, C., Bramke, S., Morawietz, H., et al. (2013). Stress reaction in outer segments of photoreceptors after blue light irradiation. *PLoS One* 8:e71570. doi: 10.1371/journal.pone.0071570

Roehlecke, C., Schumann, U., Ader, M., Knels, L., and Funk, R. H. (2011). Influence of blue light on photoreceptors in a live retinal explant system. *Mol. Vis.* 17, 876–884.

Rollag, M. D., Berson, D. M., and Provencio, I. (2003). Melanopsin, ganglion-cell photoreceptors and mammalian photoentrainment. *J. Biol. Rhythm.* 18, 227–234. doi: 10.1177/0748730403018003005

Rózanowska, M., and Sarna, T. (2005). Light-induced damage to the retina: role of rhodopsin chromophore revisited. *Photochem. Photobiol.* 81, 1305–1330. doi: 10.1562/2004-11-13-ir-371

Salas-Estrada, L. A., Leioatts, N., Romo, T. D., and Grossfield, A. (2018). Lipids alter rhodopsin function via ligand-like and solvent-like interactions. *Biophys. J.* 114, 355–367. doi: 10.1016/j.bpj.2017.11.021

SanGiovanni, J. P., and Chew, E. Y. (2005). The role of omega-3 long-chain polyunsaturated fatty acids in health and disease of the retina. *Prog. Retin. Eye Res.* 24, 87–138. doi: 10.1016/j.preteyeres.2004.06.002

Sani, M., Sebaï, H., Gadacha, W., Boughattas, N. A., Reinberg, A., and Mossadok, B. A. (2006). Catalase activity and rhythmic patterns in mouse brain, kidney and liver. *Comp. Biochem. Physiol. B Biochem. Mol. Biol.* 145, 331–337. doi: 10.1016/j.cbpb.2006.08.005

Scibior, D., and Czeczot, H. (2006). [Catalase: structure, properties, functions]. *Postepy Hig. Med. Dosw.* 60, 170–180.

Scott, B. L., and Bazan, N. G. (1989). Membrane docosahexaenoate is supplied to the developing brain and retina by the liver. *Proc. Natl. Acad. Sci. U S A* 86, 2903–2907. doi: 10.1073/pnas.86.8.2903

Semple-Rowland, S. L., and Dawson, W. W. (1987). Retinal cyclic light damage threshold for albino rats. *Lab. Anim. Sci.* 37, 289–298.

Shang, Y. M., Wang, G. S., Sliney, D., Yang, C. H., and Lee, L. L. (2014). White light-emitting diodes (LEDs) at domestic lighting levels and retinal injury in a rat model. *Environ Health Perspect.* 122, 269–276. doi: 10.1289/ehp.1307294

Shear, C. R., O'Steen, W. K., and Anderson, K. V. (1973). Effects of short-term low intensity light on the albino rat retina. An electron microscopic study. *Am. J. Anat.* 138, 127–132. doi: 10.1002/aja.1001380108

Sikka, G., Hussmann, G. P., Pandey, D., Cao, S., Hori, D., Park, J. T., et al. (2014). Melanopsin mediates light-dependent relaxation in blood vessels. *Proc. Natl. Acad. Sci. U S A* 111, 17977–17982. doi: 10.1073/pnas.1420258111

Sperling, H. G., Johnson, C., and Harwerth, R. S. (1980). Differential spectral photic damage to primate cones. *Vis. Res.* 20, 1117–1125. doi: 10.1016/0042-6989(80)90049-8

Sung, C. H., and Chuang, J. Z. (2010). The cell biology of vision. *J. Cell Biol.* 190, 953–963. doi: 10.1083/jcb.201006020

Wheeler, T. G., Benolken, R. M., and Anderson, R. E. (1975). Visual membranes: specificity of fatty acid precursors for the electrical response to illumination. *Science* 188, 1312–1314. doi: 10.1126/science.1145197

Wiegand, R. D., Giusto, N. M., Rapp, L. M., and Anderson, R. E. (1983). Evidence for rod outer segment lipid peroxidation following constant illumination of the rat retina. *Invest. Ophthalmol. Vis. Sci.* 24, 1433–1435.

Yusifov, E. Y., Kerimova, A. A., Atalay, M., and Kerimov, T. M. (2000). Light exposure induces antioxidant enzyme activities in eye tissues of frogs. *Pathophysiology* 7, 203–207. doi: 10.1016/s0928-4680(00)00051-1

Zolfaghari, R., and Ross, A. C. (2003). Recent advances in molecular cloning of fatty acid desaturase genes and the regulation of their expression by dietary vitamin A and retinoic acid. *Prostaglandins Leukot. Essent. Fatty Acids* 68, 171–179. doi: 10.1016/s0952-3278(02)00267-3

# 16

# The C-terminus of NMDAR GluN1-1a Subunit Translocates to Nucleus and Regulates Synaptic Function

*Liang Zhou [1]* and Jingjing Duan [2]*

*[1] Department of Pharmacology, College of Pharmaceutical Sciences, Soochow University, Jiangsu, China, [2] Department of Anatomy and Neurobiology, Zhongshan School of Medicine, SunYat-sen University, Guangzhou, China*

***Correspondence:**
*Liang Zhou*
*liangzhou@suda.edu.cn*

NMDARs, the $Ca^{2+}$ permeable channels, play central roles in synaptic plasticity, brain development, learning, and memory. NMDAR binding partners and associated signaling has been extensively studied in synapse-to-nucleus communications. However, whether NMDARs could directly regulate synapse-to-nucleus communications is largely unknown. Here, we analyze the four alternative splicing of the C-terminus isoforms of GluN1 (1a, 2a, 3a, and 4a), and find that C1 domain of GluN1 is necessary for nuclear localization. Besides, we find that the 10 basic amino acids in C1 domain determine the nuclear localization of GluN1 C-terminus. Further investigating the expression patterns of the full length of GluN1 four isoforms shows that only GluN-1a exhibits the cytoplasmic and nucleus distribution in primary hippocampal neurons. Electrophysiological analyses also show that over-expression of GluN1 C-terminus without C1 domain doesn't affect synaptic transmission, whereas GluN1 C-terminus containing C1 domain potentiates NMDAR-mediated synaptic transmission. Our data suggested that the 10 basic amino acids in C1 domain determine translocation of GluN1 C-terminus into nucleus and regulate synaptic transmission.

**Keywords: NMDA receptor, GluN1, synapse-to-nucleus communication, synapse transmission, cLTP**

## INTRODUCTION

NMDA receptors (NMDARs) are ionotropic glutamate receptors, which are important for neuronal development, synaptic plasticity, learning, and memory (Tsien et al., 1996). The NMDARs are composed of two GluN1 and two GluN2/3 subunits, which are located at excitatory synapses (Paoletti et al., 2013). The intracellular GluN1 C-terminus contains distinct domains, binds to different proteins, and activates different downstream signaling pathways (Horak and Wenthold, 2009; Gu et al., 2016b). Due to the alternative splicing of the C-terminus, there are four GluN1 isoforms, GluN1-1a, 2a, 3a, 4a (Horak and Wenthold, 2009; Ferreira et al., 2011). The GluN1-1a is the dominant isoform (Laurie and Seeburg, 1994), and the expression levels of GluN1 isoforms are regulated by synaptic activity (Mu et al., 2003; Paoletti et al., 2013).

The synaptic activity modulates the immediate early genes (IEGs) expression in the nucleus (Yang et al., 2014), which is called synapse-to-nucleus communication (Deisseroth et al., 1996, 2003). The synapse-to-nucleus communication is essential for learning and memory (Lim et al., 2017). NMDARs antagonist can block synaptic activation induced IEGs expressions, which demonstrates NMDARs are required for synapse-to-nucleus communication (Mokin and Keifer, 2005; Lonergan et al., 2010). It has been reported that NMDAR associated proteins

(Panayotis et al., 2015; Herbst and Martin, 2017) and $Ca^{2+}$ signaling (Hagenston and Bading, 2011) can lead to the activation of downstream signaling pathways during synaptic activity and regulate synapse-to-nucleus communication (Fainzilber et al., 2011; Lim et al., 2017). NMDAR associated proteins, such as Calmodulin (Deisseroth et al., 1998), Jacob (Dieterich et al., 2008), CRTC1 (Ch'ng et al., 2012), JAKMIP1 (Berg et al., 2015), have been extensively studied in synapse-nucleus communication. Calmodulin could translocate to neuronal nuclei upon synaptic stimulation (Deisseroth et al., 1998), and the translocation of calmodulin from cytoplasm to nucleus is mediated by γCaMKII (Ma et al., 2014). The Jacob translocates to neuronal nuclei through binding to importin α upon NMDARs activation (Dieterich et al., 2008), which could be regulated by ERK activity (Karpova et al., 2013). NMDARs activation also promotes the translocation of CRTC1 to neuronal nuclei, which could selectively increase the CREB-mediated transcription upon synapse activity (Ch'ng et al., 2012, 2015; Nonaka et al., 2014). However, whether NMDAR could directly regulate synapse-to-nucleus communication is largely unknown. Here, we found that the C-terminus of GluN1-1a translocates to neuronal nuclei, regulates synaptic transmission. Furthermore, the translocation of GluN1 C-terminus to nuclei could be regulated by neuronal activity.

## MATERIALS AND METHODS

### Plasmids

The plasmids of full-length GluN1-1a,-2a,-3a, and -4a were described preciously (Gu et al., 2016b). C2′oligonucleotides (top and bottom strands) are annealed and directly inserted into pEGFP-N3 vector at Nhe I/Sal I sites. The other truncated and full-length plasmids of GluN1 were created by standard PCR methods: PCR products were amplified from pCAGGS-GluN1-1a,−2a,−3a, and−4a using the relative primers, and subsequently inserted into pEGFP-N3 vector at Nhe I/Sal I sites. All GluN1 mutants were generated by overlapping PCR and cloned into pEGFP-N3 vector at Nhe I/Sal I sites. The primers used for the subclones in this study were provided in the **Supplementary Material.**

### Cell Culture and Animals

Human embryonic kidney 293A (HEK293A) cells were cultured in DMEM containing 10% FBS (Gibco). For DNA transfection, Effectene Transfection Reagent (QIAGEN) was used in HEK293 cells, DNA-In® Neuro Transfection Reagent (Thermo Fisher Scientific) was used in primary hippocampal neuron. 24–48 h after transfection, the cells were subjected to immunocytochemistry assay. The mice were housed under the standard conditions of temperature and humidity. All animal procedures in this study were approved by Institutional Animal Care and Use Committee of Soochow University.

### Primary Hippocampal Neurons Culture

Hippocampal primary dissociated neuronal culture was performed as previously described (Gu et al., 2016b). Briefly, the mouse hippocampi were dissected from E18 mouse embryos, and then digested using papain (Worthington) and DNase I (Worthington) to get individual neurons. After centrifuged at 800 rpm for 5 min, the pellet was resuspended in Hanks solution mixed with trypsin inhibitor (Sigma) and BSA, and then centrifuged at 800 rpm for 10 min. The pellet was resuspended in Neurobasal plating media containing 2% FBS, 2% B27 supplements, and 2 mM L-glutamine. Hippocampal neurons were plated at 200,000 cells/well on coverslips coated with poly-D-lysine in 24-well plates. Neurobasal culture media containing 2% B27 supplements, and 2 mM L-glutamine were used to replaced the culture media each other day.

### Organotypic Hippocampal Slice Culture

The mouse hippocampi were dissected from P6–P8 wild-type mice as previously described (Gu et al., 2016a), and transfected biolistically with plasmids in DIV3-4. Slices were cultured for an additional 2 days before recording. For recording evoked EPSCs in slice cultures, the extracellular solution is artificial cerebrospinal fluid (ACSF) containing (in mM) KCl 2.5, $CaCl_2$ 4, $MgCl_2$ 4, $NaH_2PO4$ 1.25, $NaHCO_3$ 25, glucose 7, sucrose 210. 15 μM 2-chloroadenosine and 100 μM picrotoxin were added into ACSF to dampen epileptiform activity and block the $GABA_A$ receptors. The supplier of pharmacological reagents is Abcam.

### Neuronal Stimulation

DIV 12–14 dissociated hippocampal neurons were used to perform neuronal stimulation experiments. After bath application of the relative chemicals, all samples were transferred to the solution without the related reagents for 15–20 min, and then the samples were subjected to immunocytochemistry assay. For neuronal membrane depolarization induction, 50 mM KCl was used to treat hippocampal neurons for 5 min. For NMDARs activation induction, 100 μM NMDA (Abcam) and 2 μM glycine was given by bath application for 5 min. For chemical long-term potentiation (cLTP) induction, 200 μM glycine in ACSF was briefly applied for 3 min to stimulate synaptic NMDARs, which is described as previously study (Lu et al., 2001). For chemical long-term depression (cLTD) induction, 50 μM NMDA (Abcam) was given by bath application for 3 min. Ten micromoles MG-132 (Sigma) was used to block the proteasome. Fifty micromoles DHPG (Abcam) was given by bath application for 5 min to induce group 1 metabotropic glutamate receptor-mediated LTD.

### Immunocytochemistry Assay

HEK293A cells or hippocampal neurons grown on coverslips were rinsed with PBS twice and fixed in 4% paraformaldehyde (PFA) for 15 min at room temperature, permeabilized with 0.2% TritonX-100 in PBS for 5 min, after blocking with 5% normal goat serum (NGS) in PBS for 1 h, the primary antibodies anti-GluN1 (mouse,1:1,000, NeuroMab, N308/48), anti-GluN1 (rabbit, 1:1,000, Millipore, AB9864) were used at room temperature for 3 h, and then the second antibodies Alexa Fluor 405-conjugated goat anti-mouse and Alexa Fluor 555-conjugated goat anti-rabbit (Invitrogen, Molecular Probes) were incubated for 1 h. Coverslips were mounted with Fluoromont

G (Southern Biotech). Fluorescent images were acquired on a Zeiss510 laser scanning confocal microscope and Olympus IX71 inverted microscope with identical settings for each group. For image quantification analysis, maximal projection images were generated by LSM510 browser software, the integrated fluorescent intensity of GluN1 was measured with ImageJ software (NIH, Bethesda). Statistical analysis was conducted with GraphPad Prism6 software using one-way analysis of variance (ANOVA).

## Synaptic Electrophysiology

The AMPA EPSCs and NMDA EPSCs were recorded by stimulating Schaffer collaterals pathway with monopolar glass electrodes filled with ACSF. GFP-positive pyramidal neurons at the CA1 region were visualized with GFP fluorescence. GFP-positive neuron and the neighboring GFP-negative neuron were chose to perform the paired whole-cell recordings. AMPA EPSCs were recorded at −70, and NMDA EPSCs were recorded at +40 mV. The NMDA EPSCs were measured at 100 ms after stimulation. The components of intracellular solution were (in mM) $CsMeSO_4$ 135, NaCl 8, HEPEs 10, $Na_3GFP$ 0.3, MgATP 4, EGTA 0.3, QX-314 5, and spermine 0.1. The 3–5 MΩ borosilicate glass pipettes were used for recording.

## Statistics

All data were given as mean ± s.e.m. Statistical significance between means was calculated using Student's *t*-test.

# RESULTS

## C1 Domain of GluN1 C-terminus Is Necessary for Nuclear Translocation

Our previous study shows the C-terminus of GluN1 play a crucial role in GABAergic synapses formation (Gu et al., 2016b), indicating that the C-terminus of GluN1 is important for NMDARs-mediated biological functions. Due to alternative splicing of the C-terminus, there are four GluN1 isoforms, GluN1-1a, 2a, 3a, and 4a (**Figure 1A**). They are composed of four domains, C0, C1, C2, and C2' (**Figure 1B**). Firstly, we investigated the cellular distribution of these four domains in HEK293A. The results showed that C1-GFP mainly localized in nucleus, while the other domains showed the whole cell diffuse distribution (**Figure 1C**). To verify whether C1 domain is required for nuclear localization, we over expressed 4 isoforms of GluN1 C-terminus in HEK293A cells and primary hippocampal neurons. We found that only the 1a-CT-GFP and 3a-CT-GFP containing the C1 domain showed nuclear localization in HEK293A cells (**Figure 1D**) and primary hippocampal neurons (**Supplementary Figure S1**). Thus, our data demonstrated that C-terminus of GluN1 containing C1 domain was necessary for nuclear translocation.

## Ten Basic Amino Acids in C1 Domain Determines the Nuclear Localization of GluN1 C-terminus

Previously, it is suggested that C1 domain contains a bi-particle nuclear localization signal (NLS) by the protein subcellular localization prediction tool (PSORT) (Holmes et al., 2002; Jeffrey et al., 2009) (**Figure 2A**). To verify whether the C1 domain contains NLS, we constructed several mutants of 1a-CT (**Figure 2B**). We found that the bi-particle 7 basic amino acids [1a-CT-GFP(7A)] were not necessary for the nuclear localization of GluN1 C-terminus, but the 10 basic amino acids in the C1 domain 1a-CT-GFP(10A) regulated the nuclear localization of GluN1 C-terminus in HEK293A cells and primary hippocampal neurons (**Figures 2C,D**).

## GluN1 C-terminus Translocates to Nucleus in Primary Neurons

To explore the nuclear localization of full-length GluN1, we transfected the full-length four isoforms of GluN1 fused to GFP into cells. Our data showed that the full-length of GluN1 showed diffuse cytoplasmic distribution in HEK293A cells (**Supplementary Figure S2**). In primary hippocampal neurons, we found that the full-length of GluN1-1a exhibited cytoplasmic and nuclear distribution, while the GluN1-2a, GluN1-3a, GluN1-4a, and GluN1-1a(10A) isoforms showed diffuse cytoplasmic distribution (**Figures 3A,B**). Given that single GluN1 subunit could not form the functional NMDARs in HEK293A cells (Cao et al., 2011; Hansen et al., 2014), we transfected GluN1 and GluN2A subunits in HEK293A cells to examine whether GluN2 is required for the translocation of GluN1-1a C terminus, the results showed the full-length GluN1-1a still showed cytoplamic distribution in HEK293A cells (**Supplementary Figure S3**), which suggests that the intrinsic genetic determinants of neuronal form determine the translocation of GluN1 C-terminus to nucleus in primary hippocampal neurons.

There were three possibilities to explain the whole cell diffuse distribution of GluN1-1a-GFP. Firstly, the full-length of GluN1-1a-GFP could translocate to nucleus because of artificial phenomena of over-expression; secondly, the GFP protein can be detached or auto-cleaved from GluN1-1a-GFP in neurons for some unknown reasons; the third possibility is that the C-terminus of GluN1-1a can be detached or cleaved from GluN1-1a-GFP in neurons, so the C-terminus contained GFP fused C1 domain can translocate to nucleus. To test these hypotheses, two commercial antibodies were used (**Figure 3C**). The N-terminus antibody is a mouse antibody that can recognize the N-terminus of GluN1 extracellular domain (amino acids 42–361); the C-terminus antibody is a rabbit antibody that can only recognize the C2 domain part of GluN1 C-terminus (LQNQKDTVLPRRAIEREEGQLQLCSRHRES) (**Figure 3C**). To test the specificity of the antibodies, we over expressed the full-length of GluN1-1a, 2a, 3a, and 4a in HEK293A cells. The results showed that N antibody could recognize all four full-length isoforms, whereas the C antibody could only recognize the full-length GluN1-1a and GluN1-2a containing C2 domain (**Supplementary Figure S4A**). We also used the C-terminus of four isoforms to test these two commercial antibodies. The results showed the N antibody couldn't recognize the C-terminus, while the C antibody could recognize the GluN1-1a-CT and 2a-CT containing C2 domain (**Supplemental Figure S4B**). Therefore,

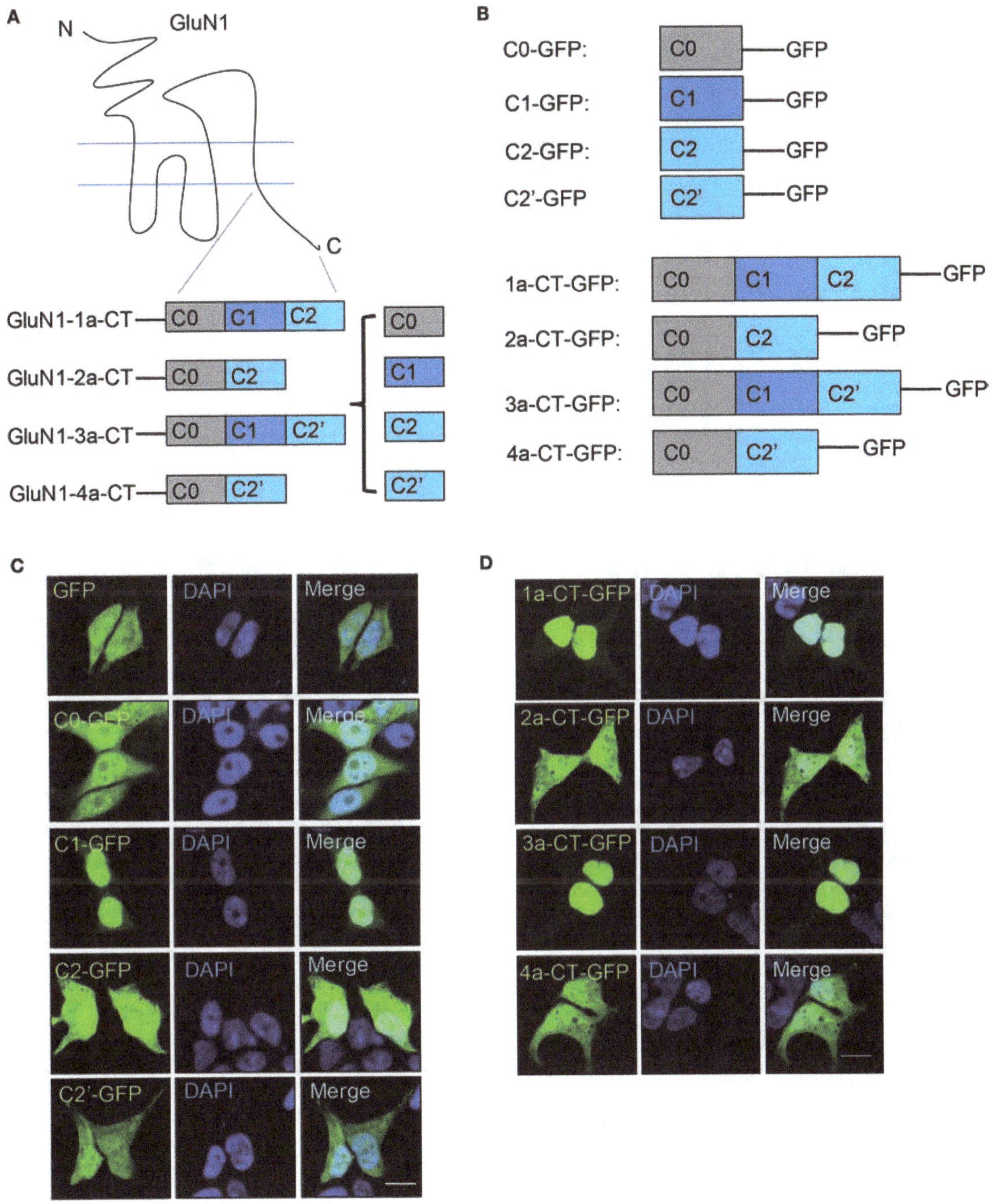


**FIGURE 1 |** C1 domain determines the nuclear localization of GluN1 C-terminus in HEK293A cells. **(A)** Schematic diagram of GluN1 C-terminus. **(B)** The plasmids of truncated GluN1 C-terminus were used in this study. **(C)** HEK293A cells were transfected with GFP, C0-GFP, C1-GFP, C2-GFP, or C2'-GFP for 24 h, and then the cells were subjected to immunocytochemistry assay. DAPI was used to visualize the cell nuclei. Scale bar: 10 μm. **(D)** The C-terminus of four GluN1 isoforms were transfected in HEK293A cells for 24 h, and then the cells subjected to immunocytochemistry assay. DAPI was used to visualize the cell nuclei. Scale bar: 10 μm.

our data showed the two antibodies could specifically recognize the immunogenic regions.

In cultured hippocampal neurons, the immunocytochemistry assays showed that the nuclear fluorescence of GluN1-1a-GFP could be identified by the C antibody (**Figures 3D–F**). Because the C antibody also recognizes the endogenous GluN1, the red fluorescence in the nucleus is weaker than in the cytoplasm (**Figure 3D**). Thus, our data support the third hypothesis that C-terminus of GluN1-1a can be detached or cleaved from GluN1-1a-GFP in neurons,

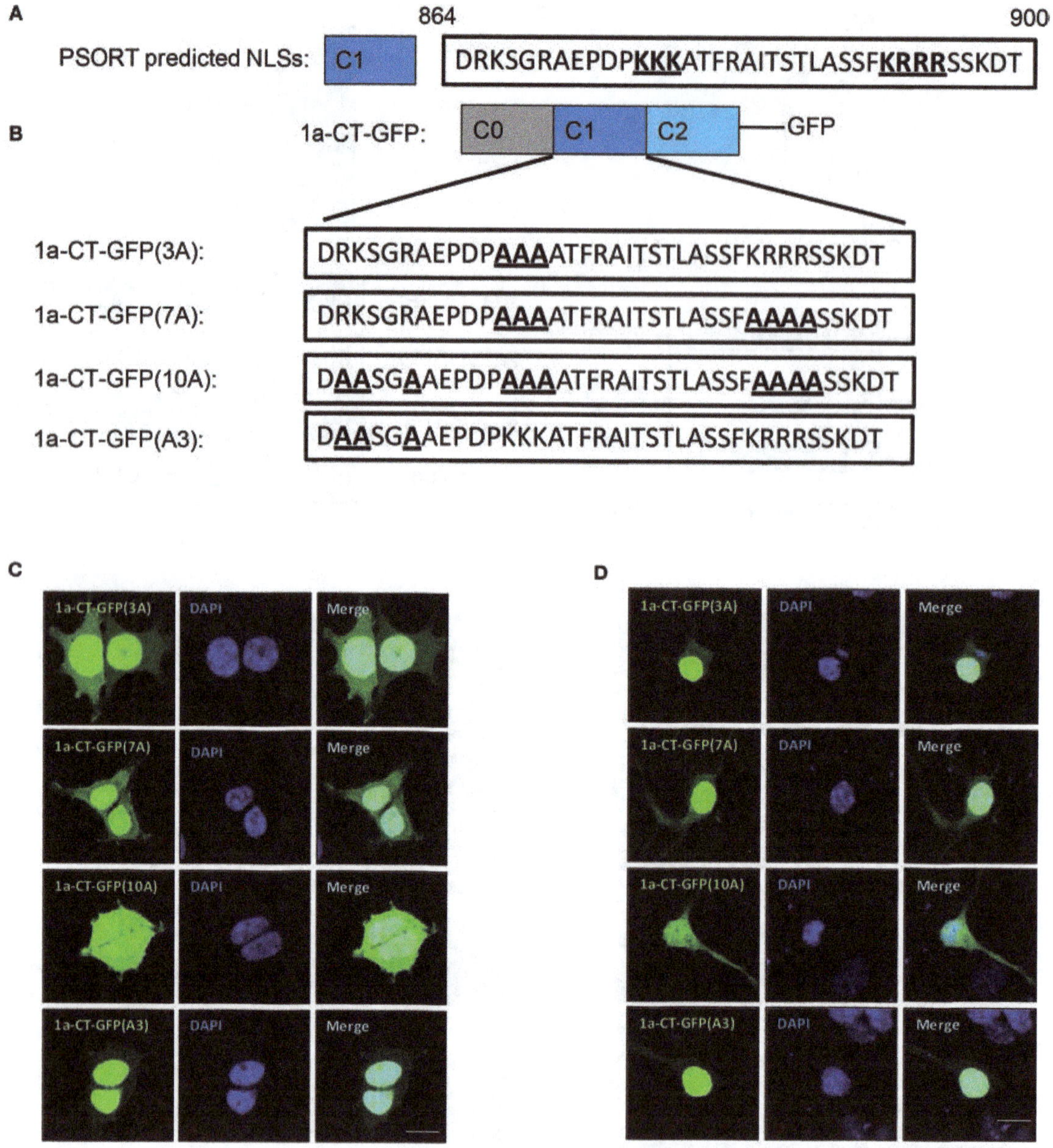


**FIGURE 2 |** Ten amino acid in C1 domain determines the nuclear localization of GluN1 C-terminus. **(A)** the protein subcellular localization prediction tool (PSORT) predicted nuclear localization signal in C1 domain. **(B)** Indicated mutation for 1a-CT-GFP (3A), 1a-CT-GFP (7A), 1a-CT-GFP (10A), or 1a-CT-GFP (A3). **(C,D)** The HEK293A (**C**) and primary hippocampal neurons **(D)** were transfected with 1a-CT-GFP (3A), 1a-CT-GFP (7A), 1a-CT-GFP (10A), or 1a-CT-GFP (A3) for 24 h, and then the cells were subjected to immunocytochemistry assay. DAPI was used to visualize the cell nuclei. Scale bar: 10 μm.

and the C-terminus including GFP can translocate to nuclei.

## Chemical LTP Regulates the Translocation of C-terminus of GluN1 to Nucleus

To explore the relationship of nuclear translocation and neuronal activity, we treated the neurons with KCl to depolarization the neuron, NMDA and glycine to activate NMDARs, glycine to induce chemical LTP (cLTP), NMDA to induce chemical LTD (cLTD), MG-132 to block the proteasome, DHPG to induce group 1 metabotropic glutamate receptor-mediated LTD. Using C antibody to detect C-terminus of GluN1, N antibody to detect total GluN1, we calculated the nuclear fluorescence'ratio of C antibody to N antibody. The results show that the chemical long-term potentiation (cLTP) treatment could significantly decrease the nuclear fluorescence intensity of GluN1 (**Figures 4A,B**).There is no significant difference in the ratios of cytoplasmic and dendritic fluorescence intensity after cLTP treatment (**Figures 4C,D**). Taken together, these data demonstrates that

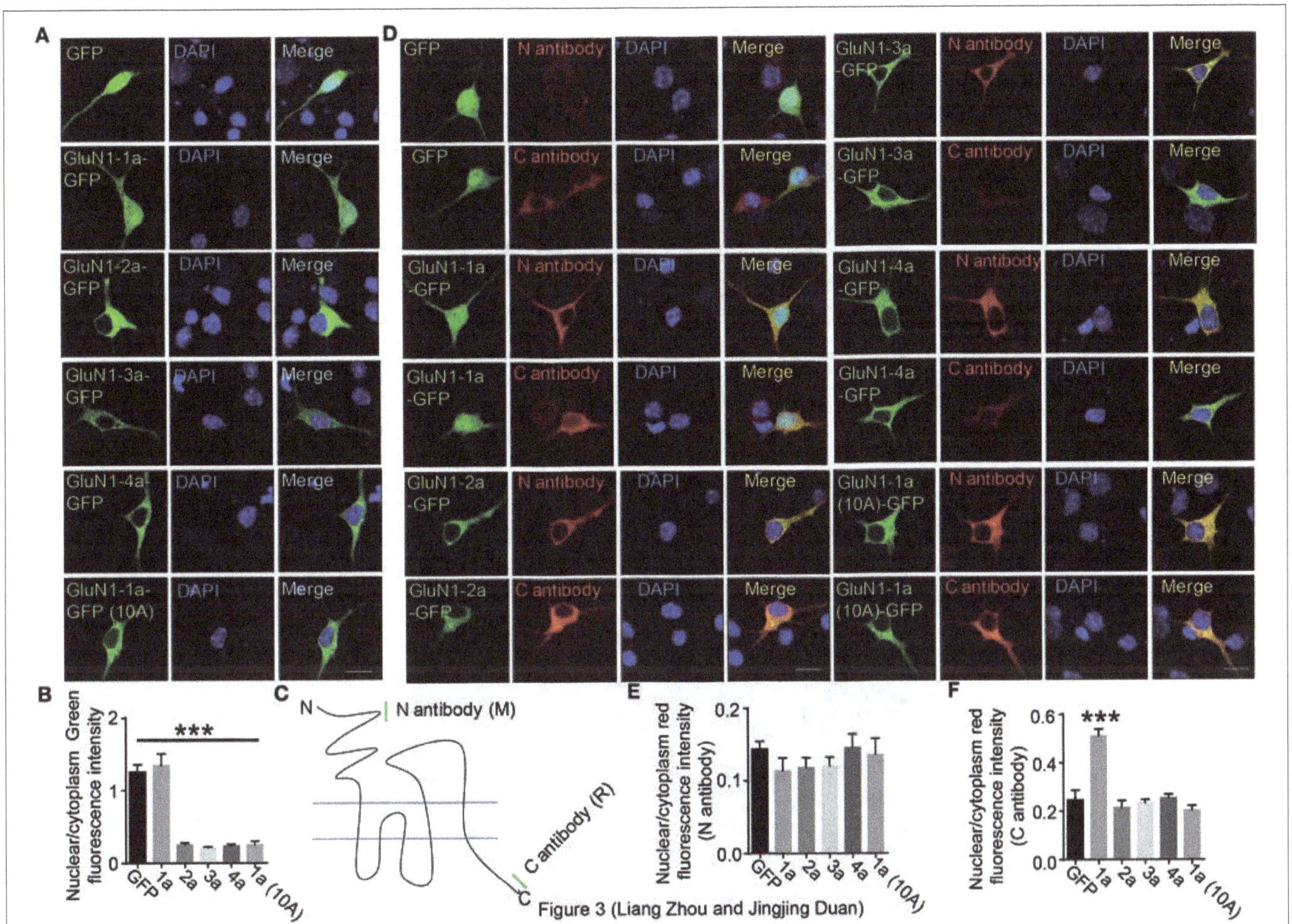

**FIGURE 3 |** The C-terminus of GluN1-1a translocates to nucleus in primary hippocampal neuron. **(A)** The primary hippocampal neurons were transfected with GFP, GluN1-1a-GFP, GluN1-2a-GFP, GluN1-3a-GFP, GluN1-4a-GFP, or GluN1-1a-GFP (10A) for 24 h, and then the cells were subjected to immunocytochemistry assay. DAPI was used to visualize the cell nuclei. Scale bar: 10 μm. **(B)** Quantitative data (mean ± SEM) of **(A)** from three independent experiments. ***$P < 0.001$, Student's *t*-test. **(C)** Two GluN1 antibodies were used in this study. The mouse N antibody recognizes the N terminus amino acids 42–361 of GluN1 extracellular domain, and the rabbit C antibody recognizes the C2 domain of GluN1. **(D)** The primary hippocampal neurons were transfected with GFP, GluN1-1a-GFP, GluN1-2a-GFP, GluN1-3a-GFP, GluN1-4a-GFP, or GluN1-1a-GFP (10A) for 24 h, and then stained with the N and C antibodies of GluN1 for immunofluorescence measurement. DAPI was used to visualize the nuclei. Scale bar: 10 μm. **(E,F)** Quantitative data (mean ± SEM) of **(D)** from three independent experiments. ***$P < 0.001$, Student's *t*-test.

cLTP could affect the translocation of GluN1 C-terminus to nucleus.

## The C-terminus of GluN1-1a Potentiates Glutamate Transmission

Given the crucial role of NMDARs in synaptic functions, we then investigated the regulation of GluN1-1a C terminus on synaptic transmission. We transfected GluN1 C-terminus into neurons, and then did the electrophysiological recording. We found that over-expression of 2a-CT-GFP without C1 domain didn't change AMPA EPSCs or NMDA EPSCs, whereas 1a-CT-GFP containing C1 domain could potentiate NMDAR-mediated synaptic transmission (**Figure 5A**). No change of paired-pulse ratio (PPR) of GluN1-1a-CT-GFP and GluN1-2a-CT-GFP suggested that C1 domain of GluN1 did not affect presynaptic neurotransmitter release probability (**Figure 5B**).

# DISCUSSION

NMDARs are widely expressed in neurons throughout the central nervous system with distinct pharmacological and electrophysiological properties because of diversity of subunit composition (Paoletti et al., 2013; Hansen et al., 2014). Once the synaptic plasticity happens, the neuronal nucleus must be informed to activate the IEGs expression, which is mediated by the synapse-to-nucleus signaling pathway (Deisseroth et al., 1996, 2003). Several proteins binding to NMDARs or forming the complex with NMDARs in the postsynaptic density have been reported that can relay the information between synapses and nucleus, such as Calmodulin (Deisseroth et al., 1998), nuclear factor-κB (NF-κB) (Meffert et al., 2003), importins (Ch'ng and Martin, 2011), and Jacob (Dieterich et al., 2008).

Here we found that NMDARs subunit GluN1-1a involved in synapse-to-nucleus communication. Our results showed that the

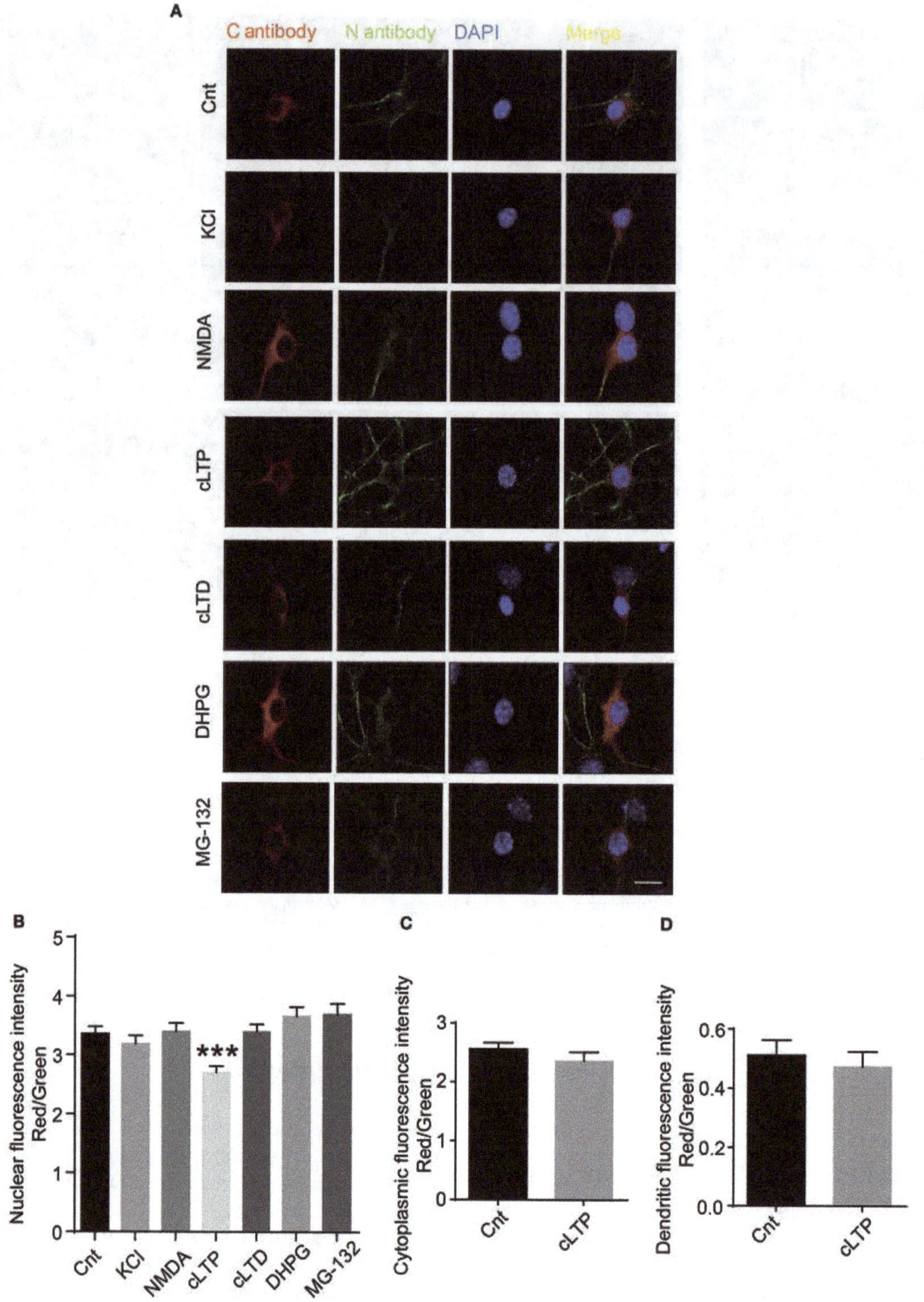


**FIGURE 4 |** Neuronal activity regulates the cleavage of GluN1. **(A)** The primary hippocampal neurons were treated with several reagents to activate the different signal pathways. 50 mM KCl was used to depolarize the neuronal membrane. One hundred micromoles NMDA (Abcam) and 2 μM glycine was used to activate NMDARs. Two hundred micromoles glycine was used to induce cLTP. Fifty micromoles NMDA was used to induce cLTD. Fifty micromoles DHPG was used to induce group 1 metabotropic glutamate receptor-mediated LTD. Ten micromoles MG-132 was used to block the proteasome. **(B)** The quantitative data were presented with the nuclear fluorescence intensity of GluN1 by measuring ratio of nuclear red fluorescence (rabbit C antibody) to nuclear green fluorescence (mouse N antibody). (Number of neurons in each group: Cnt: $n = 39$, KCl: $n = 38$, NMDA: $n = 36$, cLTP: $n = 42$, cLTD: $n = 41$, DHPG: $n = 48$, MG-132: $n = 35$). Student's t test, ***$P < 0.001$. **(C,D)** The quantitative data was presented with the cytoplasmic fluorescence intensity of GluN1 **(C)** or dendritic fluorescence intensity **(D)** by measuring ratio of cytoplamic or dendritic red fluorescence (rabbit C antibody) to cytoplamic or dendritic green fluorescence (mouse N antibody). (Number of neurons in each group: Cnt: $n = 39$, cLTP: $n = 42$). Student's $t$-test, cytoplamic fluorescence $p = 0.2899$, dendritic fluorescence $p = 0.5989$.

C-terminus of GluN1-1a could translocate to neuronal nucleus (**Figures 1–3**) and the 10 basic amino acids in C1 domain determined the nuclear localization of GluN1 C terminus. The electrophysiological recording showed that C1 domain of GluN1 affected the NMDAR-mediated synaptic transmission (**Figure 5**). Taken together, these data indicated that the 10 basic amino acids in C1 domain determined the translocation of GluN1 C-terminus into neuronal nucleus, and this translocation is highly related to synaptic transmission (**Figure 5**).

In our study, although the GluN1-1a and GluN1-3a both contained C1 domain in the C-terminus, only the GluN1-1a showed nuclear fluorescence in neurons (**Figure 3**), which suggested that the adjacent alternatively spliced C2'domain affects this process, as the C2' domain can suppresses the function of C1 domain (Standley et al., 2000).

The neuronal activity regulates the localization of NMDARs (Rao and Craig, 1997). Here, we found that cLTP regulated the translocation of C-terminus of GluN1 (**Figure 4**). However, the

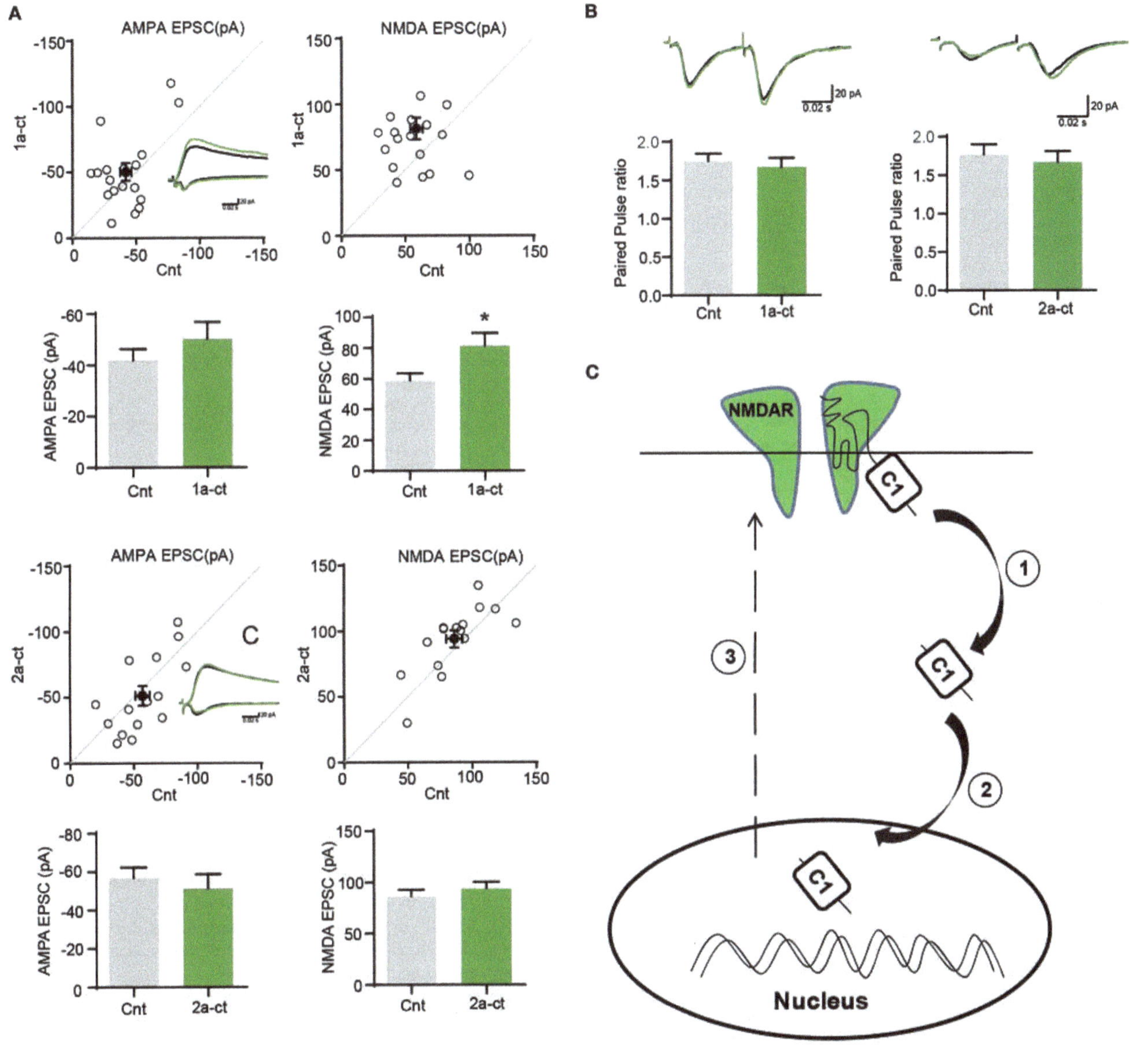


**FIGURE 5 |** The C terminus of GluN1 regulates synaptic functions. **(A)** The AMPA EPSCs and NMDA EPSCs were recorded after over expressing the 1a-CT-GFP or 2a-CT-GFP. (Amplitude of AMPA EPSCs: Cnt, 41.97 ± 4.403; 1a-CT-GFP, 50.24 ± 6.659, $n = 18$. $p = 0.1911$; Amplitude of NMDA EPSCs: Cnt, 58.84 ± 4.795; 1a-CT-GFP, 81.42 ± 8.345, n = 19. $^*p = 0.0169 < 0.05$; Amplitude of AMPA EPSCs: Cnt, 57.05 ± 5.471; 2a-CT-GFP, 51.26 ± 7.547, $n = 15$. $p = 0.3183$; Amplitude of NMDA EPSCs: Cnt, 86.42 ± 6.226; 2a-CT-GFP, 94.00 ± 6.685, $n = 15$. $p = 0.1146$; Amplitude of AMPA EPSCs: Cnt, 34.38 ± 4.166). **(B)**There were no differences in PPRs after over expressing 1a-CT-GFP or 2a-CT-GFP. (PPR control, 1.750 ± 0.09609 and PPR 1a-CT-GFP, 1.673 ± 0.1146, $n = 14$, $p = 0.3147$; PPR control, 1.767 ± 0.1343 and PPR 2a-CT-GFP, 1.673 ± 0.1380, $n = 13$, $p = 0.4804$). **(C)** A schematic diagram showing the translocation of GluN1 C-terminus to neuronal nucleus. The GluN1-1a C-terminus containing C1 domain could be cleaved by protease ①, and then translocates to neuronal nucleus ②, which eventually potentiates NMDAR-mediated synaptic transmission ③.

proteins that lead to the detachment or cleavage of C-terminus from the full-length of GluN1-1a are needed to be further identified. The calcium-dependent protease calpain could be a candidate, as calpain and NMDARs can regulate the functions of each other (Hell et al., 1996; Wu et al., 2005; Szydlowska and Tymianski, 2010). The LTP coordinates the homeostasis of synapses (Vitureira and Goda, 2013) and normalization of synapses (Hardingham et al., 2007), whether the translocation of GluN1-1a C-terminus to neuronal nuclei mediates the LTP associated these physiological functions, which are needed to be further investigated.

In summary, we found that the C-terminus of GluN1-1a can translocate to neuronal nuclei, and regulate the synaptic activity, which could be affected by cLTP.

## AUTHOR CONTRIBUTIONS

LZ supervised the research. LZ and JD performed the experiments. LZ and JD wrote and revised the manuscript.

## FUNDING

This work was supported by the National Natural Science Foundation of China (81703535), China Postdoctoral Science Foundation (2017M611895), Jiangsu Province Postdoctoral Science Foundation (1701130C), Natural Science Foundation of Jiangsu Higher Education Institutions of China (17KJD180005).

## ACKNOWLEDGMENTS

We are grateful to Dr. Wei Lu from National Institutes of Health (NIH) for generously providing the GluN1 and GluN2A plasmids.

## REFERENCES

Berg, J. M., Lee, C., Chen, L., Galvan, L., Cepeda, C., Chen, J. Y., et al. (2015). JAKMIP1, a novel regulator of neuronal translation, modulates synaptic function and autistic-like behaviors in mouse. *Neuron* 88, 1173–1191. doi: 10.1016/j.neuron.2015.10.031

Cao, J.-Y., Qiu, S., Zhang, J., Wang, J.-J., Zhang, X.-M., and Luo, J.-H. (2011). Transmembrane region of N-Methyl-D-Aspartate Receptor (NMDAR) subunit is required for receptor subunit assembly. *J. Biol. Chem.* 286, 27698–27705. doi: 10.1074/jbc.M111.235333

Ch'ng, T. H., Desalvo, M., Lin, P., Vashisht, A., Wohlschlegel, J., and Martin, K. (2015). Cell biological mechanisms of activity-dependent synapse to nucleus translocation of CRTC1 in neurons. *Front. Mol. Neurosci.* 8:48. doi: 10.3389/fnmol.2015.00048

Ch'ng, T. H., and Martin, K. C. (2011). Synapse to nucleus signaling. *Curr. Opin. Neurobiol.* 21, 345–352. doi: 10.1016/j.conb.2011.01.011

Ch'ng, T. H., Uzgil, B., Lin, P., Avliyakulov, N. K., O'dell, T. J., and Martin, K. C. (2012). Activity-dependent transport of the transcriptional coactivator CRTC1 from synapse to nucleus. *Cell* 150, 207–221. doi: 10.1016/j.cell.2012.05.027

Deisseroth, K., Bito, H., and Tsien, R. W. (1996). Signaling from synapse to nucleus: postsynaptic CREB phosphorylation during multiple forms of hippocampal synaptic plasticity. *Neuron* 16, 89–101. doi: 10.1016/S0896-6273(00)80026-4

Deisseroth, K., Heist, E. K., and Tsien, R. W. (1998). Translocation of calmodulin to the nucleus supports CREB phosphorylation in hippocampal neurons. *Nature* 392, 198–202. doi: 10.1038/32448

Deisseroth, K., Mermelstein, P. G., Xia, H., and Tsien, R. W. (2003). Signaling from synapse to nucleus: the logic behind the mechanisms. *Curr. Opin. Neurobiol.* 13, 354–365. doi: 10.1016/S0959-4388(03)00076-X

Dieterich, D. C., Karpova, A., Mikhaylova, M., Zdobnova, I., König, I., Landwehr, M., et al. (2008). Caldendrin–Jacob: a protein liaison that couples NMDA receptor signalling to the nucleus. *PLoS Biol.* 6:e34. doi: 10.1371/journal.pbio.0060034

Fainzilber, M., Budnik, V., Segal, R. A., and Kreutz, M. R. (2011). From synapse to nucleus and back again—communication over distance within neurons. *J. Neurosci.* 31, 16045–16048. doi: 10.1523/JNEUROSCI.4006-11.2011

Ferreira, J. S., Rooyakkers, A., She, K., Ribeiro, L., Carvalho, A. L., and Craig, A. M. (2011). Activity and protein kinase C regulate synaptic accumulation of N-Methyl-D-Aspartate (NMDA) receptors independently of GluN1 splice variant. *J. Biol. Chem.* 286, 28331–28342. doi: 10.1074/jbc.M111.222539

Gu, X., Mao, X., Lussier, M. P., Hutchison, M. A., Zhou, L., Hamra, F. K., et al. (2016a). GSG1L suppresses AMPA receptor-mediated synaptic transmission and uniquely modulates AMPA receptor kinetics in hippocampal neurons. *Nat. Commun.* 7:10873. doi: 10.1038/ncomms10873

Gu, X., Zhou, L., and Lu, W. (2016b). An NMDA receptor-dependent mechanism underlies inhibitory synapse development. *Cell Rep.* 14, 471–478. doi: 10.1016/j.celrep.2015.12.061

Hagenston, A. M., and Bading, H. (2011). Calcium signaling in synapse-to-nucleus communication. *Cold Spring Harb. Perspect. Biol.* 3:a004564. doi: 10.1101/cshperspect.a004564

Hansen, K. B., Ogden, K. K., Yuan, H., and Traynelis, S. F. (2014). Distinct functional and pharmacological properties of triheteromeric GluN1/GluN2A/GluN2B NMDA receptors. *Neuron* 81, 1084–1096. doi: 10.1016/j.neuron.2014.01.035

Hardingham, N. R., Hardingham, G. E., Fox, K. D., and Jack, J. J. B. (2007). Presynaptic efficacy directs normalization of synaptic strength in layer 2/3 rat neocortex after paired activity. *J. Neurophysiol.* 97, 2965–2975. doi: 10.1152/jn.01352.2006

Hell, J. W., Westenbroek, R. E., Breeze, L. J., Wang, K. K., Chavkin, C., and Catterall, W. A. (1996). N-methyl-D-aspartate receptor-induced proteolytic conversion of postsynaptic class C L-type calcium channels in hippocampal neurons. *Proc. Nat. Acad. Sci. U.S.A.* 93, 3362–3367. doi: 10.1073/pnas.93.8.3362

Herbst, W. A., and Martin, K. C. (2017). Regulated transport of signaling proteins from synapse to nucleus. *Curr. Opin. Neurobiol.* 45, 78–84. doi: 10.1016/j.conb.2017.04.006

Holmes, K. D., Mattar, P., Marsh, D. R., Jordan, V., Weaver, L. C., and Dekaban, G. A. (2002). The C-terminal C1 cassette of the N-methyl-D-aspartate receptor 1 subunit contains a bi-partite nuclear localization sequence. *J. Neurochem.* 81, 1152–1165. doi: 10.1046/j.1471-4159.2002.00865.x

Horak, M., and Wenthold, R. J. (2009). Different roles of C-terminal cassettes in the trafficking of full-length NR1 subunits to the cell surface. *J. Biol. Chem.* 284, 9683–9691. doi: 10.1074/jbc.M807050200

Jeffrey, R. A., Ch'ng, T. H., O'dell, T. J., and Martin, K. C. (2009). Activity-dependent anchoring of importin alpha at the synapse involves regulated binding to the cytoplasmic tail of the NR1-1a subunit of the NMDA receptor. *J. Neurosci.* 29, 15613–15620. doi: 10.1523/JNEUROSCI.3314-09.2009

Karpova, A., Mikhaylova, M., Bera, S., Bär, J., Reddy, P. P., Behnisch, T., et al. (2013). Encoding and transducing the synaptic or extrasynaptic origin of NMDA receptor signals to the nucleus. *Cell* 152, 1119–1133. doi: 10.1016/j.cell.2013.02.002

Laurie, D. J., and Seeburg, P. H. (1994). Regional and developmental heterogeneity in splicing of the rat brain NMDAR1 mRNA. *J. Neurosci.* 14, 3180–3194. doi: 10.1523/JNEUROSCI.14-05-03180.1994

Lim, A. F., Lim, W. L., and Ch'ng, T. H. (2017). Activity-dependent synapse to nucleus signaling. *Neurobiol. Learn. Mem.* 138, 78–84. doi: 10.1016/j.nlm.2016.07.024

Lonergan, M. E., Gafford, G. M., Jarome, T. J., and Helmstetter, F. J. (2010). Time-dependent expression of arc and Zif268 after acquisition of fear conditioning. *Neural Plast.* 2010:139891. doi: 10.1155/2010/139891

Lu, W., Man, H., Ju, W., Trimble, W. S., Macdonald, J. F., and Wang, Y. T. (2001). Activation of synaptic NMDA receptors induces membrane insertion of new AMPA receptors and LTP in cultured hippocampal neurons. *Neuron* 29, 243–254. doi: 10.1016/S0896-6273(01)00194-5

Ma, H., Groth, R. D., Cohen, S. M., Emery, J. F., Li, B., Hoedt, E., et al. (2014). gammaCaMKII shuttles $Ca^{2+}$/CaM to the nucleus to trigger CREB phosphorylation and gene expression. *Cell* 159, 281–294. doi: 10.1016/j.cell.2014.09.019

Meffert, M. K., Chang, J. M., Wiltgen, B. J., Fanselow, M. S., and Baltimore, D. (2003). NF-κB functions in synaptic signaling and behavior. *Nat. Neurosci.* 6, 1072–1078. doi: 10.1038/nn1110

Mokin, M., and Keifer, J. (2005). Expression of the immediate-early gene–encoded protein Egr-1 (zif268) during *in vitro* classical conditioning. *Learn. Mem.* 12, 144–149. doi: 10.1101/lm.87305

Mu, Y., Otsuka, T., Horton, A. C., Scott, D. B., and Ehlers, M. D. (2003). Activity-dependent mRNA splicing controls ER export and synaptic delivery of NMDA receptors. *Neuron* 40, 581–594. doi: 10.1016/S0896-6273(03)0 0676-7

Nonaka, M., Kim, R., Fukushima, H., Sasaki, K., Suzuki, K., Okamura, M., et al. (2014). Region-specific activation of CRTC1-CREB signaling mediates long-term fear memory. *Neuron* 84, 92–106. doi: 10.1016/j.neuron.2014. 08.049

Panayotis, N., Karpova, A., Kreutz, M. R., and Fainzilber, M. (2015). Macromolecular transport in synapse to nucleus communication. *Trends Neurosci.* 38, 108–116. doi: 10.1016/j.tins.2014.12.001

Paoletti, P., Bellone, C., and Zhou, Q. (2013). NMDA receptor subunit diversity: impact on receptor properties, synaptic plasticity and disease. *Nat. Rev. Neurosci.* 14, 383–400. doi: 10.1038/nrn3504

Rao, A., and Craig, A. M. (1997). Activity regulates the synaptic localization of the NMDA receptor in hippocampal neurons. *Neuron* 19, 801–812. doi: 10.1016/S0896-6273(00)80962-9

Standley, S., Roche, K. W., Mccallum, J., Sans, N., and Wenthold, R. J. (2000). PDZ domain suppression of an ER retention signal in NMDA receptor NR1 splice variants. *Neuron* 28, 887–898. doi: 10.1016/S0896-6273(00) 00161-6

Szydlowska, K., and Tymianski, M. (2010). Calcium, ischemia and excitotoxicity. *Cell Calcium* 47, 122–129. doi: 10.1016/j.ceca.2010.01.003

Tsien, J. Z., Huerta, P. T., and Tonegawa, S. (1996). The essential role of hippocampal CA1 NMDA receptor–dependent synaptic plasticity in spatial memory. *Cell* 87, 1327–1338. doi: 10.1016/S0092-8674(00)81827-9

Vitureira, N., and Goda, Y. (2013). The interplay between Hebbian and homeostatic synaptic plasticity. *J. Cell Biol.* 203, 175–186. doi: 10.1083/jcb.201306030

Wu, H.-Y., Yuen, E. Y., Lu, Y.-F., Matsushita, M., Matsui, H., Yan, Z., et al. (2005). Regulation of N-methyl-D-aspartate receptors by calpain in cortical neurons. *J. Biol. Chem.* 280, 21588–21593. doi: 10.1074/jbc.M501603200

Yang, J., Ruchti, E., Petit, J.-M., Jourdain, P., Grenningloh, G., Allaman, I., et al. (2014). Lactate promotes plasticity gene expression by potentiating NMDA signaling in neurons. *Proc. Natl. Acad. Sci. U.S.A.* 111, 12228–12233. doi: 10.1073/pnas.1322912111

# 17

# Plasma Membrane $Ca^{2+}$ Pump PMCA4z is More Active Than Splicing Variant PMCA4x

*Gerardo R. Corradi*, Luciana R. Mazzitelli, Guido D. Petrovich, Felicitas de Tezanos Pinto, Lucia Rochi and Hugo P. Adamo**

*Departamento de Química Biológica, Instituto de Química y Fisicoquímica Biológicas, Facultad de Farmacia y Bioquímica, Consejo Nacional de Investigaciones Científicas y Técnicas-Universidad de Buenos Aires, Buenos Aires, Argentina*

***Correspondence:***
*Gerardo R. Corradi*
*gcorradi@qb.ffyb.uba.ar*
*Hugo P. Adamo*
*hpadamo@qb.ffyb.uba.ar*

***In Memoriam:***
*This paper is dedicated to the memory of Dr. Alcides F. Rega.*

The plasma membrane $Ca^{2+}$ pumps (PMCA) are P-ATPases that control $Ca^{2+}$ signaling and homeostasis by transporting $Ca^{2+}$ out of the eukaryotic cell. Humans have four genes that code for PMCA isoforms (PMCA1-4). A large diversity of PMCA isoforms is generated by alternative mRNA splicing at sites A and C. The different PMCA isoforms are expressed in a cell-type and developmental-specific manner and exhibit differential sensitivity to a great number of regulatory mechanisms. PMCA4 has two A splice variants, the forms "x" and "z". While PMCA4x is ubiquitously expressed and relatively well-studied, PMCA4z is less characterized and its expression is restricted to some tissues such as the brain and heart muscle. PMCA4z lacks a stretch of 12 amino acids in the so-called A-M3 linker, a conformation-sensitive region of the molecule connecting the actuator domain (A) with the third transmembrane segment (M3). We expressed in yeast PMCA4 variants "x" and "z", maintaining constant the most frequent splice variant "b" at the C-terminal end, and obtained purified preparations of both proteins. In the basal autoinhibited state, PMCA4zb showed a higher ATPase activity and a higher apparent $Ca^{2+}$ affinity than PMCA4xb. Both isoforms were stimulated by calmodulin but PMCA4zb was more strongly activated by acidic lipids than PMCA4xb. The results indicate that a PMCA4 intrinsically more active and more responsive to acidic lipids is produced by the variant "z" of the splicing site A.

**Keywords: calcium transport, calcium ATPase, PMCA isoforms, neuronal PMCA, heart PMCA**

## INTRODUCTION

The $Ca^{2+}$ transporting P-ATPases known as $Ca^{2+}$ pumps are key elements for the control of intracellular $Ca^{2+}$ homeostasis (Chen et al., 2020). Animal cells possess three types of $Ca^{2+}$ pumps, the endoplasmic-sarcoplasmic reticulum (SERCA), the secretory pathway (SPCA), and the plasma membrane $Ca^{2+}$ pump (PMCA). By taking $Ca^{2+}$ out of the cell, the PMCA modulates the resting cytosolic $Ca^{2+}$ and is fundamental for shaping and ending the $Ca^{2+}$ signals (Lopreiato et al., 2014; Stafford et al., 2017). The relative contribution of the PMCA to these processes depends on the cell type and the activity of other $Ca^{2+}$ transporters. In excitable cells, the SERCA pump and the plasma membrane $Na^{+}/Ca^{2+}$ exchanger (NCX) are mostly responsible for removing $Ca^{2+}$ from the cytosol, while the function of PMCA seems more suited for the control of $Ca^{2+}$ dependent microdomain processes (Strehler, 2015). Consistent with this idea, in excitable cells, PMCA is a part of protein networks that by including voltage-gated $Ca^{2+}$ channels, couple influx, and clearance of $Ca^{2+}$ (Müller et al., 2010). The loss of PMCA function has been associated with several human diseases, including neurologic pathologies, such as familial spastic paraplegia (Mohamed et al., 2011, 2016; Li et al., 2014).

In humans four genes code for PMCA proteins (PMCA1-4) with a calculated molecular mass of 135 kDa and an average sequence identity of about 80% (Lopreiato et al., 2014). The expression profile of the PMCA isoforms varies depending on the tissue and the stage of development. PMCA1 and PMCA4 have ubiquitously expressed forms while the expression of PMCA2 and PMCA3 is more restricted and particularly abundant in nervous tissues (Strehler and Zacharias, 2001). While neurons are rich in all PMCA isoforms and variants, PMCA4 constitutes a major one at the early stages of the differentiation process and is markedly enriched, together with PMCA1, and PMCA2 at the postsynaptic membrane through the interaction with the postsynaptic density protein 95 (Kim et al., 1998; Boczek et al., 2019).

Recently, the Cryo-EM structure of the human PMCA1 in complex with neuroplastin was reported (Gong et al., 2018). As expected, the general architecture of the PMCA protein closely resembles that of other P-ATPases with the characteristic N, nucleotide binding, P phosphorylation, and A, action domain (**Figure 1A**). PMCA forms heteromers with the glycoproteins neuroplastin or basigin in different cell types (Korthalsa et al., 2017; Schmidt et al., 2017). Contacts between PMCA and neuroplastin were observed at the PMCA extracellular M8-M9 linker and with the M10 transmembrane segment. The interaction of the PMCA with neuroplastin takes place in the ER and affects PMCA stability, function, and plasma membrane targeting. These findings open the interesting possibility that the activity of the PMCA can influence neuroplastin functions, for example, synaptic plasticity and neuritogenesis (Beesley et al., 2014).

A distinctive characteristic of the PMCA family of $Ca^{2+}$ pumps is the autoinhibitory mechanism and the direct stimulation by calmodulin (CaM) (Hegedus et al., 2020). Autoinhibition is mediated by the interaction of the regulatory domain, located in the extended C-terminal tail with the central catalytic core of the protein. The binding of $Ca^{2+}$-CaM to the C-terminal regulatory domain releases the PMCA from the autoinhibition (Adamo and Grimaldi, 1998; Bredeston and Adamo, 2004; Corradi and Adamo, 2007; Mazzitelli and Adamo, 2014; Hegedus et al., 2020).

A second important mechanism of PMCA regulation is the $Ca^{2+}$-independent activation by acidic lipids (Niggli et al., 1981; Enyedi et al., 1987; Brodin et al., 1992; Filoteo et al., 1992; de Tezanos Pinto and Adamo, 2002, 2006). Although this mechanism has not been explained, part of the stimulatory effect of acidic lipids is due to their interaction with the C-terminal regulatory domain (Brodin et al., 1992; Filoteo et al., 1992). However, because some acidic lipids, in particular phosphoinositides, were found more effective than calmodulin to activate the PMCA at low concentrations of $Ca^{2+}$ (Enyedi et al., 1987) a second site was proposed, the so-called acidic lipid ($A_L$) responsive region, in the segment that links domain A with the transmembrane helix M3 (Brodin et al., 1992; Filoteo et al., 1992; de Tezanos Pinto and Adamo, 2002, 2006).

Besides the four PMCA genes, many PMCA variants are generated by the combination of the products of alternative splicing of mRNAs at the two sites called sites A and C. While these splice variations do not affect the basic $Ca^{2+}$ transport function, they are strategically located in the regulatory regions of the PMCA molecule and hence they may affect the maximal transport capacity and $Ca^{2+}$ affinity as well as the interaction of the PMCA with the other regulatory proteins (Strehler and Zacharias, 2001; Lopreiato et al., 2014). Splicing at site C changes the C-terminal regulatory tail, generating the most common variants "a" and "b" and others identified as "c" through "g", some of which have not yet been confirmed at the protein level. The degree of autoinhibition and the kinetics of CaM activation are unique features of each PMCA isoform and are modified by the alternative C-terminal sequences of each isoform variant (Enyedi et al., 1994; Strehler, 2015).

In humans, splicing at site A results in three PMCA variants, the forms "z", "x", and "w", which have insertions of 0, 12, and 45 extra amino acids in the $A_L$ region, respectively. PMCA1 contains only the "x" variant, while in PMCA2-4 variants "x" and "z" have been detected. In humans, only PMCA2 has the longest "w" insertion (Strehler and Zacharias, 2001; Hegedus et al., 2020) while in the rat in addition to "w", an "y" variant with the insertion of the first 31 residues has been detected (Adamo and Penniston, 1992). Because these insertions modify the $A_L$ region, previous studies have suggested that different splice A variants may differ in their sensitivity to acidic lipid activation (Brodin et al., 1992; Filoteo et al., 1992; de Tezanos Pinto and Adamo, 2002, 2006).

At present, only few PMCA forms have been individually characterized and the functional consequences of some splice variants are still controversial. Furthermore, the effect of the splicing variants may depend on the context of the particular PMCA isoform considered. In this study, we have characterized the enzymatic activity of purified preparations of the site A splice variants of PMCA4 which comprise two forms (**Figure 1B**), the ubiquitously expressed form "x" and the shorter variant "z" showing a more restricted expression profile, particularly, in the brain and heart. We found that PMCA4z is more active and more responsive to activation by acidic lipids than the PMCA4x.

**Abbreviations:** PMCA, plasma membrane $Ca^{2+}$ pump; PMCA4xb, plasma membrane $Ca^{2+}$ pump derived from the human gene 4, spliced form ***x*** at the splicing site "A" and spliced form ***b*** at the splicing site "C"; PMCA4zb, plasma membrane $Ca^{2+}$ pump derived from the human gene 4, spliced form z at the splicing site "A" and spliced form ***b*** at the splicing site "C"; GFP, green fluorescent protein, CaM, calmodulin; PC, phosphatidylcholine; PI, phosphatidylinositol; PS phosphatidylserine, PA, phosphatidic acid; $C_{12}E_{10}$, polyoxyethylene10-laurylether; $E_1$ and $E_2$, conformers of the $Ca^{2+}$-ATPase; EP, phosphoenzyme; SDS-PAGE, sodium dodecyl sulfate-polyacrylamide gel electrophoresis; BE, extract from bovine brain containing acidic lipids.

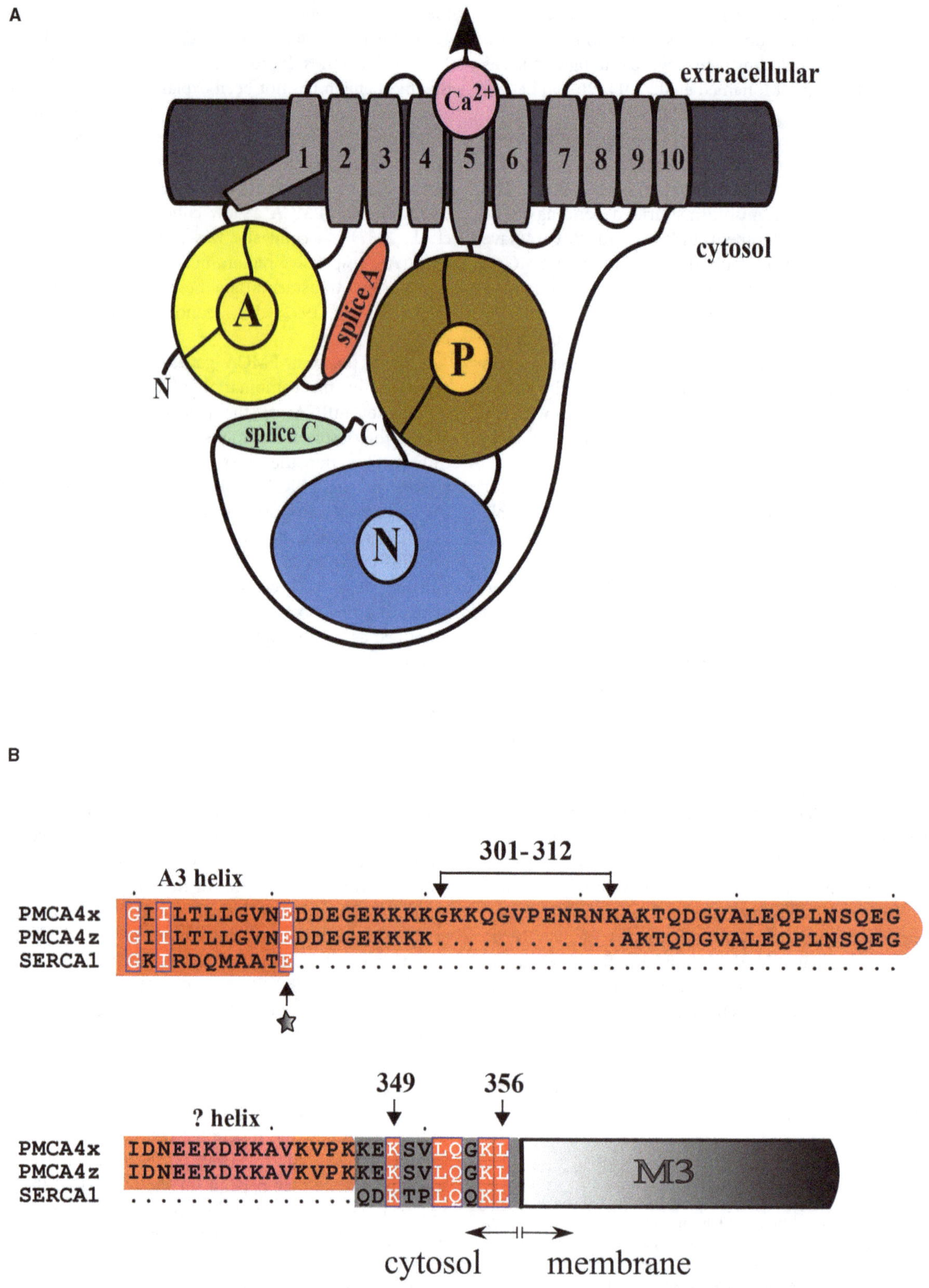


**FIGURE 1 | (A)** General architecture of the plasma membrane Ca$^{2+}$ (PMCA) P-ATPase. Only the catalytic subunit is represented. Helices M1-M6 constitute the transport domain. The action domain (A) is shown in yellow, the phosphorylation domain (P) is brown and the nucleotide-binding domain (N) is light blue. The A-M3 *(Continued)*

**FIGURE 1 |** linker, which is modified by mRNA splicing at site A, is shown in red and the regulatory C-terminal domain, which is modified by mRNA splicing at site C, is shown in green. **(B)** Alignment of the amino acid sequence of the A-M3 linker of PMCA4x, PMCA4z, and SERCA1. Conserved residues are in white bold. The "x" insertion of amino acids 301–312 is shown. The position of the A3 (red) and $A_L$ helices which are predicted by modeling (pink) are indicated. The transmembrane M3 helix is colored gray and its membrane inserted portion is shown as a box. The site of SERCA mutational insertion (site 1) described by Nyholm Holdensen and Andersen (2009) is indicated by a star.

# MATERIALS AND METHODS

## Chemicals

Yeast synthetic drop-out media supplement without leucine, yeast nitrogen base without amino acids, dextrose, polyoxyethylene 10 lauryl ether ($C_{12}E_{10}$), L-α-phosphatidylcholine type XVI-E (Sigma) from fresh egg yolk, brain extract (BE) Type I Folch Fraction I from bovine brain containing approximately (w/w) 10% PI, 50% PS, and other lipids, phosphodiesterase 3′, 5′ cyclic nucleotide activator (calmodulin) from bovine brain, calmodulin-agarose, ATP (disodium salt, vanadium-free), sodium dodecyl sulfate (SDS), and all other chemicals were obtained from Sigma.

## Construction of DNA Coding for PMCA4zb

The cDNA coding for PMCA4zb was obtained by a two-step PCR using Pfu DNA polymerase and the PMCA4xb cDNA as template. During the first step, two PCR reactions were run, one using primer His: 5′CTGGAGGTCGACATGACGCAT CACCATCACCATCACAACCCATCAGACCGTGTCTTGCCT GCCAA3′, and N-term 5′TTTCTTCTTTTTCTCCCCTTC GTCATC3′, and the other using primer 2096: 5′TGACAA CATCAACACAGCCCGGGCCATTGCCACCA3′ and C-term 5′GATGACGAAGGGGAGAAAAAGAAAGCAAAGACCCAA GACGGAGTG3′. The primer His contains a restriction site for nuclease SalI that matches a unique site for SalI at the 5′position of the PMCA4xb cDNA, while primer 2096 anneals to the PMCA4xb DNA downstream of a naturally occurring BspEI unique site. The 930-bp His-N-term and 1210-bp C-term-2096 products were combined in the next PCR step along with primers His and 2096. The amplified 2119-bp His-2096 fragment was digested with SalI and BspEI and used to replace the corresponding sequence of PMCA4xb GFP DNA cloned into pMP625 (Bredeston and Adamo, 2004) or pYX112 (Mazzitelli and Adamo, 2014) expression vectors.

## Complementation Assay on K616 *Saccharomyces cerevisiae* Strain

K616 cells (MATα pmr1::HIS3 pmc::TRP1 cnb1::LEU2, ura3) (Cunningham and Fink, 1994) were transformed using a lithium acetate/polyethylene glycol method (Elble, 1992) with expression vector pYX112 containing different PMCA constructs, and the transformants were selected for their ability to grow in the absence of uracil on plates containing 6.7% YNB, 0.67% complete supplemented medium minus Ura (Ura-), 2.2% dextrose, 0.05% 2N-morpholino-ethanesulfonic acid (MES) pH = 6.0, 10 mM $Cl_2Ca$, and 1.5% agar. For complementation studies, 15 μl of log-phase was streaked onto plates lacking uracil and containing either 10 mM $Cl_2Ca$ or 10 mM ethylene glycol-bis-N,N,N′,N′-tetra acetic acid (EGTA). The plates were allowed to grow for 72 h at 28°C.

## Plasma Membrane $Ca^{2+}$ Pump Expression and Purification

*Saccharomyces cerevisiae* strain DBY2062 (MATa his4-619 leu2-3,112) (Bauer and Kolling, 1996) was used for expression and purification. Yeast cells were transformed with vector pMP625 containing a $Leu^+$ marker and the PMA1 promoter. Yeast cells were transformed and selected in the absence of leucine. PMCA4xb-GFP and PMCA4zb-GFP were purified as described previously (Bredeston and Adamo, 2004; Mazzitelli and Adamo, 2014). Briefly, 4 L of yeast (A600 ∼ 4.0–5.0) were solubilized with $C_{12}E_{10}$ and the solubilizate was loaded onto a calmodulin-agarose chromatography column. After washing with a purification buffer containing $Ca^{2+}$, the PMCA protein was eluted with EGTA. Lipids were not added during the purification.

## Calcium-ATPase Activity

The $Ca^{2+}$-ATPase activity of the purified preparations of PMCA4xb-GFP and PMCA4zb-GFP was estimated from the release of [$^{32}$P]Pi from [γ-$^{32}$P]ATP at 28°C as described previously (Mazzitelli and Adamo, 2014). The reaction medium contained 20 mM HEPES-K (pH = 7.2 at 28°C), 100 mM KCl, 4 mM $MgCl_2$, 3 mM ATP, 500 μM EGTA, and enough $CaCl_2$ to give the $Ca^{2+}$ concentrations indicated in each experiment. The concentration of free $Ca^{2+}$ in the reaction medium was calculated using the WebmaxC Standard program. Before starting the ATPase reaction, 1 μg of the enzyme (50 μl) was gently stirred for 5 min with 5 μl of a sonicated mixture of 57 mg/ml $C_{12}E_{10}$ with 29 mg/ml PC or the indicated amount of BE. The suspension was thoroughly mixed and preincubated for at least 10 min on ice before being added to the ATPase reaction. The PMCA was incubated for 3 min at 37°C with the reaction medium before the initiation of the reaction by adding 3 mM [γ-32P]ATP. The reaction was finished by acid denaturation after 30 min. During this period, the amount of Pi released from ATP increased linearly with time.

## Sodium Dodecyl Sulfate–Polyacrylamide Gel Electrophoresis, Protein Quantitation and Western Blotting

Proteins were electrophoresed on a 7.5% acrylamide gel according to Laemmli (Laemmli, 1970) and revealed by Coomassie Blue staining as previously described (Mazzitelli and Adamo, 2014). The protein concentration was initially estimated by the method of Bradford (Bradford, 1976) using bovine

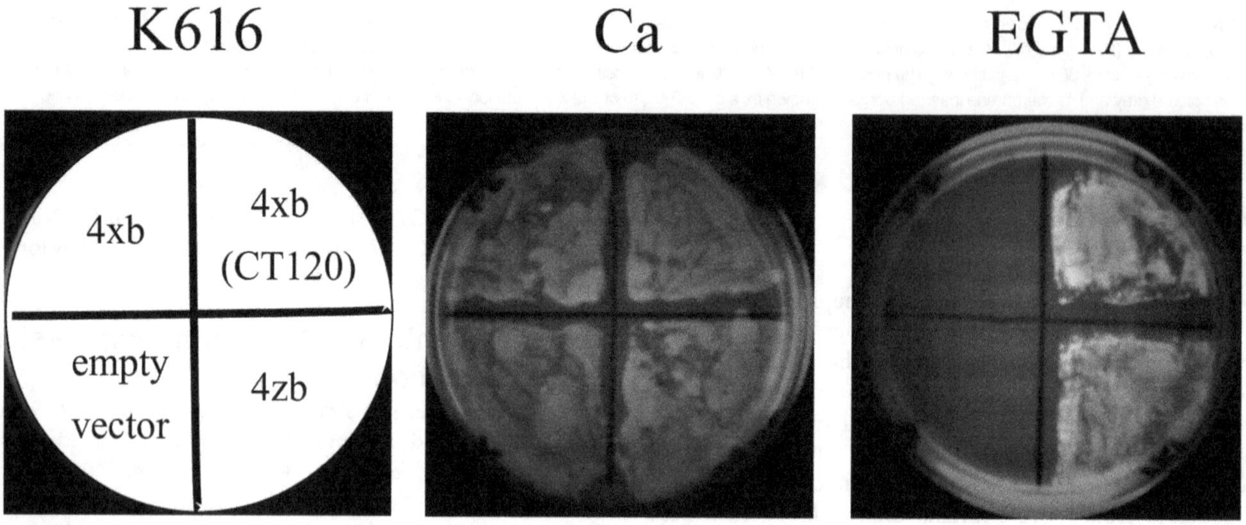


**FIGURE 2 |** PMCA4xb-GFP complements the K616 yeast strain lacking endogenous $Ca^{2+}$ ATPases. K616 cells were transformed with the empty pYX112 vector, or vector containing PMCA4xb-GFP, PMCA4zb-GFP, or the hyperactive mutant PMCA4x(CT120)-GFP lacking the C-terminal 120 amino acids segment containing the autoinhibitory domain. Cultures of K616 yeast expressing the recombinant PMCA proteins were grown for 72 h at 28°C on SC-Ura⁻ plates containing 10 mM $CaCl_2$ or 10 mM EGTA.

serum albumin as standard. The content of PMCA protein in each preparation was estimated by SDS–PAGE comparing the intensity of the bands of PMCA protein with different amounts of bovine serum albumin as standard, stained with Coomassie Blue.

Western blotting was performed as previously described (Cura et al., 2008). Briefly, after SDS–PAGE the proteins were electrotransferred onto Millipore Immobilon P membranes and the non-specific binding was blocked by incubating the membranes overnight at 4°C in a solution of 160 mM NaCl, 0.05% Tween 20, and 1% non-fat dry milk. The membranes were incubated for 1 h with anti-PMCA monoclonal antibodies (Adamo et al., 1992; Caride et al., 1996) from ascitic fluid (dilution 1:1,000) and developed using biotinylated antimouse immunoglobulin G and avidin-horseradish peroxidase conjugate.

### Data Analysis

Data presented in this work are representative of at least three independent experiments performed in duplicate. The kinetic data were analyzed by non-linear curve fitting using the SigmaPlot 10 scientific data analysis and graphing software (Systat Software Inc.). The same model based on the Hill equation was fitted to PMCA4xb and PMCA4zb and the statistical significance of the difference between datasets was assessed by the $F$-test as determined by the OriginLab2019 software.

## RESULTS

### The Isoform h4z Complements the Mutant Yeast K616

In the *S. cerevisiae* strain K616, the genes coding for $Ca^{2+}$ ATPases PMR1, PMC1, and the regulatory subunit of calcineurin (CNB) have been inactivated (Cunningham and Fink, 1994). K616 cells cannot proliferate in media containing low concentrations of $Ca^{2+}$ (10 mM EGTA), but this phenotype can be rescued by the expression of a high-affinity $Ca^{2+}$ transport system. We have previously shown that the expression of PMCA4xb does not allow the growth of K616 cells in $Ca^{2+}$ depleted media and successful complementation requires the expression of hyperactive forms of the protein, in which the autoinhibitory mechanism has been disrupted Activated versions of PMCA4xb can be produced either by introducing mutations in the A domain or by the removal of the C-terminal autoinhibitory segment, as in the case of the mutant CT120 lacking the C-terminal 120 amino acid residues (Enyedi et al., 1993; Bredeston and Adamo, 2004; Mazzitelli and Adamo, 2014). As shown in **Figure 2**, K616 cells transformed with the empty vector, and a vector containing DNA coding for PMCA4xb, PMCA4xCT120, and PMCA4zb, successfully grew in selective media containing 10 mM $CaCl_2$. However, only cells transformed with PMCA4xCT120 and PMCA4zb were able to grow in the presence of 10 mM EGTA. This result suggested that, such as the PMCA4xCT120 mutant, the PMCA4zb is hyperactive and has a higher $Ca^{2+}$ pumping activity than PMCA4xb.

### Subcellular Localization of the Human PMCA4xb and PMCAzb Expressed in Yeast Cells

Using the GFP fusions, we determined the localization of the expressed PMCA4 proteins by confocal microscopy. As shown in **Figure 3A,** both PMCA4xb and PMCA4zb exhibited a similar pattern of fluorescence intensity in the cell periphery and around the nucleus, suggesting that they localized in the membranes of the endoplasmic reticulum. Confirming this idea,

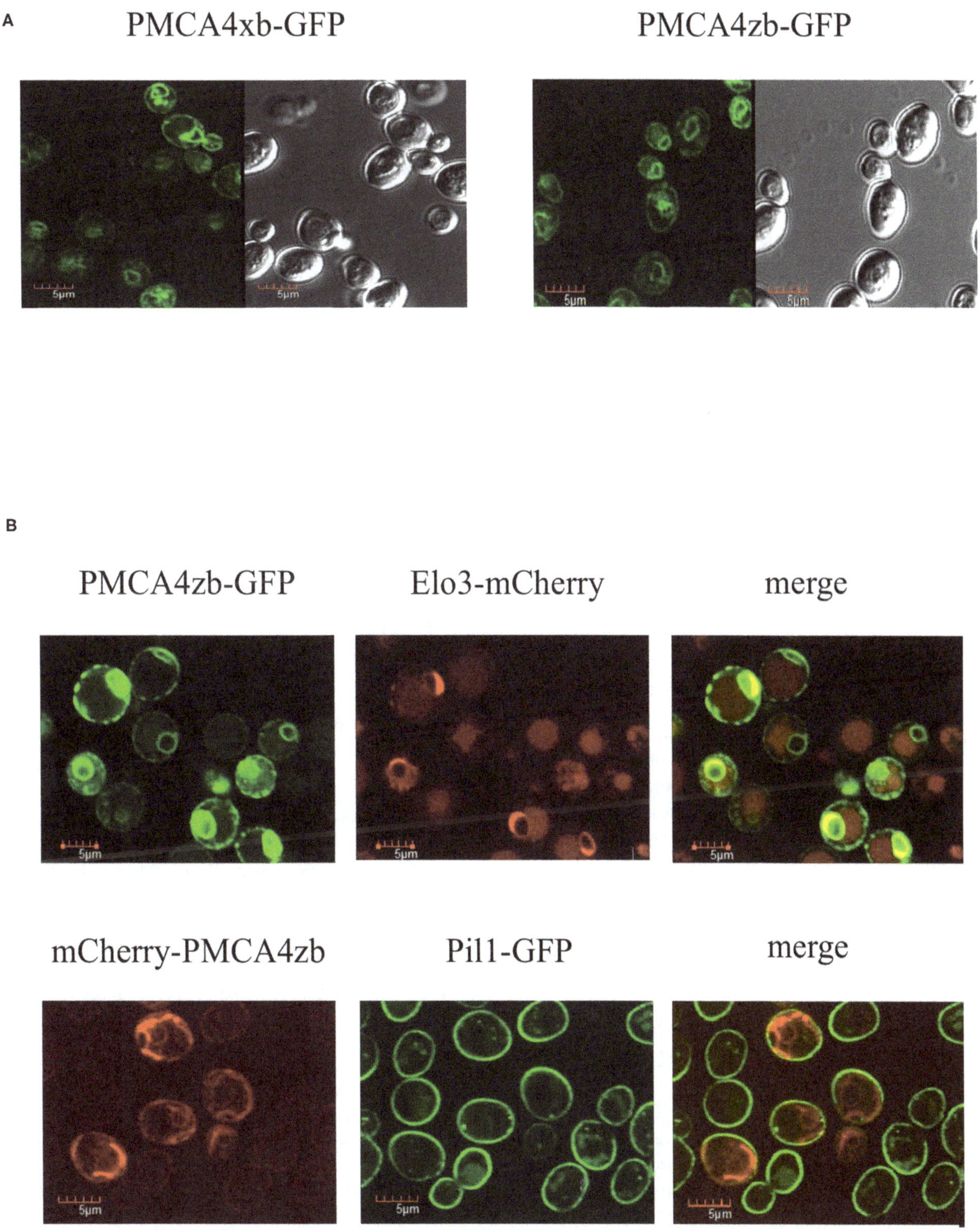


**FIGURE 3 | (A)** Expression of PMCA4xb and PMCA4zb-GFP in yeast cells. *Saccharomyces cerevisiae* cells (strain DBY2062) were transformed with the pMP625 vector containing the DNA coding for PMCA4xb-GFP and PMCA4zb-GFP and selected in a Leu⁻ media. The confocal fluorescent image (EGFP filter, LUT 2300, amplification x60) is shown on the left. The prominent yeast vacuoles can be distinguished in the visible image shown on the right. **(B)** Intracellular localization of the

*(Continued)*

**FIGURE 3 |** expressed PMCA4zb. *On top*, PMCA4zb-GFP was coexpressed with the ER membrane protein Elo3-mCherry. The observed distribution suggests that both proteins localize in the perinuclear and peripheral ER membranes. Some background mCherry fluorescence is also detected in vacuoles. *On the bottom*, mCherry-PMCA4zb was coexpressed with the plasma membrane protein Pil1-GFP. The mCherry fluorescence suggests that most of the PMCA protein in the cell periphery does not reach the plasma membrane.

PMCA fluorescence showed significant colocalization with the endoplasmic reticulum protein-membrane ELO3 and very little with PIL1 at the plasma membrane (**Figure 3B**).

## Purified Preparations of PMCA4xb and PMCA4zb

The PMCA proteins were purified from *S. cerevisiae* membranes by calmodulin affinity chromatography as described previously (Bredeston and Adamo, 2004; Corradi and Adamo, 2007; Cura et al., 2008; Mazzitelli and Adamo, 2014). Analysis by SDS–PAGE showed that both purified preparations contained a major peptide of an estimated Mr 180 kDa corresponding to the PMCA-GFP fusions and small amounts of two faster-migrating fragments of about 140 and 125 kDa. These shorter fragments were likely the result of the PMCA-GFP proteolysis at the C-terminal region because they lacked GFP fluorescence (**Figure 4A**). Both PMCA4xb-GFP and PMCAzb-GFP showed similar proteolytic peptides. We further analyzed the purified preparations by Western blot using anti-PMCA specific antibodies 5F10, JA3, and JA9 (Adamo et al., 1992; Caride et al., 1996). The 5F10 epitope is between PMCA4xb residues 719–738 in the central cytosolic loop of the molecule, while JA3 and JA9 recognize the C and N-terminal segments at residues 1156–1180 and 51–75, respectively. **Figure 4B** shows that antibodies 5F10 and JA3 detected three PMCA peptides that, based on their migration, corresponded to the full-length PMCA-GFP and two shorter proteolytic products. JA9 recognized the PMCA-GFP full-length peptide and only the larger proteolytic fragment. This proteolysis pattern suggests that the large proteolytic fragment of 140 kDa that was recognized by the three antibodies corresponded to the PMCA proteins and was produced by the removal of GFP from the PMCA-GFP. The proteolytic peptide of 125 kDa, would be produced by the cleavage of a segment from the N-terminal region of PMCA because it was no longer detected by JA9.

## Adenosine Triphosphatase Activity and $Ca^{2+}$ Dependency of PMCA4xb and PMCA4zb

The purified and partially delipidated PMCA4xb and PMCAzb were reactivated by the addition of phosphatidylcholine before the $Ca^{2+}$-ATPase activity was measured at increasing concentrations of $Ca^{2+}$. As shown in **Figure 5**, the activity of PMCA4zb was higher than that of PMCA4xb in all the range of $Ca^{2+}$ concentrations tested. Kinetic analysis indicated that the higher activity of PMCA4zb was a consequence of the increase of the Vmax and the apparent affinity for $Ca^{2+}$ (**Table 1**). The addition to the reaction media of a high saturating amount of CaM increased the Vmax and decreased the $Ca^{2+}$ apparent affinity of PMCA4xb and PMCA4zb. Both, in basal conditions and the CaM-activated state, PMCA4zb exhibited 1.5–2-fold higher maximal activity than PMCA4xb. However, in the CaM-activated state, the apparent affinity for $Ca^{2+}$ of both variants was similar.

## Dependence With Acidic Lipids

To compare the responses of PMCA4xb and PMCAzb to acidic lipids, we supplemented the purified proteins with different amounts of a mixture of acidic lipids extracted from the porcine brain (BE) before measuring the $Ca^{2+}$-ATPase activity. As shown in **Figure 6**, the activity of both PMCA4xb and PMCAzb increased with increasing amounts of BE following a sigmoidal curve. At saturating, amounts of BE PMCA4zb had about two times the activity of PMCAxb, an increment somewhat similar to that obtained with calmodulin. However, at lower amounts of acidic lipids, PMCA4zb was nearly 8-fold more active than PMCA4xb, and its activity increased steeply, reaching maximal activity at lower amounts of BE.

# DISCUSSION

The existence of a great diversity of PMCA isoforms and splice variants is likely the result of cell-specific requirements for controlling the spatial and temporal magnitude of the cytosolic $Ca^{2+}$ signaling. Most cells express simultaneously a variety of PMCA variants, and for understanding the role of PMCA, it is necessary to advance the knowledge of each PMCA protein, their basal activity and how they respond to activators (Brini et al., 2003; Streheler et al., 2007). PMCA4 is a ubiquitously expressed isoform. Previous studies of PMCA4 used the protein from natural sources, for example, red blood cells which in addition contain PMCA1, or with the recombinant PMCA4x protein (Enyedi et al., 1994; Adamo and Grimaldi, 1998; de Tezanos Pinto and Adamo, 2002, 2006; Bredeston and Adamo, 2004; Corradi and Adamo, 2007; Cura et al., 2008; Mazzitelli and Adamo, 2014). In this study, we have focused on the two PMCA4 variants "x" and "z" produced by the splice at site A, we compared the kinetics properties of purified micellar preparations of the PMCA4xb and PMCA4zb obtained by expression in yeast cells.

Recent studies showed that PMCA associates with IgG-domain proteins neuroplastin and basigin (Korthalsa et al., 2017; Schmidt et al., 2017). The interaction with these auxiliary subunits influences PMCA function, stability, and membrane targeting. The PMCA-neuroplastin interaction seems quite sensitive to the detergents used for PMCA purification, a fact that may explain why the neuroplastin peptide was not previously identified in purified preparations of PMCA despite the proposed equimolar association PMCA-neuroplastin (Schmidt et al., 2017). In this work, as in previous studies of recombinant PMCA, we expressed only the catalytic PMCA4 polypeptide.

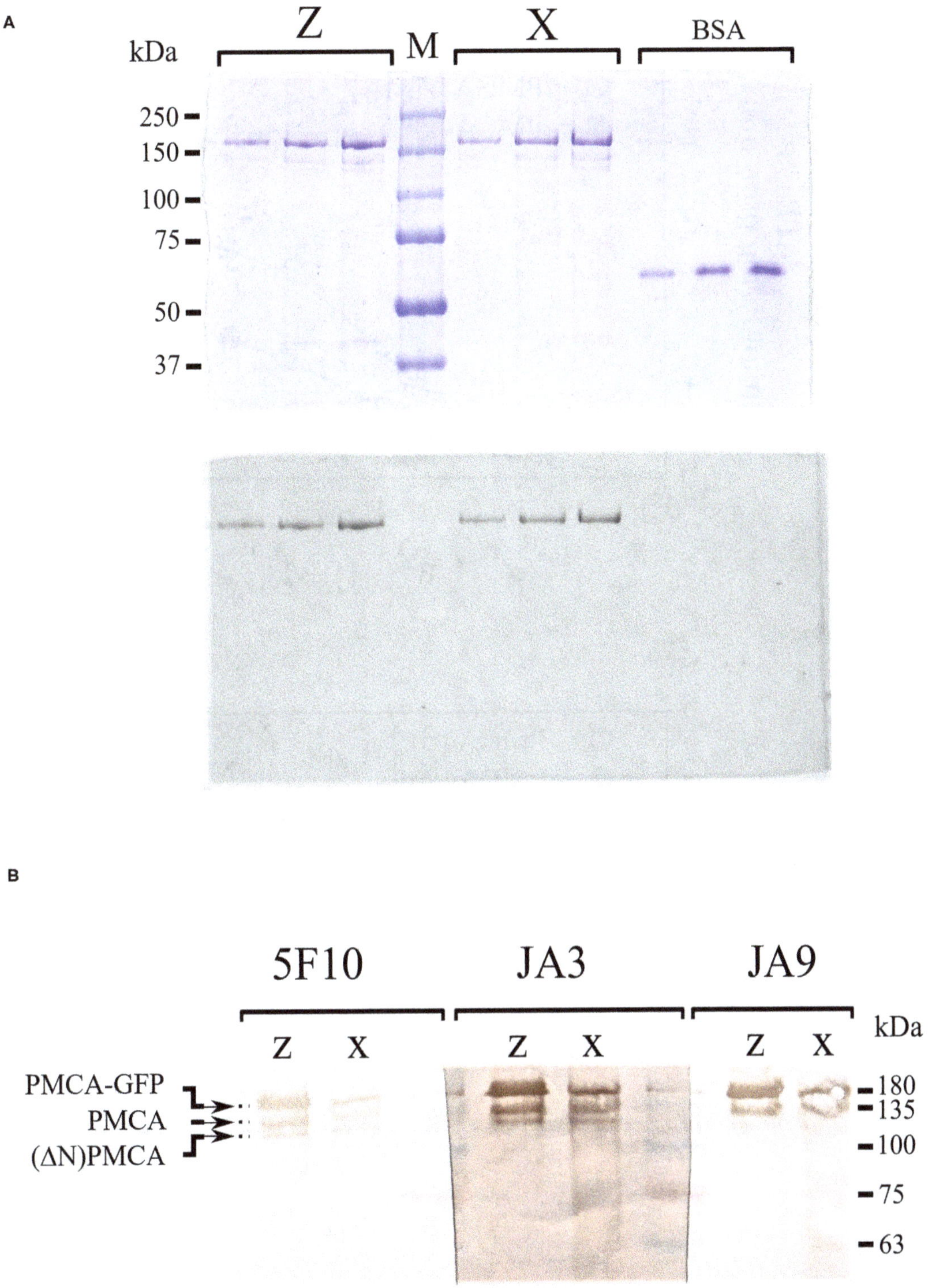


**FIGURE 4 | (A)** Sodium dodecyl sulfate-polyacrylamide gel electrophoresis (SDS-PAGE) of purified PMCA4xb-GFP and PMCA4zb-GFP. The recombinant PMCA proteins were purified as described in "Materials and methods." Aliquots of the eluate containing the purified proteins were submitted to electrophoresis in a 7.5% SDS–PAGE. Three lanes containing 0.25, 0.5, and 0.75 μg of PMCA4xb-GFP and PMCA4zb-GFP are shown. For comparison 0.3, 0.6, and 0.9 μg of bovine serum albumin were run on the right side of the gel. *On top*, the gel was stained with Coomassie-blue. *On the bottom*, the GFP-fluorescence of the same gel is shown. **(B)** Western blots of purified PMCA4xb-GFP and PMCA4zb-GFP. Western blots of purified PMCA4 preparations with antibodies 5F10, JA3, and JA9. Aliquots of 6 μl (about 1 μg of protein) of PMCA4xb-GFP and PMCA4zb-GFP eluates were loaded.

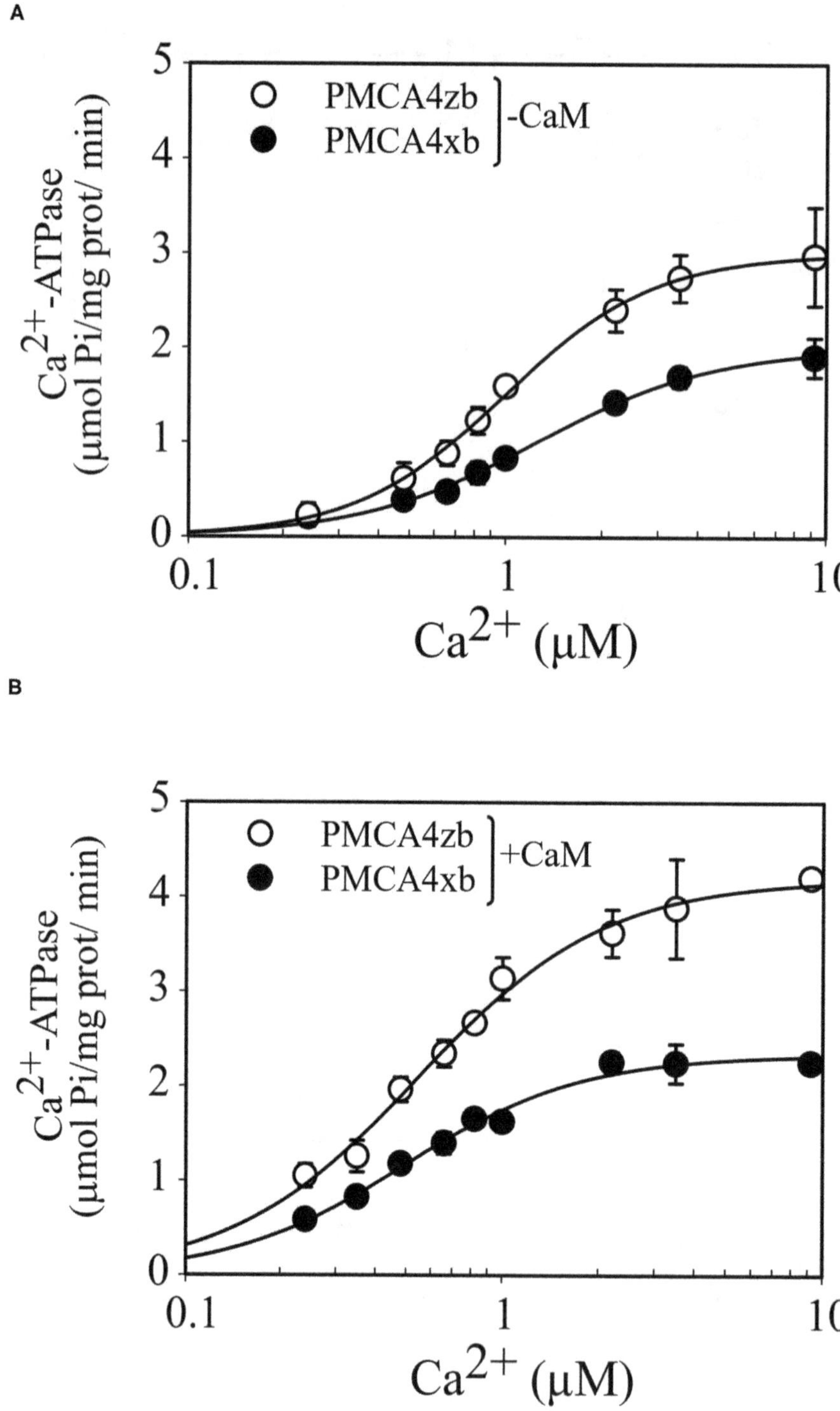


**FIGURE 5 |** $Ca^{2+}$ dependence of the $Ca^{2+}$-ATPase activity of purified PMCA4zb-GFP and PMCA4xb-GFP in the absence **(A)** and the presence of calmodulin **(B)**. The ATPase reaction was measured at 28°C as described previously (Mazzitelli and Adamo, 2014). The reaction media contained 1 µg of PMCA supplemented with PC, 50 mM HEPES-K (pH = 7.2 at 28°C), 100 mM KCl, 4 mM $MgCl_2$, 3 mM ATP, 500 µM EGTA, and enough $CaCl_2$ to give the indicated concentrations of $Ca^{2+}$. When calmodulin was present its final concentration was 200 nM. The reaction time was 15 min. The data points are from a representative experiment conducted in duplicate. *Error bars* show the SD. The lines are the best fit to the data given by the Hill equation $v = \text{Vmax} \, {}^{*}[\text{Ca}]^{nH}/([K_{0.5Ca}]^{nH} + [\text{Ca}]^{nH})$ using the values of the parameters shown in **Table 1**.

**TABLE 1** | Comparison of the $Ca^{2+}$ dependency of purified PMCA4 isoforms.

| | $K_{0.5Ca}$ (μM) | Vmáx (μmol/mg/min) | nH | Catalytic efficiency ($\mu M.s^{-1}$) |
|---|---|---|---|---|
| PMCA4xb-GFP | 1.26 ± 0.08 | 2.01 ± 0.06 | 1.6 ± 0.1 | 35 |
| PMCA4zb-GFP | 0.99 ± 0.03 | 3.00 ± 0.06 | 1.8 ± 0.1 | 68 |
| PMCA4xb-GFP+CaM | 0.50 ± 0.01 | 2.33 ± 0.07 | 1.6 ± 0.2 | 105 |
| PMCA4zb-GFP+CaM | 0.55 ± 0.04 | 4.19 ± 0.12 | 1.5 ± 0.2 | 172 |

*The kinetic constants were estimated by the non-linear fitting of the Hill equation to the data of $Ca^{2+}$-ATPase activities shown in **Figure 4**. The values of the parameters ± SE as given by the fitting program are shown. The catalytic efficiency was estimated by the ratio $Vmax/K_{0.5Ca}$. According to the F-test, at the 0.05 significance level, the datasets of PMCA4xb and PMCA4zb are statistically different.*

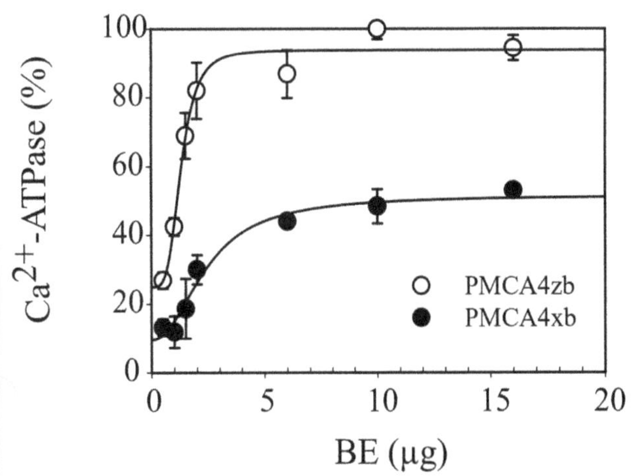


**FIGURE 6** | Activation of purified PMCA4xb-GFP and PMCA4zb-GFP by acidic lipids. The $Ca^{2+}$-ATPase activity was measured as indicated in **Figure 5**. PMCA4xb-GFP and PMCA4zb-GFP proteins (1 μg) were supplemented with the indicated amount of acidic lipid brain extract (BE). The concentration of $Ca^{2+}$ was 10 μM. The continuous lines represent the best fitting of the data to a Hill equation $v = v_0 + v_{BE} * [BE]^{nH} / ([K_{0.5BE}]^{nH} + [BE]^{nH})$ with the following parameters. For PMCA4xb, $v_0 = 9 \pm 5\%$, $v_{BE} = 42 \pm 8\%$, $K_{0.5BE} = 2.4 \pm 0.5$ μg, nH = 2 ± 1; for PMCA4zb; $v_0 = 25 \pm 7\%$, $v_{BE} = 69 \pm 7\%$, $K_{0.5BE} = 1.3 \pm 0.1$ μg, nH = 4 ± 1.

## PMCA Expression in Yeast

As we reported previously, yeasts are capable of functional PMCA expression (Bredeston and Adamo, 2004; Cura et al., 2008; Mazzitelli and Adamo, 2014). Active PMCA can complement the K616 yeast, and the purified recombinant protein is fully functional. This seems somewhat puzzling because yeasts lack an obvious neuroplastin homolog. However, we observed that expressed PMCA4xb and PMCA4zb localized in the yeast ER membrane, a fact that might be related to the lack of yeast neuroplastin. Further studies of the importance of neuroplastin for PMCA targeting, function, and regulation seem necessary.

The expression of the wild-type autoinhibited PMCA4xb does not rescue the yeast K616 phenotype (Bredeston and Adamo, 2004; Mazzitelli and Adamo, 2014). Successful K616 complementation requires the activation of PMCA4xb by mutations that disrupt the autoinhibitory mechanism. On the contrary, we found that K616 cells expressing the variant PMCA4zb did proliferate in $Ca^{2+}$ depleted media. Thus, according to the K616 complementation assay, PMCA4zb has a higher $Ca^{2+}$ transporting activity than PMCA4xb in the yeast cell. In addition, we determined that the purified PMCA4zb had higher $Ca^{2+}$-ATPase activity and higher apparent affinity for $Ca^{2+}$ than PMCA4xb in the absence of any activator, confirming the idea that PMCA4zb is a naturally hyperactive PMCA4 variant. Calmodulin activated both PMCA4 variants and increased their affinity for $Ca^{2+}$ to a high and similar value. This result suggests that the different $Ca^{2+}$ affinity of the two variants in the absence of calmodulin should be related to the mechanism of autoinhibition and does not involve the modification of the intrinsic affinity of the $Ca^{2+}$ binding site.

## Acidic–Lipid stimulation

Yeast expression provides preparations of purified PMCA, which are very sensitive to acidic lipids (Cura et al., 2008). We found that acidic lipids stimulated both yeast recombinant PMCA4 variants but the activity of PMCA4zb increased much more rapidly with low amounts of acidic lipids. The activation by acidic lipids would involve the interaction at two distinct sites of the PMCA molecule, one in the calmodulin-binding site at the C-terminal regulatory segment, and the second in the $A_L$ region of the A-M3 linker (Enyedi et al., 1994; de Tezanos Pinto and Adamo, 2002, 2006). In PMCA4xb, the linker A-M3 region comprises the segment of amino acid residues 300–356. A peptide from this region (residues 339–363) binds acidic lipids, although with a lower affinity than the calmodulin-binding site (Brodin et al., 1992; Filoteo et al., 1992). Thus, the primary site of acidic lipid activation would overlap with that of calmodulin.

We have previously characterized mutants of PMCA4xb containing deletions in the $A_L$ region using microsomes of CHO cells expressing the recombinant proteins (de Tezanos Pinto and Adamo, 2002, 2006). The deletion mutant d300-314, with a sequence similar to the natural splicing A variant PMCA4zb, exhibited a higher $Ca^{2+}$ transport activity due to the higher apparent affinity for $Ca^{2+}$. On the contrary, deletion of the downstream region (residues 339–360), which was indicated as the acidic lipid-binding site (Brodin et al., 1992), did not promote the activation of the PMCA. While the results presented here show that splice A alters the acidic–lipid stimulation of PMCA4, there is no conclusive evidence that this effect was mediated by the direct binding of lipids to residues 339–360.

The atomic model of PMCA1d was recently reported, but unfortunately, the structure of the A-M3 linker could not be determined (Gong et al., 2018). This segment is enriched in polar and charged residues, and as judged by its susceptibility to protease cleavage, is unusually accessible (Brodin et al., 1992). In this line, it is worth considering that PMCA is very sensitive to cellular proteases and most PMCA preparations exhibit some proteolysis (Adamo et al., 2000), a fact that has led to propose that proteolysis is a natural mechanism for regulating

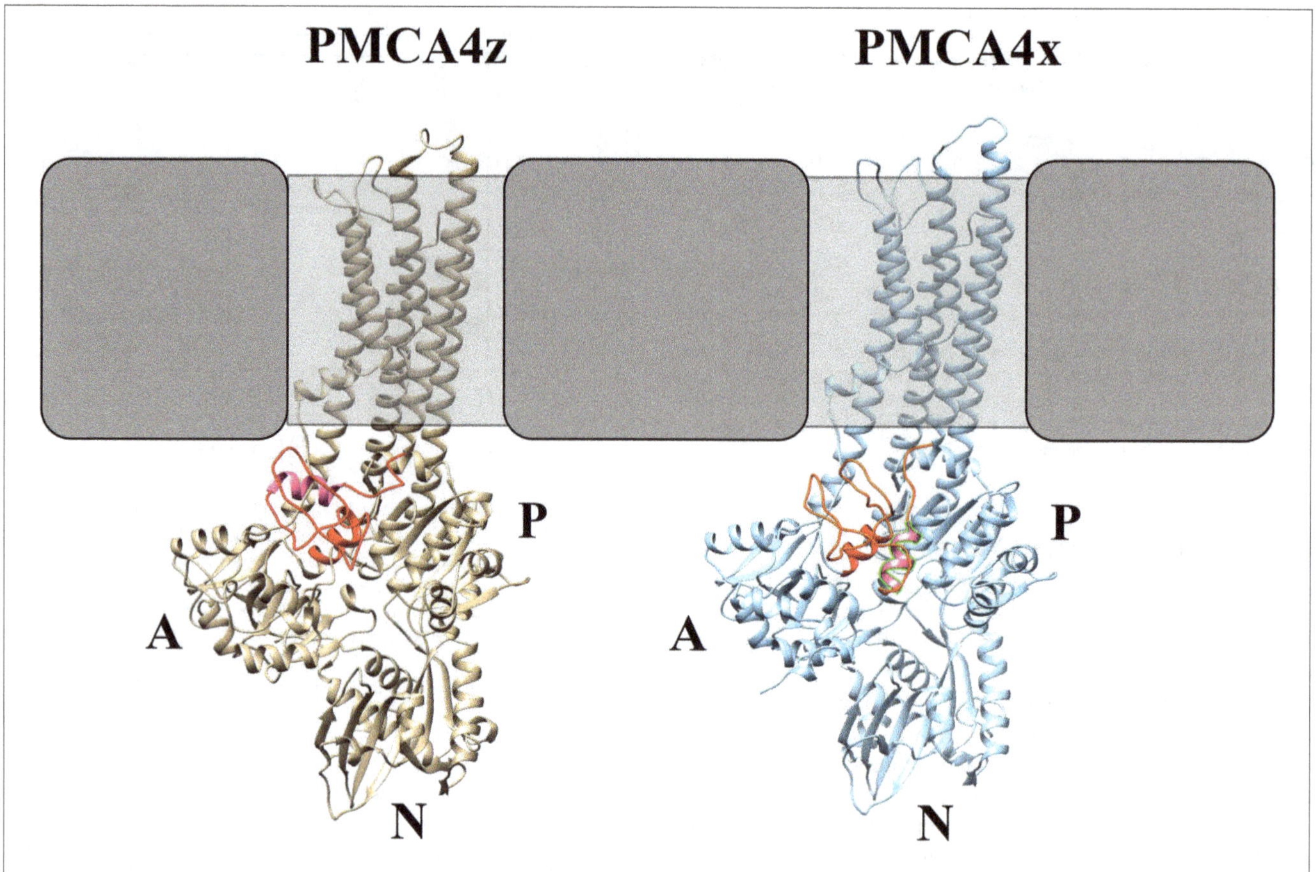


**FIGURE 7 |** Molecular modeling of PMCA4x and PMCA4z. Homology models of PMCA4 were obtained using the partial structure of PMCA1d (Gong et al., 2018) as a template. Only the portion of the PMCA from the amino-terminal region to the end of M6 was modeled. The tertiary structure and contact prediction model of the A-M3 linker were obtained using the RaptorX web service (Källberg et al., 2012). The SERCA-conserved A3 helix is colored red while the putative $A_L$ helix in PMCA is colored pink.

PMCA (Filoteo et al., 1997). We detected a small number of proteolytic fragments in both the PMCA4xb and the PMCAzb preparations. By using the GFP fusions and antibodies with defined epitopes, we observed that the endogenous proteolytic pattern of the PMCA4xb and the PMCA4zb was similar. In addition, the main proteolytic fragment corresponded to the full-length proteins lacking GFP suggesting that a cleavage near the C-terminus of the protein occurred without affecting the C-terminal regulatory region.

It seems appropriate to notice that the variability produced by the splicing site A may have different consequences depending on the PMCA isoform considered. Indeed, in polarized cells, the splice variant "w" targets PMCA2 to apical membranes, while variants "x" and "z" remain basolateral (Chicka and Strehler, 2003; Antalffy et al., 2012). On the other hand, PMCA4x is targeted to apical membranes in pancreatic acinar cells indicating that the targeting capacity of splice A variants may be isoform and cell-specific (Baggaley et al., 2007). Furthermore, membranes from CHO cells expressing PMCA2wb and PMCA2xb exhibit similar $Ca^{2+}$-ATPase activity and acidic lipid stimulation suggesting that the "w" insertion in PMCA2 had minimal functional consequences (Brini et al., 2010). Interestingly, the PMCA2zb was recognized as a very active pump capable of decreasing the $Ca^{2+}$ signal peak in about half the time needed by the PMCA2wb (Ficarella et al., 2007).

## A Possible Molecular Mechanism of PMCA4zb Activation

The A-M3 linker where the splicing A variants of PMCA occur is an important functional region of the P-ATPases. Indeed, the rotation of the A domain that accompanies the formation of an intramembrane exit pathway of the bound transported substrate is triggered by the strain of the A-M3 (Nagarajan et al., 2012). The functional consequences of the A-M3 linker length were analyzed in detail in SERCA (Nyholm Holdensen and Andersen, 2009). SERCA possesses a shorter A-M3 linker compared with the PMCA (refer to **Figure 1**). A series of insertional SERCA mutants containing up to 41 glycine and proline residues at the corresponding site of splicing A of PMCA, decreased the SERCA turnover to 30% of the WT. These results show that, in analogy with SERCA, the length of the A-M3 linker influenced the activity of the PMCA and made PMCAzb with a shorter linker more active than PMCA4x.

In comparison with SERCA, the PMCA A-M3 linker shows, in addition to the conserved A3 helix, a possible helical structure highly enriched in charged amino acids formed by PMCA4x residues E335-V342. By using a combination of homology modeling and structure prediction (Källberg et al., 2012), it can be observed that in PMCA4x these helical structures are deeply inserted in the catalytic core, where they may impair the interaction of the A and P domains while in PMCA4z these helices would move toward the surface of the protein (**Figure 7**).

A clear difference between SERCA and PMCA pumps is the C-terminal autoinhibitory domain of PMCA that binds to the A and N domains. A lower affinity of the autoinhibitory domain for its sites in the core of the protein may explain the basal activated state of PMCA4zb. It seems reasonable to consider that two activating mechanisms, one involving the modification of the A-M3 linker (splice site A) and the other resulting in the release of the C-terminal autoinhibition (splice site C) are not independent but cooperate for regulating the activity of the PMCA.

In this study, we found that PMCA4z a previously not characterized variant of PMCA originated by splicing at site A is more active and more sensitive to activation by acidic lipids than the more common form of PMCA4x. Future work will be needed to assess the relevance of this finding for the control of the $Ca^{2+}$ signal in cells expressing the variant "z" in normal and pathological conditions.

## AUTHOR CONTRIBUTIONS

GRC, LRM, GDP, LR, and FTP performed experiments and analyzed data. GRC, FTP, LRM, and HPA designed research and analyzed data. HPA conceived the project and wrote the manuscript with comments from all the authors. All authors contributed to the article and approved the submitted version.

## FUNDING

We acknowledge funding from Agencia Nacional de Promoción Científica y Tecnológica PICT 2017-1690, Consejo Nacional de Investigaciones Científicas y Tecnológicas PIP 2015-773 and Universidad de Buenos Aires UBACyT.

## ACKNOWLEDGMENTS

We thank Dr. Pablo S. Aguilar at the Institut Pasteur, Uruguay for the gift of yeasts expressing Elo3-mCherry and Pil1-GFP.

## REFERENCES

Adamo, H. P., Caride, A. J., and Penniston, J. T. (1992). Use of expression mutants and monoclonal antibodies to map the erythrocyte $Ca^{2+}$ pump. *J. Biol. Chem.* 267, 14244–14249. doi: 10.1016/S0021-9258(19)49704-4

Adamo, H. P., and Grimaldi, M. E. (1998). Functional consequences of relocating the C-terminal calmodulin-binding autoinhibitory domains of the plasma membrane $Ca^{2+}$ pump near the N-terminus. *Biochem. J.* 331, 763–766. doi: 10.1042/bj3310763

Adamo, H. P., Grimaldi, M. E., and Bredeston, L. M. (2000). The N-terminal region of the plasma membrane $Ca(^{2+})$ pump does not separate from the main catalytic fragments after proteolysis. *Biochim. Biophys. Acta.* 1464, 127–134. doi: 10.1016/S0005-2736(99)00253-9

Adamo, H. P., and Penniston, J. T. (1992). New $Ca^{2+}$ pump isoforms generated by alternative splicing of rPMCA2 mRNA. *Biochem. J.* 283, 355–359. doi: 10.1042/bj2830355

Antalffy, G., Mauer, A. S., Pászty, K., Hegedus, L., Padányi, R., Enyedi, A., and Strehler, E. E. (2012). Plasma membrane calcium pump (PMCA) isoform 4 is targeted to the apical membrane by the w-splice insert from PMCA2. *Cell Calcium* 51, 171–178. doi: 10.1016/j.ceca.2011.12.010

Baggaley, E., McLarnon, S., Demeter, I., Varga, G., and Bruce, J. I. E. (2007). Differential regulation of the apical plasma membrane $Ca^{2+}$-ATPase by protein kinase A in parotid acinar cells. *J. Biol. Chem.* 282, 37678–37693. doi: 10.1074/jbc.M703416200

Bauer, A., and Kolling, R. (1996). The SAC3 gene encodes a nuclear protein required for normal progression of mitosis. *Yeast* 12, 965–975. doi: 10.1002/(SICI)1097-0061(199608)12:10<965::AID-YEA999>3.0.CO;2-Q

Beesley, P. W., Herrera-Molina, R., Smalla, K. H., and Seidenbecher, C. (2014). The neuroplastin adhesion molecules: key regulators of neuronal plasticity and synaptic function. *J. Neurochem.* 131, 268–283. doi: 10.1111/jnc.12816

Boczek, T., Radzik, T., Ferenc, B., and Zylinska, L. (2019). The puzzling role of neuron-specific PMCA isoforms in the aging process. *Int. J. Mol. Sci.* 20:6338. doi: 10.3390/ijms20246338

Bradford, M. (1976). A rapid and sensitive method for the quantitation of microgram quantities of protein utilizing the principle of protein-dye binding. *Anal. Biochem.* 72, 248–256. doi: 10.1016/0003-2697(76)90527-3

Bredeston, L. M., and Adamo, H. P. (2004). Loss of autoinhibition of the plasma membrane $Ca^{2+}$ pump by substitution of Aspartic 170 by Asparagine: Activation of plasma membrane calcium ATPase 4 without disruption of the interaction between the catalytic core and the C-terminal regulatory domain. *J. Biol. Chem.* 279, 41619–41625. doi: 10.1074/jbc.M403116200

Brini, M., Coletto, L., Pierobon, N., Kraev, N., Guerini, D., and Carafoli, E. (2003). A comparative functional analysis of plasma membrane $Ca^{2+}$ pump isoforms in intact cells. *J. Biol. Chem.* 278, 24500–24508. doi: 10.1074/jbc.M300784200

Brini, M., Di Leva, F., Ortega, C. K., Domi, T., Ottolini, D., Leonardi, E., Tosatto, S. C., and Carafoli, E. (2010). Deletions and mutations in the acidic lipid-binding region of the plasma membrane $Ca^{2+}$ pump: a study on different splicing variants of isoform 2. *J. Biol. Chem.* 285, 30779–30791. doi: 10.1074/jbc.M110.140475

Brodin, P., Falchetto, R., Vorherr, T., and Carafoli, E. (1992). Identification of two domains which mediate the binding of activating phospholipids to the plasma-membrane $Ca^{2+}$ pump. *Eur. J. Biochem.* 204, 939–946. doi: 10.1111/j.1432-1033.1992.tb16715.x

Caride, A. J., Filoteo, A. G., Enyedi, A., Verma, A. K., and Penniston, J. T. (1996). Detection of isoform 4 of the plasma membrane calcium pump in human tissues by using isoform-specific monoclonal antibodies. *Biochem. J.* 316, 353–359. doi: 10.1042/bj3160353

Chen, J., Sitsel, A., Benoy, V., Sepúlveda, M. R., and Vangheluwe, P. (2020). Primary active $Ca^{2+}$ transport systems in health and disease. *Cold Spring Harb. Perspect. Biol.* 12:a035113. doi: 10.1101/cshperspect.a035113

Chicka, M. C., and Strehler, E. E. (2003). Alternative splicing of the first intracellular loop of plasma membrane $Ca^{2+}$-ATPase isoform 2 alters its membrane targeting. *J. Biol. Chem.* 278, 18464–18470. doi: 10.1074/jbc.M301482200

Corradi, G. R., and Adamo, H. P. (2007). Intramolecular fluorescence resonance energy transfer between fused autofluorescent proteins reveals rearrangements of the N- and C-terminal segments of the plasma membrane

$Ca^{2+}$ pump involved in the activation. *J. Biol. Chem.* 282, 35440–35448. doi: 10.1074/jbc.M703377200

Cunningham, K. W., and Fink, G. R. (1994). Calcineurin-dependent growth control in Saccharomyces cerevisiae mutants lacking PMC1, a homolog of plasma membrane $Ca^{2+}$ ATPases. *J.Cell. Biol.* 124, 351–363 doi: 10.1083/jcb.124.3.351

Cura, C. I., Corradi, G. R., Rinaldi, D. E., and Adamo, H. P. (2008). High sensibility to reactivation by acidic lipids of the recombinant human plasma membrane $Ca^{2+}$-ATPase isoform 4xb purified from Saccharomyces cerevisiae. *Biochim. Biophys. Acta Biomembr.* 1778, 2757–2764. doi: 10.1016/j.bbamem.2008.08.020

de Tezanos Pinto, F., and Adamo, H. P. (2002). Deletions in the acidic lipid-binding region of the plasma membrane $Ca^{2+}$ pump. A mutant with high affinity for $Ca^{2+}$ resembling the acidic lipid-activated enzyme. *J. Biol. Chem.* 277, 12784–12789. doi: 10.1074/jbc.M111055200

de Tezanos Pinto, F., and Adamo, H. P. (2006). Deletions in the $A_L$ region of the h4xb plasma membrane $Ca^{2+}$ pump. High apparent affinity for $Ca^{2+}$ of a deletion mutant resembling the alternative spliced form h4zb. *FEBS Lett.* 580, 1576–1580. doi: 10.1016/j.febslet.2006.01.088

Elble, R. (1992). A simple and efficient procedure for transformation of yeasts. *Biotechnology* 13, 18–20.

Enyedi, A., Flura, M., Sarkadi, B., Gardos, G., and Carafoli, E. (1987). The maximal velocity and the calcium affinity of the red cell calcium pump may be regulated independently. *J.Biol. Chem.* 262, 6425–6430. doi: 10.1016/S0021-9258(18)45587-1

Enyedi, A., Verma, A. K., Adamo, H. P., Filoteo, A. G., Streheler, E. E., and Penniston, J. T. (1994). The $Ca^{2+}$ affinity of the plasma membrane $Ca^{2+}$ pump is controlled by alternative splicing. *J. Biol. Chem.* 269, 41–43. doi: 10.1016/S0021-9258(17)42307-6

Enyedi, A., Verma, A. K., Filoteo, A. G., and Penniston, J. T. (1993). A highly active 120-kDa truncated mutant of the plasma membrane $Ca^{2+}$ pump. *J. Biol. Chem.* 268, 10621–10626. doi: 10.1016/S0021-9258(18)82243-8

Ficarella, R., Di Leva, F., Bortolozzi, M., Ortolano, S., Donaudy, F., Petrillo, M., et al. (2007). A functional study of plasma-membrane calcium-pump isoform 2 mutants causing digenic deafness. *Proc. Natl. Acad. Sci. U. S. A.* 104, 1516 1521. doi: 10.1073/pnas.0609775104

Filoteo, A. G., Elwess, N. L., Enyedi, A., Caride, A., Aung, H. H., and Penniston, J. T. (1997). Plasma membrane $Ca^{2+}$ pump in rat brain. Patterns of alternative splices seen by isoform-specific antibodies. *J. Biol. Chem.* 272, 23741–23747. doi: 10.1074/jbc.272.38.23741

Filoteo, A. G., Enyedi, A., and Penniston, J. T. (1992). The lipid-binding peptide from the plasma membrane $Ca^{2+}$ pump binds calmodulin, and the primary calmodulin-binding domain interacts with lipid. *J. Biol. Chem.* 267, 11800–11805. doi: 10.1016/S0021-9258(19)49769-X

Gong, D., Chi, X., Ren, K., Huang, G., Zhou, G., Yan, N., Lei, J., and Zhou, Q. (2018). Structure of the human plasma membrane Ca2+-ATPase 1 in complex with its obligatory subunit neuroplastin. *Nat. Commun.* 9:3623. doi: 10.1038/s41467-018-06075-7

Hegedus, L., Zámb,ó, B., Pászty, K., Padányi, R., Varga, K., Penniston, J. T., and Enyedi, Á. (2020). Molecular diversity of plasma membrane $Ca^{(2+)}$ transporting ATPases: their function under normal and pathological conditions. *Adv. Exp. Med. Biol.* 1131, 93–129. doi: 10.1007/978-3-030-12457-1_5

Källberg, M., Wang, H., Wang, S., Peng, J., Wang, Z., Lu, H., and Xu, J. (2012). Template-based protein structure modeling using the RaptorX web server. *Nat. Protoc.* 7, 1511–1522. doi: 10.1038/nprot.2012.085

Kim, E., DeMarco, S. J., Marfatia, S. M., Chishti, A. H., Sheng, M., and Strehler, E. E. (1998). Plasma membrane $Ca^{2+}$-ATPase isoform 4b binds to membrane-associated guanylate kinase (MAGUK) proteins via their PDZ (PSD-95/Dlg/ZO-1) domains. *J. Biol. Chem.* 273, 1591–1595. doi: 10.1074/jbc.273.3.1591

Korthalsa, M., Langnaese, K., Smalla, K. H., Kähne, T., Herrera-Molina, R., Handschuh, J., et al. (2017). A complex of neuroplastin and plasma membrane calcium ATPase controls T cell activation. *Sci. Rep.* 7:8358. doi: 10.1038/s41598-017-08519-4

Laemmli, U. K. (1970). Cleavage of structural proteins during the assembly of the head of bacteriophage T4. *Nature* 227, 680–685. doi: 10.1038/227680a0

Li, M., Ho, P. W., Pang, S. Y., Tse, Z. H., Kung, M. H., Sham, P. C., and Ho, S. L. (2014). PMCA4(ATP2B4) mutation in familial spastic paraplegia. *PLoS ONE* 9:e104790. doi: 10.1371/journal.pone.0104790

Lopreiato, R., Giacomello, M., and Carafoli, E. (2014). The plasma membrane calcium pump: new ways to look at an old enzyme. *J. Biol. Chem.* 289, 10261–10268. doi: 10.1074/jbc.O114.555565

Mazzitelli, L. R., and Adamo, H. P. (2014). Hyperactivation of the human plasma membrane $Ca^{2+}$ pump PMCA h4xb by mutation of Glu99 to Lys". *J. Biol. Chem.* 289, 10761–10768. doi: 10.1074/jbc.M113.535583

Mohamed, T. M., Abou-Leisa, R., Stafford, N., Maqsood, A., Zi, M., Prehar, S., et al. (2016). The plasma membrane calcium ATPase 4 signaling in cardiac fibroblasts mediates cardiomyocyte hypertrophy. *Nat. Commun.* 7:11074. doi: 10.1038/ncomms11074

Mohamed, T. M., Oceandy, D., Zi, M., Prehar, S., Alatwi, N., Wang, Y., et al. (2011). Plasma membrane calcium pump (PMCA4)-neuronal nitric-oxide synthase complex regulates cardiac contractility through modulation of a compartmentalized cyclic nucleotide microdomain. *J. Biol. Chem.* 286, 41520–41529. doi: 10.1074/jbc.M111.290411

Müller, C. S., Haupt, A., Bildl, W., Schindler, J., Knaus, H.-G., Meissner, M., et al. (2010). Quantitative proteomics of the Cav2 channel nano-environments in the mammalian *Brain* 107, 14959–14957. doi: 10.1073/pnas.1005940107

Nagarajan, A., Andersen, J. P., and Woolf, T. B. (2012). The role of domain:domain interactions vs domain:water interactions in the coarse-grained simulations of the E1P to E2P transitions in Ca-ATPase (SERCA). *Proteins* 80, 1929–1947. doi: 10.1002/prot.24070

Niggli, V., Adunyah, E. S., Penniston, J. T., and Carafoli, E. (1981). Purified (Ca2+-Mg2+)-ATPase of the erythrocyte membrane. Reconstitution and effect of calmodulin and phospholipids. *J. Biol. Chem.* 256, 395–401. doi: 10.1016/S0021-9258(19)70149-5

Nyholm Holdensen, A., and Andersen, J. P. (2009). The length of the A-M3 linker is a crucial determinant of the rate of the $Ca^{2+}$-transport cycle of sarcoplasmic reticulum Ca2-ATPase. *J. Biol. Chem.* 284, 12258–12265. doi: 10.1074/jbc.M900977200

Schmidt, N., Kollewe, A., Constantin, C. E., Henrich, S., Ritzau-Jost, A., Bildl, W., Saalbach, A., Hallermann, S., Kulik, A., Fakler, B., and Schulte, U. (2017). Neuroplastin and basigin are essential auxiliary subunits of plasma membrane $Ca^{2+}$ ATPases and key regulators of $Ca^{2+}$ clearance. *Neuron* 96, 827–838. doi: 10.1016/j.neuron.2017.09.038

Stafford, N., Wilson, C., Oceandy, D., Neyses, L., and Cartwright, E. J. (2017). The plasma membrane calcium ATPases and their role as major new players in human disease. *Physiol. Rev.* 97, 1089–1125. doi: 10.1152/physrev.00 028.2016

Streheler, E. E., Caride, A. J., Filoteo, A. G., Xiong, Y., Penniston, J. T., and Enyedi, A. (2007). Plasma membrane $Ca^{2+}$ ATPases as dynamic regulators of cellular calcium handling. *Ann. N. Y. Acad. Sci.*1099, 226–236. doi: 10.1196/annals.1387.023

Strehler, E. E. (2015). Plasma membrane calcium ATPases: from generic $Ca^{2+}$ sump pumps to versatile systems for fine-tuning cellular $Ca^{2+}$. *Biochem. Biophys. Res. Commun.* 460, 26–33. doi: 10.1016/j.bbrc.2015. 01.121

Strehler, E. E., and Zacharias, D. A. (2001). Role of alternative splicing in generating isoform diversity among plasma membrane calcium pumps. *Phys. Rev.* 81, 21–49. doi: 10.1152/physrev.2001.81.1.21

# 18

# The Potential Relationship Between HIF-1α and Amino Acid Metabolism After Hypoxic Ischemia and Dual Effects on Neurons

*Kexin Li, Yang Zheng and Xiaoming Wang**

*Department of Radiology, Shengjing Hospital of China Medical University, Shenyang, China*

***Correspondence:***
*Xiaoming Wang*
*wangxm024@163.com*

Hypoxia inducible factor (HIF) is one of the major transcription factors through which cells and tissues adapt to hypoxic-ischemic injury. However, the specific mechanism by which HIF regulates amino acid metabolism and its effect on neurons during hypoxic ischemia (HI) have remained unclear. This study analyzed the changes in cerebral metabolism of amino acids after HI by using $^1$H-MRS and investigated the relationship between the changes in cerebral metabolism of amino acids and HIF-1α as well as the potential effects on neurons. Newborn pigs were used as an HI model in this study. Twenty-eight newborn Yorkshire pigs (male, 1.0–1.5 kg) aged 3–5 days were selected and randomly divided into experimental groups tested at 0–2 h ($n$ = 4), 2–6 h ($n$ = 4), 6–12 h ($n$ = 4), 12–24 h ($n$ = 4), 24–48 h ($n$ = 4), and 48–72 h ($n$ = 4) after HI, and a control group ($n$ = 4). After the modeling was completed, $^1$H-MRS imaging was conducted, followed by immunohistochemical staining of HIF-1α, NeuN, and doublecortin (DCX), and immunofluorescence of glutamic oxaloacetic transaminase (GOT)-1, GOT2, glutathione synthase (GS), glutamate-cysteine ligase catalytic subunit (GCLC), and glutamate-cysteine ligase modifier subunit (GCLM) in brain tissues. The expression of HIF-1α exhibited two increases after HI injury. The first time was opposite to the trends of change of GOT2, aspartic acid, and the number of neurons, while the second was consistent with these trends, suggesting that HIF-1α may have a two-way induction effect on neurons by regulating GOT2 after HI. HIF-1α was closely related to GCLM expression, and GSH level was correlated with the number of hippocampal neurons, indicating that HIF-1α may regulate GCLM to promote GSH synthesis and additionally play a neuroprotective role.

**Keywords: hypoxic-ischemic injury, hypoxia inducible factor, amino acid metabolism, neurogenesis, neural plasticity**

---

**Abbreviations:** α-KG, α-ketoglutarate; γ-GC, γ-glutamylcysteine; Asp, aspartic acid; DCX, doublecortin; ETC, electronic transport chain; GCLC, glutamate-cysteine ligase catalytic subunit; GCLM, glutamate; cysteine ligase modifier subunit; Gln, glutamine; GLS, glutaminase; Glu, glutamate; GOT, glutamic oxaloacetic transaminase; GS, glutathione synthase; GSH, glutathione; HI, hypoxic ischemia; HIE, hypoxic-ischemic encephalopathy; HIF, hypoxia inducible factor; MAS, malate-aspartate shuttle; OAA, oxaloacetic acid; OD, optical density; PHD, prolyl 4-hydroxylase; ROS, reactive oxygen species; TCA, glycolytic or tricarboxylic acid.

## INTRODUCTION

Neonatal hypoxic ischemic encephalopathy (HIE) refers to neonatal brain injury caused by perinatal asphyxia or decreased placental perfusion, the main pathogenesis of which is hypoxic ischemia (HI). HI can lead to energy failure and in turn triggers a cascade of injury and causes disorders of nervous system structure and function (Douglas-Escobar and Weiss, 2015; Millar et al., 2017). While the neonatal brain has a strong inherent capacity to recover, after HI injury, the nervous system can promote nerve recovery and reduce nerve injury through multiple pathways, including regulating signal transduction as well as neurotransmitter transmission, etc. (Ismail et al., 2017).

Hypoxia inducible factor (HIF) is a kind of transcription factor responsible for regulating oxygen homeostasis, which is composed of α and β subunits. After HI, HIF-1α promotes nerve recovery by regulating angiogenesis, neurogenesis, glucose transport, and metabolism (Chen et al., 2009; Vetrovoy and Rybnikova, 2019; Zhu et al., 2019). Under hypoxic conditions, prolyl 4-hydroxylase (PHD) activity is inhibited, which reduces the degradation of HIF-1α and increases HIF-1α expression, further promoting the transcription of HIF-1α target genes. This in turn boosts the expression of EPO and VEGF, among others, and facilitates angiogenesis (Chu and Jones, 2016; Yang et al., 2018). HIF-1α affects the differentiation and neurogenesis of neural stem cells by regulating Notch and Wnt/β-catenin signaling pathways (Chen et al., 2018), and it also reprograms cell metabolism to maintain cell energy homeostasis under hypoxia by upregulating many metabolic enzymes, including glucose and lactate transporters, and pyruvate dehydrogenase kinase (Parks et al., 2017; Kierans and Taylor, 2021; Paredes et al., 2021).

In recent years, the regulation of amino acid metabolism by HIF has gradually attracted increasing attention. It has been reported that HIF-1α promoted the synthesis of glutathione (GSH) in a bone regeneration model by upregulating glutaminase (GLS), reduced the damage of reactive oxygen species (ROS), thus promoting the survival of osteogenic cells, and further provided a new therapeutic strategy for stem cell therapy (Stegen et al., 2016). Besides, HIF-1α can contribute to the conversion of glutamine (Gln) to α-ketoglutarate (α-KG), which can be used in the glycolytic or tricarboxylic acid (TCA) cycle to generate energy (Jiang et al., 2017; Stegen et al., 2019).

After HI injury, complex change in the cerebral metabolism of amino acids occurs. It can affect the transmission of neurotransmitters and regulate the signal transduction of nerve cells (Blaise et al., 2017; Pregnolato et al., 2019), for example, the increase of glutamic oxaloacetic transaminase (GOT) after neonatal HI injury helps to reduce the excitotoxicity of glutamate (Glu) (Perez-Mato et al., 2016). The malate-aspartate shuttle (MAS) process includes amino acid conversion and is also coupled to the electron transport chain to facilitate energy homeostasis (Satrustegui and Bak, 2015; Beckervordersandforth, 2017). In addition, the increase of cerebral GSH after HI may play a neuroprotective role, the synthesis of which requires the participation of glutathione synthase (GS), glutamate-cysteine ligase catalytic subunit (GCLC) and glutamate-cysteine ligase modifier subunit (GCLM) (Lian et al., 2018; Li et al., 2021). However, it remains unclear the relationship between HIF-1α and the metabolism of amino acids after HI, and whether neuronal changes are due to the metabolism of amino acids by HIF-1α regulation. $^1$H-MRS imaging is a non-invasive strategy to determine the levels of cerebral metabolites, and it can be used to assess the changes in metabolites and the degree of injury after HI (Shibasaki et al., 2018; Dhamala et al., 2019). This study was established to analyze the changes in the metabolism of amino acids after HIE by using $^1$H-MRS and to investigate the relationship between the changes in the metabolism of amino acids and HIF as well as the potential effects of HIF on neurons.

## MATERIALS AND METHODS

### Experimental Animals and HI Modeling

Newborn pigs ($n$ = 28) aged 3–5 days (bodyweight 1.0–1.5 kg, male) were used as experimental animals in this study. They were randomly divided into experimental groups, namely, 0–2 h ($n$ = 4), 2–6 h ($n$ = 4), 6–12 h ($n$ = 4), 12–24 h ($n$ = 4), 24–48 h ($n$ = 4), and 48–72 h groups ($n$ = 4), according to the different times after HI, and a control group ($n$ = 4). The procedures to which the experimental animals were subjected were approved by the Animal Care and Use Institutional Committee of China Medical University (approval number 2015PS337K), and performed in accordance with the *Laboratory Animal Care and Use Guidelines* issued by the National Research Council. The modeling process is shown in **Figure 1**. The drugs and equipment used were as follows: sumianxin (Changchun Institute of Military Medical Research, Changchun, China) used in animal anesthesia; a mixture of 6% oxygen and 94% nitrogen (Dalian Special Gas, Dalian, China); U-25T bi-level airway pressure ventilator (BMC Medical Co., Ltd., Tianjin, China); and Heal Force pulse oximeter (Hexin Zondan Medical Equipment Co., Ltd., Shenzhen, China).

### $^1$H-MRS Scan and Data Postprocessing

An Achieva 3.0T magnetic resonance scanner (Philips Healthcare, Netherlands) was employed as the MR equipment, with a gradient coil transmission and 8-channel RF coil reception. A single-voxel PRESS sequence was used for $^1$H-MRS. The scanning parameters were as follows: TR = 2,000 ms, TE = 37 ms, NSA = 64, and VOI = 10 × 10 × 10 mm, with the basal ganglia being manually outlined as the region of interest (ROI) (Zheng and Wang, 2018). Shimming and fluid attenuation were conducted automatically by the scanner. LCModel software package was employed for further processing of the $^1$H-MRS results (metabolites included Glu at 2.04–2.35 ppm and 3.75 ppm, Gln at 2.35 ppm, Asp at 2.71 ppm, and GSH at 2.95 ppm; Moss et al., 2018).

### Immunohistochemistry and Immunofluorescence Staining

The brain tissue was fixed with formaldehyde and sliced into 4-mm-thick coronal sections incorporating the hippocampus, basal ganglia, and cortex. A Leica BOND-MAX$^{TM}$ automatic

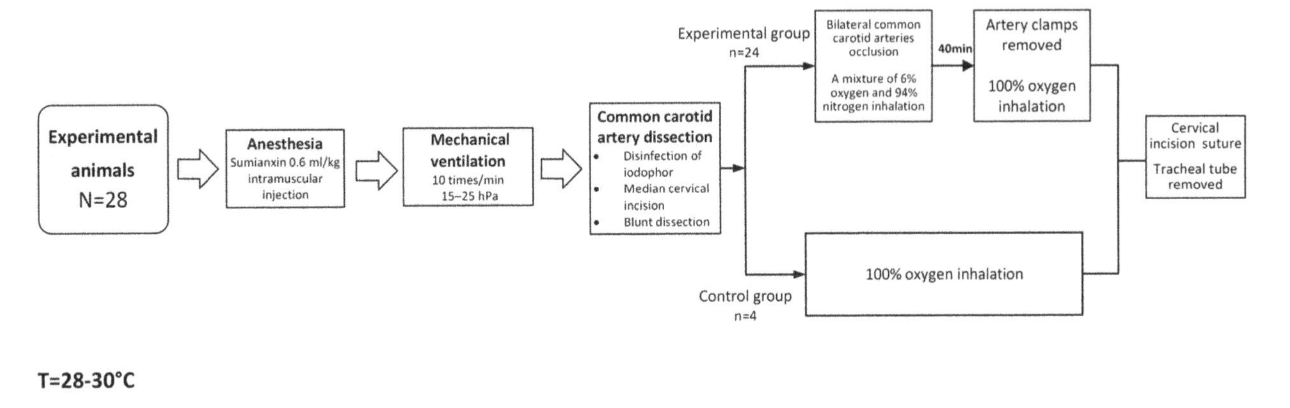


**FIGURE 1** | Flow chart of animal modeling.

staining machine (Leica, Germany) was used to conduct the immunohistochemical staining for HIF-1α (1:500; ab16066; Abcam), the neuronal marker NeuN (1:2,000; ab128886; Abcam), and neuronal migration protein doublecortin (DCX) (1:100; YP1091; Immunoway).

For GS, GCLC, GCLM, GOT1, and GOT2, immunofluorescent staining was performed. The staining steps were as follows: deparaffinization with xylene and alcohol hydration with gradient concentrations; antigen repair (0.01 M citrate buffer, pH 6.0, microwave for 37 min); blocking of endogenous peroxidase activity and non-specific antibody binding (3% hydrogen peroxide and normal goat serum, incubated at room temperature for 40 min); incubation with primary antibody overnight at 4°C (primary antibodies used: anti-GCLC antibody, 1:100, ab53179; anti-GCLM antibody, 1:100, ab154017; anti-GS antibody, 1:100, ab124811; anti-GOT1 antibody, 1:100, 60317-1-Ig; anti-GOT2 antibody, 1:100, 14800-1-AP); incubation with secondary antibody at room temperature for 4 h (secondary antibodies used: Alexa Fluor 488-labeled goat anti-mouse IgG 1:100, Immunoway, RS3208; Alexa Fluor 488-labeled goat anti-rabbit IgG 1:100, Immunoway, RS3211); and finally nuclear staining by incubation with 4,6-diamidino-2-phenylindole dihydrochloride (DAPI) for 5 min.

The immunohistochemistry images were collected using NIS-Elements F software (version 4.6; Nikon, Japan). The immunofluorescence images were collected using a confocal laser scanning microscope (LSM880; Zeiss, Göttingen, Germany) (×400). Three high-magnification (×400) fields from parietal cortical and hippocampal region were randomly and manually selected. Each image was analyzed automatically by ImageJ software (Java1.6.0; National Institutes of Health). The mean optical density (OD) of three fields was used to represent the staining intensity of the section.

## Statistical Analysis

One-way analysis of variance and LSD-*t*-*t*est were employed to analyze the differences between the subgroups, while Pearson's correlation analysis was used to evaluate the correlations, with $P < 0.05$ being considered statistically significant. All statistical analyses were conducted by SPSS (version 22.0; IBM, Armonk, New York) and GraphPad Prism (version 8.0.2; GraphPad Software, San Diego, California).

# RESULTS

## Changes in Asp, GSH, Glu, and Gln Content Observed by $^1$H-MRS After HI Injury

$^1$H-MRS was used to observe the changes in the cerebral metabolism of amino acids at different time points after HI, as shown in **Figure 2**. Asp exhibited a tendency to initially decrease and then increase after HI; the Asp content at 0–2 h after HI was significantly reduced compared with that in the control group ($P = 0.032$, LSD-*t*-*t*est). GSH content at 12–24 h after HI was significantly higher than that in the other groups ($P < 0.05$, LSD-*t*-*t*est). Glu content at 24–48 h after HI was significantly higher than that in the control group ($P = 0.002$, LSD-*t*-*t*est). Finally, Gln content initially decreased and then significantly increased at 6–12 h after HI ($P < 0.05$, LSD-*t*-*t*est).

## Changes in GOT1, GOT2, GS, GCLC, and GCLM Expression After HI Injury

The trends of change of GOT1, GOT2, GS, GCLC, and GCLM expression over time after HI injury are shown in **Figure 3**. GOT1 and GOT2 were significantly decreased at 2–6 h and 6–12 h after HI (both $P < 0.01$, LSD-*t*-*t*est), and significantly increased at 6–12 h and 12–24 h after HI, respectively ($P < 0.01$, $P < 0.05$, LSD-*t*-test). Peaks in the expression of GCLC and GCLM occurred at 2–6 h and 6–12 h after HI, respectively, and such expression was significantly higher than that in the other groups ($P < 0.01$, $P < 0.05$, LSD-*t*-*t*est). There was a tendency for an initial increase and then a decrease in GS expression after HI injury, which significantly increased at 6–12 h ($P = 0.047$, LSD-*t*-test).

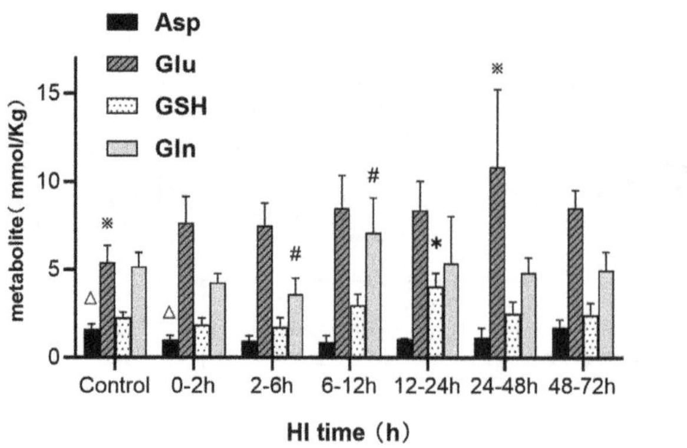


**FIGURE 2** | Changes in Asp, Glu, Gln, and GSH after HI injury (△, ※, ∗, # indicate a significant difference in a pairwise comparison, $P < 0.05$). The data are expressed as mean ± SD.

## HIF-1α Expression in Brain Tissue After HI Injury and Its Relationship With the Expression of GS, GCLC, GCLM, GOT1, and GOT2

**Figure 4** shows the changes in HIF-1α expression in brain tissue over time after HI injury. There were two peaks in the HIF-1α expression level after HI, namely, at 6 − 12 h and 48–72 h ($P < 0.01$, LSD-*t*-*test*). In the HI group, the HIF-1α expression level was significantly positively correlated with the GCLM expression level ($r = 0.537$, $P = 0.007$), while it was not significantly correlated with GCLC and GS ($P = 0.917$ and 0.055, respectively). The HIF-1α expression level was significantly negatively correlated with the GOT2 expression level in control group and at 0–12 h after HI ($r = -0.542$, $P = 0.037$), which reversed to a significant positive correlation at 12–72 h after HI ($r = 0.762$, $P = 0.004$). There was no significant correlation between the expression levels of HIF-1α and GOT1 ($P = 0.549$).

## Changes in the Numbers of Hippocampal and Cortical Neurons After HI Injury

The numbers of hippocampal and cortical neurons exhibited significant differences compared with those in the control group ($P < 0.001$ and $P = 0.034$, ANOVA). The numbers of hippocampal and cortical neurons both initially decreased and then increased. The number of neurons increased at 12–24 h ($P < 0.01$, LSD-*t*-*test*) and 48–72 h ($P < 0.01$, LSD-*t*-*test*), respectively (**Figure 5** and **Supplementary Figure**).

## Changes in DCX Expression After HI Injury

The expression of hippocampal and cortical DCX exhibited significant differences among the HI groups and the control group ($P < 0.001$, respectively, ANOVA). The expression of hippocampal DCX decreased at 0–2 h ($P < 0.01$, LSD-*t*-*test*) and increased at 12–24 h ($P < 0.01$, LSD-*t*-*test*), while the expression of cortical DCX increased at 48–72 h ($P < 0.01$, LSD-*t*-*test*) (**Figure 6** and **Supplementary Figure**).

# DISCUSSION

Hypoxia is a trigger of many pathological conditions such as HIE, which is usually accompanied by insufficient synthesis or increased consumption of glucose and amino acids. HIF is one of the major transcription factors through which cells and tissues adapt to hypoxia. By participating in the regulation of metabolic reprogramming, HIF can meet the body's biosynthetic and energy requirements under hypoxic conditions (Semenza, 2012; Chen and Sang, 2016). Research performed to date on the mechanism by which HIF regulates cell metabolism has mainly focused on glucose and fatty acid metabolism (Bouthelier and Aragones, 2020), while the specific mechanism by which amino acid metabolism is regulated remains to be studied. In addition, owing to a large number of downstream target genes of HIF and its extensive effects, HIF-1α after HI injury can activate not only neuroprotection but also the signal pathways after HI injury (e.g., apoptosis), resulting in a dual effect of neuroprotection and nerve injury (Chen et al., 2007, 2009). In this study, we used $^{1}$H-MRS imaging to observe the dynamic changes of cerebral metabolites after HI injury and analyzed their correlations with HIF-1α expression and changes in the number of neurons to investigate the mechanisms by which HIF-1α regulates amino acid metabolism and neurons after HI injury.

## Correlation Between GSH Synthesis and HIF-1α Expression After HI Injury and the Effect of HIF-1α on Neurons

The neural synthesis of GSH involves the Glu, cysteine, and glycine as precursors. Glu is mainly derived from the transport by excitatory amino acid carrier 1 and the Glu-Gln shuttle (Aoyama et al., 2008; Sedlak et al., 2019). The first synthesis step of GSH is the formation of γ-glutamylcysteine (γ-GC), which is catalyzed by GCL, a heterodimer composed of GCLC and GCLM. GCLC acts as the catalyst, while the synthesis process modified and regulated by GCLM. In the second step, GSH is synthesized in a manner catalyzed by GS (Chen et al., 2005; Lian et al., 2018).

The $^{1}$H-MRS results in this study showed that Gln increased at 6–12 h and decreased rapidly at 12–24 h after HI, at which time the GSH content increased significantly. The immunofluorescence staining results of synthetases showed that GCLC reached its peak at 2–6 h after HI injury, and GCLM and GS reached their peaks at 6–12 h after HI, indicating that the synthesis of GSH was activated after HI injury. However, this study found that the changes of GCLC and GCLM were not synchronized, and the GCLC expression increased earlier than that of GCLM, suggesting that GCLC may have catalyzed the whole reaction. The 5′end of GCLM mRNA has an HIF-1α binding site, which can be used to induce GCLM expression by HIF-1α (Lu et al., 2015; Stegen et al., 2016). This study found that the HIF-1α expression was significantly positively correlated with the GCLM expression, but not significantly correlated with the GCLC and GS expression after HI injury, indicating that HIF-1α mainly promotes GSH synthesis by upregulating the GCLM expression after HI.

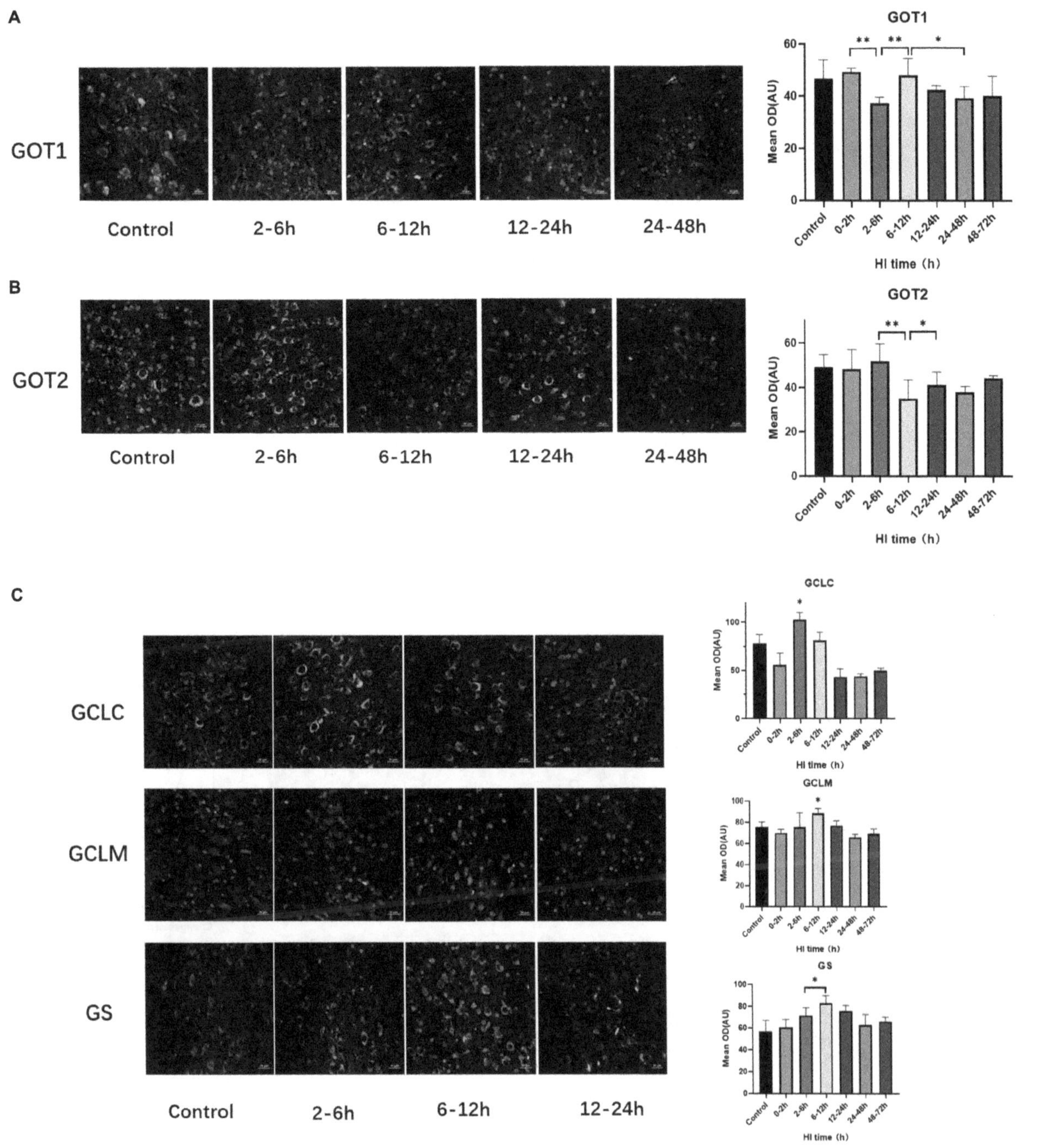


**FIGURE 3 |** Changes in the expression of GOT1, GOT2, GCLC, GCLM, and GS after HI injury (×400). **(A)** Tendency chart for cerebral GOT1 staining and mean optical density in the control group and HI groups at 2–6, 6–12, 12–24, and 24–48 h after HI. Green fluorescence represents GOT1. The fluorescence intensity of GOT1 decreases at 2–6 h, then increases at 6–12 h, and significantly decreases again at 24–48 h after HI. **(B)** Tendency chart for cerebral GOT2 staining and mean optical density in the control group and HI groups at 2–6, 6–12, 12–24, and 24–48 h after HI. Green fluorescence represents GOT2. The fluorescence intensity of GOT2 decreases at 6–12 h and then increases at 12–24 h after HI. **(C)** Tendency chart for the cerebral GCLC, GCLM, and GS staining, and mean optical density in the control group and the groups at 2–6, 6–12, and 12–24 h after HI. Green fluorescence represents GCLC, GCLM, and GS. The fluorescence intensity of GCLC, GCLM, and GS peaks at 2–6 h and 6–12 h after HI. $^{**}P < 0.01$, $^{*}P < 0.05$; data are expressed as mean ± SD.

GSH is the most abundant antioxidant in cells, the increased content of which in cells can further reduce ROS production and alleviate oxidative stress injury (Moss et al., 2018). The decreased GSH content can enhance the cytotoxicity induced by glutamate or NO, resulting in neuronal injury (Ibi et al., 1999). Previous assessment of neuronal damage after HI by our team found that the main pathological change of neurons at 0–24 h was edema, which was a

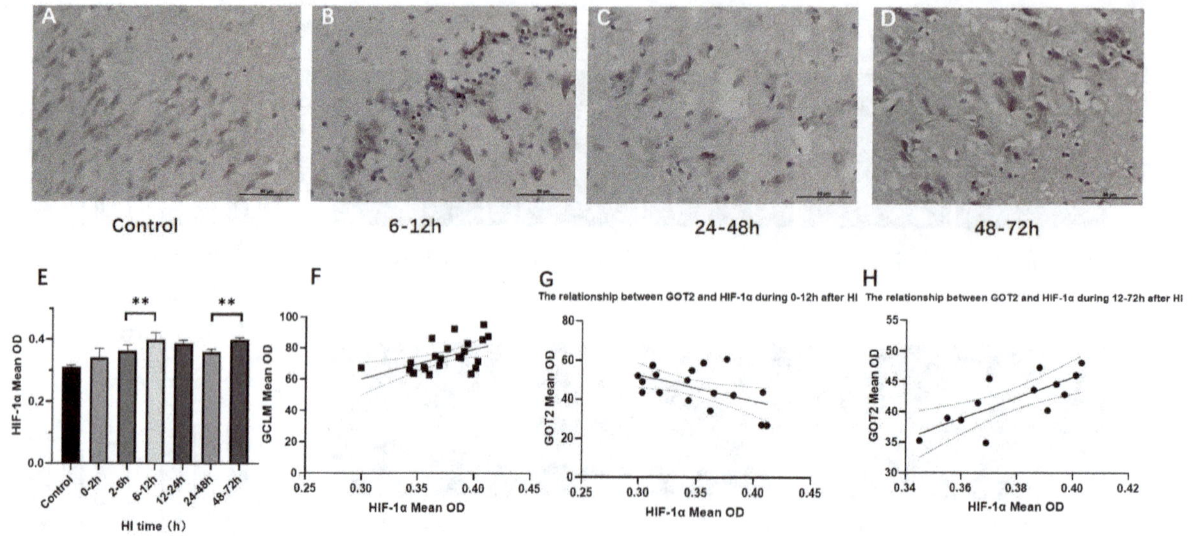


**FIGURE 4 |** Changes in HIF-1α expression (×400) and scatter plot of correlation with GCLM and GOT2 after HI. **(A–D)** Immunohistochemical staining for HIF-1α in the control group and HI groups at 6–12, 24–48, and 48–72 h after HI. **(E)** HIF-1α expression level gradually increases after HI, reaching the first peak in the 6–12 h group, significantly decreases in the 24–48 h group, and increases again in the 48–72 h group. **(F)** Scatter plot of the correlation between HIF-1α and GCLM expression. There is a significant positive correlation. **(G,H)** Scatter plot of the correlation between HIF-1α and GOT2 expression. In the control group and HI groups at 0–2, 2–6, and 6–12 h after HI, HIF-1α expression and GOT2 expression show a significant negative correlation. In the groups at 12–24, 24–48, and 48–72 h after HI, they instead show a significant positive correlation. $^{**}P < 0.01$; data are expressed as mean ± SD.

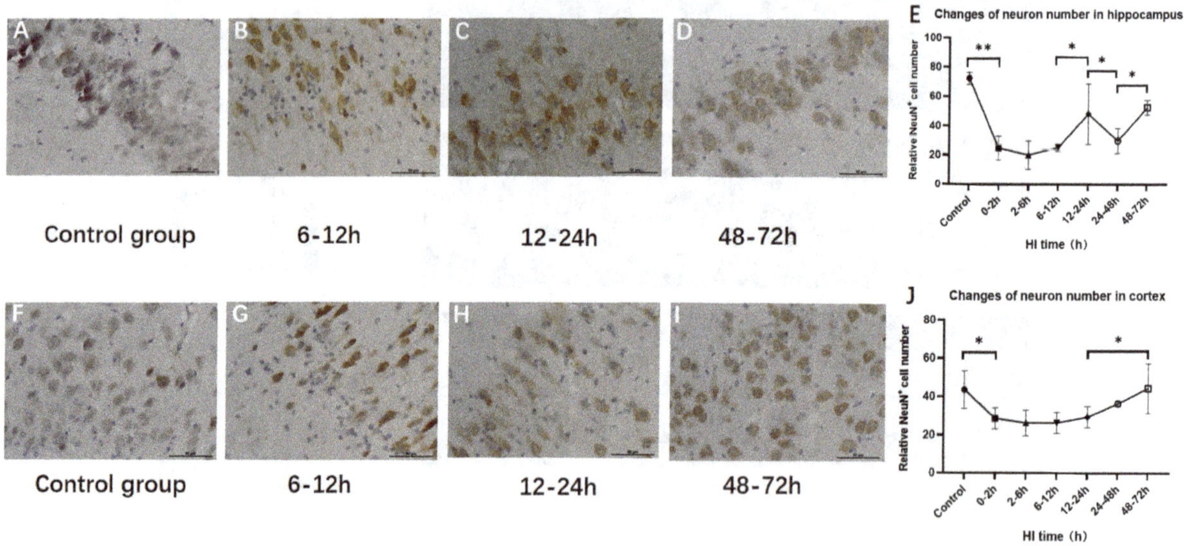


**FIGURE 5 |** Changes in the number of NeuN-positive cells in the hippocampus and cortex after HI (×400). **(A)** NeuN immunohistochemical staining of the hippocampus in the control group. **(B–D)** NeuN immunohistochemical staining of the hippocampus in HI groups at 6–12, 12–24, and 48–72 h after HI. **(E)** The number of NeuN-positive cells in the hippocampus decreases at 0–12 h and significantly increases at 12–24 h after HI injury. **(F)** NeuN immunohistochemical staining of the cortex in the control group. **(G–I)** NeuN immunohistochemical staining of the cortex in groups at 6–12, 12–24, and 48–72 h after HI. **(J)** Compared with the control group, there is a significant decrease in the number of NeuN-positive cells in the cortex at 0–2 h after HI injury, and the number of NeuN-positive cells at 48–72 h after HI is significantly increased. $^{**}P < 0.01$, $^{*}P < 0.05$; data are expressed as mean ± SD.

kind of mild reversible injury (Zheng and Wang, 2018; Dang and Wang, 2020). In this study, histopathological analysis confirmed that the number of hippocampal NeuN-positive cells initially decreased, which may due to neural antigen injury and diminishing the ability to bind anti-NeuN antibodies (Gusel'Nikova and Korzhevskiy, 2015). Then the number of the hippocampal NeuN-positive cells rebounded at 12–24 h after HI, consistent with the expression of DCX and the peak time of GSH, which probably means neurogenesis and neuroprotective effect of GSH in this period. GSH content decreased at 24–48 h after HI,

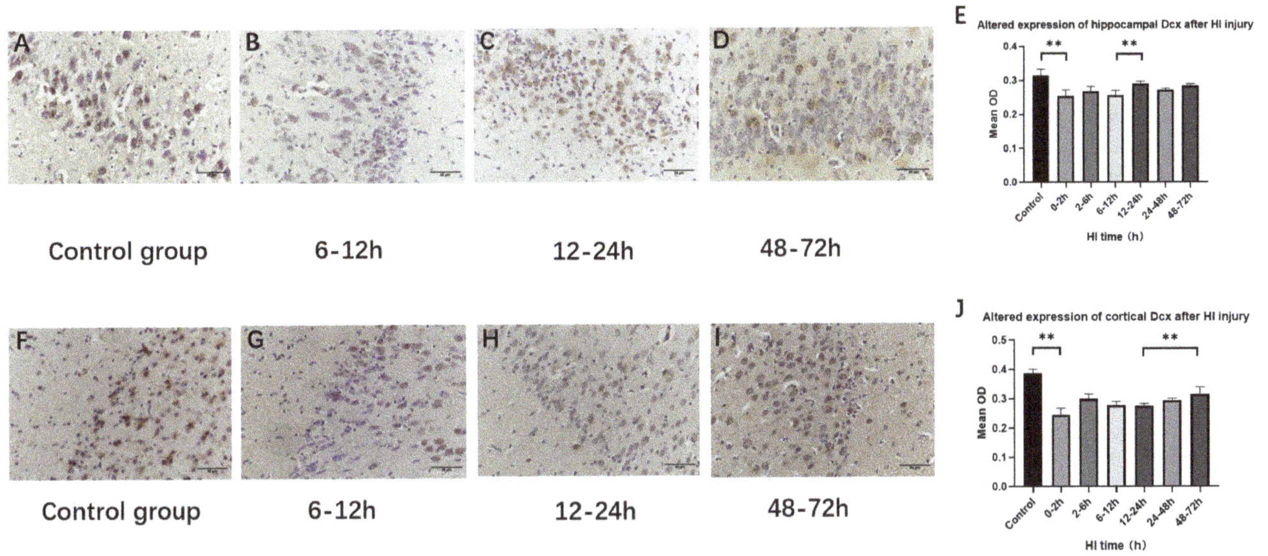


**FIGURE 6 |** Changes in DCX expression in the hippocampus and cortex after HI (×400). **(A)** DCX immunohistochemical staining of the hippocampus in the control group. **(B–D)** DCX immunohistochemical staining of the hippocampus in HI groups at 6–12, 12–24, and 48–72 h after HI. **(E)** The expression of DCX in the hippocampus decreases at 0–2 h and significantly increases at 12–24 h after HI injury. **(F)** DCX immunohistochemical staining of the cortex in the control group. **(G–I)** DCX immunohistochemical staining of the cortex in groups at 6–12, 12–24, and 48–72 h after HI. **(J)** Compared with the control group, DCX expression significant decrease in the cortex at 0–2 h after HI injury, and the expression of DCX at 48–72 h after HI is significantly increased. $^{**}P < 0.01$; data are expressed as mean ± SD.

at which time the number of neurons decreased again, suggesting that the changes of GSH after HI can reflect neuronal injury and recovery to a certain extent.

## The Relationship Between HIF-1α and Asp Metabolism After HI Injury and the Effect of HIF-1α on Neurons

Asp functions in regulating neurometabolism and biosynthesis; the MAS is one of the ways in which Asp participates in metabolic regulation. GOT is an important part of the MAS, which includes two isoenzymes: GOT1 and GOT2. The former is mainly present in the cytoplasm and is used to transform Asp and α-KG into oxaloacetic acid (OAA) and Glu in normal cells. The latter is present in the mitochondrial matrix and is employed to generate Asp and α-KG (Birsoy et al., 2015), which can transform Glu into α-KG to form part of the TCA cycle, and finally replenish the lost energy and reduce the nerve injury caused by Glu during ischemic stroke (Rink et al., 2017). Previous studies found that the electronic transport chain (ETC) is inhibited after hypoxia, Asp production is decreased (Garcia-Bermudez et al., 2018), and HIF-1α inhibits Asp metabolism by downregulating GOT expression (Melendez-Rodriguez et al., 2019; Bouthelier and Aragones, 2020). This study analyzed the relationships between HIF-1α, GOT, and Asp after HI, with the results showing that there were two peaks of HIF-1α expression after HI. The HIF-1α expression gradually increased at 0–12 h after HI, and reached its first peak at 6–12 h, while GOT2 expression decreased. There was a significant negative correlation between HIF-1α and GOT2 expression, and the Asp content also showed a downward trend during this period. At 12–72 h after HI, there was a significant positive correlation between HIF-1α and GOT2. The second peak of HIF-1α appeared at 48–72 h after HI, the GOT2 expression increased, as did the Asp content. This indicates that HIF-1α may affect Asp production by regulating GOT2 expression, and that HIF-1α has various effects during different recovery periods after HI. Previous studies also confirmed the "biphasic activation" phenomenon of HIF-1α after cerebral ischemia, which may cause dual effects of protection of and damage to neurons (Baranova et al., 2007; Arumugam et al., 2018). However, the specific mechanism by which HIF-1α regulates GOT and whether there is synergistic activation of multiple transcription factors remain to be studied (Chen and Sang, 2016).

In addition, this study found that HIF-1α had no significant correlation with GOT1, and the changes of GOT1 and GOT2 were not synchronized, which may be related to the difference in regulation between them. After ETC inhibition, GOT1 can catalyze the reductive carboxylation pathway of Gln alone to produce Asp, but this cannot completely compensate for the loss of Asp synthesis in mitochondria (Fendt et al., 2013; Perez-Mato et al., 2014; Birsoy et al., 2015). This study found that Gln increased significantly at 6–12 h after HI, GOT1 expression increased, and Asp showed an upward trend, suggesting that the Gln-dependent Asp synthesis may be one of the reasons for the increase in Asp content. However, further experiments are needed to clarify the degree of ETC inhibition after HI injury and the dynamic changes in intermediate metabolites.

The MAS plays an important role in the electron transfer process of the neuronal oxidative transport chain, and is involved in maintaining neuronal metabolism and synaptic function after cerebral ischemia (Juaristi et al., 2019; Xu et al., 2020). This study analyzed the effects of Asp metabolism and MAS changes on the number of neurons using histopathology. The results showed that there was an upward trend in the numbers of hippocampal and cortical neurons at 12–24 h after HI. At this time, GOT2 expression increased and GOT1 expression decreased, indicating the increased production of Asp and α-KG in the mitochondrial matrix, which can provide energy for neurons and reduce Glu excitotoxicity. Asp is the main raw material for pyrimidine synthesis (Lane and Fan, 2015) and participates in amino acid metabolism during cell proliferation. This study found that Asp, DCX and cortical neurons shared the same trends of change, suggesting that Asp may provide synthetic precursors during the neurogenesis, migration and recovery process of cortical neurons.

## CONCLUSION

The expression of HIF-1α exhibits two increases after HI injury. The first time is opposite to the trends of change of GOT2, Asp, and the number of neurons, while the second is consistent with these trends, suggesting that HIF-1α may have a two-way induction effect on neurons by regulating GOT2 after HI. HIF-1α is closely related to GCLM expression, and the GSH level was correlated with the number of hippocampal neurons, suggesting that HIF-1α may regulate GCLM to promote GSH synthesis and further play a neuroprotective role.

## AUTHOR CONTRIBUTIONS

KL: investigation, data curation, and writing-original draft. YZ: validation, resources, and supervision. XW: conceptualization, methodology, writing-review and editing, and project administration. All authors participated sufficiently to take public responsibility for its content, read and approved the submitted version.

## FUNDING

This study was supported by the National Natural Science Foundation of China (Nos. 81871408 and 81271631), the National Science Foundation for Young Scientists of China (No. 81801658), Outstanding Scientific Fund of Shengjing Hospital (No. 201402), and 345 Talent Support Project of Shengjing Hospital (No. 30B).

## REFERENCES


Aoyama, K., Watabe, M., and Nakaki, T. (2008). Regulation of neuronal glutathione synthesis. *J. Pharmacol. Sci.* 108, 227–238. doi: 10.1254/jphs.08r01cr

Arumugam, T. V., Baik, S. H., Balaganapathy, P., Sobey, C. G., Mattson, M. P., and Jo, D. G. (2018). Notch signaling and neuronal death in stroke. *Prog. Neurobiol.* 16, 103–116. doi: 10.1016/j.pneurobio.2018.03.002

Baranova, O., Miranda, L. F., Pichiule, P., Dragatsis, I., Johnson, R. S., and Chavez, J. C. (2007). Neuron-specific inactivation of the hypoxia inducible factor 1 alpha increases brain injury in a mouse model of transient focal cerebral ischemia. *J. Neurosci.* 27, 6320–6332. doi: 10.1523/JNEUROSCI.0449-07.2007

Beckervordersandforth, R. (2017). Mitochondrial metabolism-mediated regulation of adult neurogenesis. *Brain Plast.* 3, 73–87. doi: 10.3233/BPL-170044

Birsoy, K., Wang, T., Chen, W. W., Freinkman, E., Abu-Remaileh, M., and Sabatini, D. M. (2015). An essential role of the mitochondrial electron transport chain in cell proliferation is to enable aspartate synthesis. *Cell* 162, 540–551. doi: 10.1016/j.cell.2015.07.016

Blaise, B. J., Schwendimann, L., Chhor, V., Degos, V., Hodson, M. P., Dallmann, G., et al. (2017). Persistently altered metabolic phenotype following perinatal excitotoxic brain injury. *Dev. Neurosci.* 39, 182–191. doi: 10.1159/000464131

Bouthelier, A., and Aragones, J. (2020). Role of the HIF oxygen sensing pathway in cell defense and proliferation through the control of amino acid metabolism. *Biochim. Biophys. Acta Mol. Cell. Res.* 1867:118733. doi: 10.1016/j.bbamcr.2020.118733

Chen, C., Hu, Q., Yan, J., Lei, J., Qin, L., Shi, X., et al. (2007). Multiple effects of 2ME2 and D609 on the cortical expression of HIF-1alpha and apoptotic genes in a middle cerebral artery occlusion-induced focal ischemia rat model. *J. Neurochem.* 102, 1831–1841. doi: 10.1111/j.1471-4159.2007.04652.x

Chen, S., and Sang, N. (2016). Hypoxia-inducible factor-1: a critical player in the survival strategy of stressed cells. *J. Cell. Biochem.* 117, 267–278. doi: 10.1002/jcb.25283

Chen, W., Ostrowski, R. P., Obenaus, A., and Zhang, J. H. (2009). Prodeath or prosurvival: two facets of hypoxia inducible factor-1 in perinatal brain injury. *Exp. Neurol.* 216, 7–15. doi: 10.1016/j.expneurol.2008.10.016

Chen, X., Zhou, B., Yan, T., Wu, H., Feng, J., Chen, H., et al. (2018). *Peroxynitrite enhances* self-renewal, proliferation and neuronal differentiation of neural stem/progenitor cells through activating HIF-1alpha and Wnt/beta-catenin signaling pathway. *Free Radic. Biol. Med.* 117, 158–167. doi: 10.1016/j.freeradbiomed.2018.02.011

Chen, Y., Shertzer, H. G., Schneider, S. N., Nebert, D. W., and Dalton, T. P. (2005). Glutamate cysteine ligase catalysis: dependence on ATP and modifier subunit for regulation of tissue glutathione levels. *J. Biol. Chem.* 280, 33766–33774. doi: 10.1074/jbc.M504604200

Chu, H. X., and Jones, N. M. (2016). Changes in hypoxia-inducible factor-1 (HIF-1) and regulatory prolyl hydroxylase (PHD) enzymes following hypoxic-ischemic injury in the neonatal rat. *Neurochem. Res.* 41, 515–522. doi: 10.1007/s11064-015-1641-y

Dang, Y., and Wang, X. (2020). Evaluation of altered glutamatergic activity in a piglet model of hypoxic-ischemic brain damage using (1)h-mrs. *Dis. Markers.* 2020:8850816. doi: 10.1155/2020/8850816

Dhamala, E., Abdelkefi, I., Nguyen, M., Hennessy, T. J., Nadeau, H., and Near, J. (2019). Validation of in vivo MRS measures of metabolite concentrations in the human brain. *NMR Biomed.* 32:e4058. doi: 10.1002/nbm.4058

Douglas-Escobar, M., and Weiss, M. D. (2015). Hypoxic-ischemic encephalopathy: a review for the clinician. *JAMA Pediatr.* 169, 397–403. doi: 10.1001/jamapediatrics.2014.3269

Fendt, S. M., Bell, E. L., Keibler, M. A., Olenchock, B. A., Mayers, J. R., Wasylenko, T. M., et al. (2013). Reductive glutamine metabolism is a function of the alpha-ketoglutarate to citrate ratio in cells. *Nat. Commun.* 4:2236. doi: 10.1038/ncomms3236

Garcia-Bermudez, J., Baudrier, L., La, K., Zhu, X. G., Fidelin, J., Sviderskiy, V. O., et al. (2018). Aspartate is a limiting metabolite for cancer cell proliferation under hypoxia and in tumours. *Nat. Cell. Biol.* 20, 775–781. doi: 10.1038/s41556-018-0118-z

Gusel'Nikova, V. V., and Korzhevskiy, D. E. (2015). Neun as a neuronal nuclear antigen and neuron differentiation marker. *Acta Naturae* 7, 42–47. doi: 10.32607/20758251-2015-7-2-42-47

Ibi, M., Sawada, H., Kume, T., Katsuki, H., Kaneko, S., Shimohama, S., et al. (1999). Depletion of intracellular glutathione increases susceptibility to nitric oxide in mesencephalic dopaminergic neurons. *J. Neurochem.* 73, 1696–1703. doi: 10.1046/j.1471-4159.1999.731696.x

Ismail, F. Y., Fatemi, A., and Johnston, M. V. (2017). Cerebral plasticity: windows of opportunity in the developing brain. *Eur. J. Paediatr. Neurol.* 21, 23–48. doi: 10.1016/j.ejpn.2016.07.007

Jiang, Z. F., Wang, M., Xu, J. L., and Ning, Y. J. (2017). Hypoxia promotes mitochondrial glutamine metabolism through HIF1alpha-GDH pathway in human lung cancer cells. *Biochem. Biophys. Res. Commun.* 483, 32–38. doi: 10.1016/j.bbrc.2017.01.015

Juaristi, I., Contreras, L., Gonzalez-Sanchez, P., Perez-Liebana, I., Gonzalez-Moreno, L., Pardo, B., et al. (2019). The response to stimulation in neurons and astrocytes. *Neurochem. Res.* 44, 2385–2391. doi: 10.1007/s11064-019-02803-7

Kierans, S. J., and Taylor, C. T. (2021). Regulation of glycolysis by the hypoxia-inducible factor (HIF): implications for cellular physiology. *J. Physiol.* 599, 23–37. doi: 10.1113/JP280572

Lane, A. N., and Fan, T. W. (2015). Regulation of mammalian nucleotide metabolism and biosynthesis. *Nucleic Acids Res.* 43, 2466–2485. doi: 10.1093/nar/gkv047

Li, K., Zheng, Y., and Wang, X. (2021). Self-regulation of cerebral metabolism and its neuroprotective effect after hypoxic-ischemic injury: evidence from 1H-MRS. *Front. Neuroanat.* 15:45.

Lian, G., Gnanaprakasam, J. R., Wang, T., Wu, R., Chen, X., Liu, L., et al. (2018). Glutathione de novo synthesis but not recycling process coordinates with glutamine catabolism to control redox homeostasis and directs murine T cell differentiation. *Elife* 7:e36158. doi: 10.7554/eLife.36158

Lu, H., Samanta, D., Xiang, L., Zhang, H., Hu, H., Chen, I., et al. (2015). Chemotherapy triggers HIF-1-dependent glutathione synthesis and copper chelation that induces the breast cancer stem cell phenotype. *Proc. Natl. Acad. Sci. U.S.A.* 112, E4600–E4609. doi: 10.1073/pnas.1513433112

Melendez-Rodriguez, F., Urrutia, A. A., Lorendeau, D., Rinaldi, G., Roche, O., Bogurcu-Seidel, N., et al. (2019). HIF1alpha suppresses tumor cell proliferation through inhibition of aspartate biosynthesis. *Cell Rep.* 26, 2257–2265. doi: 10.1016/j.celrep.2019.01.106

Millar, L. J., Shi, L., Hoerder-Suabedissen, A., and Molnar, Z. (2017). Neonatal hypoxia ischaemia: mechanisms, models, and therapeutic challenges. *Front. Cell Neurosci.* 11:78. doi: 10.3389/fncel.2017.00078

Moss, H. G., Brown, T. R., Wiest, D. B., and Jenkins, D. D. (2018). N-Acetylcysteine rapidly replenishes central nervous system glutathione measured via magnetic resonance spectroscopy in human neonates with hypoxic-ischemic encephalopathy. *J. Cereb. Blood Flow Metab.* 38, 950–958. doi: 10.1177/0271678X18765828

Paredes, F., Williams, H. C., and San, M. A. (2021). Metabolic adaptation in hypoxia and cancer. *Cancer Lett.* 502, 133–142. doi: 10.1016/j.canlet.2020.12.020

Parks, S. K., Cormerais, Y., and Pouyssegur, J. (2017). Hypoxia and cellular metabolism in tumour pathophysiology. *J. Physiol.* 595, 2439–2450. doi: 10.1113/JP273309

Perez-Mato, M., Iglesias-Deus, A., Rujido, S., Da, S. A., Sobrino, T., Couce, M. L., et al. (2016). Potential protective role of endogenous glutamate-oxaloacetate transaminase against glutamate excitotoxicity in fetal hypoxic-ischaemic asphyxia. *Dev. Med. Child Neurol.* 58, 57–62. doi: 10.1111/dmcn.12851

Perez-Mato, M., Ramos-Cabrer, P., Sobrino, T., Blanco, M., Ruban, A., Mirelman, D., et al. (2014). Human recombinant glutamate oxaloacetate transaminase 1 (GOT1) supplemented with oxaloacetate induces a protective effect after cerebral ischemia. *Cell Death Dis.* 5:e992. doi: 10.1038/cddis.2013.507

Pregnolato, S., Chakkarapani, E., Isles, A. R., and Luyt, K. (2019). Glutamate transport and preterm brain injury. *Front. Physiol.* 10:417. doi: 10.3389/fphys.2019.00417

Rink, C., Gnyawali, S., Stewart, R., Teplitsky, S., Harris, H., Roy, S., et al. (2017). Glutamate oxaloacetate transaminase enables anaplerotic refilling of TCA cycle intermediates in stroke-affected brain. *FASEB J.* 31, 1709–1718. doi: 10.1096/fj.201601033R

Satrustegui, J., and Bak, L. K. (2015). Fluctuations in cytosolic calcium regulate the neuronal malate-aspartate NADH shuttle: implications for neuronal energy metabolism. *Neurochem. Res.* 40, 2425–2430. doi: 10.1007/s11064-015-1652-8

Sedlak, T. W., Paul, B. D., Parker, G. M., Hester, L. D., Snowman, A. M., Taniguchi, Y., et al. (2019). The glutathione cycle shapes synaptic glutamate activity. *Proc. Natl. Acad. Sci. U.S.A.* 116, 2701–2706. doi: 10.1073/pnas.1817885116

Semenza, G. L. (2012). Hypoxia-inducible factors in physiology and medicine. *Cell* 148, 399–408. doi: 10.1016/j.cell.2012.01.021

Shibasaki, J., Aida, N., Morisaki, N., Tomiyasu, M., Nishi, Y., and Toyoshima, K. (2018). Changes in brain metabolite concentrations after neonatal hypoxic-ischemic encephalopathy. *Radiology* 288, 840–848. doi: 10.1148/radiol.2018172083

Stegen, S., Laperre, K., Eelen, G., Rinaldi, G., Fraisl, P., Torrekens, S., et al. (2019). HIF-1alpha metabolically controls collagen synthesis and modification in chondrocytes. *Nature* 565, 511–515. doi: 10.1038/s41586-019-0874-3

Stegen, S., van Gastel, N., Eelen, G., Ghesquiere, B., D'Anna, F., Thienpont, B., et al. (2016). HIF-1alpha promotes glutamine-mediated redox homeostasis and glycogen-dependent bioenergetics to support postimplantation bone cell survival. *Cell Metab.* 23, 265–279. doi: 10.1016/j.cmet.2016.01.002

Vetrovoy, O., and Rybnikova, E. (2019). Neuroprotective action of PHD inhibitors is predominantly HIF-1-independent: an editorial for 'sex differences in neonatal mouse brain injury after hypoxia-ischemia and adaptaquin treatment' on page 759. *J. Neurochem.* 150, 645–647. doi: 10.1111/jnc.14822

Xu, J., Khoury, N., Jackson, C. W., Escobar, I., Stegelmann, S. D., Dave, K. R., et al. (2020). Ischemic neuroprotectant PKCepsilon restores mitochondrial glutamate oxaloacetate transaminase in the neuronal NADH shuttle after ischemic injury. *Transl. Stroke Res.* 11, 418–432. doi: 10.1007/s12975-019-00729-4

Yang, X., Zhong, M., Chen, J., Li, T., Cheng, Q., and Dai, Y. (2018). HIF-1 <alpha> repression of PTEN transcription mediates protective effects of BMSCs on neurons during hypoxia. *Neuroscience* 392, 57–65. doi: 10.1016/j.neuroscience.2018.09.024

Zheng, Y., and Wang, X. M. (2018). Expression changes in lactate and glucose metabolism and associated transporters in basal ganglia following hypoxic-ischemic reperfusion injury in piglets. *AJNR Am. J. Neuroradiol.* 39, 569–576. doi: 10.3174/ajnr.A5505

Zhu, L., Qi, B., and Hou, D. (2019). Roles of HIF1alpha- and HIF2alpha-regulated BNIP3 in hypoxia-induced injury of neurons. *Pathol. Res. Pract.* 215, 822–827. doi: 10.1016/j.prp.2019.01.022

# Permissions

All chapters in this book were first published by Frontiers; hereby published with permission under the Creative Commons Attribution License or equivalent. Every chapter published in this book has been scrutinized by our experts. Their significance has been extensively debated. The topics covered herein carry significant findings which will fuel the growth of the discipline. They may even be implemented as practical applications or may be referred to as a beginning point for another development.

The contributors of this book come from diverse backgrounds, making this book a truly international effort. This book will bring forth new frontiers with its revolutionizing research information and detailed analysis of the nascent developments around the world.

We would like to thank all the contributing authors for lending their expertise to make the book truly unique. They have played a crucial role in the development of this book. Without their invaluable contributions this book wouldn't have been possible. They have made vital efforts to compile up to date information on the varied aspects of this subject to make this book a valuable addition to the collection of many professionals and students.

This book was conceptualized with the vision of imparting up-to-date information and advanced data in this field. To ensure the same, a matchless editorial board was set up. Every individual on the board went through rigorous rounds of assessment to prove their worth. After which they invested a large part of their time researching and compiling the most relevant data for our readers.

The editorial board has been involved in producing this book since its inception. They have spent rigorous hours researching and exploring the diverse topics which have resulted in the successful publishing of this book. They have passed on their knowledge of decades through this book. To expedite this challenging task, the publisher supported the team at every step. A small team of assistant editors was also appointed to further simplify the editing procedure and attain best results for the readers.

Apart from the editorial board, the designing team has also invested a significant amount of their time in understanding the subject and creating the most relevant covers. They scrutinized every image to scout for the most suitable representation of the subject and create an appropriate cover for the book.

The publishing team has been an ardent support to the editorial, designing and production team. Their endless efforts to recruit the best for this project, has resulted in the accomplishment of this book. They are a veteran in the field of academics and their pool of knowledge is as vast as their experience in printing. Their expertise and guidance has proved useful at every step. Their uncompromising quality standards have made this book an exceptional effort. Their encouragement from time to time has been an inspiration for everyone.

The publisher and the editorial board hope that this book will prove to be a valuable piece of knowledge for researchers, students, practitioners and scholars across the globe.

# List of Contributors

**Guojie Qu, Boqiang Fan, Xin Fu and Yuguo Yu**
State Key Laboratory of Medical Neurobiology, School of Life Science, Human Phenome Institute, Institute of Brain Science, Institute of Science and Technology for Brain-Inspired Intelligence, Fudan University, Shanghai, China

**Jie Zhu, Li-Kun Yang, Wei-Liang Chen, Wei Lin, Yu-Hai Wang and Tao Chen**
Department of Neurosurgery, The 101th Hospital of PLA, School of Medicine, Anhui Medical University, Wuxi, China

**Yanel A. Volonté, Harmonie Vallese-Maurizi, Marcos J. Dibo, Victoria B. Ayala-Peña, Andrés Garelli, Samanta R. Zanetti, Axel Turpaud, Nora P. Rotstein, Luis E. Politi and Olga L. German**
Instituto de Investigaciones Bioquímicas de Bahía Blanca, Departamento de Biología, Bioquímica y Farmacia, Universidad Nacional del Sur - National Research Council of Argentina (CONICET), Bahía Blanca, Argentina

**Cheryl Mae Craft**
Department of Ophthalmology, USC Roski Eye Institute, Keck School of Medicine of the University of Southern California, Los Angeles, CA, United States
Department of Integrative Anatomical Sciences, Keck School of Medicine of the University of Southern California, Los Angeles, CA, United States

**Natalia P. Alza**
Instituto de Investigaciones Bioquímicas de Bahía Blanca, Consejo Nacional de Investigaciones Científicas y Técnicas, Universidad Nacional del Sur, Bahía Blanca, Argentina
Departamento de Química, Universidad Nacional del Sur, Bahía Blanca, Argentina

**Pablo A. Iglesias González**
Instituto de Investigaciones Bioquímicas de Bahía Blanca, Consejo Nacional de Investigaciones Científicas y Técnicas, Universidad Nacional del Sur, Bahía Blanca, Argentina

**Suangsuda Supasai**
Department of Nutrition and Department of Environmental Toxicology, University of California, Davis, CA, United States
Department of Molecular Tropical Medicine and Genetics, Faculty of Tropical Medicine, Mahidol University, Bangkok, Thailand

**Melisa A. Conde, Romina M. Uranga and Gabriela A. Salvador**
Instituto de Investigaciones Bioquímicas de Bahía Blanca, Consejo Nacional de Investigaciones Científicas y Técnicas, Universidad Nacional del Sur, Bahía Blanca, Argentina
Departamento de Biología, Bioquímica y Farmacia, Universidad Nacional del Sur,Bahía Blanca, Argentina

**Katarzyna Kośla, Elżbieta Płuciennik, Ewa Styczeń-Binkowska, Magdalena Nowakowska, Magdalena Orzechowska and Andrzej K. Bednarek**
Department of Molecular Carcinogenesis, Medical University of Łódź, Łódź, Poland

**Ana M. Adamo and Patricia Mathieu**
Department of Biological Chemistry and IQUIFIB (UBA-CONICET), Facultad de Farmacia y Bioquimica, Universidad de Buenos Aires, Buenos Aires, Argentina

**Xiuzhen Liu, Johnathan R. Nuttall and Patricia I. Oteiza**
Department of Nutrition and Department of Environmental Toxicology, University of California, Davis, Davis, CA, United States

**Horacio Uri Saragovi**
Lady Davis Institute, Montreal, QC, Canada
Jewish General Hospital, Montreal, QC, Canada
Department of Ophthalmology and Visual Sciences, McGill University, Montreal, QC, Canada

**Alba Galan**
Lady Davis Institute, Montreal, QC, Canada
Jewish General Hospital, Montreal, QC, Canada

**Leonard A. Levin**
Department of Ophthalmology and Visual Sciences, McGill University, Montreal, QC, Canada
McGill University Health Centre, Montreal, QC, Canada
Montreal Neurological Institute, Mcgill University, Montreal, QC, Canada

**Paula V. Subirada, María C. Paz, Magali E. Ridano, Gustavo A. Chiabrando and María C. Sánchez**
Departamento de Bioquímica Clínica, Facultad de Ciencias Químicas, Universidad Nacional de Córdoba, Córdoba, Argentina
Consejo Nacional de Investigaciones Científicas y Técnicas (CONICET), Centro de Investigaciones en Bioquímica Clínica e Inmunología (CIBICI), Córdoba, Argentina

**Valeria E. Lorenc**
Nanomedicine and Vision Group, Facultad de Ciencias Biomédicas, Instituto de Investigaciones en Medicina Traslacional, Universidad Austral, Consejo Nacional de Investigaciones en Ciencia y Tecnología (CONICET), Pilar, Argentina

**Claudio M. Fader**
Facultad de Odontología Mendoza, Universidad Nacional de Cuyo, Mendoza, Argentina
Instituto de Histología y Embriología (IHEM), Facultad de Ciencias Médicas, Universidad Nacional de Cuyo, Consejo Nacional de Investigaciones Científicas y Técnicas (CONICET), Mendoza, Argentina

**Vicente Bermúdez, Paula Estefanía Tenconi, Norma María Giusto and Melina Valeria Mateos**
Instituto de Investigaciones Bioquímicas de Bahía Blanca (INIBIBB), Consejo Nacional de Investigaciones Científicas y Técnicas (CONICET), Bahía Blanca, Argentina
Departamento de Biología, Bioquímica y Farmacia (DBByF), Universidad Nacional del Sur (UNS), Bahía Blanca, Argentina

**Luis Pedro Morera**
Instituto de Organizaciones Saludables, Universidad Siglo 21, Córdoba, Argentina

**Georgina Noel Marchiori and María Daniela Defagó**
Instituto de Investigaciones en Ciencias de la Salud (INICSA), CONICET, Universidad Nacional de Córdoba, Córdoba, Argentina
Escuela de Nutrición, Facultad de Ciencias Médicas, Universidad Nacional de Córdoba, Córdoba, Argentina

**Leonardo Adrián Medrano**
Department of Pyschology, Pontificia Universidad Católica Madre y Maestra, Santiago de los Caballeros, Dominican Republic

**Amalia Perna**
Department of Medicine, University of Fribourg, Fribourg, Switzerland

**Lavinia Auber Alberi**
Department of Medicine, University of Fribourg, Fribourg, Switzerland
Swiss Integrative Center for Human Health, Fribourg, Switzerland

**Alexandra Bouscary, Cyril Quessada, Althéa Mosbach and Jean-Philippe Loeffler**
Université de Strasbourg, UMR_S 1118, Fédération de Médecine Translationnelle, Strasbourg, France
INSERM, U1118, Mécanismes Centraux et Périphériques de la Neurodégénérescence, Strasbourg, France

**Noëlle Callizot**
Neuro-sys SAS, Gardanne, France

**Michael Spedding**
Spedding Research Solutions SAS, Le Vesinet, France

**Casey N. Barber and Daniel M. Raben**
Department of Biological Chemistry, The Johns Hopkins University School of Medicine, Baltimore, MD, United States

**Alexandre Henriques**
Université de Strasbourg, UMR_S 1118, Fédération de Médecine Translationnelle, Strasbourg, France
INSERM, U1118, Mécanismes Centraux et Périphériques de la Neurodégénérescence, Strasbourg, France
Spedding Research Solutions SAS, Le Vesinet, France

**Ferenc Deák**
Department of Geriatric Medicine, Reynolds Oklahoma Center on Aging, University of Oklahoma Health Sciences Center, Oklahoma City, OK, United States
Oklahoma Center for Neurosciences, University of Oklahoma Health Sciences Center, Oklahoma City, OK, United States
Harold Hamm Diabetes Center, University of Oklahoma Health Sciences Center, Oklahoma City, OK, United States

**Robert E. Anderson**
Department of Geriatric Medicine, Reynolds Oklahoma Center on Aging, University of Oklahoma Health Sciences Center, Oklahoma City, OK, United States
Oklahoma Center for Neurosciences, University of Oklahoma Health Sciences Center, Oklahoma City, OK, United States
Dean McGee Eye Institute, University of Oklahoma Health Sciences Center, Oklahoma City, OK, United States
Department of Ophthalmology, University of Oklahoma Health Sciences Center, Oklahoma City, OK, United States
Department of Cell Biology, University of Oklahoma Health Sciences Center, Oklahoma City, OK, United States

**David M. Sherry**
Oklahoma Center for Neurosciences, University of Oklahoma Health Sciences Center, Oklahoma City, OK, United States
Department of Cell Biology, University of Oklahoma Health Sciences Center, Oklahoma City, OK, United States
Department of Pharmaceutical Sciences, University of Oklahoma Health Sciences Center, Oklahoma City, OK, United States

**Jennifer L. Fessler**
Department of Cell Biology, University of Oklahoma Health Sciences Center, Oklahoma City, OK, United States

**Maria M. Benedetto and Maria A. Contin**
Departamento de Química Biológica Ranwel Caputto, Facultad de Ciencias Químicas, Universidad Nacional de Córdoba, Córdoba, Argentina
Centro de Investigaciones en Química Biológica de Córdoba (CIQUIBIC), CONICET, Universidad Nacional de Córdoba, Córdoba, Argentina

**Liang Zhou**
Department of Pharmacology, College of Pharmaceutical Sciences, Soochow University, Jiangsu, China

**Jingjing Duan**
Department of Anatomy and Neurobiology, Zhongshan School of Medicine, SunYat-sen University, Guangzhou, China

**Gerardo R. Corradi, Luciana R. Mazzitelli, Guido D. Petrovich, Felicitas de Tezanos Pinto, Lucia Rochi and Hugo P. Adamo**
Departamento de Química Biológica, Instituto de Química y Fisicoquímica Biológicas, Facultad de Farmacia y Bioquímica, Consejo Nacional de Investigaciones Científicas y Técnicas-Universidad de Buenos Aires, Buenos Aires, Argentina

**Kexin Li, Yang Zheng and Xiaoming Wang**
Department of Radiology, Shengjing Hospital of China Medical University, Shenyang, China

# Index

www.ingramcontent.com/pod-product-compliance
Lightning Source LLC
LaVergne TN
LVHW082204200926
848484LV00008B/2212